TEXTBOOK OF GYNECOLOGY

VOLUME 1: FOUNDATIONS OF FEMALE REPRODUCTIVE HEALTH

Dr. Beatriz Lezama

ALLIED HEALTH PRESS

Textbook of Gynecology

Volume 1: Foundations of Female Reproductive Health

Author: **Dr. Beatriz Lezama**

Allied Health Press
4164 Lakeshore Road
Burlington ON L7L 1A4
Canada
www.alliedhealthpress.com
Email: orders@arclereducation.com

ISBN: 978-1-77956-847-2

ABOUT THE AUTHOR

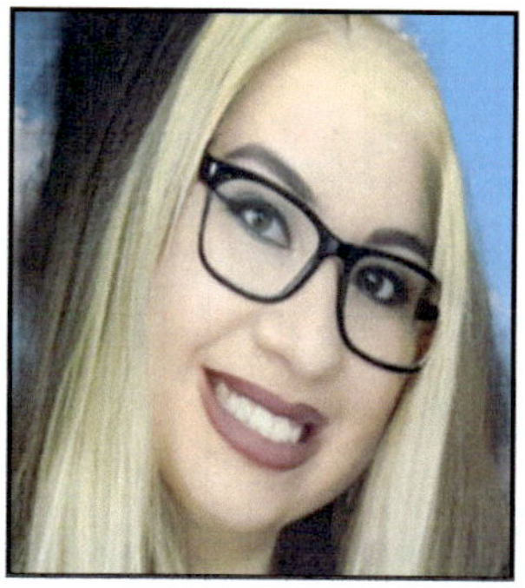

Dr. Beatriz Lezama is a pediatric specialist and fellow in neonatology, with a strong clinical foundation and a passion for early-life care. She holds certifications in general ultrasound, vascular Doppler, and maternal-fetal Doppler, enhancing her diagnostic and perinatal care skills. In addition to her clinical work, Dr. Lezama is an active health communicator and blog writer, with several health-focused articles published on LinkedIn. Her work bridges expert pediatric knowledge with accessible public education, promoting wellness and informed care for families and communities.

Brief Table of Contents

Getting Started with This Book

Chapter Openers

A list of Chapter Outline is presented providing a brief Introduction to what will be covered in the chapter.

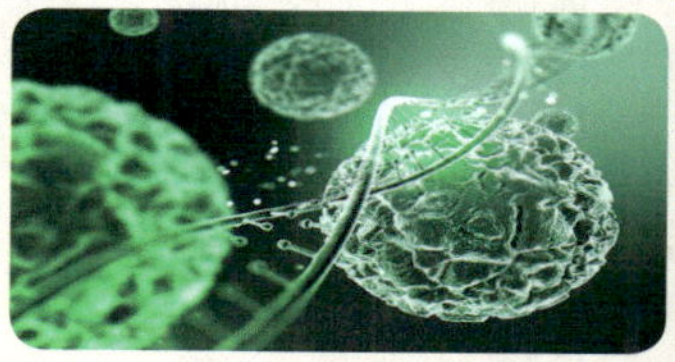

Introduction

Often referred to as the science of life, biology is a broad field of study aimed at comprehending the several kinds of life on Earth, from tiny creatures to sophisticated multicellular entities. Comprising several subfields, including molecular biology, ecology, and evolutionary biology, each of which advances our knowledge of living systems, this field clarifies the mechanisms controlling life events, including development, reproduction, and interaction with the surroundings, which is the central goal of biology. Moreover, biology fills in the void between the natural sciences and medicine by offering a necessary understanding of health, illness, and the interactions between organisms and their environments. Dealing with urgent global issues such as climate change, biodiversity loss, and new diseases depends on an awareness of these complex biological interactions, therefore highlighting the critical part biology plays in modern civilization. Fundamentally, biology explores and tests ideas about the living world using the scientific method. Through methodical observation and experimentation,

LEARNING OBJECTIVES

After studying this chapter, you will be able to:

1. Discuss the scientific method in biology;
2. Explain the cell theory;
3. Discuss the genetics and heredity;
4. Evolution and natural selection;
5. Focus on ecology and ecosystems;
6. Learn about human biology;
7. Evaluate the plant biology;
8. Explain the microbiology;
9. Focus on current trends in biology.

1.1. The Scientific Method in Biology

Learning Outcome

1. Describe the steps of the scientific method;
2. Focus on hypothesis formation;
3. Learn about experimental design.

Learning Outcomes

The beginning of each section of every chapter contains a set of Learning Outcomes that inform students of concepts they should understand. These outcomes help students understand what they should be able to do if they have mastered the material in that section.

Test Your Knowledge

Throughout each chapter, Test Your Knowledge cues you to note which topics have been covered and to self-test your understanding of the material presented.

Test Your Knowledge

1. Explain why correlation does not imply causation in scientific experiments.
2. How does the scientific method help reduce the influence of personal opinions in research?

Chapter Summary

The Summary Section appear at the end of each chapter and summarize main concepts covered throughout the chapter. These points provide key concepts in an engaging and meaningful way.

Summary

The investigation of biological principles highlights the importance of a comprehensive view of life by reflecting the intricate interactions that occur within living systems. The complexity of biology goes beyond individual species or systems, as this essay highlights; it also includes the interactions that mold ecosystems and affect biodiversity. Researchers can conduct in-depth analyses of metabolomic data using sophisticated technologies like MetaboAnalyst, which offer insights into the molecular mechanisms underlying these interactions. As demonstrated by the developments in MetaboAnalyst, for example, the integration of diverse omics data promotes a thorough understanding of metabolic pathways and helps identify important biological markers necessary for research on development and disease (Chong et al., 2018). Additionally, the phenomenon of ecological invasions is a key component of biological research and a vital field of study. The introduction of non-native species into unfamiliar habitats has significant ramifications and calls for multidisciplinary management strategies. Examining the origins and effects of these biological incursions, invasion science has become a crucial field that highlights the need to comprehend ecological dynamics and community interactions. As interest in biological invasions increases, new findings are emerging that put conventional ecological theories and practices to the test. The importance of incorporating various scientific viewpoints is shown by this developing discipline, which also highlights how invasive species shape ecosystems and advances our knowledge of ecological resilience (David et al., 2013). When taken as a whole, these discoveries from invasion science and metabolomics highlight the value of multidisciplinary biology research. Fostering cross-disciplinary collaboration and utilizing technological breakthroughs to improve our comprehension of intricate biological interactions are crucial as we look to the future of biological research. In addition to deepening our understanding of the complexities of life, this method lays the groundwork for tackling urgent environmental issues. Future studies can ensure the continued relevance of biology in a world that is constantly changing by acknowledging the interconnection of biological systems and opening the door to creative solutions that support sustainability and biodiversity conservation. We might imagine a thorough comprehension of life that serves both academia and society at large through ongoing investigation and integration of scientific knowledge.

Knowledge Assessment

The chapter includes material designed to review and reinforce each content. It includes Critical Thinking Questions to help test of your understanding of information presented in the chapter and Short answer Questions to review your understanding of the key concepts presented in the chapter.

Critical Thinking Questions

1. **Who is known as the "Father of Modern Biology"?**
   a. Aristotle
   b. Charles Darwin
   c. Gregor Mendel
   d. Louis Pasteur
2. **What is the basic unit of life?**
   a. Atom
   b. Molecule
   c. Cell
   d. Organism
3. **Which branch of biology studies the interaction of organisms with their environment?**
   a. Genetics
   b. Ecology
   c. Physiology
   d. Botany
4. **Which macromolecule is the main source of energy for living organisms?**
   a. Proteins
   b. Lipids
   c. Carbohydrates
   d. Nucleic acids
5. **DNA is primarily responsible for which function in living organisms?**
   a. Energy production
   b. Protein synthesis
   c. Storing genetic information
   d. Regulating body temperature

Short Answer Questions

1. What is biology, and why is it important to study biology?
2. What are the three main domains of life, and how are they different from one another?
3. Define homeostasis and give an example of how it works in living organisms.
4. What is the cell theory, and why is it fundamental to biology?
5. How do autotrophs and heterotrophs differ in the way they obtain energy?
6. What is the scientific method, and how is it applied in biological research?
7. Discuss how biology helps address global challenges such as climate change, disease, and food security.
8. Explain the levels of biological organization from the smallest unit to the largest. Provide examples at each level.
9. Describe the relationship between structure and function in biology, giving specific examples from cells or organs.
10. How has the discovery of genetics shaped our understanding of inheritance and variation among organisms?

Supplementary Materials

Key Terms: A list of key terms is given for quick reference

KEY TERMS FROM THIS CHAPTER

Annotation enrichment analysis	Biological structure	Cell
Cell theory	Cellular structure	Ecology
Ecosystems	Genetics	Human biology
Microbiology	Natural selection	Organism
Plant biology		

Further Resources: Recommendations for additional readings, websites, and multimedia resources.

References

1. Argelaguet, R., Velten, B., Arnol, D., Dietrich, S., Zenz, T., Marioni, J. C., Buettner, F., et al. (2018). Multi-omics factor analysis—A framework for unsupervised integration of multi-omics data sets. *Molecular Systems Biology, 14*. https://doi.org/10.15252/msb.20178124.
2. Bacher, S., Blackburn, T. M., Essl, F., & Genovesi, P. (2017). *Socio-Economic Impact Classification of Alien Taxa (SEICAT)*. https://core.ac.uk/download/286567949.pdf (accessed on 8th March 2025).
3. Barnett, R., Brace, S., Cucchi, T., & Dobney, K. (2013). *Divergent Evolutionary Processes Associated with Colonization of Offshore Islands*. https://core.ac.uk/download/20664364.pdf (accessed on 8th March 2025).

Detailed Table of Contents

CHAPTER 3

Puberty Normal and Abnormal 67

CHAPTER 4

Menopause 101

LIST OF FIGURES

PREFACE

Gynecology is at the center of medical practice, ranging from the inspection of the female reproductive organs in both states of normalcy and disease. Its history dates back to ancient reports of menstruation and delivery, but it has become a scientific discipline that covers anatomy, physiology, endocrinology, and pathology. Physicians and scientists both desire to understand not only the organs and tissues but also the complex hormonal systems and cellular interactions that govern reproduction, menstrual cyclicity, and transition through life stages. Imaging, molecular biology, and minimal access surgery have extended our diagnostic and treatment capabilities, allowing patients to have more precise and less intrusive interventions than previously possible. Over the past century, the study of women's reproductive health has progressed from qualitative, general descriptions to highly specialized subdisciplines.

Experts now diagnose today from congenital malformations of the genital tract to menstrual cycle disorders, from treatment of benign lesions to detection of systemic endocrine disease with gynecologic presentations. Advances such as these are as much a function of technology as they are of a greater recognition of the interconnectingness of reproductive health and overall status—the latter affecting cardiovascular status, bone density, metabolic equilibrium, and even psychiatric well-being. With increasing ages in our population, post-reproductive health and menopause are as important to understand as puberty and fertility, paralleling the lifespan context that characterizes contemporary gynecologic practice.

In *Textbook of Gynecology: Volume 1,* we integrate essential topics that all clinicians, trainees, and students must be competent in. The book offers a sequential journey through normal development and anatomy, the physiological milestones of puberty and menstrual physiology, and the important disorders that disrupt them. Special focus is given to hormonal regulation and clinical significance, in order to enable readers to correlate symptomatology with the underlying pathophysiology. The text reflects both didactic progression—from function and form to clinical syndromes—and clinical utility, with chapters structured to permit intense study or easy reference in the care of patients.

Chapter 1 offers a complete description of female genital tract anatomy, both external and internal structures, blood supply, and innervation. Chapter 2 is dedicated to the development of the embryologic gonad and the genital organs, following the genetic and hormonal cues that form the male and female phenotypes. Chapter 3 addresses puberty in both normal and pathologic states, offering criteria for discrimination between constitutional delay and pathologic causes of premature or delayed onset.

Chapter 4 discusses menopause's endocrine changes and clinical presentation, as well as guidelines for assessment and management of its systemic effect. Chapter 5 discusses the mechanisms and phases of normal menstruation, providing the foundation for appreciating deviation. Chapter 6 discusses the many causes and classifications of amenorrhea, from functional hypothalamic suppression to ovarian failure.

Chapter 7 addresses abnormal uterine bleeding, including use of the FIGO PALM-COEIN classification to guide diagnosis and management. Chapter 8 presents a complete discussion of polycystic ovarian syndrome, including metabolic sequelae and fertility interventions. Chapter 9 covers causes and treatment of dysmenorrhea and premenstrual syndrome with emphasis on both pharmacologic and lifestyle treatments.

Chapter 10 clarifies benign lesions of the vulva, vagina, and cervix, with histologic correlations and operative considerations. Chapter 11 updates reproductive tract infections, ranging from common bacterial vaginosis to rare parasitic and viral pathogens, with diagnostic tests and antimicrobial therapy. Finally, Chapter 12 addresses endocrine disorders in gynecology, ranging from thyroid disease to adrenal disease, emphasizing the relationship between systemic glands and reproductive well-being.

This book is written for medical students seeking a step-by-step introduction, residents refining clinical skills, practicing obstetricians updating knowledge, and allied health professionals in women's health. It is also a guide for investigators who require clear, concise definitions of basic concepts. As a primary text or used in conjunction with the bedside, the book aspires to enable informed decision-making and enhance outcomes across the spectrum of gynecologic practice.

ANATOMY OF THE FEMALE REPRODUCTIVE SYSTEM

1

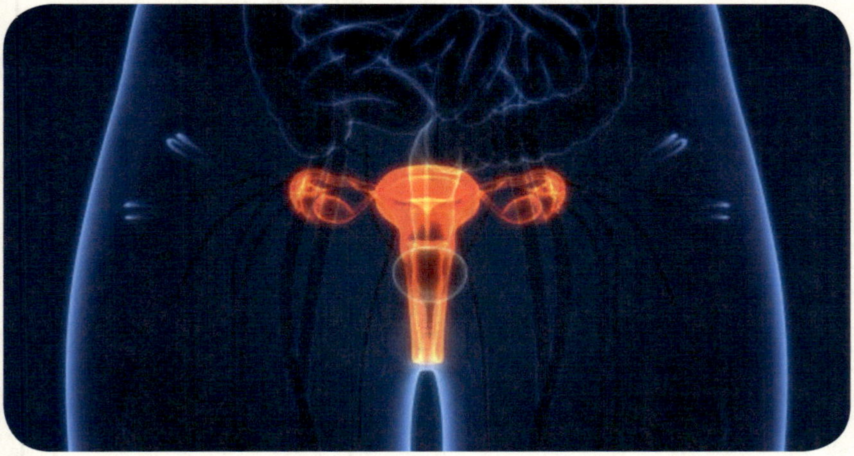

LEARNING OBJECTIVES

After studying this chapter, you will be able to:

1. Describe the external and internal structures of the female reproductive system
2. Understand the menstrual cycle
3. Define fertilization and pregnancy
4. Discuss the common disorders of the female reproductive system

Introduction

Understanding the anatomy of the female reproductive system is important not only for medical students but also for practitioners who work with women's health. The system plays a vital role in reproductive functions, including ovulation, menstruation, and childbirth. Understanding its anatomical structures, including the ovaries, fallopian tubes, uterus, and vagina, provides insight into how every organ operates independently and in conjunction. Besides, precise examination of the physiological mechanisms underlying such structures can reveal their significance in healthy and pathological conditions. Such information is required to address inequalities in health and improve reproductive health outcomes among women of diverse backgrounds, and guide the need for a comprehensive discussion that unites anatomical, biological, and societal perspectives of women's reproductive health. Apart from the anatomical profile, it is significant to consider the implications of variations in the female reproductive system, particularly on intersex and disorders of sexual development

(DSD) conditions. Parental feelings and emotional undertones in coping with these intersex conditions have increasingly become more foregrounded, testifying to an expanded gender identity and medical ethics debate. The experience of an intersex diagnosis by the family can be very much influenced by what healthcare professionals inform them about. As underlined by recent research, it is important to learn about the needs and concerns of the parents in those critical moments in order to deliver empathic and informed medical intervention.

This intersection of anatomy, genetics, and patient experience is essential to the maintenance of an inclusive model of women's reproductive health, relevant both to the clinical setting and to gender and identity norms more generally (McCarthy *et al.*, 2008). Furthermore, the physiology of female reproductive anatomy is shaped by knowledge obtained through comparative study with animal models, particularly the mouse, which is an appropriate experimental subject. While mice and humans share enormous anatomical and hormonal differences, patterns of development underlie a fundamental understanding that can be utilized in developing an understanding of human reproductive tract development. Scientists must traverse the subtleties of extrapolating knowledge from mouse models to human disease with caution in regard to both convergent and divergent features between species (Baskin *et al.*, 2019). Such an understanding is particularly valid when viewed in the context of women's reproductive disorders, and therefore puts a high value on such research that aims to cross-pollinate developmental biology and clinical application. In putting the anatomy of the female reproductive system in such broader discourses, this chapter aims to contribute to the debate a holistic model for such understanding of women's reproductive health and its multifaceted challenges.

Definition of the Female Reproductive System

It is crucial to be familiar with the female reproductive system in order to comprehend many biological processes and fertility. The female reproductive system consists of multiple structures that co-exist in synergy to maintain reproduction, hormonal regulation, and sexuality. The core of the system is the ovaries, whose function is to produce ova and secrete hormones such as estrogen and progesterone. These hormones are crucial in regulating the menstrual cycle, influencing ovulation, and preparing the uterus for potential implantation of an ovum fertilized during intercourse. The interaction of these components not only signifies the anatomical complexity of the system but also recognizes it as a key component to female well-being and biological function. In addition to the ovaries, the female reproductive system includes the fallopian tubes, uterus, and vagina, all of which have specific functions in the reproduction process. The fallopian tubes transport the ova from the ovaries to the uterus and are typically the location where fertilization takes place. The muscular uterus is found in the pelvic cavity and provides a fertile environment for a fetus during pregnancy. The vagina is also the birth canal and the passage through which the sperm travels during intercourse. This positioning of the vagina in anatomy implies that the female system is not merely a series of distinct structures but an integrated system designed to allow reproduction, balance hormones, and maintain overall health throughout a woman's life. Besides, understanding the female reproductive system extends beyond anatomy to include the socio-cultural aspects that shape health education and consequences. Effective comprehensive sexual education, particularly in institutions like public schooling, is vital towards empowering individuals with knowledge regarding their reproductive health. Based on research, most schools do not provide adequate and accurate information on the female reproductive system, causing health practice and anatomy misconceptions (Yager *et al.*, 2012). Poor education has long-term effects on health behaviors and outcomes, not just for the individual but also for society as a whole. Closing these gaps in knowledge with improved standards of education can function well to improve the appreciation and comprehension of the female reproductive system, with improved health awareness and decision-making. The canvas of female reproductive health thus needs not only anatomical awareness, but also cultural awareness that informs perceptions and reproductive health practices.

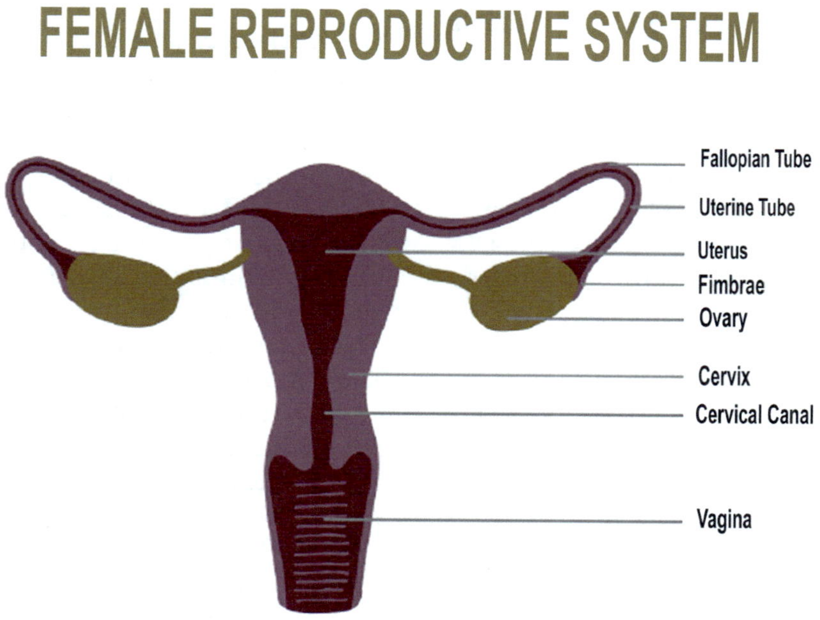

Figure 1.1. Illustration of female human reproductive system.

Source: https://static.vecteezy.com/system/resources/previews/023/548/875/original/illustration-of-female-human-reproductive-system-free-png.png

Importance of Understanding Female Anatomy

Knowledge of the female anatomy is a fundamental part of sexual education and reproductive health, one that is usually left in insufficiently covered areas, particularly through public education systems. There exists an overwhelming amount of educational material that fails to correctly and fully detail female reproductive anatomy, as noted in the report 'Birds, Bees and Bias: How Absent Sex Ed Standards Fail New York's Students'(Yager *et al.*, 2012). This confusion can create myths and misinformation and make it difficult for young people to make educated decisions regarding their health.

By pointing out the various structures of the female reproductive system, such as the ovaries, fallopian tubes, uterus, and vagina, students can be empowered and have a clearer concept of the human body. Furthermore, this knowledge facilitates appreciation and respect for the woman's body, which is the precondition for building a society that respects educated sex-related health discourse. Apart from the promotion of well-informed decision-making, knowledge of female anatomy is required for the delivery of efficient health care. Accurate knowledge allows doctors to interpret information to patients clearly, leading to better diagnosis and treatment. For instance, understanding the normal anatomy and physiology of the female reproductive system allows clinicians to identify anomalies or conditions such as endometriosis or fibroids. Development of electronic health record (EHR) data, as expounded in the article on the Obstetric and Neonatal Ontology (OntONeo), makes normal anatomical knowledge even more critical across health systems. By ensuring that health professionals have a rational understanding of female anatomy, continuity of care during vulnerable reproductive phases can be significantly enhanced, ultimately benefiting the wellbeing of both mother and baby. Moreover, knowledge of female anatomy transcends individual physical health and enters social and cultural awareness. Increased awareness engenders greater receptiveness to conversation about women's health issues, which have long been a taboo subject. Through the revelation of the diverse experiences and complications faced by women concerning their reproductive systems, society can provide a framework that allows for advocacy and education. Honest conversation about these issues can diminish the barriers that stand in the way of women receiving care and assistance. Female anatomy knowledge facilitates logical discussion regarding reproductive rights and health care access, thereby promoting social equality. An educated populace is thus indispensable to advise on policy reform initiatives aimed at improving women's health, for more education, and to allow female reproductive health to receive the consideration it so rightfully deserves in public health settings.

1.1. External Structures

Learning Outcome

1. Define the vulva and its components
2. Discuss the clitoris and its role in sexual arousal
3. Describe the labia majora and labia minora functions

The external organs of the female reproductive system play an important role in sexual and reproductive well-being. These organs, such as the vulva, clitoris, and outer labia, play very important protective functions and are fundamental in the sexual arousal and birth processes of physiology. The vulva consists of various components with varying functions, which include the protection of the internal organs and the stimulation of sexual intercourse. The outer labia, or labia majora, are soft, fleshy folds that help shield the more sensitive inner structures from external stimuli. Knowledge of these exterior characteristics is crucial not merely for an overall comprehension of female anatomy but also for the recognition of potential abnormalities that can affect reproductive health. One of the most significant components of the external reproductive anatomy is the clitoris, not just a source of sexual pleasure but also a significant marker of sexual identity and health. The clitoris has been described as a complex organ, with architecture radiating beyond the surface glans into significant internal structures that are often underappreciated. It is highly innervated with nerve endings, rendering it incredibly sensitive and vital to female sexual arousal. Researchers point out that the clitoris is an exemplar of the intricacy between anatomy and sexuality, highlighting the importance of taking into account the internal and external organs in studies of reproduction. Information and education regarding the clitoris can facilitate sexual health and empower people in their reproductive lives. The interactions between the external structures and hormonal influences point toward the necessity of understanding how development, as well as exposure to a range of substances, might affect these reproductive structures. The environmental influences, such as endocrine disruptors, can profoundly affect the physical characteristics of the reproductive system, including the external anatomy. For instance, studies have established that prenatal exposure to hormone-modulating chemicals is responsible for causing malformations, which impact the formation of structures like the labia and clitoris. Such studies are significant, given that they emphasize the vulnerability of the reproductive anatomy in females to environmental stimulation, as revealed in studies examining the effects of anti-androgens on reproductive structures (Baskin *et al.*, 2019; Baskin *et al.*, 2017). By combining anatomical data and endocrine science, researchers can develop an overall view of the vulnerabilities and intricacies of women's external reproductive organs.

1.1.1. Vulva and Its Components

The vulva, an external female reproductive system organ, consists of a number of different structures that serve important physiological functions collectively. These principal structures are the mons pubis, labia majora, labia minora, clitoris, and vestibule, which all serve protection and sexual arousal functions. The mons pubis, fatty covering of the pubic symphysis, cushions, while the labia majora and labia minora serve as cover folds that shield inner structures from microbes and mechanical damage. The labia minora, being also more fragile and better supplied with blood, are a significant component of sexual stimulation, contributing to sexual pleasure due to their heightened sensitivity. Peculiar at the center of the vulva's sexual and reproductive functionality is the clitoris, an organ which is extremely innervated and composed of a great deal of erectile tissue. The main job of this organ is sexual stimulation for women and is included in the sexual response cycle. Although small by external visibility, the clitoris is internally large, contributing to precipitate an elaborate network of pleasures. Understanding the anatomy of the clitoris is key to appreciating female sexual function and health.

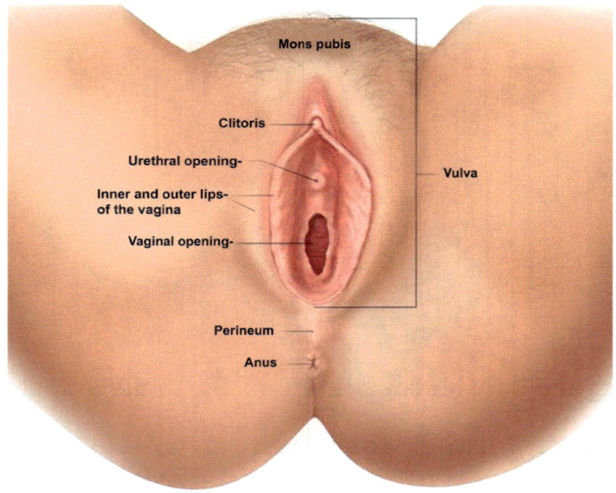

Figure 1.2. Vulva anatomy.

Source: https://visualsonline.cancer.gov/retrieve.cfm?imageid=9472&dpi=72&fileformat=jpg

The vestibule, which covers the vulva and vagina openings, also plays a central function in sexual intercourse and childbearing, indicating the dependency of the vulva's components in female reproduction. Besides, the linings of the vulva are made up of stratified squamous epithelium that varies in thickness based on hormonal fluctuation during menstruation. It is a dynamic system that allows flexibility and changes that accommodate the physiological demands of the female body. As noted, the organization and anatomy of the vulva, including the mucosal covering, allow for multiple functions, including protection during coitus as well as those during pregnancy and parturition. In discussing the vulva's structures, it is evident that intricate relationships between these structures are vital to female and reproductive health and provide the foundation for the argument that an extensive understanding of the female body is integral to addressing concerns of health and promoting sexual education (Whittier *et al.*, 1993; Ali *et al.*, 2020).

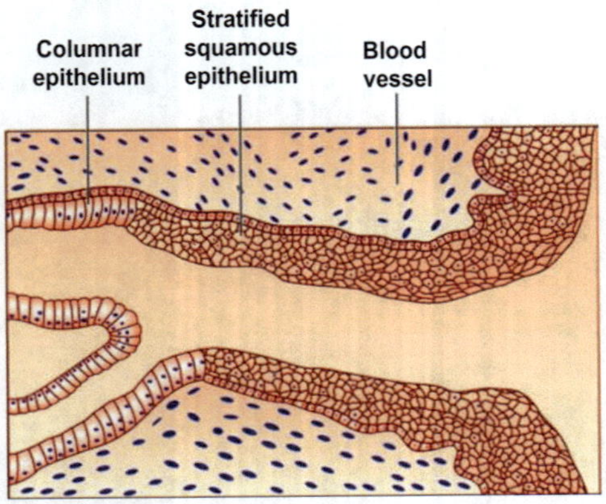

Figure 1.3. Mucous lining of Bartholin's duct.

Source: https://oshimu.com/wp-content/uploads/2021/07/Gynaecology-DC-Dutta.pdf

1.1.2. Clitoris and Its Role in Sexual Arousal

The tiny but vital clitoris at the tip of the vulva is an erectile organ that has a central role to play in women's sexual excitement and satisfaction. Made up of erectile tissue that is similar to that of the male, the clitoris is richly innervated—precisely 8,000 of them—with nerve endings, thus quite possibly the most sensitive area on the human body. Its primary function is the excitation of sexual pleasure, which plays a crucial role in sexual arousal and overall sexual health. Its anatomical function, as explained above, is generally not referred to in educational texts addressing female sexuality. The majority of undergraduate anatomy and physiology courses deal with reproductive functions to the detriment of the value of sexual pleasure, so that there is a significant knowledge deficit among future healthcare professionals, which is emphasized in the report on the representation of sexual pleasure in A&P textbooks (Ganeng *et al.*, 2022).

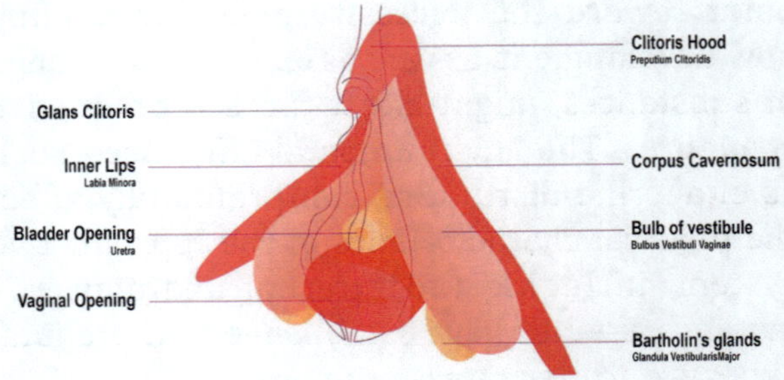

Figure 1.4. The clitoris.

Source: https://www.wmhp.com.au/sites/default/files/the-clitoris.jpg

Sexual arousal is triggered by the chain of bodily events made possible to a great degree through the clitoris. Stimulation of it induces blood flow to the area that causes swelling and heightened sensitivity that paralleled physiological changes in the female body, e.g., vaginal engorgement and lubrication. The bond between the clitoris and sexual pleasure is not only biological but also has an emotional and psychological component. Positive sex is essential to a woman's sexual health, and understanding this intricate connection can give women the power to look after their sexual health. Understanding this organ can eliminate the age-old stereotypes and social taboos about women's sexual pleasure, bringing about much-needed debate on the importance of the clitoris in women's sexuality and health (Phillips *et al.*, 2015). In addition to that, the clitoris' function goes beyond functional anatomy itself; it has profound connotations of emotional and relational processes of intimacy. Access to sexual pleasure not only encourages positive experiences but also feelings of belonging and being included amongst women. Mainly because the sex education made accessible to healthcare professionals does not emphasize sexual pleasure and intimacy as a focus, not many may be prepared with the knowledge or expertise required to effectively cater to the needs. The language of women's sexuality must also shift, including the extent of the clitoris and its associated functions in sexual pleasure within medical school curricula. This helps empower women to own their sexuality and also helps healthcare professionals practice more whole-person, educated, and compassionate sex-positive care that addresses sexual pleasure as well as reproductive health (Ganeng *et al.*, 2022).

1.1.3. Labia Majora and Labia Minora Functions

Labia majora and labia minora are vital components of the external female genitalia and contribute immensely to the female reproductive system's form and function. Labia majora, the outer major folds, have protective roles of encasing and safeguarding the more delicate structures of the vulva, which include the clitoris, the urethra, and the opening of the vagina. This protective function is significant because it prevents pathogens from reaching the internal reproductive tract and helps maintain the overall hygiene of the area. The labia majora also have adipose tissue, which not only serves as padding and protection but also helps in sexual arousal because of sensitivity to touch, thus enhancing sexual pleasure and responsiveness. In contrast, the labia minora, which are located within the labia majora, have specific anatomical and functional characteristics. These inner folds of smaller sizes are rich in nerve endings and highly vascularized, making them highly sensitive to touch. Research indicates that the labia minora have a function in sexual arousal and pleasure through increased vulvar sensitivity since they fill with blood and swell during sexual arousal. Furthermore, labia minora help protect the vaginal opening and lubricate, preparing for a conducive environment for sexual function and reproduction. Understanding these intricate functions reveals the significance of these structures in the female sexual response and their function in overall reproductive health, particularly in the aspect of aesthetic value and surgery such as labiaplasty, focusing on the morphology and function of the labia minora (Ali *et al.*, 2024).

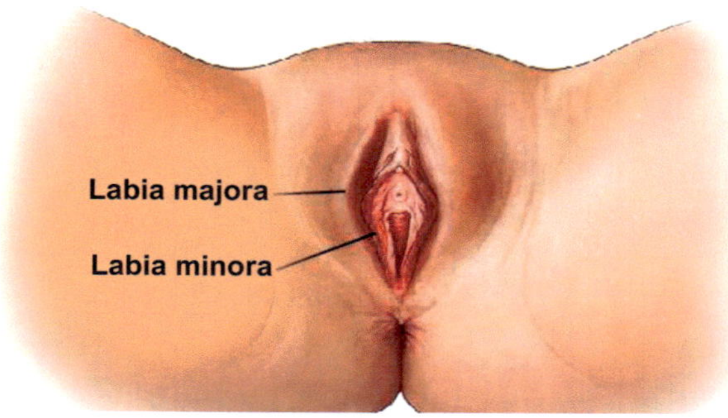

Figure 1.5. External to the labia minora are the labia majora.

Source: https://www.yourpelvicfloor.org/conditions/labiaplasty/

Additionally, the labia majora and labia minora play important roles in some physiological processes of the female reproductive system. They are responsible for the upkeep of effective functioning of the reproductive tract, particularly during pregnancy and delivery. The histological and structural features of the labia provide support and facilitate an adaptation to the changes in the woman's body during various stages of life. As the reproductive systemundergoes cycles of hormonal changes, the labia majora and minora also experience adaptations in structure that collaborate to serve the global function of the vulva throughout various phases of reproduction (Ali *et al.*, 2020). Such a functional capacity is supportive of why such recognition and value of the complexity of female genital anatomy, as well as its importance to health, wellbeing, and surgical planning, are essential.

Test Your Knowledge

1. What anatomical structures make up the vulva?
2. What is the function of the clitoris in the female sexual response?

1.2. Internal Structures

Learning Outcome

1. Understand the vagina and its anatomical features
2. Explain the uterus: structure and layers
3. Define ovaries and their functions

The internal organs of the female reproductive system reveal a high level of complexity that operates in concert to facilitate reproduction, control by hormones, and health. Of these structures, the ovaries are two-in-one organs, which are responsible for producing oocytes and hormone secretion, such as estrogen and progesterone. Ovarian follicles undergo cyclical reproduction, culminating in ovulation, while hormonal secretion synchronizes the menstrual cycle and readies the endometrium for the potential of implantation. The uterine tubes, or fallopian tubes, also play a crucial role in capturing and transporting the oocyte after ovulation, where fertilization will typically occur. Successful reproduction relies on the intricate interaction of these organs, and their operations are regulated by hormonal feedback mechanisms. Understanding these dynamics gives more insight into various reproductive disorders and highlights the importance of exploring both the anatomical and physiological aspects of female reproductive function. Leaving the ovaries behind, the uterus is the other major internal organ, characterized by its multilayered architecture made up of the endometrium, myometrium, and perimetrium. The endometrium, the innermost layer, is at the core of the menstrual cycle, and its cyclical changes as a response to the hormonal fluctuations. During the secretory phase, the endometrium thickens to create a site for the reception of an implanted embryo, whereas sloughing off during menstruation illustrates the two-way control of the reproductive process by hormones. The myometrium, a muscular layer, plays an important role in expelling the fetus at parturition, illustrating functional specialization of individual layers. In addition, perimetrium is a covering that lines the exterior of reproductive organs and keeps them intact. By studying the structural and functional functions of the uterus, one can understand diseases such as endometriosis and fibroids, which have an immense influence on women's health. Along with the ovaries and uterus, the cervix and vagina form the essential internal reproductive organs. The cervix is the pathway between the vagina and uterus, and it has a significant function during labor and menstruation. Its anatomy allows dilation and effacement in order for the fetus to exit through it during labor. The cervical canal also produces mucus with different consistencies during the menstrual cycle, which affects sperm transport and storage. The vagina, especially as a muscular, elastic organ, is not only the canal of birth entry but also the female receptacle for the penis during copulation. Its dual use underscores the vagina's adaptive role, calling for reproductive and protective functions. Cumulatively, the interplay of these internal structures sheds more light on the female reproductive system's complex design, which can be greatly affected by hormonal imbalance and extrinsic factors, further highlighting the importance of extensive studies in reproductive health (Baskin *et al.*, 2019; Baskin *et al.*, 2017).

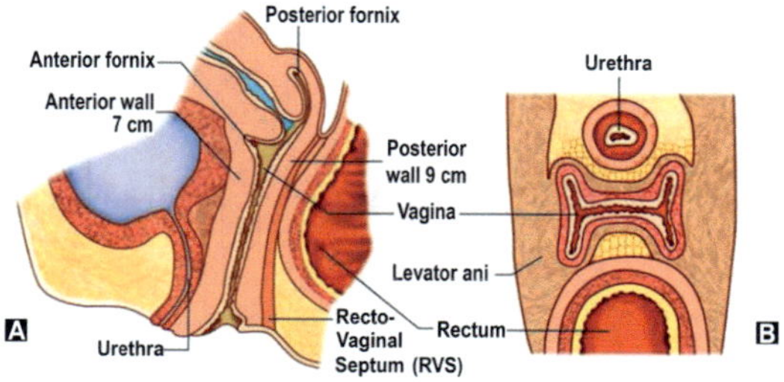

Figure 1.6. (A) Relation of the anterior and posterior vaginal wall; (B) 'H' shaped on cross-section.

Source: https://oshimu.com/wp-content/uploads/2021/07/Gynaecology-DC-Dutta.pdf

1.2.1. Vagina and Its Anatomical Features

The vagina is a critical female reproductive anatomy that serves as a conduit between the external environment and the internal reproductive system. The vagina is an elastic, muscular tube extending from the vulva to the cervix and serves multiple functions in sexual intercourse, labor, and menstrual fluid expulsion. Vaginal walls are made up of layers like mucosa, muscularis, and adventitia that give vaginal walls unprecedented flexibility and stretch during various physiological occurrences. The vaginal mucosal lining also contains rugae or folds that further enhance the vaginas capacity to retain structures during sex and childbirth. In addition, the vaginal microbiome, which is primarily made up of *Lactobacillus* species, is responsible for pH balance, and hence infection prevention—a physical property that is indicative of the vaginas function not just in reproduction but also in health.

The physical structure of the vagina is also supplemented by its closeness to crucial female reproductive organs, particularly the ovary and uterus. The vaginal environment should be understood with consideration for the hormonal factors that control its development and functioning. Hormones such as estrogen are used to maintain the thickness and elasticity of the vaginal walls in response to cellular requirements at various stages in life, from puberty to menopause. This interaction of hormones is fundamental to the health of the vagina, particularly in the context of background anatomical features that influence susceptibility to such conditions as vaginal atrophy or infection. Recognizing these hormonal influences is not only fundamental to the clinic but serves as a reminder of why the vagina is a part of core female reproductive anatomy that illustrates its dynamic nature responsive to systemic hormonal change.

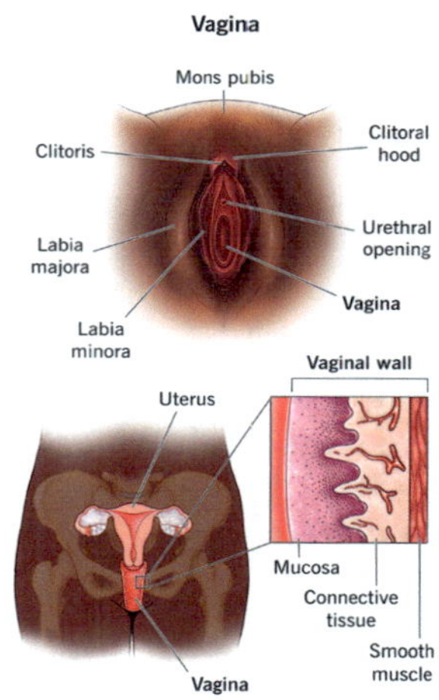

Figure 1.7. Your vagina is just one organ that's part of your reproductive and sexual health.

Source: https://my.clevelandclinic.org/health/body/22469-vagina

Furthermore, vaginas' interactions with neighboring anatomical structures include not only physiological functions but also stimulus and condition response, indicating their significance within the reproductive health continuum. With the vagina being the portal of the reproductive system, it would interact with different systems, including the neurovascular and endocrine, which further elucidate its total role in regards to sexuality and reproduction. For instance, the rich vascular supply to the vaginal canal supports sexual responsiveness and lies at the heart of the process of arousal. Additionally, the vaginal canal possesses large structural differences among individuals, depending on genetic, hormonal, and environmental factors. Understanding these structures of the anatomy not only assists in an understanding of the vagina's role in reproduction and sexual health but also the intricacy of its function, setting the stage for more research on the female reproductive system and its intricate relationships.

1.2.2. Uterus: Structure and Layers

The uterus, one of the female reproductive organs, is characterized by its complex structure, which plays a critical role in menstruation, pregnancy, and childbearing. The uterus is anatomically divided into three primary layers: endometrium, myometrium, and perimetrium. The innermost structure, the endometrium, is made up of a mucous lining that varies cyclically with hormonal fluctuations and is hence an integral part of the implantation of the fertilized ovum and maintenance of pregnancy.

The endometrium is shed every month in the absence of a fertilization process, during menstruation, thereby illustrating the uterus's dynamic nature. The fluctuating thickness and texture of the endometrium during the menstrual cycle demonstrate its plasticity and fundamental functions in reproductive health and fertility. Surrounding the endometrium is the myometrium, a thick smooth muscle layer responsible for an important function in uterine contractions. The muscular layer provides the capability for labor during delivery, permitting the passage of the fetus through rhythmic, coordinated contractions.

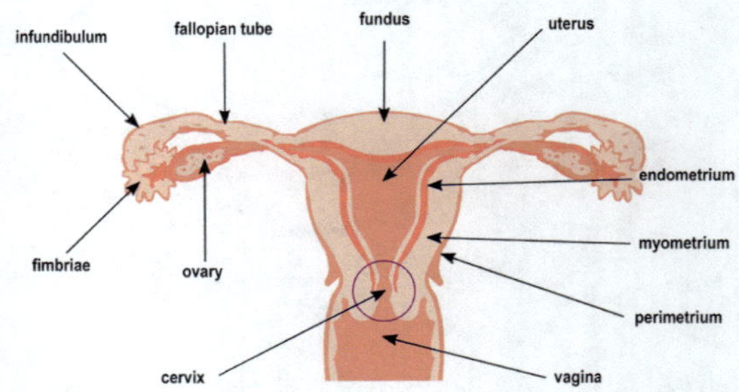

Figure 1.8. Human uterus and surrounding structures.

Source: https://upload.wikimedia.org/wikipedia/commons/7/72/Illu_cervix.svg

The myometrium is also characterized by the fact that it is capable of generating massive force, and its production is based on hormonal changes, particularly estrogen and oxytocin. Understanding the intricacy of the functioning of the myometrium explains the role of this layer in normal reproduction as well as in potential complications, such as uterine atony, where the uterus fails to contract adequately following delivery. The muscular structure of the myometrium also accounts for its defining contractile properties, underscoring its crucial function in reproductive health during and outside of pregnancy. Over the myometrium lies the perimetrium, a sheath of serous tissue that protects and supports the uterus. Its external cover is composed primarily of connective tissue and epithelial cells that firmly hold the uterus in the pelvic cavity. The perimetrium serves to maintain the location of the uterus in its position throughout the changes the uterus goes through during a woman's lifetime, such as hormonal changes concerning menstruation, pregnancy, and menopause. Additionally, awareness of the anatomic association between the perimetrium and other pelvic organs is significant in the understanding of numerous pathologies, such as adenomyosis or pathologies outside the uterus.

An integrative approach to the uteruss structure and layers is concerned with the multifunctional character of the organs role and its position in the general context of the anatomy of the female reproductive system, as outlined in previous research of emphasis on these aspects and their function in reproductive health (Elliott *et al.*, 2006; Baskin *et al.*, 2019).

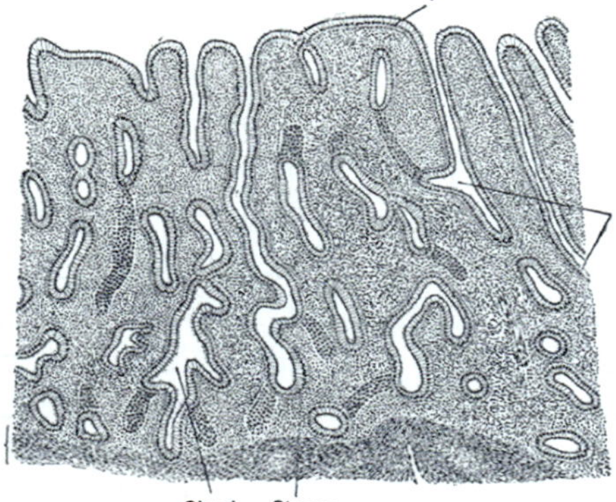

Figure 1.9. Vertical section of mucous membrane of human uterus.

Source: https://en.wikipedia.org/wiki/Uterus#/media/File:Gray1169.png

1.2.3. Ovaries and Their Functions

The two tiny almond-shaped organs in the female pelvic cavity, the ovaries, play a central role in female reproductive anatomy and function. The ovaries secrete oocytes, or eggs, on which reproduction is based. Each ovary contains numerous structures called follicles in which there is an immature egg. Throughout a woman's reproductive life, typically from puberty to menopause, a collection of follicles ripens with each menstrual cycle, peaking with ovulation—when a single or multiple mature eggs are secreted into the fallopian tubes for potential fertilization. This hormonal message-controlled monthly cyclical process keeps the female body prepared for possible pregnancy monthly, highlighting the key role of the ovaries in fertility and reproductive health. In addition to their contribution to gamete formation, the ovaries secrete hormones that are crucial to the body, i.e., estrogen and progesterone. Estrogen, which is primarily released by mature follicles, is essential in the regulation of the menstrual cycle and in the development of secondary sexual characteristics such as breast enlargement and pubic hair. Progesterone, released from the corpus luteum after ovulation, prepares the endometrium for a fertilized ovum to implant and maintains early pregnancy. The balance between these hormones is important since their imbalance can lead to irregular menstrual cycles and impact reproductive well-being. Pertinent research shows the complex interaction of ovarian hormones with the uterine environment, influencing such disease states as endometrial hyperplasia or associated pathologies, and the central role the ovaries play in maintaining a healthy reproductive system (Chatdarong *et al.*, 2003).

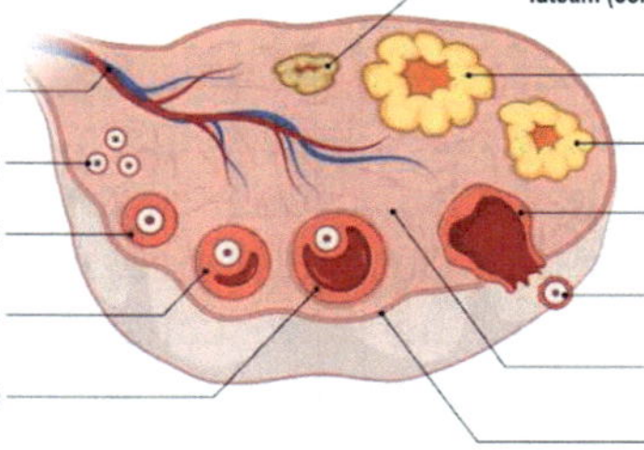

Figure 1.10. Ovary anatomy.

Source: https://biologynotesonline.com/ovaries-definition-structure-hormones-functions/

Furthermore, the ovaries are anatomically significant organs that have interactions with much of the female reproductive system. They not only secrete eggs and hormones but also contribute to regulating cervical and uterine function throughout the various phases of the menstrual cycle. Current studies highlight that physiology and morphology of the uterus are adjusted to the ovarian function, with uterine contractions and motility of the cervix being regulated by ovarian steroid hormones (Elliott *et al.*, 2006). This interaction outlines the importance of ovaries not just for the formation of gametes but also for regulating the whole reproductive process. Disruptions of ovarian activity can thus chain into a chain of reproductive difficulties, ranging from infertility to menstrual dysfunction, highlighting the importance of in-depth understanding and exploration of these organs of significance in the female reproductive system.

Test Your Knowledge

1. What are the key anatomical features of the vagina and their roles?
2. What are the main structural layers of the uterus, and what is the function of each?

1.3. The Menstrual Cycle

Learning Outcome

1. Define phases of the menstrual cycle
2. Focus on the hormonal regulation of the cycle
3. Identify the impact of the menstrual cycle on female health

The menstrual cycle is a complex physiological process characterized by a sequence of physical and hormonal alterations that prepare the female body for potential pregnancy. Taking around 28 days, the cycle consists of a series of unique stages, including the follicular phase, ovulation, luteal phase, and menstruation. During the follicular phase, the pituitary gland secretes follicle-stimulating hormone (FSH), which stimulates ovarian follicles to grow. As follicles ripen, they secrete estrogen, and the uterine lining is thickened in preparation for implantation. This orchestration of hormonal interaction illustrates how delicate the mechanism is to achieve fertility in an effort to ensure species reproduction. Following the follicular phase is ovulation, a pivotal occurrence in the menstrual cycle. Triggered by a surge of luteinizing hormone (LH), ovulation occurs on day 14 when a mature follicle releases an ovum into the fallopian tube. Increased fertility lasts for about 24 hours, providing optimal opportunity for fertilization if sperm are available. The physiological readiness of the female body at this time is remarkable, with the uterine lining becoming even more profound, creating a fertile ground for a fertilized egg. Understanding ovulation timing and its biological purpose is crucial in women who may wish to become pregnant or adopt natural methods of family planning, recognizing the relevance of understanding the menstrual cycle as part of reproductive health education (Fehring *et al.*, 2004). Unless fertilization occurs, the menstrual cycle progresses into the luteal phase, with progesterone production, solidifying and holding the uterine lining in place. Without implantation, the hormone levels would then decrease eventually, leading to the shedding of this lining during menstruation. This is a pivotal phase not only signaling the end of one but also readying for the other. The process of menstruation can be traced back to broader health implications in terms of the ways in which environmental forces and endocrine disruptors could influence menstrual control. Studies with chemicals like diethylstilbestrol (DES) point to the significance of understanding how endocrine disruptors impact reproductive health across generations and emphasize the complex relationship between natural bodily processes and external forces (Cunha *et al.*, 1999).

1.3.1. Phases of the Menstrual Cycle

The menstrual cycle, a complex interplay of physiological processes, consists of four principal phases: the menstrual phase, follicular phase, ovulation, and luteal phase. The cycle lasts approximately 28 days, although variations exist between individuals. The menstrual phase is where the cycle begins, with the uterine lining being shed when the process of fertilization is unsuccessful, with or without menstrual bleeding. This phase is typically three to seven days in duration and is critical in making way for potential new ovulation. The release of stimulation hormones by the hypothalamus initiates the cycle, appreciating the delicate control of the female reproductive system. Understanding this phase is significant to appreciate how the cycle renews itself for potential conception in the subsequent cycle, encapsulating the importance of reproductive health. Entering the follicular phase, beginning after menstruation, the body prepares for ovulation.

The phase is characterized by the maturation of ovarian follicles, stimulated by follicle-stimulating hormone (FSH), which leads to a boost in estrogen. The increasing estrogen aids in the regeneration of the endometrial lining within the uterus in preparation for potential implantation of a fertilized ovum. Concurrently, follicles are selected in the ovaries, where typically a single follicle matures and others degenerate. This shows that female reproductive biology is dynamic because it has a direct impact on reproductive potential. Significantly, the follicular phase illustrates the body's intricate hormonal feedback processes, emphasizing how minuscule changes in hormones have profound repercussions for overall reproductive well-being, especially as it applies to natural family planning procedures, which rely on intimate knowledge of these cycles and their function in women's health (Fehring *et al.*, 2004).

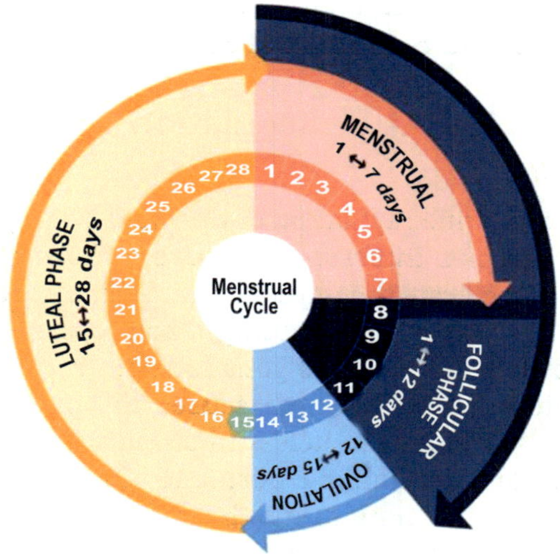

Figure 1.11. Menstrual cycle phases.

Source: https://www.cityfertility.com.au/wp-content/uploads/2025/03/Topic-1-Menstrual-Cycle-Phases-1-1-554x660.png

Ovulation is the climax of the menstrual cycle, occurring at approximately the midpoint of the cycle, frequently at day 14. The process involves the release of a mature egg from the ovary, triggered by a sudden surge in luteinizing hormone (LH). Not only does the sudden hormone shift mark the highest level of reproductive ability, but it also engages the uterus in potential pregnancy. Following ovulation, the luteal phase begins with the formation of the corpus luteum, which secretes progesterone to maintain the uterine lining in readiness for implantation. If there is no fertilization, progesterone will reduce, which will return the cycle to the menstrual phase. Existing studies have examined cognitive processes associated with fluctuating hormones throughout the cycle; however, evidence suggests discrepancies in such associations, and there should be caution when interpreting the findings on the correlation between hormone levels and cognitive capacity (Egli *et al.*, 2017). Each phase, therefore, reflects an integral part of the menstrual cycle that encompasses the interconnection of hormone function and reproductive capacity.

1.3.2. Hormonal Regulation of the Cycle

The endocrine regulation of the menstrual cycle is a complex interaction of several hormones that orchestrate the physiological events needed for reproduction. Starting each cycle, the hypothalamus releases gonadotropin-releasing hormone (GnRH), which causes the pituitary gland to release follicle-stimulating hormone (FSH) and luteinizing hormone (LH). FSH is essential in stimulating the development of the follicles in the ovaries, leading to increased levels of estrogen. With rising estrogen levels, they give negative feedback to the pituitary gland, regulating FSH and LH release. This delicate balance is not only crucial for follicular growth but also for preparing the uterine lining for potential implantation, emphasizing the intricate regulatory systems involved in the progression of cycles. With progression of the cycle into the luteal phase, hormonal communication undergoes a dramatic change. After ovulation, the ruptured follicle turns into the corpus luteum, which secretes progesterone. This hormone maintains the endometrial lining, creating a fertile ground for a fertilized egg. High levels of progesterone also suppress the secretion of GnRH, FSH, and LH, so that no other follicles grow during this period. Conversely, if not leading to fertilization, the corpus luteum collapses, and progesterone and estrogen levels drop. This hormone withdrawal leads to the sloughing of the uterine lining and subsequent menstruation and return to the follicular phase, illustrating how the hormones exhibit a cyclical trend in the reproductive cycle. Coordination between hormonal systems is not only essential for reproductive success but also has significant implications for women's health. It was discovered that hormonal contraceptives could interfere with this natural rhythm, affecting womens hormonal communication and potentially causing behavioral and physiological changes. For instance, HBC has been linked to variation in stress response and HPA axis function, and thus further research on its long-term impact on women's health (Perry *et al.*, 2023).

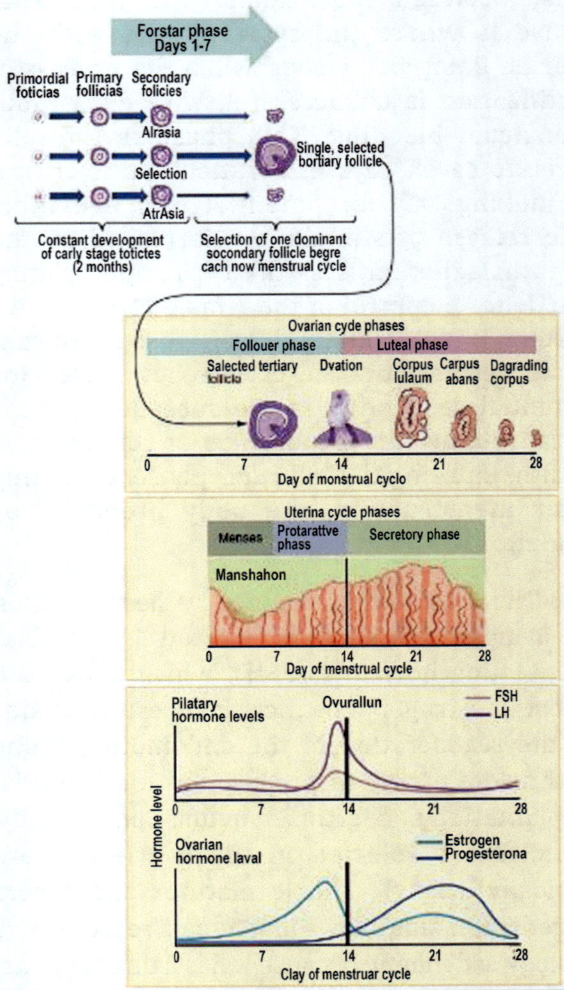

Figure 1.12. Hormone levels in ovarian and menstrual cycles.

Source: https://iastate.pressbooks.pub/app/uploads/sites/43/2021/02/ovarian-uterine-cycles.jpg

The variation in hormonal action between users and non-users can promote enhanced understanding of how hormonal control modifies physical and mental health outcomes in women (Perry *et al.*, 2023). Hence, proper education regarding hormonal functions and their overall implication is important in facilitating women's right to health decisions.

The variation in hormonal action between users and non-users can promote enhanced understanding of how hormonal control modifies physical and mental health outcomes in women (Perry *et al.*, 2023). Hence, proper education regarding hormonal functions and their overall implication is important in facilitating women's right to health decisions.

1.3.3. Impact of the Menstrual Cycle on Female Health

The article discusses the menstrual cycle, a dynamic equilibrium of hormonal shifts, with tremendous influence upon most aspects of women's health. Throughout each phase, varying concentrations of estrogen and progesterone hormones exert powerful influences upon physical as well as psychological well-being. For instance, estrogen has been suggested to stimulate mood and mental processes during the follicular phase, and progesterone, whose levels are at their peak during the luteal phase, is typically associated with premenstrual syndrome (PMS) and mood swings.

These cyclical changes are capable of inducing fluctuating symptoms that disrupt daily functioning and thereby impact the quality of life. Moreover, the co-existence of menstrual cycles and conditions like Irritable Bowel Syndrome (IBS) shows that hormonal fluctuations can further exacerbate gastrointestinal symptoms, hence drawing the connection between the reproductive and the digestive system, as evidenced by the cyclical pattern of IBS and menstrual cycle symptoms (Linson *et al.*, 2013).

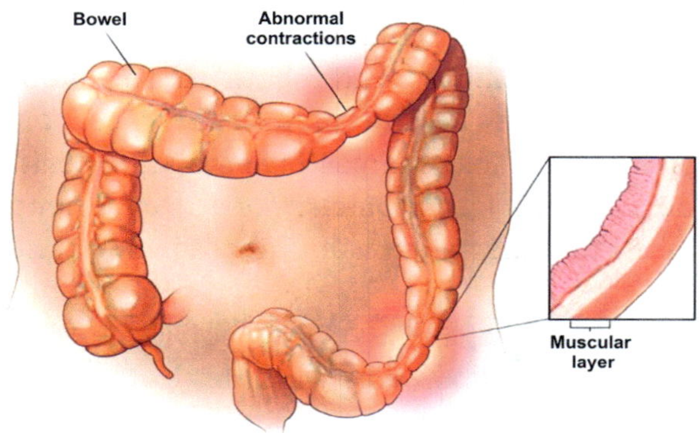

Figure 1.13. Irritable bowel syndrome (IBS).

Source: https://drrohitgoyalgastro.com/wp-content/uploads/2024/06/Untitled-design-1170x684.png

Significant here is that the significance of the menstrual cycle extends beyond reproductive health to influence other systems within the broader body that are responsive to hormonal change. As one example, cardiovascular health can be impacted by the changes in estrogen levels, which gives protective shielding during reproductive years but may contribute to increased risk after menopause. The role of endocrine disruptors in this context cannot be overruled. Their interference with hormonal cascades can further entangle health implications throughout the menstrual cycle. Developmental profiles and risk assessment for certain cancers are affected by low-dose exposures, particularly those that are estrogenic or androgenic (Cunha *et al.*, 1999). Lastly, knowledge about such effects is crucial in order to develop an efficient management plan to minimize discomfort and promote general well-being during the menstrual cycle. Aside from physical health, the menstrual cycle can also exert significant effects on mental health and emotional balance. Many women report experiencing increased levels of depression or anxiety with some parts of their cycles, most typically in the luteal phase, when progesterone acts. This correlation emphasizes the need to treat women's health in a holistic manner that incorporates both the hormonal consequences of the menstrual cycle and psychosocial factors impacting emotional health. The variability in women's health experience affirms that the reaction to changes in hormones can be greatly disparate, necessitating specific healthcare interventions. As the intricate relationship between the menstrual cycle and overall health consequences continues to be learned more about, it is significant that such elements of female health be dealt with in terms of female health perception and care.

Test Your Knowledge

1. What are the main phases of the menstrual cycle, and what occurs in each phase?
2. How do hormones like estrogen and progesterone regulate the menstrual cycle?

1.4. Fertilization and Pregnancy

Learning Outcome

1. Explain the process of fertilization
2. Describe the stages of embryonic development
3. Define changes in the female body during pregnancy

Fertilization is a key turning point in the female reproductive system anatomy that initiates the complex process culminating in pregnancy. Fertilization normally occurs in the fallopian tubes and is the union between the sperm and ovum, forming a zygote. The anatomical mechanisms are centrally important; the fallopian tube fimbriae assist in the trapping of the emitted ovum, while tubal conditions are ideal for sperm survival. Fertilization initiates a sequence of developmental processes that the zygote will go through, such as cell division and differentiation, as it makes its way to the uterus. It is necessary to understand these initial phases, as any disruption can cause infertility or ectopic pregnancy, which is very dangerous for health. This initial occurrence determines the course of the other stages of gestation. Following successful fertilization, the zygote goes through some rapid divisions known as cleavage, which becomes a multicellular organism known as a blastocyst. This phase of development is important as it leads the way to implantation into a prepared uterine endometrial lining. The fallopian tubes facilitate the passage of the blastocyst as well as provide conditions for initial embryonic development. The zygote to blastocyst transition is a dynamic process of intricate signaling and hormonal changes within the female reproductive tract that optimizes the uterine environment for implantation. The hCG hormone, secreted by the implanting blastocyst, plays a central role in maintaining the pregnancy by ongoing progesterone secretion. This hormonal interaction is indicative of the dynamic role of the reproductive anatomy and the reproductive system's capacity to adjust during early pregnancy as it conforms to the demands of the growing embryo.

The female reproductive system anatomy, over the duration of the pregnancy, significantly modifies to accommodate the expanding fetus. One of the significant changes is uterine enlargement since it becomes enormously large and voluminous. Another is increased vascularization, which facilitates the efficient delivery of nutrients and oxygen to the fetus.

The cervix, too, is altered, becoming softer and more vascularized to accommodate labor once the time is ripe. Lastly, the female body also experiences enormous hormonal alterations, primarily in progesterone and estrogen, to facilitate maternal health as well as fetal development.

These physical changes not only reflect the flexibility of the reproductive system but also reiterate the core interaction between function and anatomy throughout pregnancy. The culmination of these processes epitomizes the core significance of a healthy reproductive system in facilitating efficient fertilization and gestation throughout the entire process of pregnancy, laying the foundation for an effective birth outcome (Baumgartner *et al.*, 2020; Speiser *et al.*, 2018).

1.4.1. Process of Fertilization

Fertilization is a highly evolved interaction of biochemical and physiological events, the culmination of the cyclical phenomena of the female reproductive organs. Following ovulation, an oocyte that has been matured within the ovary departs and, for a specific period, is available for fertilization, typically 12 to 24 hours. Sperm inserted into the canal of the female reproductive tract will need to travel through the cervix and uterus to reach the oviduct, where fertilization occurs. This is facilitated by a number of postulated factors, including muscular contractions and biochemical signals that guide the sperm to their destination.

Sperm-oocyte interaction is important; not only must numerous sperm reach the site of fertilization, but they must be capacitated, a process that renders them penetrable through the protective oocyte coat. Upon reaching the oocyte, one sperm tends to enter to achieve fertilization.

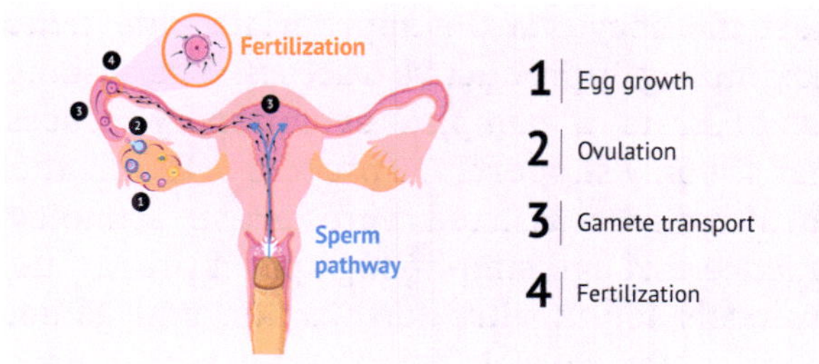

Figure 1.14. The steps of fertilization.

Source: https://www.invitra.com/en/wp-content/uploads/2019/12/natural-fertilization-process.png

The oocyte itself is surrounded by the zona pellucida, a glycoprotein covering that provides protection as well as a polyspermic barrier. Once a sperm manages to stick to and penetrate this covering, it causes a series of events that include the cortical reaction, which prevents other sperm from penetrating the oocyte. The sperm-oocyte membrane fusion leads to the activation of the oocyte, leading to the attainment of the second meiotic division and formation of a diploid zygote. This critical event not only initiates the pattern of development of the embryo but highlights the importance of each component of the fertilization process in congruence with the anatomical structure and function of the female reproductive system. The understanding of fertilization not only applies to the initial sperm-oocyte interaction but also to the significance of the female reproductive tract in maintaining the viability of sperm and providing optimal conditions for fertilization. In mammals such as pigs, there is a store of differentiated sperm within the utero-tubal junction that maintains viability over extended periods prior to ovulation. This reservoir is controlled by the composition of the oviductal fluid and by the presence of glycosaminoglycans, which are also involved in sperm capacitation and storage. These physiological remodelings ensure that the healthiest sperm are only released to meet the oocyte at the appropriate time, hence maximizing reproductive success. The findings demonstrate a complex evolutionary process that not only supports the process of fertilization but also directs assisted reproductive technology practice through simplifying sperm preparation protocols for in vitro fertilization and gamete conservation, as well as in porcine reproduction research (Tienthai *et al.*, 2003).

1.4.2. Stages of Embryonic Development

The journey through the embryonic stages of development is a marvelous and highly organized process that begins at fertilization, when a sperm and an egg unite to form a zygote. This single cell undergoes a rapid series of divisions and forms a morula, a compact ball of cells. With ongoing cleavage, the morula develops into a blastocyst that subsequently implants in the uterine wall, signaling the onset of the most critical period of development after differentiation has begun. The fate of these cells is decided by internal signals and cell-to-cell interactions, and the germ layers develop: the ectoderm, the mesoderm, and the endoderm. Each layer will then give rise to the numerous tissues and organ systems, including the reproductive organs, as exponential growth in complexity occurs in the embryo over this period (Davies, 2016). This initial phase sets the foundation for the elaborate anatomy that constitutes the female reproductive system. As development continues, the embryo is in the organogenesis stage, during which major structures of the reproductive system begin forming. During weeks five to six of pregnancy, the primordial germ cells migrate into the gonads forming at this stage. Differentiation into testes or ovaries is decided by specific genetic and hormone signals present. In females, the ovaries produce estrogen, which is essential for further differentiation of reproductive organs like the uterus and the fallopian tubes. This process is not only decided by predetermined genetic pathways but also by environmental forces that are interacting with the forming tissues. With the continued progression of embryonic development, endoderm and mesoderm contribute significantly to the establishment of the intricate architecture of the female reproductive system (Creek, 2009). Finally, embryonic complexity is comprehended in detail employing Waddington's model of epigenetic landscape, in which cellular differentiation is explained to occur along diverging paths.

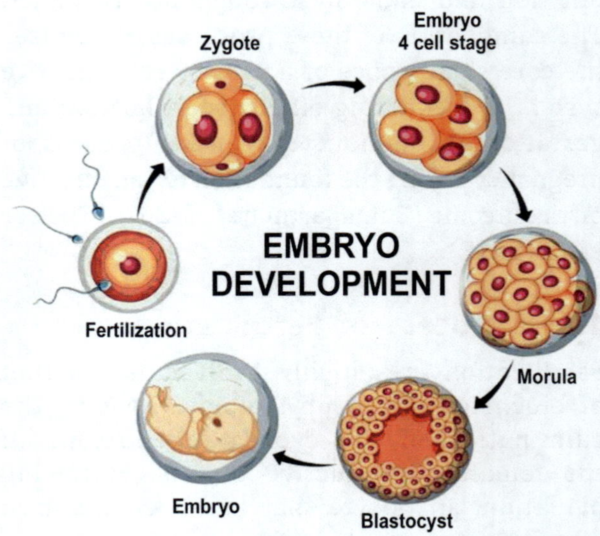

Figure 1.15. The four stages of embryonic development.

Source: https://www.ferty9.com/blog/the-four-stages-of-embryonic-development

Throughout the process of development of the embryo, the relation between genes and environment leads to an increase in cellular variety, finally yielding characteristic features of a reproductive system. Evidence indicates that the formation of varying cell types in the reproductive system follows an exponential process at this phase of development (Davies, 2016). Once complete, this intricate process ends with the formation of a fully operational anatomical structure with the ability to support later reproductive processes. It is here that perhaps we can better appreciate the awe-inspiring complexity and dynamism of embryonic development, particularly with regard to the anatomy of the female reproductive system.

1.4.3. Changes in the Female Body During Pregnancy

Pregnancy leads to profound physiological changes in the woman's body, reflective of the complex interplay of hormonal control and anatomical modification. The most pertinent among these alterations is the increase in blood volume, up to 50% of its non-pregnant state. This rise ensures adequate oxygen and nutritional supply to the fetus forming within, as well as prepares the mother to withstand the stresses associated with childbirth. Furthermore, the cardiac system counteracts this through increased cardiac output so that the heart is able to pump blood in larger quantities per minute. This not only supports fetal development but also changes the mother's physiology, at times leading to such conditions as gestational hypertension. Modifications to blood flow are echoed throughout the rest of the organs' systems, indicating a concerted action by the female body to nurture the developing life within, which points to the simultaneous interdependence of anatomical structure and reproductive role (Didoruc *et al.*, 2025).

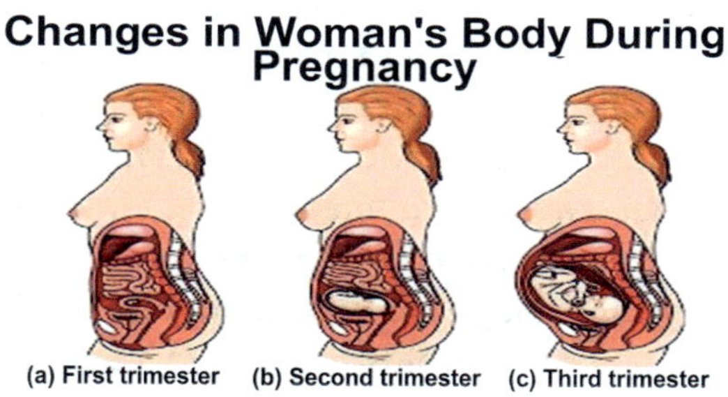

Figure 1.16. Body Changes during Pregnancy.

Source: https://cdn2.momjunction.com/wp-content/uploads/2014/04/Typical-Body-Changes-During-Pregnancy-1.jpg

The endocrine system is significantly altered during pregnancy, with the majority of the changes caused by the effect of hormones such as human chorionic gonadotropin (hCG), estrogen, and progesterone. hCG is important shortly after conception, as it instructs the ovaries to continue secreting progesterone, which is required to help maintain the uterine lining and also prevent menstruation. Later in pregnancy, rising estrogen and progesterone levels induce numerous changes, including enlargement of breast tissue and changes in metabolism. Further, these hormonal alterations are also accountable for the body's adaptation to support fetal growth, influencing mood, energy, and overall health.

Moreover, the hormonal milieu acts to dampen the mother's immune system to prevent rejection of the fetus, an indicator of the critical function of endocrine alterations during this period (Mathyk *et al.*, 2024). This delicate hormonal balance is not only necessary for the support of pregnancy but also for facilitating the female body's preparation to lactate after giving birth. In addition to physiological changes, profound anatomical modifications occur within the female reproductive system throughout pregnancy. The uterus undergoes extreme enlargement, from a minute pear-shaped organ to a gigantic organ with the capacity to hold a developing fetus.

This growth is followed by changes in the uterine musculature and blood supply that adapt to accommodate the needs of pregnancy. Simultaneously, the cervix becomes softer and more open to accommodate giving birth. The ligaments of the pelvis also stretch to permit the movement of the fetus and to prepare the body for delivery. Besides, the additional weight gained during pregnancy alters the mother's center of gravity and leads to postural adjustments and, at times, pain or discomfort. These anatomical changes are important to facilitate successful delivery and overall mother and infant health, indicating the dynamic nature of the womanly form during this development process (Didoruc *et al.*, 2025).

Test Your Knowledge

1. What are the key steps involved in the process of fertilization?
2. What are the main stages of embryonic development from zygote to fetus?

1.5. Common Disorders

Learning Outcome

1. Discuss the polycystic ovary syndrome (PCOS)
2. Understand endometriosis and its effects
3. Define uterine fibroids and treatment options

The female reproductive system is susceptible to a wide variety of disorders that can have a significant impact on a woman's quality of life and well-being. One such common disorder is endometriosis, where tissue similar to the lining of the uterus develops outside the uterus and causes chronic pain, heavy bleeding, and infertility. Not only does this impact usual reproductive function, but it also causes long-term problems such as psychological disturbance and lowered work performance. Accurate diagnosis is paramount since many of the symptoms overlap with other gynecologic diseases; imaging methods, particularly magnetic resonance imaging (MRI), have proven helpful in outlining the degree of endometriosis because of their better contrast and resolution. With increasing awareness of this condition, so does the importance of early and precise diagnostics in addressing women's health issues (Anastasi *et al.*, 2015).

Another widespread disorder of the female reproductive system is polycystic ovary syndrome (PCOS), an endocrine disorder characterized by irregular menses, high levels of androgens, and polycystic ovaries. PCOS women tend to develop multiple metabolic complications such as obesity, insulin resistance, and risk of type 2 diabetes. The disease also complicates pregnancy because abnormal menstruation prevents ovulation. Treatment of PCOS involves changes in lifestyle such as diet and exercise, as well as medical treatment aimed at hormonal control. A clear understanding of PCOS is necessary for healthcare professionals, as the disorder acts to describe the interrelatedness between endocrine and reproductive health. Identification and treatment of PCOS effectively is key to enhancing the overall health status of such women (Gilbert *et al.*, 2021).

Last but not least, uterine fibroids are another prevalent issue in the female reproductive disorders arena. These benign uterine tumors can produce a wide range of symptoms, including excessive menstrual flow, pelvic discomfort, and pressure on nearby organs. The pathogenesis of fibroids remains multifactorial with contributions from genetic, hormonal, and environmental factors. Imaging studies like ultrasound or MRI are predominantly employed for diagnosis, which not only confirm the presence of fibroids but also evaluate their size and impact on uterine well-being. Treatment varies from watchful waiting in asymptomatic cases to medical treatment and surgery in severe cases. Education and enlightenment regarding uterine fibroids are the order of the day, as the majority of women may not realize they have the condition until complications arise, and this further underscores the importance of regular check-ups with a gynecologist (Anastasi *et al.*, 2015).

1.5.1. Polycystic Ovary Syndrome (PCOS)

Polycystic ovary syndrome (PCOS) is a complex endocrine disorder with considerable impact on the anatomy and physiology of the female reproductive system. The condition is defined by hormonal disturbances and is predominantly expressed in terms of irregular menstrual cycles, which can have significant impacts on reproductive health. PCOS is frequently associated with high androgen levels, resulting in manifestations like hirsutism and acne. Not only do these expressions disrupt physiological processes, but they also disrupt psychological well-being. It has been learned through studies that the majority of women with PCOS attest to a lowered quality of life due to these symptoms, which shows why learning about this disorder is essential as part of female reproductive anatomy and health (Srour *et al.*, 2024).

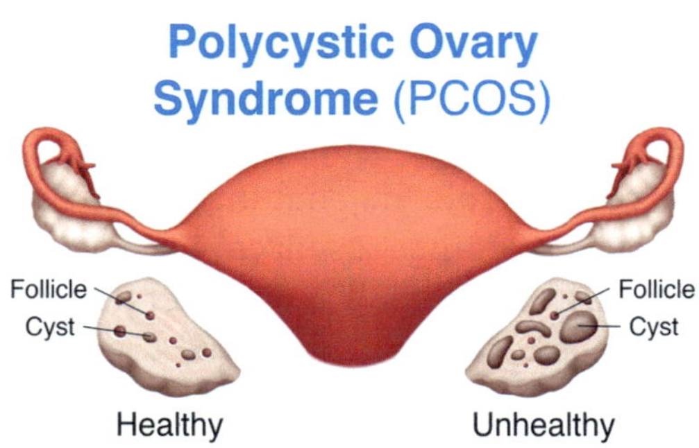

Figure 1.17. Polycystic Ovary Syndrome (PCOS).

Source: https://static.acne.org/ipb_uploads/monthly_2018_08/02-polycystic-ovary-syndrome-pcos.jpg.92a2e229cfe22f2517bda8879751c5d3.jpg

The prevalence of PCOS is notable, affecting a substantial number of women in the childbearing population. The estimated prevalence suggests that a substantial percentage of females are diagnosed with or manifest compatible signs of the syndrome. A study reported that approximately half of a group of female nurses were suspected to have PCOS and did not know they had the condition, even though they had presented common symptoms (Srour *et al.*, 2024). These findings reflect an alarming lack of education and knowledge about PCOS. Given the syndromes' complex nature, health professionals must promote education and early diagnosis in an effort to improve the quality of life for those afflicted with this disease.

Effective management procedures coupled with lifestyle modification and medical intervention will be required to minimize long-term health repercussions of PCOS. PCOS has numerous treatment options, and the most important aspect of management is an approach that is multipronged. Exercise, in the form of aerobic activity, is usually a part of a complete program for management, having a favorable impact on hormonal balance, weight control, and general well-being. Exercise has been said to significantly influence insulin sensitivity and metabolic control in women with PCOS and improve their quality of life accordingly. In addition, exercise intervention has been associated with symptom reductions such as mood disturbance and weight gain, which are prevalent in this population. Therefore, the integration of exercise as a core component of PCOS management not only addresses metabolic and reproductive conditions but also increases well-being, which shows the intricate association between endocrine function and lifestyle in the physiology of the female reproductive tract.

1.5.2. Endometriosis and Its Effects

Endometriosis, a state of endometrial tissue being found outside the uterus, greatly influences the anatomy and physiology of the female genital tract. The illness can lead to various pelvic abnormalities, including pain, menorrhagia, and formation of adhesions that alter the usual anatomical relations in the pelvis. Symptomatic manifestations of endometriosis also have a tendency to reach beyond the genital tract and impact overall health and quality of life. Pelvic pain is particularly disabling, generally precipitating increased absenteeism from work and school and therefore disrupting the social and economic functioning of women. Moreover, the psychological effects of living with a chronic illness may lead to anxiety, depression, and reduced self-esteem and contribute to the overall impact of this disease on women's lives. Endometriosis diagnosis is critical because it informs management and allows early treatment of symptoms. Laparoscopy has traditionally been the gold standard for endometriosis diagnosis since it allows direct visualization of the ectopic endometrium. The last few years have witnessed ultrasound and magnetic resonance imaging (MRI) modalities playing a more significant role. MRI in particular has been shown to be very accurate in the diagnosis of endometriosis and its extent, with good details of associated conditions like adenomyosis. Advances in imaging techniques show a better understanding of the disease, allowing for diagnosis and treatment of endometriosis by medical practitioners more effectively, lessening its detrimental effect on women's reproductive health and overall well-being (Anastasi *et al.*, 2015).

Management of endometriosis is typically a multi-modal experience including medical therapy, surgery, and changes in lifestyle. Hormonal therapies like oral contraceptives or GnRH agonists are employed to reduce menstrual pain and bleeding, whereas surgical techniques—via laparoscopy—can be employed to remove endometrial lesions and adhesions. Using a combination of these treatment modalities can not only alleviate symptoms but also improve the fertility potential for the women involved.

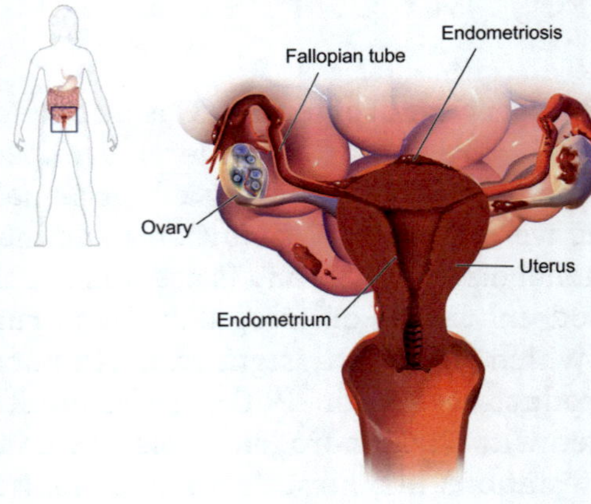

Figure 1.18. Endometriosis occurs when the uterine tissue (endometrium) grows outside of the uterus, usually around the pelvic area.

Source: https://www.drnavdeepfertility.com/wp-content/uploads/2022/03/1.-Endometriosis-graphic-pic-copy.jpg

Notably, addressing the psychological and emotional dimensions of coping with endometriosis is equally important for overall care; support groups, counseling, and education play a central role in enabling such holistic care. With ongoing research improvements continuously expanding our understanding of endometriosis, further initiatives are required to give the best possible care and support to impacted women during their reproductive life (Bosteels *et al.*, 2007).

1.5.3. Uterine Fibroids and Treatment Options

Uterine fibroids, or leiomyomas, are benign smooth muscle tumors representing the most common pathologic abnormality within the female reproductive tract. Epidemiologic information indicates that these tumors occur in 20 to 50% of women older than 30 years, with mixed manifestations ranging from asymptomatic status to disabling complications such as abnormal vaginal bleeding, urinary problems, and infertility (N/A, 2021). The cause of uterine fibroids is still somewhat mysterious; predispositions may include genetic ones, hormonal factors, and environmental influences. A knowledge of the anatomy and physiology of the uterine organ is fundamental to an understanding of the significance of fibroids, which can profoundly affect women's health and their reproductive function. With respect to uterine fibroid treatments, medical and surgical approaches both lie on a spectrum of measures depending on the symptoms and reproductive goals of the patient. Pharmacologic interventions include hormonal therapy and gonadotropin-releasing hormone agonists that treat symptoms but do not remove fibroids entirely. Surgical interventions vary from myomectomy, where the uterus is not removed, to hysterectomy, where it is completely removed (N/A, 2021). With long-term implications of all of the available treatments in mind, particularly the patient's future desire for fertility and the impact of surgery on normal reproductive function, over the years, a trend has been to pursue minimally invasive treatments that reduce recovery time and rates of complications. New non-invasive therapies such as Magnetic Resonance-guided Focused Ultrasound Surgery (MRgFUS) are revolutionizing the treatment of uterine fibroids. This technology uses ultrasound waves to ablate fibroid tissue by heating it without incising, thereby reducing risks related to traditional surgery, such as bleeding and infection (Zaher *et al.*, 2010). In addition to the advantages of outpatient procedure status and preservation of the uterus, MRgFUS is meeting not only symptom relief that patients pursue but also their concerns about future childbearing and recovery time. Initial studies have reported substantial relief from symptoms and long-term reduction in fibroid size, holding out hope for a new option for those who were not willing to attempt conventional treatments in the past. These developments represent a shift towards patient-centered treatment of uterine fibroids, ultimately improving quality of life for women.

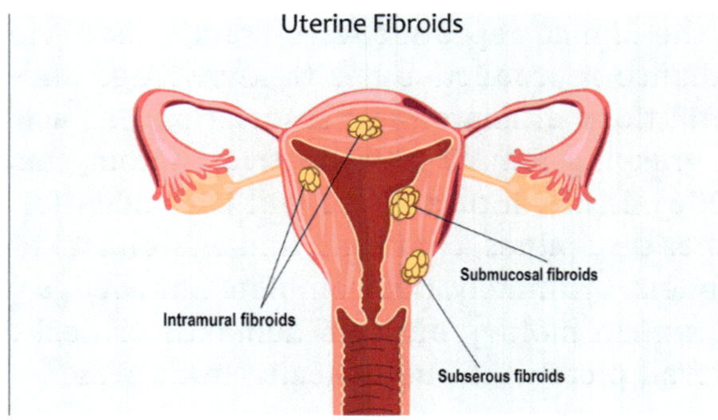

Figure 1.19. Uterine Fibroids.

Source: https://preferredvasculargroup.com/wp-content/uploads/2020/01/Preferred-Vascular_Uterine-Fibroids.png

Test Your Knowledge

1. How does endometriosis affect the reproductive system and overall health?
2. What are uterine fibroids, and what treatment options are available?

SUMMARY

The anatomy of the female reproductive system is the key to understanding not only the reproduction physiology but also more universal health and disease concepts. This complex system comprises various structures, each with its own function that collectively makes conception, gestation, and childbirth possible. Ovaries, oviducts, uterus, and vagina all play important parts in the cyclical female process of reproduction, in which hormonal interaction regulates oocyte and uterine lining development for potential implantation. Awareness of the coordinated interaction of the anatomical structures enhances knowledge regarding reproductive health and the significance of continued study of the normal processes and pathological aberrations within this system. Besides, integration of reproductive knowledge into common health care practice can ensure better clinical outcomes for women. As seen in the case of native turkeys, where experiential knowledge of reproductive management is declining, it is crucial to accord a very high priority to education and training in reproductive health among various populations (Cuca-García *et al.*, 2025). Understanding the female reproductive system is not only a matter of biology but also social, cultural, and economic dimensions that influence how women perceive and care for their reproductive health. By developing an environment conducive to learning and support, healthcare providers are able to manage the unique concerns of women with varying backgrounds in such a manner that reproductive health care becomes attainable and informed. As we put together our understanding of the female reproductive system, it is obvious that we require a multi-disciplinary approach to enhance reproductive health knowledge and therapeutic management. Formalizations of precise definitions of anatomical associations, as achieved in certain biomedical ontologies, can assist us in grasping female reproductive anatomy and clinical correlates more effectively (Bittner *et al.*, 2006). In the future, there will be a need for interdisciplinary co-operation between scientists of other disciplines, clinicians, and anatomists to fill in the gaps in knowledge and improve healthcare models. Ultimately, this complete knowledge of this anatomy not only increases our understanding of human biology but also demands critical discourse about the worth of women's health in the overall picture of public health initiatives.

The anatomy of the female reproductive system is a complex arrangement of structures that plays a central function in reproduction, overall well-being, and the regulation of the hormones. The foundation of the system lies with the ovaries, which are responsible for the production of oocytes as well as hormones like estrogen and progesterone. Not only does the menstrual cycle control these hormones, but secondary sexual characteristics and pregnancy rely on them. Moreover, the fallopian tubes, the uterus, and the vagina are contiguous tubes, which carry sperm and oocytes through, again highlighting the complex correspondence between these organs. Understanding the nuances of these organs is important to gaining insight into how they function within reproductive health and highlighting where medical intervention might be required, as in more general discussions both of hormonal equilibrium and of reproductive anatomy (Arnold *et al.*, 2002). The other key aspect of the female reproductive system is the influence of various hormonal signals on its functioning and development. Menstruation, follicular phase, ovulation, and the luteal phase are controlled by hormonal changes in the menstrual cycle. Each stage is marked by specific hormonal changes in anticipation of potential conception. Disruptions of this hormonal equilibrium may result in disease states like polycystic ovary syndrome or endometriosis, which not only affect fertility but also have general health implications for women's health. Examination of the hormonal interdependencies illustrates the delicate balance required for successful reproduction and general health and demonstrates the importance of hormonal research in dictating female physiology (Baskin *et al.*, 2017). In addition to control at the hormonal level, interplay among genetic, environmental, and developmental factors also shapes the anatomy and physiology of the female reproductive system. For instance, prenatal exposure to certain substances may lead to congenital anomalies, which in females can manifest as structural and functional differences in girls and women. The adolescent anatomical alterations form the basis of adult reproductive wellness, and the prospective activity of certain genetic markers could possibly provide insight into susceptibility to reproductive sickness. Of note, investigations into conditions such as hypospadias have demonstrated how disruptions during periods of critical development can have lasting effects. Hence, extensive research into these diverse factors gives us a greater understanding of the female reproductive system and offers areas for investigation and possible treatments (Arnold *et al.*, 2002; Baskin *et al.*, 2017).

KEY TERMS FROM THIS CHAPTER

Oocyte	Follicle
Corpus luteum	Fallopian tube
Fimbriae	Uterus
Endometrium	Myometrium
Perimetrium	Cervix
Cervical canal	Vagina
Hymen	Vulva
Labia majora	Labia minora
Clitoris	Vestibule

CRITICAL THINKING QUESTIONS

1. **Which of the following is the site of fertilization in the female reproductive system?**
   a. Uterus
   b. Vagina
   c. Ovary
   d. Fallopian tube
2. **What is the function of the ovaries in the female reproductive system?**
   a. Transport of the egg
   b. Fertilization of the egg
   c. Production of eggs and hormones
   d. Implantation of the embryo
3. **Which structure connects the uterus to the external environment?**
   a. Fallopian tube
   b. Vagina
   c. Cervix
   d. Urethra
4. **What is the name of the inner lining of the uterus that sheds during menstruation?**
   a. Myometrium
   b. Endometrium
   c. Perimetrium
   d. Epithelium
5. **The narrow passage forming the lower end of the uterus is called the:**
   a. Fallopian tube
   b. Cervix
   c. Vagina
   d. Fundus

Short Answer Questions

1. What are the main internal organs of the female reproductive system?
2. Which external structure protects the vaginal and urethral openings?
3. What hormone triggers ovulation during the menstrual cycle?
4. Where in the female reproductive system does fertilization typically occur?
5. What is the term for the developing human during the first 8 weeks of pregnancy?
6. Name one common disorder of the female reproductive system that can affect fertility.

Answer to Critical Thinking Questions

1. (d) 2. (c) 3. (b) 4. (b) 5. (b)

REFERENCES

1. Ali, M., & Sikandar, A. (2020). *Micro-Architecture of The Female Reproductive System*. https://core.ac.uk/download/322580266.pdf (accessed on 14th June 2025).
2. Ali, R., Lei, R., & Xu, J. (2024). *Research Progress of Applied Anatomy of Labia Minora in Plastic Surgery*. https://core.ac.uk/download/616936497.pdf (accessed on 14th June 2025).
3. Almeida, M., Elkin, P., Farinelli, F., *et al.* (2016). *OntONeo: The Obstetric and Neonatal Ontology*. https://core.ac.uk/download/131214730.pdf (accessed on 14th June 2025).
4. Anastasi, E., Ballesio, L., Bernardo, S., *et al.* (2015). *Endometriosis: 10 Keys Points for MRI*. https://core.ac.uk/download/54518026.pdf (accessed on 14th June 2025).
5. Arnold, K., Lloyd, E., Mitchell, S. D., *et al.* (2002). *Session 2: Female Orgasms and Evolutionary Theory*. https://core.ac.uk/download/11920462.pdf (accessed on 14th June 2025).
6. Baskin, L. S., Cao, M., Cunha, G. R., *et al.* (2019). *Reproductive Tract Biology: Of Mice and Men*. https://core.ac.uk/download/323311356.pdf (accessed on 14th June 2025).
7. Baskin, L., Cao, M., Cunha, G. R., *et al.* (2017). *Flutamide-Induced Hypospadias in Rats: A Critical Assessment*. https://core.ac.uk/download/323311348.pdf (accessed on 14th June 2025).
8. Baumgartner, H., De Backer, J., Babu-Narayan, S. V., Budts, W., Chessa, M., Diller, G. P., Lung, B., *et al.* (2020). 2020 ESC Guidelines for the management of adult congenital heart disease. *European Heart Journal, 42*, 563–645. https://doi.org/10.1093/eurheartj/ehaa554 (accessed on 14th June 2025).
9. Bittner, T., Donnelly, M., & Rosse, C. (2006). *A Formal Theory for Spatial Representation and Reasoning in Biomedical Ontologies*. https://core.ac.uk/download/pdf/9412351.pdf (accessed on 14th June 2025).
10. Bosteels, J., D'Hooghe, T., Van Herendael, B., *et al.* (2007). *The Position of Diagnostic Laparoscopy in Current Fertility Practice*. https://core.ac.uk/download/55795844.pdf (accessed on 14th June 2025).
11. Chatdarong, K. (2003). *Reproductive Physiology of The Female Cat*. https://core.ac.uk/download/11694645.pdf (accessed on 14th June 2025).
12. Creek, G. A. (2009). The reproductive system and embryology of the snail *Pomatiids elegans* (Müller). *Volume (121)*, 599–640. https://www.semanticscholar.org/paper/186eeefc694cca313835be1a8abc9c623514adac (accessed on 14th June 2025).
13. Cuca-García, J. M., Gallegos-Sánchez, J., Herrera-Barragán, J. A., *et al.* (2025). *Reproductive Characterization of The Female Mexican Turkey (Meleagris gallopavo L.)*. https://core.ac.uk/download/647994365.pdf (accessed on 14th June 2025).
14. Cunha, G. R., Forsberg, J. G., Golden, R., *et al.* (1999). *New Approaches for Estimating Risk from Exposure to Diethylstilbestrol*. https://core.ac.uk/download/323072016.pdf (accessed on 14th June 2025).
15. Davies, J. (2016). *Anatomical Complexity Is Acquired at An Exponential Rate During Mouse Embryonic Development. Volume (2)*. https://www.semanticscholar.org/paper/ef1049319c697d30ee191171e247ab501edd96d0 (accessed on 14th June 2025).
16. Didoruc, S., & Enciu, V. (2025). Morphologic variations of the arterial vascular branches of the reproductive system in the female rabbits. *Medicină Veterinară: Materialele Simpozionului*

Ştiinţific Internaţional "50 Ani De Învăţământ Superior Medical Veterinar Din Republica Moldova." https://www.semanticscholar.org/paper/0d6e28632ee52e599871057b18ce5b37e022e2a0 (accessed on 14th June 2025).

17. Egli, M., Geraedts, K., Hengartner, M. P., *et al.* (2017). *Lack of Associations Between Female Hormone Levels and Visuospatial Working Memory, Divided Attention and Cognitive Bias Across Two Consecutive Menstrual Cycles.* https://core.ac.uk/download/141696144.pdf (accessed on 14th June 2025).
18. Elliott, C. J. H., Middleton, C. A., Nongthomba, U., *et al.* (2006). *Neuromuscular Organization and Aminergic Modulation of Contractions in the Drosophila Ovary.* https://core.ac.uk/download/60330.pdf (accessed on 14th June 2025).
19. Fehring, R. (2004). *The Future of Professional Education in Natural Family Planning.* https://core.ac.uk/download/213077036.pdf (accessed on 14th June 2025).
20. Franklin-Hall, L. (2020). *The Animal Sexes as Historical Explanatory Kinds.* https://core.ac.uk/download/199234750.pdf (accessed on 14th June 2025).
21. Ganeng, A., & Kucha, B. (2022). *Representations and Perceptions of Sexual Pleasure in Undergraduate Anatomy and Physiology (A&P) Courses.* https://core.ac.uk/download/643705091.pdf (accessed on 14th June 2025).
22. Linson, E. A. (2013). *The Interplay Between Hormones and Irritable Bowel Disease.* https://open.bu.edu/bitstream/2144/12149/6/Linson_Elyse_2013_nosig_nocv.pdf (accessed on 14th June 2025).
23. Mathyk, B., Imudia, A., Quaas, A. M., Halicigil, C., Karouia, F., Avci, P., Nelson, N. G., *et al.* (2024). Understanding how space travel affects the female reproductive system. *npj Women's Health.* https://www.semanticscholar.org/paper/1d1c3f6bcd7bd833d93dd645fbfbb05286429b45 (accessed on 14th June 2025).
24. McCarthy, G. L. (2008). *A Boy or A Girl? Parental, Family and Whanau Information Needs When a Child Is Born with An Intersex/DSD Condition: A Thesis Presented in Fulfilment of The Requirements for The Degree of MPHIL in Nursing at Massey University, Auckland, New Zealand.* https://core.ac.uk/download/157568810.pdf (accessed on 14th June 2025).
25. Peek, K. E. (2017). *Interview with Kathryn Peek.* https://core.ac.uk/download/80296538.pdf (accessed on 14th June 2025).
26. Perry, M. (2023). *Synthetic or Not: Implications of Hormonal Birth Control on Women's Hormones and The Cortisol Stress Response.* https://core.ac.uk/download/586154027.pdf / https://core.ac.uk/download/572707241.pdf (accessed on 14th June 2025).
27. Phillips, A., & Phillips, S. (2015). Recognizing female sexual dysfunction as an essential aspect of effective diabetes care. *Applied Nursing Research, 28*(3), 235–238. https://doi.org/10.1016/j.apnr.2015.04.007 (accessed on 14th June 2025).
28. Speiser, P., Arlt, W., Auchus, R. J., Baskin, L. S., Conway, G. S., Merke, D. P., Meyer-Bahlburg, H. F. L., *et al.* (2018). Congenital adrenal hyperplasia due to steroid 21-hydroxylase deficiency: An Endocrine Society* clinical practice guideline. *The Journal of Clinical Endocrinology & Metabolism, 103,* 4043–4088. https://doi.org/10.1210/jc.2018-01865 (accessed on 14th June 2025).

29. Srour, I. A., Salhab, S., Skaiki, H., Sakr, S., & Sheet, I. (2024). Assessment of prevalence, knowledge of polycystic ovary syndrome and health-related practices among female nurses in Lebanon. *The Open Public Health Journal*. https://www.semanticscholar.org/paper/bae735e073162096edce3a656d39b58dc39ad42f (accessed on 14th June 2025).

30. Tienthai, P. (2003). *Studies on the Sperm Reservoir of The Pig Oviduct*. https://core.ac.uk/download/11694536.pdf (accessed on 14th June 2025).

31. Trivedi, S., & Shah, A. (2024). Effect of aerobic exercises in polycystic ovarian syndrome (PCOS) females–A systematic review. *International Journal of Research and Review*. https://www.semanticscholar.org/paper/c538eb8e07eee20e4f911a81b7719e6dafb965a8 (accessed on 14th June 2025).

32. Whittier, J. (1993). *Beef Cattle Reproduction (1993)*. https://core.ac.uk/download/62788282.pdf (accessed on 14th June 2025).

33. Yager, A., Lok, E., Miller, J., Noel, K., Goodman, M., & Santamaria-Schwartz, R. (2012). *Birds, Bees and Bias: How Absent Sex ed Standards Fail New York's Students*. https://core.ac.uk/download/71361426.pdf (accessed on 14th June 2025).

34. Zaher, S. S. (2010). *Magnetic Resonance Guided Focused Ultrasound Surgery–A Novel Treatment for Uterine Fibroids*.

DEVELOPMENT OF GENITAL ORGANS AND GONADS

2

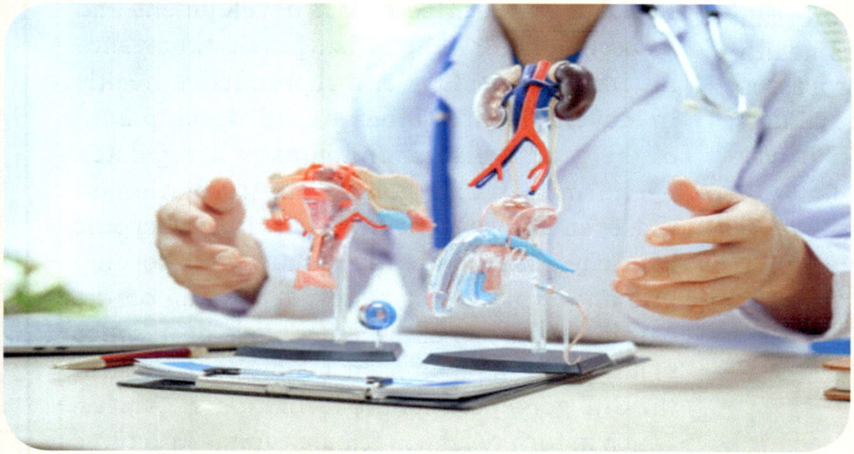

LEARNING OBJECTIVES

After studying this chapter, you will be able to:

1. Describe the embryonic development of the female reproductive system
2. Explain the processes involved in ovarian development
3. Outline the development of the uterus and vagina
4. Discuss the external genitalia development

Introduction

Development of the female genital organ and gonad is a complex, bidimensional biological process that is required for sexual identity and reproductive capacity. The development is regulated by hundreds of genetic, hormonal, and environmental factors that interact during embryonic and fetal maturation. It is crucial to know the intricate mechanisms of differentiation of these structures, particularly in light of disorders of sex development (DSD) resulting in abnormal development of chromosomal, gonadal, or genital sex. DSD encompasses an array of conditions that can result in clinical presentations such as primary amenorrhea and detection of unusual karyotypes, which underscore the necessity of an exhaustive review of present and past medical histories to ensure misdiagnosis is excluded, as in the case of a female patient with primary amenorrhea and a 46 XY karyotype (Huang *et al.*, 2016). Hormone regulation is a pivotal event in the development and function of female genital organs and gonads. Specifically, steroidogenesis, or the biochemical transformation of cholesterol into steroid hormones, is pivotal in this development. This complex biochemical process involves a series of enzymes, such as cytochrome P450 enzymes and hydroxysteroid dehydrogenases, each carrying out specific functions in hormone production. Steroidogenic enzyme regulation is not gland-specific but rather a dynamic system with complex interactions that dictate not only the quantity but also the quality of steroid hormones being synthesized. Here, knowledge of steroidogenesis is essential since it entails the entwining of genital organ structures with reproductive as well as health consequences. These developmental processes can be disrupted, leading to considerable clinical abnormalities and developmental disorders (Miller *et al.*, 2011). Beyond their function in reproductive health, the implications of normal genital organ and gonadal development include their effects on overall physiological homeostasis in women. Pathologies associated with the disruption of the developmental processes can affect multiple facets of health, such as fertility, body composition, and endocrine homeostasis. The interaction of genetic determinants, environment, and hormones underscores the complexity of the female reproductive development process. As research continues to elucidate the genes and pathways involved in these developmental processes, therapeutic regimen potential emerges. Therefore, a clear understanding of the female genital organ and gonad formation is not only central to the resolution of DSD, but central to resolving reproductive health and other health challenges on the whole, bearing witness to the centrality of this field in contemporary biological and medical research.

Definition of Genital Organs and Gonads

The definition of genital organs and gonads is vital in following the pattern of development of female reproductive organs. Genital organs, broadly categorized, are both external and internal organs involved in sexual reproduction. In females, the external genitalia are the clitoris, labia majora, and labia minora, whereas internal organs are the vagina, uterus, fallopian tubes, and ovaries. Gonads, in women specifically the ovaries, are crucial since they possess dual functions to generate gametes and to secrete hormones.

The ovaries are indispensable in regulating the menstrual cycle and influencing secondary sexual traits such as breast development and fat accumulation, emphasizing their importance in female physiology and reproductive health. In developmental biology, the development of the genital organs and gonads is regulated by hormones and genes. The formation of these structures occurs early in embryonic life, when the bipotential gonads can develop into either ovaries or testes, depending on the chromosomal sex and the presence or absence of the Y chromosome. In females, the lack of the SRY gene permits the formation of ovaries, which in turn results in female genital structures becoming mature. These organs' work is not only required for reproduction but for the entire endocrine system, as ovarian hormones such as estrogen and progesterone play a significant role in affecting the body functions throughout a woman's life span, including bone mass and reproductive function (Cools *et al.*, 2018). Understanding of genital organs and gonads also crosses over into more general implications for health and wellbeing, as with disorders of sex development (DSDs). These conditions present at birth can profoundly influence genital organ formation and function, and gonadal structure and function, and with them come multiple clinical issues as people with DSDs move through their physical and psychosocial environments. Interestingly, the treatment of such disorders requires a multidisciplinary frame that entails both medical and psychological care (Avasthi *et al.*, 2017). Such an integrated care model ensures a holistic understanding of the requirements of affected individuals, improving their healthcare outcomes. As research becomes more complex in the field of reproductive health, emphasis will remain on clear definitions and functional knowledge of genital structures and gonads for both clinical use and education of patients.

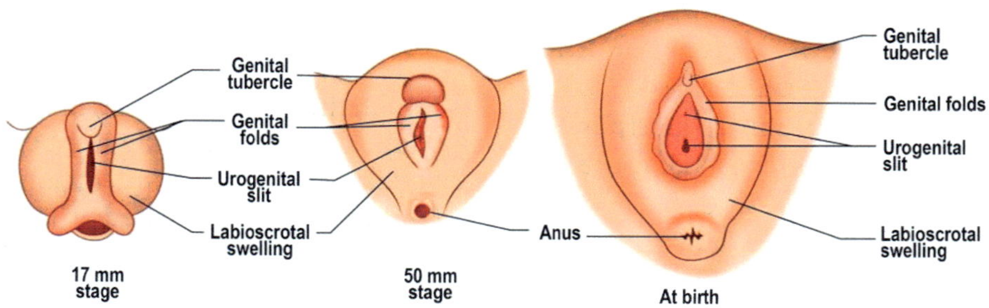

Figure 2.1. Diagrammatic representation showing differentiation of the female external genitalia.

Source: https://oshimu.com/wp-content/uploads/2021/07/Gynaecology-DC-Dutta.pdf

Importance of Studying Female Reproductive Development

Understanding female reproductive development is most significant for the advancement of medical science and societal perception of gender. The complexities of female gonadal and genital development are of critical significance not only in the context of normal development but also in the explanation of many medical disorders and intersex variation. The traditional markers of gender difference, such as chromosomes or genitals, are prone to overlooking the underlying neurologic and hormonal forces driving identity and reproductive capability. Studies have indicated that the BSTc area of the brain presents notable sex-differentiation, which, in itself, further justifies the argument that female reproductive development is researched in order to gain a better understanding of gender dysphoria and the transsexual phenomenon. By integrating conclusions from findings with implications for both biological and psychological aspects, we are able to refine our knowledge of gender, thus being able to offer better care and support to those investigating their gender (Kilty *et al.*, 2007). Also, the effects of endocrine disruptors such as atrazine reflect the sensitivity and complexity of gonad development. The evidence suggests that these types of chemicals may cause severe reproductive malformations such as hermaphroditism and unpigmented ovaries. Information on how environmental substances impact the normal progression of female reproductive development is crucial to public health and conservation concerns. The consequences of atrazine exposure demonstrate the vulnerability of developing gonads, pointing to the need for increased sensitivity in reproductive health policy. Whilst prudent in regard to environmental influences on development grows stronger, scientists are better equipped to influence legislative opinion around the use of chemicals and environmental protection policies. With a study on reproductive development, we can lobby for healthier worlds and shape educational courses that promote awareness of such effects at a wider scale (Collins *et al.*, 2006).

Lastly, the study of female reproductive development involves interdisciplinary approaches spanning biology, psychology, and sociology. The broad scope of inquiry guarantees comprehensive perspectives towards women's health, reproductive rights, and gender identity. By promoting collaborations across disciplines, scientists can address the intricate nature of female development, optimizing health outcomes, and informing best practices within the clinical setting. Perhaps most importantly for already vulnerable groups, in-depth knowledge of reproductive development offers potential for tailored healthcare approaches that honor personal needs. Moreover, this inter-disciplinary framework imposes the cultural competency of medicine to educate practitioners in the nuances of gender and reproductive health. Therefore, the applicability of research on female reproductive development extends beyond academic observation and transfers into the focus on actual social change and public health policy improvement around the globe.

2.1. Embryonic Development of the Female Reproductive System

Learning Outcome

1. Define the formation of the bipotential gonads
2. Describe the role of the Müllerian ducts
3. Discuss the influence of genetic and hormonal factors

Female reproductive system embryonic development is a complex process characterized by genetically and molecularly different routes that ultimately lead to the formation of ovarian structures and associated genital ducts. The indifferent gonad is established in the sixth week of pregnancy, and the process is regulated by coordinated gene expression and signaling cascades. One of the most important molecules of this developmental cascade is WNT4, which is crucial to the induction of ovary differentiation and simultaneously to the inhibition of male development. In vertebrates, WNT4 conservation suggests its importance in other species, and thus asserts its regulatory function in female sex determination and formation of the reproductive duct (Draper *et al.*, 2019). The mutual dependency of such cascades of signaling makes events early in embryonic development key to influencing not only reproductive anatomy but also broader implications for reproductive health and fertility. With further development, interaction between various transcription factors becomes the most critical. For instance, the transcription factor WT1 has been established as a key determinant in gonadal development. It has been found via scientific investigation that a lack of WT1 in early gonadogenesis results in substantive abnormalities within the male and female lines, destabilizing the balance required for proper gonad development (Chau *et al.*, 2025). The function of WT1 does not lie in structural integrity alone; its interaction with other genes enables somatic cell types to differentiate, which is necessary for reproductive function. Thus, the intricate interaction of gene control, pro-differentiation, and inhibitory signals guides the exact balance required for normal female reproductive anatomy development. Further, abnormalities caused by interruptions in these important pathways could lead to severe reproductive consequences. For instance, loss-of-function mutations in WNT4 and WT1 genes not only suppress the differentiation of normal gonads but also cause structural defects such as the existence of ambiguous genitalia and the absence of mature gonads. These observations are significant since they form a platform for understanding congenital disorders of the female reproductive system. When the specialized roles these genes play in embryonic development are studied, researchers can better understand the etiology of various reproductive anomalies and potential therapies. That detailed knowledge, in turn, guides clinical practice for reproductive health and corrects issues resulting from early development interference, illustrating developmental biology's role in guiding future medical treatment.

2.1.1. Formation of the Bipotential Gonads

The formation of the bipotential gonads is a critical aspect of sexual differentiation during embryonic development, and it is an essential period in the genital formation of both the male and female. All embryos initially form a batch of structures known as gonadal ridges, which are capable of developing into testes or ovaries depending on the genetic and hormonal influences to which they are exposed. The bipotential state of these gonads allows for flexibility in early embryonic life, setting the stage for sexual differentiation. At the period of 6 to 7 weeks of gestation, external and internal morphological features begin to emerge, depending on the chromosomal complement and subsequent hormonal occurrences, resulting in the development of either the male or female phenotype.

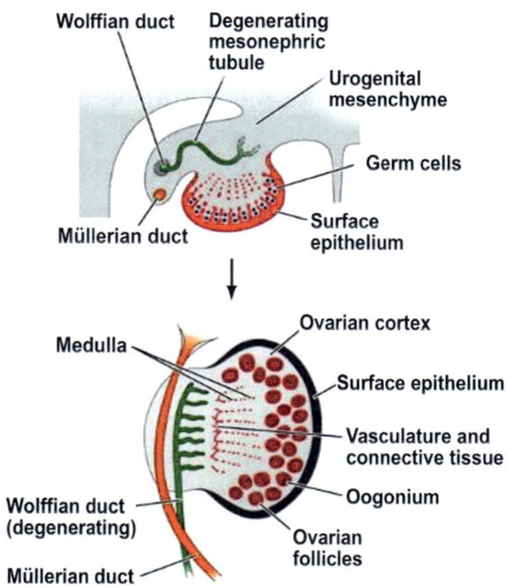

Figure 2.2. Bipotential gonads formation.

Source: https://image1.slideserve.com/2095001/bipotential-gonad-formation2-l.jpg

As the bipotential gonads develop, several factors orchestrate their differentiation. In chromosomally male embryos, the SRY gene on the Y chromosome plots the pathway to testis development. This gene initiates the induction of SOX9, a requirement for Sertoli cell differentiation, which in turn influences the nearby support cells to differentiate into Leydig cells. These events cause the release of testosterone and Müllerian inhibiting factor (MIF), which are responsible for the regression of female duct structures and induction of male secondary sex features.

In chromosomally female embryos, nevertheless, the absence of SRY allows a distinct pathway of ovarian development, wherein the absence of such male hormones allows the Müllerian ducts to develop into female reproductive features (Svingen *et al.*, 2013). Besides, bipotential gonad development not only acts as a basis for sexual differentiation but also emphasizes the intricate interplay of various signaling pathways and regulatory genes. The crucial protagonists such as WNT4 and DAX1 are well known to play key roles in ovarian development in support of ovarian follicle development and, thereby, oocyte maturation. In contrast to the male pathway, the female development remains largely hormone-independent at this point, thereby signaling the intrinsic nature of the bipotential gonads. This elementary understanding of bipotential gonad development not only adds to our vocabulary of reproductive biology but also educates us on disorders of sex development (DSD), which can provide insight into potential chromosomal defects or hormonal disruptions that can take place during this critical stage of development (Svingen *et al.*, 2013).

2.1.2. Role of the Müllerian Ducts

The Müllerian ducts, also known as the paramesonephric ducts, play a central role in the embryogenesis of the female genitalia. They arise from the urogenital ridge from around the sixth week of gestation and are accountable for the formation of major structures such as the fallopian tubes, the uterus, the cervix, and the upper two-thirds of the vagina. Unless male hormonal influences, particularly anti-Müllerian hormone (AMH), produced by Sertoli cells during the development of testicles, the ducts develop into female reproductive organs. Thus, the presence of functional Müllerian ducts is essential for the formation of a female internal reproductive system, in contrast to the regression in male embryos where testosterone and AMH induce the persistence of the Wolffian ducts and the regression of the Müllerian ducts (Díaz *et al.*, 2021).

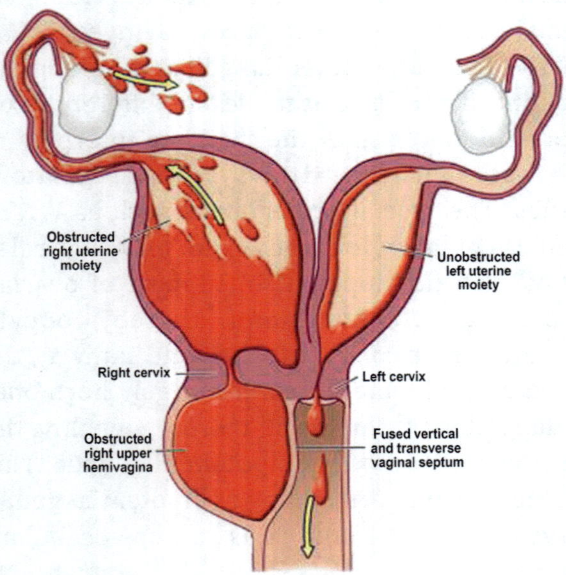

Figure 2.3. The Müllerian ducts.

Source: https://www.artfertilityclinics.com/in/en/art-blog/mullerian-duct-anomalies-causes-symptoms-treatment

Differentiation of Müllerian ducts into female reproductive organs also relies on intricate hormonal interactions during embryonic stages. In the normal XX embryo, the lack of testosterone results in the development of Müllerian ducts but simultaneously inhibits the growth of Wolffian ducts. The procedure is not a passive absence of male hormones, but specific factors such as WNT4, RSPO1, and FOXL2 play a crucial role in facilitating the development of these ducts and differentiation of the ovaries.

Abnormality in the pathways regulating Müllerian duct development can lead to numerous disorders of sex development (DSDs), highlighting the importance of this body structure in normal female sexual differentiation and reproductive health. The interplay of hormonal and genetic influences emphasizes the complex nature of the processes of development governing the female reproductive tract (Alejandro Díaz *et al.*, 2021).

Müllerian duct anomalies are a form of congenital anomaly that can have significant implications for reproductive health and function. Agenesis, duplication, or hypoplasia of Müllerian ducts may result in a variety of reproductive anomalies, including infertility, menstrual dysfunction, and pregnancy disorders.

As an example, Müllerian agenesis, or Mayer-Rokitansky-Küster-Hauser syndrome, results in rudimentary or absent development of the uterus and superior two-thirds of the vagina, with normal functioning ovaries. This is difficult for the victims in physical and psychological health. Furthermore, one must understand these anomalies through a full clinical and genetic evaluation to direct management options, such as surgery or assisted reproduction, hence emphasizing the preeminent position of the Müllerian ducts in the structure and function of the female reproductive system (Chitayat *et al.*, 2010).

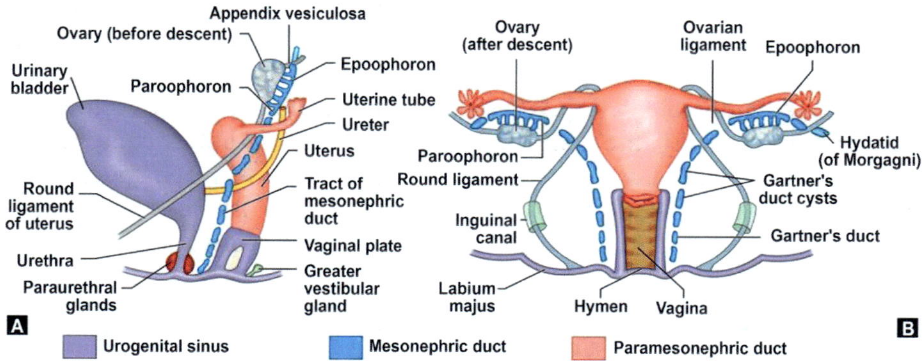

Figure 2.4. Diagrammatic representation showing the development of female reproductive systems from the primitive genital ducts. Vestigial structures are also shown. (A) Female fetus at 12 weeks; (B) Newborn female

Source: https://oshimu.com/wp-content/uploads/2021/07/Gynaecology-DC-Dutta.pdf

2.1.3. Influence of Genetic and Hormonal Factors

Sexual differentiation of the female genitalia and gonads is significantly influenced by these complex, intertwined combinations of genetic and hormonal determinants. Endogenous genetic elements of the reproductive cells are responsible for the earliest blueprints of sexual differentiation, in which some genes determine primary and secondary sexual characteristics. The SRY gene, for instance, initiates male differentiation mainly; its absence induces the formation of ovaries and associated feminine genitalia. Genetic variation can form heterogeneous states that affect genital structure and function, underscoring the significance of gene integrity to healthy reproductive development. Genetic impact is not just confined to structural outcomes since the chromosomal abnormalities also lead to disorders of sex development (DSD), producing clinical complexities regarding the diagnosis and treatment of abnormal genitalia (Ahmed *et al.*, 2017). Thus, it is necessary to understand these genetic factors for early detection and appropriate intervention strategies. Hormonal factors also play equally important roles in the development of female genitalia and gonads, well coordinated and regulated at different stages of prenatal and postnatal life. During fetal development, estrogen plays a critical role in the differentiation of the Müllerian duct to female organs like the uterus, the fallopian tubes, and the upper two-thirds of the vagina. The hormonal effect must be appropriately balanced, as any disruption could cause illnesses like congenital adrenal hyperplasia (CAH), brought on by hyperproduction of androgens that block the usual ovarian development. Furthermore, the intricate feedback loops of hormonal communication also persist in shaping reproductive function throughout a lifetime, influencing menstrual cycles, fertility, and general hormonal health. An understanding of these hormonal pathways reveals something of the fine detail of reproductive endocrinology in women, and why hormonal derangement will give rise to such maladies as polycystic ovary syndrome (PCOS), one of the most common of reproductive diseases. Also, the interaction of hormonal and genetic variables is expressed in unique ways within certain animal models, giving hints to broader concepts of reproductive health. For instance, the freemartin phenomenon in cattle illustrates how interactions within hormones combined with genetic variables can create distorted gonadal development. A freemartin, which is genetically female but masculine in character, is usually an occurrence of twin pregnancies in which a male and a female are involved; the hormones of the males disrupt the females' normal growth. The condition demonstrates not only the genetic nature of sexual differentiation but also the essential role of hormones in determining reproductive anatomy and function in abnormal situations (Gebisa *et al.*, 2021). Recognition of these interrelationships allows researchers and practitioners to better comprehend reproductive performance between species, where pertinent information is relevant for both animal husbandry practice and veterinary medicine.

Test Your Knowledge

1. What role do the Müllerian ducts play in the development of the female reproductive system?
2. How do genetic and hormonal factors influence the differentiation of the reproductive organs?

2.2. Ovarian Development

Learning Outcome

1. Differentiation of primordial germ cells
2. Define folliculogenesis and the formation of ovarian follicles
3. Explain the hormonal regulation during ovarian development

In the intricate pattern of female sexual development, ovarian development is a crucial component in establishing reproductive capacity. The ovaries arise from the genital ridges during embryogenesis and undergo a series of developmental stages that eventually yield mature functional gonads. The differentiation of these ancient germ cells into oocytes occurs in conjunction with a series of somatic cells, including granulosa and theca cells, that constitute the structural and functional integrity of the ovarian follicle. The microenvironment allows for oogenesis and supports the complex hormonal regulation necessary to enable menstrual cycling and fertility. As discussed, disruptions to ovarian development may result in aberrations of reproductive health, highlighting the significance of learning the cellular and molecular mechanisms associated with this process (Ray Coquard *et al.*, 2018).

In addition to the complexity of ovarian development, environmental influences, such as exposure to nanoparticles, further complicate the process. Recent studies focus their attention on the damaging effect these materials have on ovarian function by disrupting the protective capsules of the ovarian follicle. Nanoparticles can penetrate layers of theca and granulosa cells, ultimately disrupting hormone release and oocyte maturation as a result of oxidative stress and inflammatory mechanisms. More intriguing is the fact that hormone concentration alterations can quite forcefully interfere with the hypothalamic-pituitary-gonadal axis, with broader reproductive implications. This emerging field of research underscores the relevance of understanding how environmental exposures could interfere with ovarian integrity and function at critical points of development (Hou *et al.*, 2017). Because growth of the ovaries continues throughout a woman's life, it must also contend with the forces of age and disease, such as ovarian tumors. Non-epithelial ovarian cancer, including malignant germ cell tumors and sex cord-stromal tumors, accounts for a notable portion of ovarian cancers and can arise due to developmental anomalies in the ovarian tissue. Notably, malignant germ cell tumors have a high prevalence in young women, while sex cord-stromal tumors are more common in postmenopausal women and middle-aged women. Cognizance of the histopathological features and risk factors of such tumors enhances our diagnostic ability and targeted therapy design. Normal and abnormal ovarian development, therefore, deserves continued investigation to unlock the causative mechanisms that could be applied in clinical practice within gynecology and oncology (Ray Coquard *et al.*, 2018).

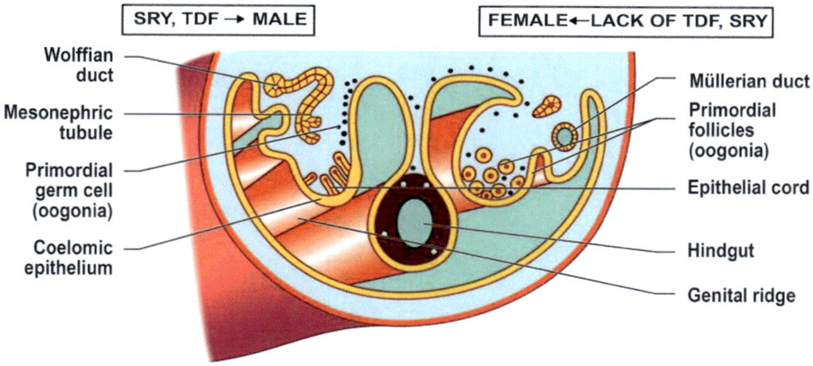

Figure 2.5. Differentiation of the indifferent gonads into ovary and testis with migration of the germ cells into the genital ridge (TDF = Testicular Determining Factor)

Source: https://oshimu.com/wp-content/uploads/2021/07/Gynaecology-DC-Dutta.pdf

2.2.1. Differentiation of Primordial Germ Cells

Primordial germ cells (PGCs) differentiation is a critical process in female genital organ and gonad development. The PGCs, which are pluripotent cells, in early embryogenesis migrate from their point of origin within the yolk sac to the point of gonad development and, in a series of developmental stages, are required for gametogenesis. The process of migration is controlled by unique signaling pathways and transcription factors required for PGC commitment to an oogenic fate. They reach this point in the cells, where they both proliferate and begin to differentiate and express differentiation markers into oocytes. Understanding these processes is very important because any disruption to them has serious reproductive health repercussions, which makes it important to understand the process of PGC differentiation within the overall context of female reproductive development. Furthermore, the role of genetic and epigenetic factors in PGC differentiation cannot be overstated. Several genes and the processes they are involved in regulate the subtle balance required for proper development of the female reproductive tract. For instance, specific signaling proteins are required to maintain the pluripotency of PGCs until they are in their right positions in the developing ovaries. Dysregulation of such genetic pathways is responsible for sex development disorders, illustrating the complexity of this differentiation stage. Refining such pathways is not only crucial for the formation of functional germ cells but also for the overall morphogenesis of the ovaries, underscoring the delicate interplay between genetic cues and physiological responses during female development. In addition to the genetic foundation, environmental factors and the surrounding cellular milieu heavily impact the differentiation of PGCs. For instance, the interaction of PGCs with neighboring somatic cells within the gonadal environment plays a significant determining role in their fate choice. Once germ cell differentiation starts, the local environment provides essential signals that initiate maturation and organization into structures for future fertility. Further, it has been suggested in research that variations in such environmental signals can lead to deviations from the predicted outcome, for example, as observed in certain intersex conditions. Identification of these interactions shines a light on the complexity of germ cell development and refers to the necessity for an integrative understanding when it comes to studying disorders that include germ cell differentiation and feminine reproductive health, as exemplified in findings related to genetic regulation of sex development in human biology (Caruso *et al.*, 2015;Indig-Weingarten *et al.*, 2012).

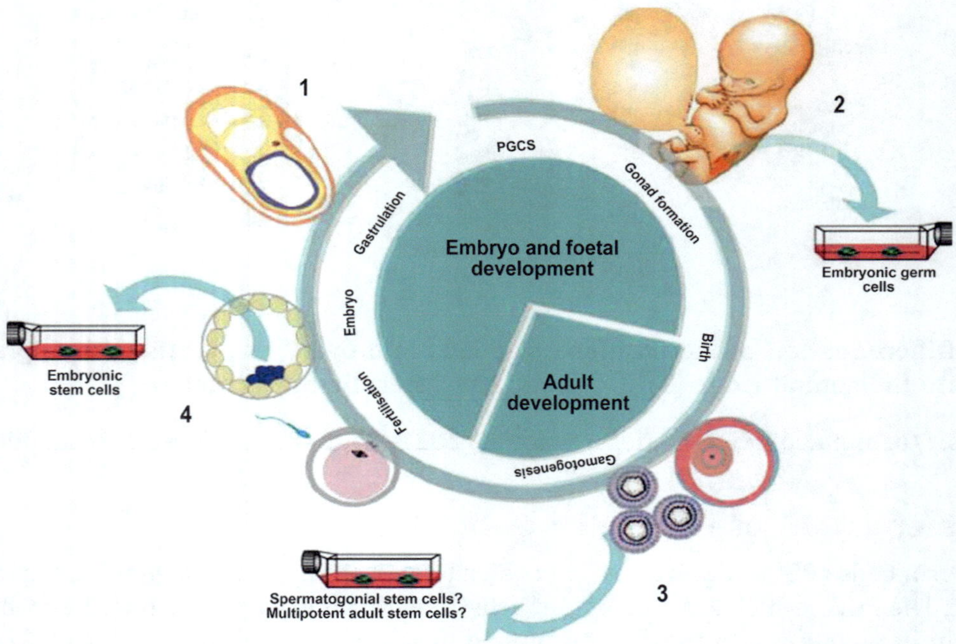

Figure 2.6. Primordial germ cells (PGCs) are first specified in the proximal epiblast (1) and migrate into the genital ridge of the developing gonad (2). Embryonic germ cell lines have been derived by transformation of PGCs in vitro. In the female, germ cells enter meiosis and remain in an arrested state until follicular development occurs after puberty (3). In the male, germ cells retain mitotic capacity for proliferation (3) and pluripotent murine spermatogonial and multipotent adult germ stem cell lines have been reported. From the inner cell mass of the pre-implantation blastocyst, pluripotent embryonic stem cells have been derived (4).

Source: https://www.researchgate.net/profile/Behrouz-Aflatoonian/publication/6724129/figure/fig1/AS:277818991759364@1443248617408/The-germ-cell-cycle-Primordial-germ-cells-PGCs-are-first-specified-in-the-proximal.png

2.2.2. Folliculogenesis and the Formation of Ovarian Follicles

The formation of ovarian follicles and folliculogenesis begins at the initial stages of development of the female reproductive organs. Primordial follicles, i.e., an oocyte surrounded by a layer of granulosa cells, are the initial phase of this intricate process of development. As females mature through various stages of life, primordial follicles are stimulated to grow into primary, secondary, and then antral follicles. Folliculogenesis is regulated by complex interactions among endocrine signals, more generally, luteinizing hormone (LH) and follicle-stimulating hormone (FSH). These gonadotropins have significant roles in inducing the proliferation and differentiation of granulosa and theca cells and affect the development and maturation of ovarian follicles. Initiation of this process marks an essential phase of female fertility because it prepares the oocytes for eventual ovulation and potential fertilization. The contribution of endocrine factors to folliculogenesis cannot be overstated. All stages of development of ovarian follicles are under tight regulation by hormonal negative feedback mechanisms, ensuring maximum maturation.

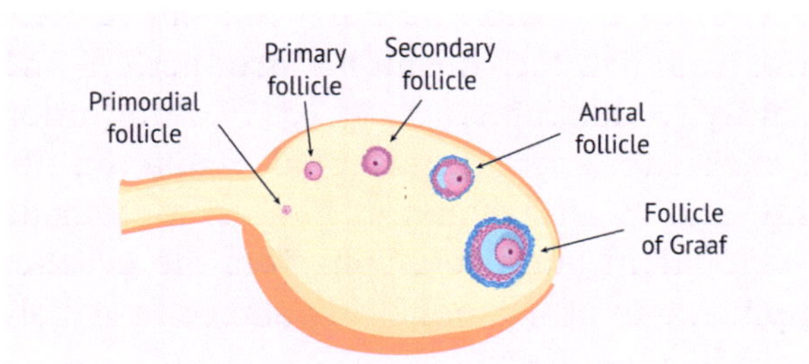

Figure 2.7. Phases of folliculogenesis.

Source: https://www.invitra.com/en/folliculogenesis/folliculogenesis-types-of-follicles/

For instance, it has been established that FSH plays a central role in stimulating the onset of early stages of follicular growth by promoting the proliferation of granulosa cells. At a larger level, research has established that imbalances in such endocrine mechanisms can result in diseases such as polycystic ovarian syndrome (PCOS), where there are abnormalities in the growth of follicles. Furthermore, newer studies indicate that gonadotropin-induced follicular growth may begin earlier than was previously thought, particularly the effects of FSH on the activation of primordial to primary follicles. The discrepancy in the current understanding underscores the necessity of ongoing studies in order to unravel the nuances of folliculogenesis and its implications in female reproductive health. Increasingly, the impact of environmental agents, with a focus on endocrine-disrupting chemicals (EDCs), on folliculogenesis is a subject of growing concern. EDCs can interfere with the hormonal messaging that regulates follicular development, and with this, disrupted reproductive health ensues.

Epidemiological evidence suggests a correlation between EDC exposure and various reproductive disorders, with potential concern regarding its impact on both wildlife and human populations. Significantly, these chemicals can have effects during windows of developmental sensitivity and have long-term impacts on ovarian function and fertility. Molecular mechanisms by which EDCs impact gonadal development are currently under investigation, reinforcing the importance of stringent regulation and public health policy to safeguard reproductive well-being. Understanding the synergistic effect of endogenous hormonal pathways and exogenous disruptors will play a key role in broadening our understanding of folliculogenesis and its broader significance in female reproductive health (Oduwole *et al.*, 2021; Géraldine Delbès *et al.*, 2021).

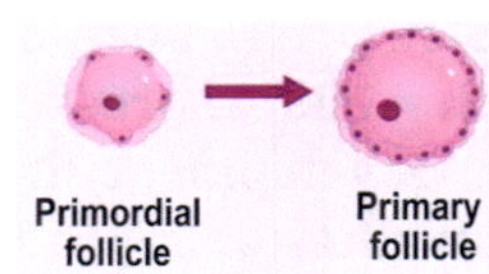

Figure 2.8. Primordial follicle to primary follicle

Source: https://www.invitra.com/en/folliculogenesis/

2.2.3. Hormonal Regulation During Ovarian Development

Hormonal regulation of ovarian development also includes a complex interplay of several endocrine factors that regulate the growth of the female reproductive system. Ovarian development is triggered by the action of gonadotropin-releasing hormone (GnRH) secreted by the hypothalamus, which stimulates the secretion of follicle-stimulating hormone (FSH) and luteinizing hormone (LH) by the anterior pituitary gland. These hormones are important in the growth and maturation of follicles in the ovaries, leading to ovulation. Furthermore, estrogens that are secreted by growing follicles stimulate not only follicular growth but also proliferation and differentiation of the neighboring granulosa and theca cells. These hormonal effects open the way for female sexual development and reproductive capacity, which forms the foundation for the needed equilibrium in normal ovarian function and fertility. In addition to FSH and LH, there also exists a critical role for androgens and estrogens in ovarian development in the establishment of the morphological and functional organization of the ovaries. Androgens, produced not only by the ovaries but also by the adrenal glands, are accountable for the early stages of folliculogenesis and for the establishment of the ovarian reserve. During the embryonic period, androgens secreted by the adrenal glands have been shown to promote differentiation of the müllerian ducts into female external genitalia. Estrogens have similarly been shown to have crucial roles in gene expression regulation during ovarian development, influencing not only the organization of reproductive organs but also broader developmental processes. Hormonal fine-tuning of such signals is essential, as dysregulation would lead to disorders of sex development, making understanding normal ovarian hormonal dynamics important (Indig-Weingarten *et al.*, 2012).

Finally, evidence has been brought to the fore recently in relation to the importance of local endocrine regulation within the ovary, which is in addition to systemic hormonal action. It entails the steroid hormone metabolic pathways in ovarian tissue, showing that ovarian health ischaracterized not only by peripheral levels of circulating hormones, but also by the action and processing of such hormones at the cellular level. Hydroxysteroid (17β) dehydrogenase 1 (HSD17B1) enzyme, for example, plays a pivotal role in the regulation of estrogen and androgen production, thereby having great reproductive function implications. In knockout models, the absence of this enzyme has been linked with impaired ovarian hormone production and fertility (Hakkarainen *et al.*, 2017). Admiration of such subtleties in hormonal regulation not only shows the dynamic nature of ovarian development but also emphasizes the broader implications of hormonal imbalance in female reproductive health.

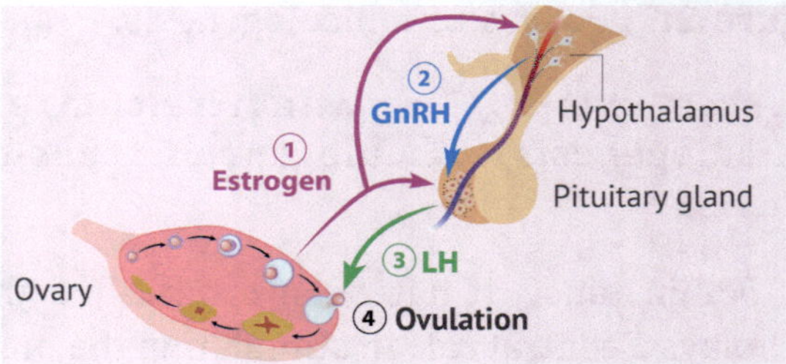

Figure 2.9. Hormonal control of ovulation.

Source: https://www.invitra.com/en/wp-content/uploads/2014/04/hormonal-contro-ovulation.png

Test Your Knowledge

1. How does folliculogenesis contribute to the formation of ovarian follicles?
2. Which hormones regulate ovarian development, and how do they influence this process?

2.3. Development of the Uterus

Learning Outcome

1. Define fusion of the müllerian ducts
2. Explain the formation of the uterine cavity
3. Discuss the structural changes during puberty

Uterine formation is a crucial aspect of female reproductive morphology, entangled with the overall context of genital organ and gonad development. In embryogenesis, the Müllerian ducts or paramesonephric ducts play a central role in the differentiation of the female genital tract. These develop during the sixth week of gestation and elongate to form the uterine body, cervix, and upper two-thirds of the vagina. Critical among these is the function of estrogen in promoting this process of development, encouraging the growth and differentiation of the Müllerian ducts towards the complex structures of the female reproductive potential. The elegant choreography of the hormonal signals during this time creates a canvas on which the future reproductive function is set, so that the development of the uterus is not just a morphogenetic one but also highly essential as a process for the orchestration of hormones. Throughout development, various environmental and genetic factors influence the accurate morphology of the uterus, resulting in anatomical variations that are necessary for reproductive health. Exposure timing to hormones, as well as genetic sex determinants that are involved in sex development, predominantly establishes the shape and function of the uterus. Normal uterine cavity formation is essential for embryo implantation, so any disruption of this pattern of development is sure to result in severe reproductive issues. If disorders of sex development or abnormal genitalia are present, the outcome can be malformations of the uterus that not only impact fertility but also complicate clinical management. These abnormalities emphasize the importance of interdisciplinary treatment for cases in which the course of development is not harmonious with the usual patterns, as has been stressed in recent texts on sex differentiation in the human being (Ahmed *et al.*, 2017).

Furthermore, recent research into intersexuality and abnormal development of the uterus is important in providing information about the complexity of the development of female genitalia. Animal model studies, as detailed in recent theses on intersexuality, reveal similar developmental processes that emphasize the universality of such processes across species (Jaggard *et al.*, 1931). These studies are critically valuable in demystifying our comprehension of abnormal uterine development and its relevance to reproductive health, as well as broader societal attitudes towards sexual development diversity. Understanding the way these conditions manifest enables clinicians to develop more effective, tailored management plans without sacrificing awareness of the evolving understandings of sex and gender. By fostering collaboration among clinicians, scientists, and families, the medical profession can more effectively negotiate the obstacles of uterine development and its associated malformations.

2.3.1. Fusion of the Müllerian Ducts

Müllerian duct fusion is a critical process in the embryologic development of female gonads and genitalia. Both males and females possess paired Müllerian ducts early in gestation, which later develop into the uterus, fallopian tubes, cervix, and proximal vagina. This is initiated during the sixth week of embryo formation when the ducts begin to grow and move towards one another in the midline of the embryo. The eventual fusion of the ducts is then important as it develops the originally separate structures into one continuous reproductive tract that is vital to female reproductive function. Disruption or abnormality in this fusion process can lead to developmental disorders such as Mayer-Rokitansky-Küster-Hauser (MRKH) syndrome, characterized by the non-existence of a functional uterus at birth, highlighting the importance of the fusion of the Müllerian duct during sexual differentiation (Paul-Holterhus *et al.*, 2023).

As development continues, the involvement of hormones is important in determining the destiny of the Müllerian ducts. With no testosterone and Anti-Müllerian Hormone (AMH), primarily active during male differentiation, the ducts of males become atrophied. In females, absence or depletion of AMH allows the Müllerian ducts to persist and eventually fuse to form the overarching structures of the reproductive apparatus. The role of specific genes, such as those controlling the regulation of WNT4 and RSPO1 expression, is essential in promoting this process. These molecular signals not only regulate the survival and union of the Müllerian ducts but also simultaneously suppress male pathway genes. This finessed cooperation between hormones and genetic direction is central to the formation of a functional female reproductive system (Alejandro Díaz *et al.*, 2021).

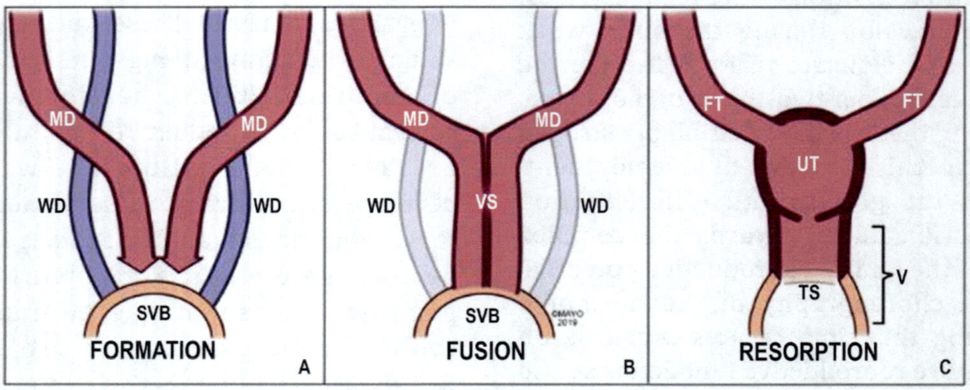

Figure 2.10. Three stages of Müllerian duct (MD) development. (a) Formation, elongation, and canalization of the MDs. (b) Fusion of the MDs in the midline and with the sinovaginal bulb (SVB) of the genitourinary sinus; regression of the Wolffian ducts (WD). (c) Resorption of the septum between the MDs to create a patent uterine cavity (UT), cervix, and upper vagina..

Source: https://www.researchgate.net/figure/Three-stages-of-Muellerian-Duct-MD-development-a-During-the-first-stage-MDs-form_fig1_339982865

The last anatomical structures that develop due to Müllerian duct union are critical for fertility and reproductive health. The united ducts develop into the uterus, where the embryo implants and grows during pregnancy. In addition, the fallopian tubes are involved in gamete transport and the site of fertilization, so they are critical in development. Abnormalities that result from the failure of proper fusion can cause obstructive states or absence of the female reproductive structures, which have serious reproductive consequences and issues, such as infertility. The understanding of Müllerian duct development, in conjunction with advances in imaging and genetic diagnosis, has important clinical applications for the assessment and management of conditions with anomalies of the female reproductive tract, providing insights into individualized treatments (Paul-Holterhus *et al.*, 2023).

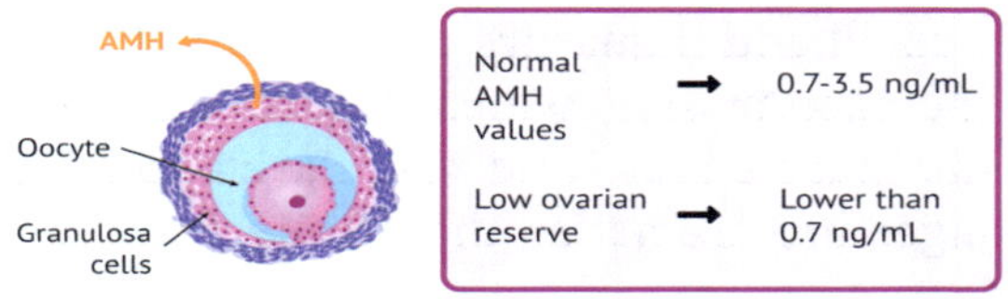

Figure 2.11. Anti-Mullerian Hormone (AMH).

Source: https://www.invitra.com/en/blood-test-egg-count/anti-mullerian-hormone-production-follicle/

2.3.2. Formation of the Uterine Cavity

Formation of the uterine cavity is a critical aspect of female genital tract development that entails a complex interplay between embryologic tissue and hormones. The uterus initially arises from the fusion of the Müllerian ducts during embryogenesis, which underlines the significance of these paired structures. As the ducts fuse, they become one uterine canal that further differentiates into the uterine body, cervix, and finally the uterine cavity itself. The growth is controlled by hormones like estrogen, which plays a very crucial role in regulating the growth and development of reproductive tissues. Appreciation of these developmental processes not only highlights the biological complexity of the female reproductive tract but also indicates the likely implications of abnormalities in the process of uterine cavity formation, potentially leading to clinical presentations like Müllerian agenesis or malformations of the uterus that have a major bearing on fertility and reproductive well-being. Uterine cavity differentiation is intimately linked with the processes of hormonal signaling during development. With rising estrogen levels, particularly at puberty, they ensure uterine tissue growth, which supports the creation of a functional endometrium. The hormonal influence continues to be an important factor in organizing the uterine space to support implantation and early pregnancy. Other factors, such as relaxin, are also involved in regulating the structural integrity in the pelvic region to enable the uterus to remodel during various reproductive stages. These endocrine interactions point out the importance of the endocrine system and its normal functioning in providing reproductive welfare and normality in uterine cavity growth. Disruption of these hormonal communications may lead to severe reproductive disorders, highlighting the interdependence of hormonal regulation and anatomical organization of the female reproductive system. Environmental influences and genetic background are also involved in uterine cavity growth and functionality, aside from hormonal effects.

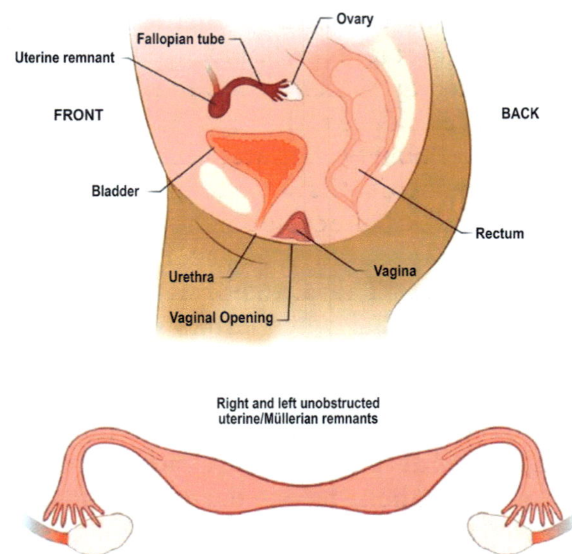

Figure 2.12. Müllerian Agenesis.

Source: https://scienceblog.cincinnatichildrens.org/mullerian-agenesis-room-for-improvement-in-care-counseling/

A number of studies show that exposure to certain environmental endocrine disruptors may have a negative impact on the trajectory of development of the Müllerian ducts, whose potential outcome could be structural abnormalities. In addition, genetic syndromes or mutations can adversely affect the pattern of normal uterine development, resulting in variations in uterine cavity morphology. Identification of these multi-dimensional factors is important to enhance our knowledge of common reproductive disorders and avoid future complications. Examining the formation of the uterine cavity through an integrative approach can add to both clinical application and future research directions in the overall area of female reproductive health, particularly as the advances of reproductive technology and intervention continue.

2.3.3. Structural Changes During Puberty

Puberty is an essential transitional phase in the development of female genitalia and gonads, during which profound structural changes are induced through alterations in hormones. Puberty initiates the release of gonadotropins from the anterior pituitary gland, which activates the development of ovaries as well as the appearance of secondary sexual characteristics. The transformation of the ovaries is essential when primordial follicles start to grow, leading to mature oocytes ready to be ovulated. This is a complicated process and not an easy maturation of existing structures; it's a complicated development of supportive tissues and vascularization, making the organs function correctly as the reproductive function comes into readiness. The interaction of hormones during this phase, especially estrogen, makes these developmental processes, which play an important role in the morphology of the gonads and related genitalia, thereby creating the groundwork for future reproductive health. With puberty development, there are profound changes in the vaginal and uterine structures. The small and immature uterus initially begins to increase in size, which reflects an increase in the muscle mass and vascularization. These changes are crucial as the uterus prepares for potential embryo implantation and pregnancy. Concurrently, the vaginal canal becomes longer and more elastic so that its role in intercourse and childbirth becomes possible. In addition, the structural changes are followed by shifts in the vaginal microbiome and pH, which aid in infection prevention and general reproductive health. The establishment of these organs is a synchronic process regulated by the hormonal milieu, specifically the increase in estrogen levels at this formative stage, highlighting the correspondence of endocrine action and anatomical development within the female reproductive tract. The role of the thyroid gland during this developmental stage cannot be overlooked as well. The effect of thyroids on growth and metabolic processes is significant, influencing the many endocrine pathways responsible for puberty regulation. Reproductive system development during normalcy, according to various epidemiological investigations, relies on the proper operation of both thyroid and gonadal hormones, as suggested by alterations observed in such turning points as puberty and pregnancy. Pathological thyroid hormones negatively affect ovarian functioning, causing disorders that may suppress normal development and overall reproductive health. Hence, understanding the structural changes during puberty involves not only looking at the gonads and genitalia but also illustrates the importance of the thyroid's role in directing such changes effectively, producing before it a complex web of interconnected systems that govern female reproductive development (Canning, 2019; Shurpyak *et al.*, 2018).

Test Your Knowledge

1. How is the uterine cavity formed during embryogenesis?
2. What structural changes occur in the female reproductive system during puberty?

2.4. Development of the Vagina

Learning Outcome

1. Define origin from the urogenital sinus
2. Describe the role of estrogen in vaginal maturation
3. Explain the anatomical features of the mature vagina

Development of the vagina is a critical process of female genital organogenesis, and it is a very well-coordinated interplay of genetic and hormonal determinants during embryogenesis. It begins around the seventh week of gestation, when the vagina is created by the fusion of the Müllerian ducts, or paramesonephric ducts, which are essential for the formation of female reproductive organs. Because these ducts grow and fuse in the midline, they create the vaginal canal as part of developing other key structures such as the uterus and the fallopian tubes. This is all delicately orchestrated through many signaling pathways and hormones, demonstrating the importance of establishing a female phenotype. Dysregulation at this development stage has been shown to lead to abnormalities like agenesis or malformation of the vagina, and thus highlights the necessity for proper comprehension of vaginal development within the context of the overall female genital anatomy. In addition to the physical build of the vagina, psychological and social dimensions begin to form, which would influence the lives of individuals quite immensely. Conditions like vaginal agenesis, due to developmental disorders, can present particular physical and psychological difficulties for the patient. The interaction between genital development and mental status is of utmost relevance; for instance, it has been demonstrated that patients with disorders/differences of sex differentiation/ development (DSD), including those involving vaginal development, have a greater frequency of mental disorders, especially in females. The acknowledgment of these ailments necessitates a multi-faceted approach, considering not just medical intervention but also psychological guidance and personalized counseling.

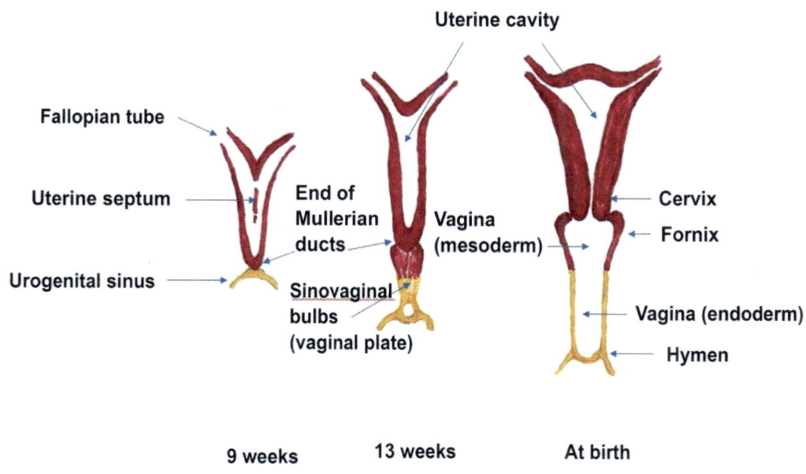

Figure 2.13. Embryological development of the internal female genitalia.

Source: https://external-content.duckduckgo.com/iu/?u=https%3A%2F%2Fvulvovaginaldisorders.org%2Fwp-content%2Fuploads%2Fembryological-vagina-1-1.jpg&f=1&nofb=1&ipt=c83d83e58f2e538be2e2ff5f5ad335c2c1aec47a9fec14a7cdf4513f21fa04dc

Through an understanding of these interdependencies, healthcare professionals are better able to help patients cope with the complexity of genital formation and its implications. Besides, the evolving social perception concerning gender and sexual health underscores the need for increased knowledge and education about vaginal development conditions. In today's clinical practice, engaging families and communities in conversation about such developmental conditions is essential since variability in social attitudes can influence medical practice. Global experts on the management of DSD emphasize the necessity for an integrated care plan, which involves medical, psychological, and sociocultural factors. This guarantees that the treatment is not just clinically effective but also patient-sensitive and responsive to family expectations. Repeated efforts at understanding and documenting the varied experiences of individuals with vaginal development disorders can contribute to a better support system, ultimately leading to improved health outcomes and improved quality of life for patients with these many different types of issues, as discussed throughout the literature regarding DSD outcomes (Ahmed *et al.*, 2017; Bajszczak *et al.*, 2020).

2.4.1. Origin From the Urogenital Sinus

The urogenital sinus plays a central role in the embryonic development of female genitalia and gonads as a prime anatomical structure in early sexual differentiation. In its role as a cloacal derivative formed by development, the sinus directly produces the urethra, bladder, and vaginoplasty. While the urogenital and anal elements separate from the cloaca, the urogenital sinus also forms structures like the distal regions of the reproductive system, i.e., the vagina and the external genitalia. The contribution of the urogenital sinus to female development cannot be overstated, as it gives rise to the platform that will be used to form the reproductive potential that will characterize the adult organism. In development research following the development of the urogenital sinus, it is observed that there are specific signaling pathways that control the transition from undifferentiated embryonal tissues to the expression of sexual characteristics. There is a hormonal balance of signals that plays a significant role in the transition, where the presence or absence of androgens will determine the fate of the gonads. In females, the lack of testosterone from the XY chromosome promotes the differentiation of the urogenital sinus to female-specific structures and ultimately leads to the development of ovaries and supporting reproductive organs.

This distinction is of paramount importance, since it designates the interdependent correlation among genetic, hormonal, and anatomical variables, which determine female sex organs during critical windows in fetal development, positioning the urogenital sinus in the key position of a required cornerstone in this regard. The development of the urogenital sinus also has a close association with a multitude of congenital malformations of female genitalia. Pathologic disruptions in the critical stages of gestation responsible for urogenital sinus development can lead to agenesis, malformations, or other urogenital reproductive system abnormalities in a woman that affect her health and fertility. Given recent developments in genetic studies that have enhanced our understanding of the complex nature of congenital anomalies, understanding the etiology and ontogeny of the urogenital sinus remains critical for maternal-fetal medicine and clinical genetics. Increased knowledge of these developmental processes and their implications bears great importance for inter-disciplinary interventions in the treatment of these malformations, like genetic counseling and certain interventions to manage concomitant risks. Hence, the thorough analysis of the role of urogenital sinus is necessary for the reinforcement of the broader context of women's reproductive health, as exemplified by the evidence that is relevant to populations with congenital differences in genital organ development (Pierpont *et al.*, 2018;Akram *et al.*, 2017).

2.4.2. Role of Estrogen in Vaginal Maturation

Estrogen is central to the process of vaginal maturation, a key milestone in the growth of female genital organs. During puberty, rising estrogen levels trigger a chain of physiological changes that transform the vaginal epithelium from a thin, immature membrane to a thicker, more resilient organ. Such remodeling is required for a functional reproductive system capable of supporting menstrual cycles and potential pregnancies. The formation of the vagina also influences the general look and use of the female reproductive tract, as well as sexual and reproductive function.

Through vaginal mucosa growth, estrogen functions to provide a healthy environment for the maintenance of flora, keeping the vagina free from infection while producing optimum conditions for the survival of sperm during reproduction. Apart from its impact on the structure, estrogen significantly influences vascularization and lubrication of the vaginal tissue. The hormone causes the development of blood vessels within the walls of the vagina, making it more blood-rich and receiving a higher supply of nutrients, which is essential for tissue health. Estrogen also causes the formation of vaginal secretions, leading to increases in vaginal canal moisture and elasticity. These changes are not only important for sexual intercourse but also play an essential role in the overall health of the reproductive system.

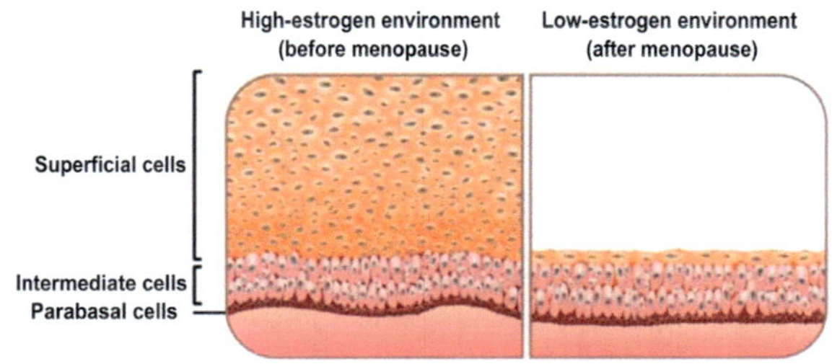

Figure 2.14. Influence of estrogen on the vaginal epithelium.

Source: https://www.researchgate.net/figure/Influence-of-estrogen-on-the-vaginal-epithelium-Notes-Before-menopause-high-levels-of_fig1_236077722

Proper lubrication avoids discomfort during intercourse, which otherwise can lead to psychological and relational issues, thereby further underlining the function of estrogen in the development process. The multifaceted role of estrogen, thus, underscores its role in encouraging physical as well as psychological ease among female adolescents in their sexual development towards adult life. The impact of estrogen on the development of the vagina transcends superficial body differences, welcoming significant psychosocial attributes as well. The process of maturation, triggered by estrogen, can have ,profound effects on a young woman's self-esteem, sexual identity, and social relations. While puberty unfolds and these physical changes take place, the role of estrogen can also serve to catalyze psychosocial development. With the increased level of estrogen, not only do the physical changes occur, but also the secondary maturation of reproductive organs can induce a change in social and personal relationships. Nurturing of these developmental aspects through appropriate education can lead to understanding and acceptance of these changes, which in turn can continue to foster healthy sexuality and reproductive health attitudes among young women. Thus, estrogen is not directly responsible for the physiological development of the vagina alone, but also for shaping the broader psychosocial context of the development of females.

2.4.3. Anatomical Features of the Mature Vagina

The adult vagina's anatomical structures are key to its function and the upkeep of female reproductive health.

The vaginal tube is fibromuscular in nature, approximately 7.5 to 10 centimeters in length, and positioned between the external genitalia and the uterus. The walls of the vagina are formed by a stratified squamous epithelium that protects and lubricates, which is needed during coitus and delivery. Also, the vaginal mucous lining is made to absorb certain materials, so it can preserve its unique flora and pH condition. This condition is very important in preventing infection, highlighting the dynamic aspect of the vagina throughout various stages of life, particularly puberty, menstruation, and menopause. Understanding the anatomical structures is vital to knowing the vaginas functional relationships with surrounding organs and overall role in reproductive health. The structure of the mature vagina is not just complicated to the eye, but a reflection of a system of structures that complicate physiological and psychological functions. Its elastic walls of smooth muscle, composing most of the muscular layer, allow high elasticity such that the vagina may be stretched for several activities like coitus and childbirth. The ability of the vaginal canals to expand and contract is augmented by the presence of the pubococcygeus muscle, one of the pelvic floor muscles, which provides support to the vagina and other organs around it. Moreover, the length and width of the vagina can be extremely variable amongst women, based on variables such as age, hormonal state, and individual anatomy. This variability lends credence to having a multidimensional conceptualization of the vagina, including clinical assessment where anatomical variability can inform hidden pathology or developmental abnormalities, as outlined in research on disorders of sex development (Ahmed *et al.*, 2017). Also, the vagina is richly innervated with blood vessels, nerve endings, and lymphatic structures, making it sensitive and operational. Vascularization of the vaginal walls is required for the supply of adequate lubrication and is also involved in sexual arousal and physiological reactions. Nerve endings within the vaginal wall are key in sexual feeling and enjoyment, demonstrating the vaginas role in feminine sexuality. In addition, the vagina is also an important pathway during delivery, which dilates to allow the baby's passage without loss of structural support. As part of the woman's reproductive system, development and anatomic features depend on hormonal status throughout life, which implies that there is an intimate relationship between vaginal health and hormonal status. Thus, the adult vagina is a dynamic interplay of hormonal, physiological, and anatomical factors that are essential to reproductive function and overall health (Jackson *et al.*, 2018).

Test Your Knowledge

1. How does estrogen influence the maturation of the vagina during development?
2. What are the main anatomical features of a mature vagina?

2.5. External Genitalia Development

Learning Outcome

1. Describe the formation of the labia and clitoris
2. Explain the influence of androgens on external structures
3. Identify common variations in external genitalia anatomy

Development of the external genitalia is a crucial aspect of complete female genital organ development and is influenced mostly by genetic, hormonal, and environmental factors during embryogenesis. The bipotential gonadal morphology is first programmed to develop into male or female genitalia and is primarily regulated by chromosomal sex.

Chromosomal female (XX) involves the absence of the SRY gene, leading to the development of ovaries instead of testes, which then generate estrogens and other hormones for the development of features typical of female external genitalia. It is characterized by the formation of labia majora, labia minora, clitoris, and other structures, which is a crucial developmental stage from ambiguous to clearly female anatomy. Understanding these mechanisms highlights the role of hormonal action during periods of key development, when any disruption leads to disorders of sex development (DSD) in relation to ambiguous or non-typical presentation of genitalia.

During the period when the external genitalia develop, the role of hormones is even more significant. Estrogens are also the cause of inducing growth and differentiation of genital structures because they direct the formation of the transformation of the cloacal membrane to the clitoris and labia. In fact, absence of androgens, e.g., in individuals with Mullerian duct anomalies, results in diminished growth of male-biased structures and increased female phenotype. The active interaction among genetic inclinations and environmental hormonal milieu can lead to superficial anatomy and function differences, and these differences are pertinent when considering clinical implications regarding gender identity and anatomical normality. The presence of unusual external genitalia requires a multidisciplinary evaluation and treatment plan, focusing on the consideration of both the biological and social histories of genital development as reflected by contemporary societal awareness and expectations of gender variation (Ahmed *et al.*, 2017).

Specialized conditions such as complete androgen insensitivity syndrome (CAIS) capture the complexity involved in external genitalia development and the importance of proper diagnosis and care. CAIS patients, despite having XY chromosomes and a genetic makeup that is male, present as females with normally developed external genitalia but lacking the internal sex organs typical of biological females. This is due to androgen receptor gene mutations leading to the body's inability to respond to androgens, which are fundamental to normal development in males. Therefore, even though a person may have a female phenotype, their internal anatomy consists of rudimentary Müllerian structures and persistent gonads. Clinical diagnosis of such abnormalities requires advanced imaging modalities and in-depth knowledge of the developmental biology of the formation of external genitalia to enable management approaches that are responsive to the patient's identity and to the medical needs (Visschere *et al.*, 2013).

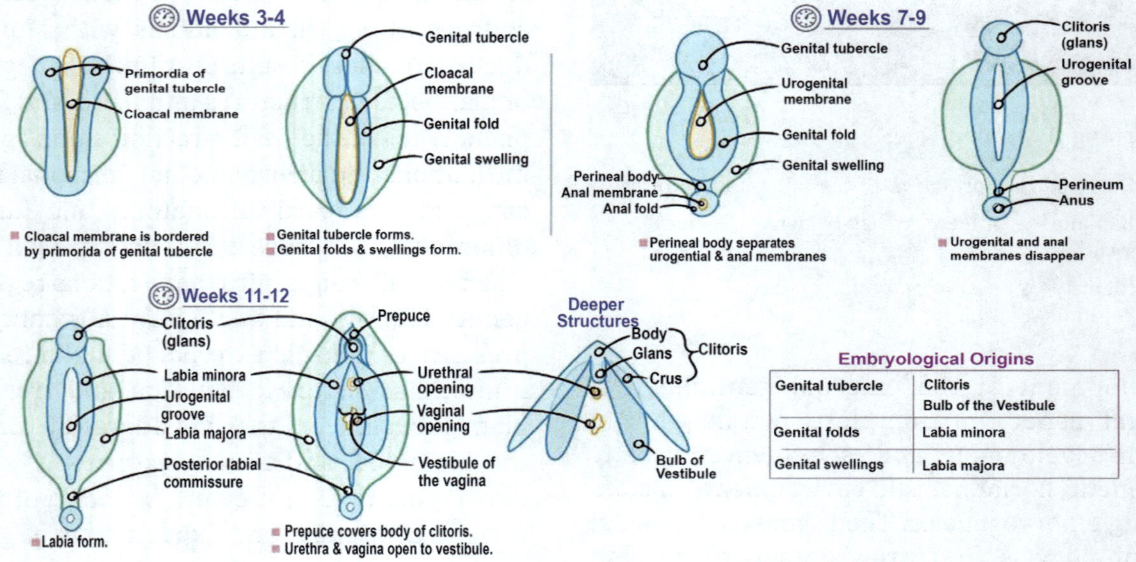

Figure 2.15. Embryology of female external genitalia.

Source: https://d1j63owfs0b5j3.cloudfront.net/term/images/development-of-the-vulva-1993.png

2.5.1. Formation of the Labia and Clitoris

Formation of the external female genitalia, or labia and clitoris development, occurs during those early stages of embryonic development. All embryos, both chromosomally male and chromosomally female, initially possess a shared system of embryonic structures that will differentiate into male or female phenotypes depending on genetic and hormonal information. In women, the genital tubercle, which plays a significant role in clitoris development, begins to elongate in week 7 of gestation. Meanwhile, the labioscrotal swellings grow up to form the labia majora, and the urogenital folds grow up to form the labia minora. This process demonstrates the importance of ectodermal and mesodermal input in the development of genital systems, demonstrating how external genitalia are created by both genetic control and hormonal environment at narrow windows of development (Georgas *et al.*, 2015). Hormonal impact, particularly the absence of androgens, plays a pivotal role in the differentiation of female external genitalia. As opposed to male development, where masculinization is facilitated by testosterone and its analogs, differentiation in females occurs mainly under conditions without these hormones. That is, the lack of testicular function leads to tissue proliferation, resulting in clitoral formation and development of labia. This bifurcation occurs in the seventh week of pregnancy when, without the SRY gene, gonads are formed into ovaries rather than testes. The external genitalia form gradually a female morphology through the development of the labia majora and minora and the clitoris, creating a complex relationship between genetic coding and hormonal signaling (Chitayat *et al.*, 2010). The interplay of genetic factors and molecular signals is responsible for the delicate development of the labia and clitoris, which can have significant implications for sexual health and reproductive biology. Such mechanisms are especially significant in the case of disorders of sexual development (DSD), which result in indeterminate genitalia and stress the need for accurate prenatal diagnosis. Interdisciplinary methodology towards DSDs ensures a holistic study of genetic, anatomical, and hormonal aspects, applying detailed studies of the urogenital systems ontology to inform clinical treatment. A strong familiarity with labial and clitoral development not only clarifies developmental biology but also integrates genetic, endocrinological, and anthropological theory to better enhance the clinical treatment of individuals with malformations of the genitalia (Georgas *et al.*, 2015).

2.5.2. Influence of Androgens on External Structures

The role of androgens in the development of the external genitalia is pivotal, particularly at significant times of development. Androgens such as testosterone have pivotal roles in male genitalia masculinization, but, although less crucial, nonetheless, equally vital roles in females. Dysfunction of androgens during significant periods of fetal development results in a range of conditions, such as congenital adrenal hyperplasia. This condition leads to an excess production of androgens, which can virilize the female fetus, resulting in ambiguous genitalia or masculinized external anatomy. It is crucial to comprehend the physiological mechanisms by which androgens influence these structures in order to gain a better insight into their role in sexual differentiation as well as the overall implications for female reproductive health. Moreover, the intricate machinery of steroidogenesis plays a central role in regulating androgen levels in the body. Steroidogenesis encompasses the enzymatic reactions by which cholesterol is converted into steroid hormones, including androgens. Various enzymes, primarily members of the cytochrome P450 family, are involved in converting the precursors into biologically active steroids. These are not only found in the ovaries but also in the adrenal glands, a fact that signifies the complexity of androgen production. Studying the enzymatic intricacies, as presented in Miller *et al.* (2011), provides valuable information regarding how dysregulation can lead to pathologies like polycystic ovary syndrome (PCOS), indicated by hyperandrogenism and its secondary outward signs. These disorders indicate the delicate balance required for normal sexual differentiation and reproductive health in women. Clinical presentations of abnormal androgen levels also illustrate their effect on the external genitalia. In conditions such as PCOS, which involves functional ovarian hyperandrogenism as reported in Rosenfield *et al.* (2016), hyperandrogen exposure would more likely cause external structure symptoms such as hirsutism and changes in skin texture. Such environmental and genetic interaction leading to excess androgen production highlights the multifactorial etiology of such conditions and their impact on female gender expression. Besides, ongoing research is continually uncovering the complex interconnections between androgenic levels and external characteristics that define female genitalia and establishing the necessity of having full knowledge of biological and environmental parameters. The ramifications extend far beyond mere physical anatomy into psychological and social dimensions of identity and health.

2.5.3. Variations in External Genitalia Anatomy

The female external genitalia are noted for dramatic variations that are crucial to the understanding of normal development as well as disorders of atypical anatomy. Such variations can be due to a number of genetic, hormonal, and environmental determinants of early fetal life. For instance, disorders of sex development (DSD) can lead to atypical external genital morphologies, which make it challenging for the conventional procedures of sex assignment. With increasing knowledge of these anatomical anomalies, clinicians are increasingly better positioned to approach the treatment of infants who are born with non-traditional genitalia with individualized care consistent with evolving societal attitudes toward gender difference. Professionals involved in the care and assessment of such infants often function within multidisciplinary teams to ensure that discussions regarding sex assignment and management are knowledgeable and respectful, based on both medical understanding and family situation (Ahmed *et al.*, 2017). Further, understanding anatomical variation in external genitalia is of utmost significance within evolutionary biology. Morphologic differences among species, like those of the primates, are informative regarding reproductive strategy and ecological fitness. For example, research has focused on gross and microscopic anatomy of the genitalia in various primate species and separated essential differences like erectile tissue morphology and prostate variations. These differences not only point towards the difference of reproductive anatomy across the primate line but also support conservation efforts in the direction of protecting species that are gifted with unique reproductive characteristics. Such comparisons can potentially help us better comprehend the evolutionary pressures that shape genital morphology and refine the approach to undertaking reproductive health studies across species (Alperin *et al.*, 2018). Finally, anatomical variations of external genitalia are both clinically and evolutionarily significant. Clinicians are forced to handle these differences on the basis of educated anatomy knowledge, genetics, and social niceties, developing tolerant medicine for patients with abnormal genitalia. On the other hand, morphological research of external genitalia in different animals presents broad prospects for investigation in reproductive ecology. A dual approach that incorporates both the clinical and evolutionary perspectives is necessary to facilitate understanding in the development of female genitalia and gonads, hence towards the broader intellectual debate of gender and sexuality within contemporary society. This extensive analysis will advance an understanding of biological variation and inform the direction of future research in the area.

Test Your Knowledge

1. What role do androgens play in shaping the external genital structures?
2. What are some common variations observed in the anatomy of external genitalia?

2.6. Disorders of Sexual Development (DSDs)

Learning Outcome

1. Define DSDs in females
2. Explain the genetic and environmental causes
3. Discuss the implications for health and reproductive function

Disorders of Sexual Development (DSDs) syndrome describes a broad range of congenital disorders of the interruption of usual genitalia and gonadal organ differentiation, primarily in female development. These disorders can arise from various genetic and hormonal factors that alter the normal sequence during embryonic development. For instance, conditions such as Congenital Adrenal Hyperplasia (CAH) in 46, XX individuals are exhibited as endocrine disturbances that lead to different degrees of virilization of the external genitalia. The complex nature of DSDs is a reflection of the entangled complexity of genetic, endocrine, and environmental components that could lead to or unusual anatomical presentation in individuals, ultimately influencing their reproductive health and gender identity (Alejandro Díaz *et al.*, 2021). DSD Classification is broad and usually allocated based on the trends of chromosomes and hormone response. Commonly encountered are complete or partial Androgen Insensitivity Syndrome (AIS), where individuals carry a 46, XY karyotype but develop near entirely female external genitalia due to a lack of response to the effects of androgens. Similarly, ovotesticular DSD and Mixed Gonadal Dysgenesis can lead to mixed gonadal structures, with profound implications for development and reproduction. The clinical implication of these disorders is not negligible, and an endocrinologist, geneticist, and psychologist team working together must offer total care that addresses the medical and psychosocial dimensions of living with DSDs (Hosseinirad *et al.*, 2021). Genetic testing has changed the therapy for DSDs, with the potential for earlier diagnosis and a precise intervention plan.

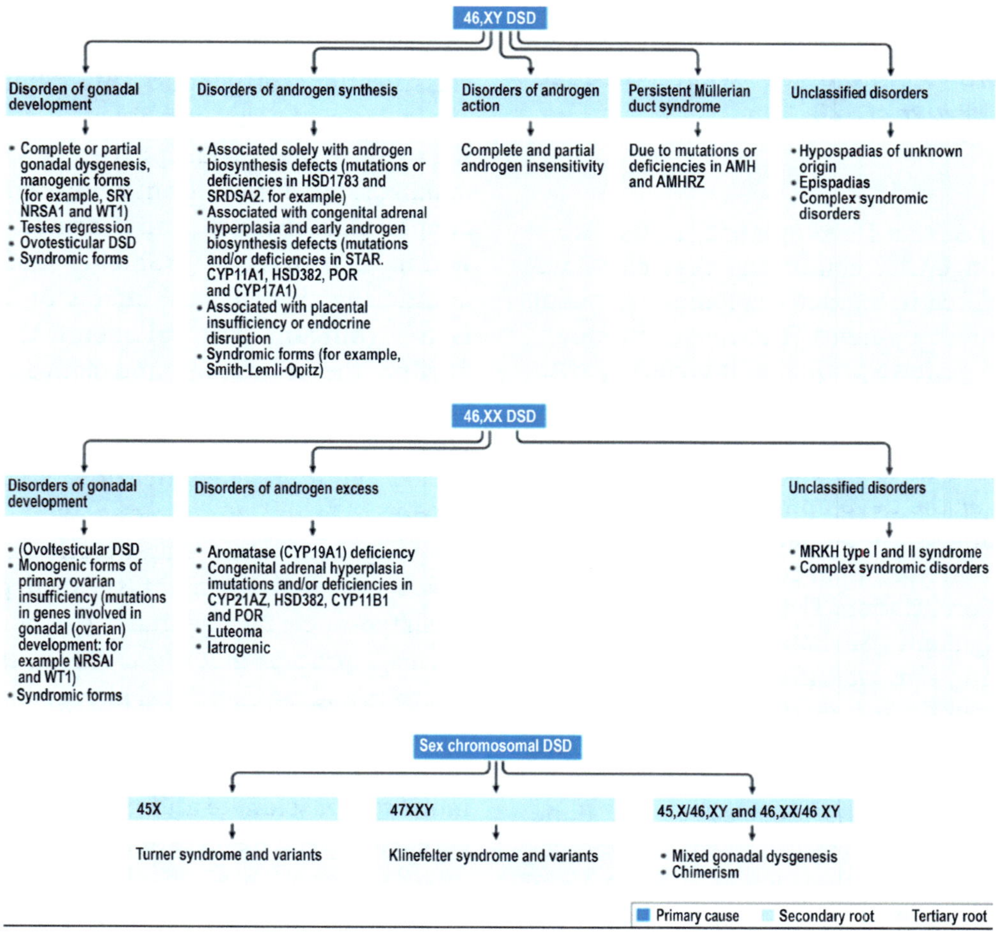

Figure 2.16. Disorders of sex development (DSDs) are classified into three main groups on the basis of the karyotype of the affected individual (primary cause). Each main group encompasses several subgroups (secondary root) that orient towards a specific diagnosis (tertiary root).

Source: https://www.researchgate.net/publication/325175641/figure/fig1/AS:626901836132352@1526476453009/classification-of-dSds-Disorders-of-sex-development-DSDs-are-classified-into-three.png

This shift is important to best practices of gender assignment and informed consent for surgical procedures in childhood, once conducted often without complete comprehension of long-term effects. With rising awareness, there is heightened emphasis on the need for delay in procedures that are irreversible until patients are able to participate in decisions regarding their care. The focus has increasingly been on creating supportive environments that embrace and affirm one's gender identity, as well as optimizing reproductive health through assisted reproductive technologies where needed (Alejandro Díaz *et al.*, 2021).

2.6.1. Overview of DSDs in Females

Disorders of Sexual Development (DSDs) are a group of congenital conditions that can have a very significant impact on female gonadal and genital development. They most commonly arise due to genetic problems interfering with the usual pathways of sexual differentiation, particularly prenatal. In females, DSDs may manifest as atypical genitalia, ovarian dysgenesis, or the development of male-related structures due to the deficient function of both the genetic and hormonal components involved in sexual differentiation. The complexity of these disorders highlights the importance of extensive understanding and classification because they range from relatively benign anomalies to more complex disorders, which need to be treated and psychologically counseled in affected individuals. Management of DSDs is most effectively done through a multiauthored platform of medical professionals so that the case of every patient is evaluated thoroughly and treated according to their personal requirements. The classification of DSDs in female patients is often based on specific anatomical, hormonal, and genetic criteria. For instance, syndromes such as Androgen Insensitivity Syndrome (AIS) and Congenital Adrenal Hyperplasia (CAH) are examples of pathways in which sexual development differs from the norm. AIS is typically brought about by mutations in the gene for the androgen receptor, yielding a female phenotype despite the presence of XY chromosomes. CAH, in contrast, arises as a result of deficiencies of enzymes taking part in the biosynthesis of cortisol, leading to heightened androgens that virilize external genitalia.

These variations not only pose challenges in terms of diagnosis but also influence the psychosocial aspects of affected individuals, as societal norms often lean heavily towards binary classifications of gender. This binary mindset can exacerbate the complexities that arise in the medical and social spheres regarding DSDs, making it imperative for healthcare providers to adopt a more inclusive and informed perspective within their practice (O'Shields *et al.*, 2013). In addition to the physical effects of DSDs, there is a significant cultural factor that extends beyond the treatment and conceptualization of the affected persons in societal contexts. Most Western cultures have a dominant, strict binary gender classification with ensuing marginalization of persons who do not fit properly into those classifications. Historical views have led to infant surgical procedures to shape uncertain genitalia based on cultural norms, a process that is growing in criticism for its ethics and psychological impact on individuals with DSDs. Understanding and tackling these implications are crucial because they allow for a more compassionate and informed approach to care. Moreover, observations of societies where intersex people are included constructively in social and legal frameworks can provide valuable evidence regarding how medical experts and society can negotiate these issues (D'Anza *et al.*, 2019). Comparative analysis across cultures underscores the imperative of rethinking norms concerning gender classification and treatment of DSD in contemporary medical practice.

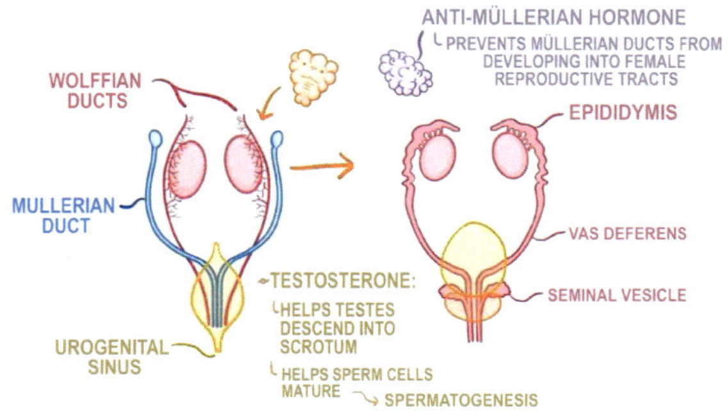

Figure 2.17. Androgen insensitivity syndrome.

Source: https://www.osmosis.org/_next/image?url=https%3A%2F%2Fd16qt3wv6xm098.cloudfront.net%2FuLm2f56gSJ6s70tb7hePk7NLQBeyoZvN%2F_.jpg&w=3840&q=75

2.6.2. Genetic and Environmental Causes

Understanding the development of genital organs and gonads in women requires attention to environmental and genetic influences on these processes. The genetic influences are responsible for determining not just the anatomical features but also the functional ability of the reproductive system. Studies have indicated that certain gene expressions can influence the formation of structures such as ovaries and fallopian tubes, which are necessary for successful conception. Genetic differences in these genes can lead to developmental abnormalities, illustrating the intricate relationships between genetics and female reproductive health. Furthermore, as studies suggest, inherited traits such as polycystic ovarian morphology might put certain individuals at risk of disruption of reproductive function and hormonal regulation, thus linking genetically determined predispositions to clinico-pathological states in female genital development. In addition to genetic considerations, environmental influences also play a significant part in the development of female genitalia and gonads. For instance, prenatal exposure to doses of androgen can disrupt normal ovarian growth and regulation. Such hormonal impacts during crucial windows of development may lead to conditions such as Polycystic Ovary Syndrome (PCOS), characterized by functional ovarian hyperandrogenism and insulin resistance. This multifactorial syndrome illustrates the manner in which environmental factors, such as nutrition and maternal health, converge with genetic susceptibility to define reproductive outcomes.

Notably, the intricate nature of these interactions is such that no one factor exists independently; rather, they work together to either facilitate normal development or lead to reproductive disorders, highlighting the value of an integrative paradigm in the investigation of female genital organ development (Rosenfield *et al.*, 2016). In addition, the recognition of environmental influences extends beyond prenatally received influences to postnatal exposures, such as lifestyle, that may affect ovarian function. Obesity, eating habits, and level of exercise have been observed to modulate hormonal equilibrium and subsequently affect reproductive organ functions.

For example, being overweight can increase insulin resistance in women with susceptibility to PCOS and trigger additional complications of gonadal function. Assessment of these environmental components in conjunction with genetic risk factors gives a holistic view of women's reproductive health. Thus, research shows that increasing understanding about these interactions can offer opportunities for intervention design to reverse the occurrence of reproductive ill-health. The above findings conclude on the point that genetic and environmental factors matter in attempting to gain a comprehensive understanding of development within the female genital and gonadal systems (Akram *et al.*, 2017).

2.6.3. Implications For Health and Reproductive Function

The development of female genitalia and gonads is a highly intricate biological process that is very reliant upon genetic, hormonal, and environmental influences. The reproductive and health implications extend far beyond mere anatomy; they consist of the very balance of endocrine systems and the potential for reproductive success throughout one's lifetime. Sex development disorders or disruptions during windows of fetal life have lifetime consequences, not only in terms of fertility but also in the vulnerability to a plethora of health conditions. The involvement of genes such as Dmrt1, now crucial in the maintenance of Sertoli cell phenotype, emphasizes the significance of genetic regulation in gonadal differentiation. This regulation can affect reproductive outcomes and overall health since abnormalities of sex determination can result in various pathologies or disease of infertility later in life (Koopman *et al.*, 2015). The prenatal environment is also important to the future health and reproductive potential of the offspring. Maternal nutrition, stress, and environmental exposure to chemicals can program neuroendocrine systems that ultimately regulate reproductive function. Exposure to exogenous hormones during pregnancy, such as androgens and estrogens, has been shown to alter the trajectory of reproductive development, and this may be followed by intergenerational effects. Sensitivity of the GnRH neurosecretory system in fetal life, as detailed in ovine models, illustrates the key interface between environmental cues and sexual differentiation. These findings underscore the importance of a healthy gestational environment in preserving the best reproductive health and suggest that interventions or pregnancy manipulations may preclude some adverse effects on future generations (Bellingham *et al.*, 2016).

With the amount of knowledge regarding the health outcomes and reproductive function increasing, there is no doubt that scrupulous care measures need to be guaranteed for the pregnant woman as well as the offspring. Public interventions that establish awareness of the functioning of prenatal determinants play an important role in promoting reproductive health outcomes. Adjusting lifestyle determinants, such as diet and stress management, plays an important role in establishing a good environment for fetal growth. Continuous studies on genetic and environmental factors determining genital organ and gonad development will inform the existing understanding of reproductive health. Lastly, those insights will assist in specific interventions against reproductive disorders and maintaining good health over generations (Koopman *et al.*, 2015; Bellingham *et al.*, 2016).

Test Your Knowledge

1. What are Disorders of Sex Development (DSDs) in females?
2. What genetic and environmental factors can cause DSDs in females?

SUMMARY

Development of the genital and gonadal system in females is a complex interaction between genetic, hormonal, and environmental factors. An understanding of it lies at the heart of the response to disorders of sex development (DSD) with significant implications for those affected by them. Such conditions as ambiguous genitalia not only have body consequences but also very profound psychological implications. Patients acquire gender dysphoria, expressed in the shape of anxiety, depression, and decreased quality of life in general. Treatment of DSD cases requires an integrative approach, as evidenced by the necessity of multidisciplinary teams consisting of several specialties, including psychiatry, endocrinology, urology, and genetics (Agung *et al.*, 2021). Emphasizing such interaction emphasizes the need for complete appreciation of both physiological and psychological processes in female genital organ development. Finally, the significance of psychiatric care in the treatment of individuals with DSD cannot be overstated. As can be observed in many case studies, such as those related to diseases like Partial Androgen Insensitivity Syndrome (PAIS), correct psychological intervention makes a significant difference to outcomes. When people are faced with incongruities between their physical statuses and social gender norms, a comprehensive support system is essential. Convergence of supportive psychotherapy, psychoeducation, and cognitive behavioral therapy has been found to promote adaptation and mitigate stress among people who face gender identity conflicts concerning DSD (Masood *et al.*, 2020). The intersection of genetics, psychology, and developmental biology thus requires attention to allow for not only medical interventions but emotional resiliency among patients, affirming their identities and improving their quality of life. Ultimately, advancing the frontiers of our understanding in female genital organ and gonadal development requires a sustained commitment to research and clinical practice. The evolving backdrop of genetic studies, cultivating greater responsiveness to the psycho-social implications of conditions like DSD, requires continuous education and sensitivity among healthcare professionals. For optimal management, there is a need to recognize the significant emotional discomfiture inherent in biological variation in genital development. As new therapies and technologies become available, it is crucial to evolve our care strategies in order to assist individuals in achieving a balance between their gender identity and their physical reality so that this can be supported with a compassionate and educated practice (Agung *et al.*, 2021; Masood *et al.*, 2020). This multidisciplinary strategy not only expands the excellence of care delivered but also contributes to the overall aims of fostering health equity and enlightenment within the medical community.

Development of female genitalia and gonads is a complex process influenced by genetics as well as the environment. Understanding the biology of this development is crucial to identifying potential reproductive health issues. Key areas in female development include the differentiation of the gonads into the ovaries, oviduct development, and development of the external genitalia. Regulation of such processes is predominantly governed by genetic signals, particularly those linked to the presence of specific sex-determining genes. In addition, disruption at pivotal phases of development might lead to congenital malformations of the genital tract, underscoring the importance of the comprehension of development processes. Research continues to delineate these mechanisms, discovering their relevance for reproductive health and general sexual differentiation. Under hormonal influence, the contributions of estrogen and progesterone to the formation of the female genitalia cannot be overemphasized. Not only are these hormones essential for the structural maturation of organs, but also for the functional development of these organs. Estrogen encourages the development of reproductive tissues, whereas progesterone readies the endometrium for possible implantation of embryos. The interaction of the hormones with the genetic components forms a cornerstone concept to understand conditions such as polycystic ovary syndrome (PCOS) or endometriosis, which could arise due to disrupted hormonal communication. Evidence from studies examining hormonal regulation in development illustrates how variations in the levels of the hormones can affect long-term health and reproductive system function. This connection highlights the necessity of an interdisciplinary approach to research in studying women's reproductive health throughout the stages of life.

Finally, the consequences of the ontogeny of female genitalia extend beyond theoretical biology and impinge on clinical practice and public health. What is discovered from studies of these developmental processes informs ideal practices in gynecologic health, contraceptive development, and reproductive technology assistance. It is of prime significance to realize that the prevention and management of reproductive health disorders require a complete appreciation of the developmental determinants and their variation across different populations. Also, the intercalation of sex and gender in health and illness, as evident in contemporary studies, suggests that biomedical research must incorporate these aspects to enhance vaccine performance and reproductive health interventions efficiently. By synthesizing the key concepts on female genital organ and gonad development, health practitioners can better deal with women's unique reproductive concerns and improve care practices in reproductive healthcare settings.

KEY TERMS FROM THIS CHAPTER

- Genital ridge
- Bipotential gonad
- Sertoli cells
- Wolffian duct
- Anti-Müllerian hormone (AMH)
- Paramesonephric duct
- Genital tubercle
- Spermatogonia
- Primordial germ cells
- SRY gene
- Leydig cells
- Müllerian duct
- Testosterone
- Urogenital sinus
- Labioscrotal swellings
- External genitalia

CRITICAL THINKING QUESTIONS

1. **Which embryonic structure gives rise to the male genital ducts (epididymis, vas deferens, seminal vesicles)?**
   a. Müllerian duct
   b. Wolffian duct
   c. Urogenital sinus
   d. Genital tubercle
2. **The gonads (ovaries or testes) are derived from which embryonic structure?**
   a. Mesonephros
   b. Endoderm
   c. Genital ridge
   d. Cloaca
3. **In the absence of testosterone, the Wolffian ducts will:**
   a. Develop into male internal genitalia
   b. Degenerate
   c. Develop into the uterus
   d. Form the urethra
4. **The SRY gene on the Y chromosome is responsible for:**
   a. Formation of ovaries
   b. Regression of Müllerian ducts
   c. Development of the female external genitalia
   d. Initiating development of testes
5. **The uterus and upper part of the vagina develop from which structure?**
   a. Wolffian ducts
   b. Cloaca
   c. Müllerian ducts
   d. Genital tubercle

Short Answer Questions

1. Which embryonic duct system primarily gives rise to female reproductive organs?
2. From which embryonic structure do the ovaries develop?
3. The uterus is formed from the fusion of which embryonic ducts?
4. Which two embryonic sources contribute to the formation of the vagina?
5. Which hormone must be absent or minimal for female external genitalia to form normally?

Answer to Critical Thinking Questions

1. (b) 2. (d) 3. (b) 4. (d) 5. (c)

REFERENCES

1. Agung, J., & Setiawati, Y. (2021). Consultation liaison psychiatry on case management of children with mixed gonadal dysgenesis mosaicism 45X (60%) and 46XY (40%). *Volume (5)*, 62–66. https://www.semanticscholar.org/paper/6e9049d6e687008840ff36dbdf39c52dd0cf7cbd (accessed on 14th June 2025).
2. Ahmed, S. F., & Markosyan, R. (2017). Sex assignment in conditions affecting sex development. https://core.ac.uk/download/150597685.pdf (accessed on 14th June 2025).
3. Akram, M., Iqbal, M., Daniyal, M., & Khan, A. U. (2017). Awareness and current knowledge of breast cancer. *Biological Research, 50*. https://doi.org/10.1186/s40659-017-0140-9 (accessed on 14th June 2025).
4. Armour, J., Boyd, R., Cunningham, C., Darwin, C., Department of Health and Human Services, Dunsworth, H. M., Fausto-Sterling, A., *et al.* (2020). Expanding the evolutionary explanations for sex differences in the human skeleton. https://core.ac.uk/download/322809885.pdf (accessed on 14th June 2025).
5. Avasthi, A., Grover, S., & Sathyanarayana Rao, T. S. (2017). Clinical practice guidelines for management of sexual dysfunction. *Indian Journal of Psychiatry, 59*, 91–91. https://doi.org/10.4103/0019-5545.196977 (accessed on 14th June 2025).
6. Bajszczak, K., Marchlewska, K., Slowikowska-Hilczer, J., *et al.* (2020). The risk of mental disorders in patients with disorders/differences of sex differentiation/development (DSD) and Y chromosome. https://core.ac.uk/download/288280195.pdf (accessed on 14th June 2025).
7. Bellingham, M., Evans, N. P., & Robinson, J. E. (2016). Prenatal programming of neuroendocrine reproductive function. https://core.ac.uk/download/42371121.pdf (accessed on 14th June 2025).
8. Calvo, A., Caprio, M. G., Escolino, M., *et al.* (2016). Laparoscopic approach for gonadectomy in pediatric patients with intersex disorders. https://core.ac.uk/download/80338153.pdf (accessed on 14th June 2025).
9. Canning, D. (2019). Re: Surgery of anomalies of gonadal and genital development in the "post-Truth Era." *Journal of Urology*. https://www.semanticscholar.org/paper/238e598cdb4085a040c7edd09421e8b8ac6d4fb3 (accessed on 14th June 2025).
10. Caruso, M., Catizone, A., Ciccarone, F., *et al.* (2015). R-spondin 1/Dickkopf-1/beta-catenin machinery is involved in testicular embryonic angiogenesis. https://core.ac.uk/download/54528318.pdf (accessed on 14th June 2025).
11. Chau, Y. Y., Martínez Estrada, O. M., Müller Sánchez, C. A., *et al.* (2025). Deletion of Wt1 during early gonadogenesis leads to differences of sex development in male and female adult mice. https://core.ac.uk/download/643237194.pdf (accessed on 14th June 2025).
12. Chitayat, D., & Glanc, P. (2010). Diagnostic approach in prenatally detected genital abnormalities. *Ultrasound in Obstetrics and Gynecology, 35*, 637–646. https://doi.org/10.1002/uog.7679 (accessed on 14th June 2025).
13. Collins, A., Hayes, T., Johnston, G., *et al.* (2006). Characterization of atrazine-induced gonadal malformations in African clawed frogs (Xenopus laevis) and comparisons with effects of an androgen antagonist (cyproterone acetate) and exogenous estrogen (17beta-estradiol): Support for the demasculinization/feminization hypothesis. https://core.ac.uk/download/323082216.pdf (accessed on 14th June 2025).

14. Cools, M., Nordenström, A., Robeva, R., Hall, J. C., Westerveld, P., Flück, C. E., Köhler, B., *et al.* (2018). Caring for individuals with a difference of sex development (DSD): A consensus statement. *Nature Reviews Endocrinology, 14*, 415–429. https://doi.org/10.1038/s41574-018-0010-8 (accessed on 14th June 2025).

15. D'Anza, E. (2019). *Genetic, Cytogenetic and Morphometric Analyses in The Study of Reproductive Problems That Affect Animal Productions in The Main Livestock and Pets Species.* https://core.ac.uk/download/328815052.pdf (accessed on 14th June 2025).

16. de Siqueira, G. H. L., Silva, F. E., & Santana, M. I. S. (2018). Morphological description of male genital organs of Marca's marmoset (*Mico marcai*). *Anatomia, Histologia, Embryologia, 47*(4), 372–384. https://doi.org/10.1111/ahe.12365 (accessed on 14th June 2025).

17. Visschere De , P., Nezzo, M., T'Sjoen, G., Villeirs, *et al.* (2013). *Role of Imaging in The Diagnosis and Management of Complete Androgen Insensitivity Syndrome in Adults.* https://core.ac.uk/download/55846159.pdf (accessed on 14th June 2025).

18. Delbès, G., Blázquez, M., Fernandino, J. I., Grigorova, P., Hales, B. F., Metcalfe, C. D., Navarro-Martín, L., *et al.* (2021). Effects of endocrine disrupting chemicals on gonad development: Mechanistic insights from fish and mammals. *Environmental Research, 204*, 112040–112040. https://doi.org/10.1016/j.envres.2021.112040 (accessed on 14th June 2025).

19. Díaz, A., & Lipman Diaz, E. G. (2021). Disorders of sex development. *Pediatrics in Review, 42*, 414–426. https://doi.org/10.1542/pir.2018-0183 (accessed on 14th June 2025).

20. Draper, B. W., Postlethwait, J. H., Kossack, M. E., Parr, R. E., Hopton, S. K., High, S. K., *et al.* (2019). Female sex development and reproductive duct formation depend on Wnt4a in zebrafish. https://core.ac.uk/download/323068109.pdf (accessed on 14th June 2025).

21. Flanagan, K. L., Fink, A. L., Plebanski, M., & Klein, S. L. (2017). Sex and gender differences in the outcomes of vaccination over the life course. *Annual Review of Cell and Developmental Biology, 33*, 577–599. https://doi.org/10.1146/annurev-cellbio-100616-060718 (accessed on 14th June 2025).

22. Gebisa, G. (2021). *Cause for the Occurrence of Freemartin and Its Influence on Livestock Reproductive Performance.* https://core.ac.uk/download/481608050.pdf (accessed on 14th June 2025).

23. Georgas, K., Armstrong, J. F., Keast, J. R., Larkins, C. E., McHugh, K. M., Southard-Smith, E. M., Cohn, M. J., *et al.* (2015). An illustrated anatomical ontology of the developing mouse lower urogenital tract. *Development, 142*, 1893–1908. https://doi.org/10.1242/dev.117903 (accessed on 14th June 2025).

24. Hakkarainen, J. (2017). *Regulation of Gonadal Steroid Synthesis and Reproduction: Novel Roles of Hydroxysteroid (17β) Dehydrogenase 1.* https://core.ac.uk/download/198011070.pdf (accessed on 14th June 2025).

25. Holterhus, P. M., Kulle, A., Busch, H., & Spielmann, M. (2023). Classic genetic and hormonal switches during fetal sex development and beyond. *Medizinische Genetik, 35*, 163–171. https://doi.org/10.1515/medgen-2023-2036 (accessed on 14th June 2025).

26. Hosseinirad, H., Yadegari, P., Mohanazadeh Falahieh, F., Nouraei, S., Paktinat, S., Afsharzadeh, N., & Sadeghi, Y. (2021). Disorders of sex development and female reproductive capacity: A literature review. *Systems Biology in Reproductive Medicine, 67*, 323–336. https://doi.org/10.1080/19396368.2021.1937376 (accessed on 14th June 2025).

27. Hou, C. C., & Zhu, J. (2017). Nanoparticles and female reproductive system: How do nanoparticles affect oogenesis and embryonic development. *Oncotarget, 8*, 109799–109817. https://doi.org/10.18632/oncotarget.19087 (accessed on 14th June 2025).

28. Huang, H., & Tian, Q. (2016). Primary amenorrhea after bone marrow transplantation and adjuvant chemotherapy misdiagnosed as disorder of sex development. *Medicine, 95*, e5190–e5190. https://doi.org/10.1097/md.0000000000005190 (accessed on 14th June 2025).

29. Indig-Weingarten, G. (2012). *Molecular Mechanism of XY Gonadal Dysgenesis*. https://core.ac.uk/download/217329305.pdf (accessed on 14th June 2025).

30. Jackson, W. P. U. (2018). *Intersexual Causes of Primary Amenorrhoea*. https://core.ac.uk/download/478313537.pdf (accessed on 14th June 2025).

31. Jaggard, I. V. (1931). *A study of Intersexuality as Exhibited in Animal Forms*. https://core.ac.uk/download/543559891.pdf (accessed on 14th June 2025).

32. Kilty, M. (2007). *Brain Gender and Transsexualism*. https://core.ac.uk/download/144579262.pdf (accessed on 14th June 2025).

33. Koopman, P., Svingen, T., Ng, T. E., Zhao, *et al.* (2015). *Female-to-Male Sex Reversal in Mice Caused by Transgenic Overexpression of Dmrt1*. https://core.ac.uk/download/43248704.pdf (accessed on 14th June 2025).

34. Madjunkov, M., Dviri, M., & Librach, C. (2020). A comprehensive review of the impact of COVID-19 on human reproductive biology, assisted reproduction care and pregnancy: A Canadian perspective. *Journal of Ovarian Research, 13*. https://doi.org/10.1186/s13048-020-00737-1 (accessed on 14th June 2025).

35. Masood, F. T., & Kiran, Z. (2020). SUN-038 Social and psychological aspects of partial androgen insensitivity syndrome, therapeutic challenges. *Journal of the Endocrine Society, 4*. https://www.semanticscholar.org/paper/8b7ea4a0837524d23c0412f9dae76da30c81f267 (accessed on 14th June 2025).

36. Miller, W. L., & Auchus, R. J. (2011). The molecular biology, biochemistry, and physiology of human steroidogenesis and its disorders. *Endocrine Reviews, 32*, 81–151. https://doi.org/10.1210/er.2010-0013 (accessed on 14th June 2025).

37. O'Shields, J. (2013). *Genetic Sex Conditions and Redefining Sex*. https://core.ac.uk/download/217162224.pdf (accessed on 14th June 2025).

38. Oduwole, O., Huhtaniemi, I., & Misrahi, M. (2021). The roles of luteinizing hormone, follicle-stimulating hormone and testosterone in spermatogenesis and folliculogenesis revisited. *International Journal of Molecular Sciences, 22*, 12735–12735. https://doi.org/10.3390/ijms222312735 (accessed on 14th June 2025).

39. Pierpont, M. E., Brueckner, M., Chung, W. K., Garg, V., Lacro, R. V., McGuire, A. L., Mital, S., *et al.* (2018). Genetic basis for congenital heart disease: Revisited: A scientific statement from the American Heart Association. *Circulation, 138*. https://doi.org/10.1161/cir.0000000000000606 (accessed on 14th June 2025).

40. Ray-Coquard, I., Morice, P., Lorusso, D., Prat, J., Oaknin, A., Pautier, P., & Colombo, N. (2018). Non-epithelial ovarian cancer: ESMO Clinical Practice Guidelines for diagnosis, treatment and follow-up. *Annals of Oncology, 29*, iv1–iv18. https://doi.org/10.1093/annonc/mdy001 (accessed on 14th June 2025).

41. Rizgalla, J. (2016). *An Investigation of The Health Status of Wild Libyan Dusky Grouper, Epinephelus Marginatus (Lowe), with Characterization of a New Disease, Dusky Grouper Dermatitis (DGD)*. https://core.ac.uk/download/77612390.pdf (accessed on 14th June 2025).

42. Rosenfield, R. L., & Ehrmann, D. A. (2016). The pathogenesis of polycystic ovary syndrome (PCOS): The hypothesis of PCOS as functional ovarian hyperandrogenism revisited. *Endocrine Reviews, 37*, 467–520. https://doi.org/10.1210/er.2015-1104 (accessed on 14th June 2025).

43. Shurpyak, S., Pyrohova, V., Malachinska, M. Y., & Gerasimenko, V. V. (2018). Reproductive health and thyroid dysfunction. *Health of Woman*. https://www.semanticscholar.org/paper/b82f3f7cd3146238e404a9747d522c7ca275efa5 (accessed on 14th June 2025).

44. Svingen, T., & Koopman, P. (2013). Building the mammalian testis: Origins, differentiation, and assembly of the component cell populations. *Genes & Development, 27*, 2409–2426. https://doi.org/10.1101/gad.228080.113 (accessed on 14th June 2025).

PUBERTY NORMAL AND ABNORMAL

3

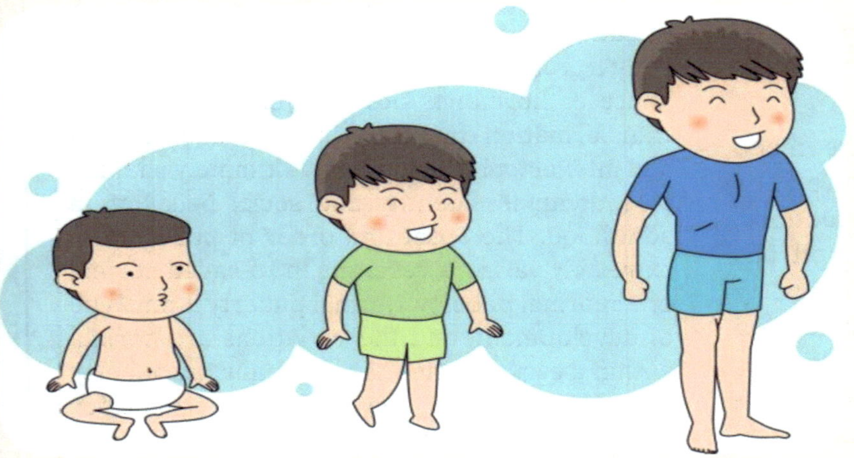

LEARNING OBJECTIVES

After studying this chapter, you will be able to:

1. Describe the key stages of normal puberty
2. Explain the hormonal changes that occur during puberty
3. Analyze the psychological and emotional development associated with puberty
4. Identify the signs of normal puberty
5. Recognize indicators of abnormal puberty
6. Evaluate the health implications related to abnormal puberty

Introduction

The onset of puberty is a critical turning point in a woman's life cycle, marking the beginning of dramatic physiological and psychological transformations that profoundly impact her health and identity. This period of development most commonly begins between the ages of 9 and 14, governed by an intricate interplay of hormonal cues controlled primarily by the hypothalamic-pituitary-gonadal axis. These procedures include the development of secondary sexual characteristics, such as breast enlargement, an increase in body fat, and the onset of menstruation. The puberty experience, however, varies extensively from person to person and leads to definitions of puberty as normal or abnormal. Normal puberty must be defined since it's what is used as the reference for medical evaluation and treatment once abnormality arises, eventually impacting long-term health status. Abnormal puberty is central to solving the complexities of deviations from normal development patterns. Precocious puberty, or early onset, and delayed puberty potentially have direct psychological as well as physiological effects. Premature maturation has the potential to bring unwanted pressure and attention at the expense of emotional and mental well-being. Delayed puberty, conversely, has been linked to higher levels of body image and self-esteem anxiety, particularly when in social contexts where peers may already be experiencing these events. Furthermore, these deviations are generally symptomatic of underlying health disorders like hormonal dysregulation or genetic illness that need to be carefully evaluated and treated with tailor-made interventions to enable normal development and minimize suffering.

Studies on female puberty have made spectacular advances, laying bare the complex interplay of hormonal fluctuations, environmental factors, and well-being. It has been established through research that puberty development is influenced by a combination of genetics, nutrition, and psychosocial development, suggesting that the socio-economic environment as well as the biological environment have important roles to play. For instance, (Gebre *et al.*, 2007) suggests that nutritional intake and nutrition levels can influence the age and speed of puberty development in a variety of populations, suggesting an alignment between economic prosperity and health.

Moreover, the effect of the use of hormonal contraceptives and the incidence of conditions such as exercise-induced anaphylaxis in women illustrates the potency of hormonal therapy to impact formation and immunity in adolescence, as evidenced by findings in Frodella *et al.* (2015). These impacts on adolescence are significant for healthcare professionals to establish properly informed approaches to handling normal and abnormal processes of development in women.

Definition of Puberty

Puberty is a critical stage in human development, with numerous physiological, psychological, and social changes. Puberty is the period of transformation from childhood to adulthood, typically beginning between the ages of 9 and 14 years for females. The body, at this time, undergoes tremendous changes based on hormonal changes, primarily in the hypothalamus, pituitary gland, and ovaries. Puberty begins with thelarche, or the growth of breast tissue, and then the initiation of menstruation, an indicator of the body's reproductive maturity. This complex dance of hormones not only initiates physical transformation but also influences emotional and intellectual development, ultimately shaping an individual's identity and social behavior in adulthood. The onset and order of puberty are extremely variable, resulting in so-called normal or abnormal puberty. Normal puberty is any type of development, and the variations are normal within a certain range of age. Abnormal puberty would encompass diagnoses of precocious puberty, where development occurs much earlier than normal, or delayed puberty, which might reflect underlying disease. Understanding the criteria for normal versus abnormal puberty is crucial for addressing potential health concerns. For instance, early onset of physical signs or delayed menstruation can necessitate medical evaluation to rule out hormonal imbalances or genetic disorders, impacting both physical health and psychological well-being. In discussing the nuances of female puberty, it is essential to consider individual variations and their implications. Genetic, dietary, and environmental influences have an impact on the timing and progression of puberty. Social and cultural pressures also have an impact on the way females view their bodies at this crucial period. The combination of these variables can have differing experiences of puberty, which may be further complicated by psychological variables such as body image and self-esteem. A correct understanding of normal and abnormal female puberty is hence a must for health professionals, educators, and parents in order to provide an environment that will ensure healthy growth at this crucial stage of life.

Importance of Understanding Female Puberty

It is crucial that diverse stakeholders like parents, educators, and doctors understand female puberty clearly. Puberty is the duration that marks a significant shift from childhood to adolescence, where a girl's physical, emotional, and psychological traits change significantly. It is crucial to value the changes so that the environment is healthy and robust. As milestones of development are reached, options between normal and abnormal puberty emerge. This realization not only warns adults to speak with young girls better but also encourages them to seek experts when aberrations from normative patterns occur. By identifying the importance of this transitional period, society is able to better meet the challenges adolescent girls face and offer more comprehensive reproductive health education, leading to an educated generation well suited to pursue their developmental trajectory. Recognition of abnormal puberty is also important, as the ability to treat it early on can significantly improve outcomes in adolescent girls. Puberty disorders may manifest as atypical presentation or timing and produce long-term psychosocial impact if unresolved. Premature menarche or delay in menarche, for instance, can coexist with both physiological and psychological outcomes. Although delayed menarche has been discovered to be associated with reduced risk of affective symptoms during adulthood, premature maturation bears another risk that is likely to lead to negative self-image and other affective disorders. With this understanding of how all these areas are interconnected, individualized management plans can be developed in a multidisciplinary environment. This level of understanding not only benefits the concerned individuals but also enhances the support groups with family and healthcare providers so that a comprehensive strategy for female puberty management under normal or abnormal conditions is provided (Gaysina *et al.*, 2015). The social consequences of being aware of female puberty extend beyond education and medical care; they attack the core of evolving expectations and norms around gender. As society's cultural norms slowly shift toward accommodation, demands for nuanced discourse around female development have never been more necessary. For instance, the complex nature of disorders of sex development (DSD) highlights the importance of interprofessional care that is responsive to different identities and experiences (Ahmed *et al.*, 2017). By playing a role in the cultural environment that is attuned to and respects diversity in pubertal experiences, physicians can foster acceptance and discourage stigma. Combining medical expertise with cultural competence is important to ensure that adolescent girls are addressed properly with care, inducing self-advocacy and empowerment in the critical period of their lives. Lastly, developing the body of knowledge regarding girls' puberty promotes a healthier dialogue that is respectful of the unique paths each girl travels while maintaining the fundamental significance of community and education in this very special phase of life.

Overview of normal vs. abnormal puberty

Puberty is the characteristic transformation in female development, which is accompanied by a sequence of physical, endocrine, and psychological changes announcing the onset of reproductive adulthood. Puberty, typically beginning between 9 and 14 years of age, initiates breast enlargement, the formation of menstruation, and other secondary sexual characteristics in females. Normal puberty is defined by a coordinated series of these events, provoked by activation of the hypothalamic-pituitary-gonadal (HPG) axis. Estrogen and progesterone are central to these events that induce growth spurts and body composition changes. Gradual and appropriate development is normal and indicates a well-functioning endocrine system with a direct influence on overall well-being and development pathways. Therefore, an understanding of normal stages of puberty is essential because it helps in the provision of a standard against which abnormal growth can be measured and managed. Abnormal puberty appears in different ways, typically with delayed or premature sexual development. Retarded puberty refers to the absence of physical manifestations of puberty at 13 years of age, whereas precocious puberty refers to the emergence of these signs before the age of 9 years. These abnormalities may be due to numerous etiologies, some of which include genetic susceptibility, nutritional deficiencies, and underlying clinical conditions that may affect hormonal balance. For delayed puberty, chronic illness or hypogonadism may be a significant factor, leading to anxieties about subsequent reproductive function and psychosocial effects of late onset of physical maturity. For precocious puberty, increased environmental exposure to estrogens or hormonal abnormalities has been shown to lead to psychological distress as well as more adverse health effects. Therefore, it is imperative to diagnose and manage these abnormalities to prevent long-term health and developmental consequences. Normal and abnormal puberty differ not just in terms of physical development but also incorporate the psychological and social connotations of such development milestones. Adolescent female teenagers experiencing puberty experience profound changes in self-concept, peer relationships, and social interaction. Although normal puberty fosters a sense of belonging and identity, abnormalities can lead to confusion, isolation, and anxiety. For instance, girls exhibiting precocious maturation may struggle with inapplicable social expectations, while girls with delayed puberty may be forced to confront low self-esteem and bullying. Developing effective assessment and intervention methods is necessary for addressing girls with these challenges, to ensure access to education about bodily changes and emotional support. Embracing the richness of adolescence allows for a richer understanding of how girls can successfully navigate this critical stage of development in a healthy and informed manner.

3.1. The Stages of Normal Puberty

Learning Outcome

1. Describe the Tanner stages of development
2. Define the average age of onset and duration
3. Discuss the physical changes during puberty

Onset of puberty is an important landmark in the life of a girl with physical, endocrine, and psychological alterations. The onset tends to occur between the ages of 8 and 13 and is prompted by the activation of the hypothalamic-pituitary-gonadal (HPG) axis. The biologic process begins with the secretion of gonadotropin-releasing hormone (GnRH), which prompts the pituitary gland to secrete luteinizing hormone (LH) and follicle-stimulating hormone (FSH). These hormones are significant to ovarian function, resulting in the secretion of estrogen, which is responsible for developing secondary sexual characteristics such as enlarged breasts and wider hips. The first sign is the development of breast buds as girls experience a spurt in growth, gaining height and body fat percentage. This stage is critical to know because it results in all subsequent advances in sexual development and reproductive health. As the puberty process continues, girls will at times pass through the menarche stage, which is the first menstruation cycle, and it will typically occur between the ages of 9 and 16. Menarche would be followed by a series of endocrine alterations, for example, fluctuating hormone levels, which induce the growth of the ovarian follicles. Around this time, girls will also experience mood swings and shifts in emotional sensitivity as a result of the Android changes in brain chemistry. Most importantly, menarche is mistakenly thought of as a definite proof of the attainment of puberty when, in fact, several physiological adjustments remain to occur afterwards. For instance, hormonal regulation still settles and stabilizes over several years following menarche, influencing overall reproductive well-being. Such intricate hormonal interactions require a deeper understanding to classify normal patterns of growth from abnormal patterns, which might be indicative of latent discrepancies. In addition to these physical developments, the psychological aspects of puberty must be taken into consideration to a great extent, as they are likely to have a great impact on a girl's self-perception and social relationships. Adolescents are likely to struggle with complex identity constructions in puberty, in accordance with peer relationships and familial obligations. Issues such as body dissatisfaction and exploration of gender identity are possible, based on external influences and personal experience. In addition, disorders like P450 oxidoreductase deficiency can make this developmental process more challenging, as evidenced by signs such as incomplete puberty and ovarian cysts due to impaired hormonal pathways (Adachi *et al.*, 2010). Physical and emotional maturation are deeply intertwined, and how they work together in determining the general picture of puberty is very important since any variation from normal growth can have serious psychological and physical consequences. Therefore, the stages of normal puberty constitute a crucial blueprint for the determination of normal and abnormal adolescent experience.

3.1.1. Tanner Stages of Development

The Tanner stages of development provide a key means of explaining the physical and hormonal processes that occur in females during puberty. This classification system includes five such specific stages, each characterized by some breast and pubic hair developments, which correspond to the initiation and advancement of the sexual maturation process.

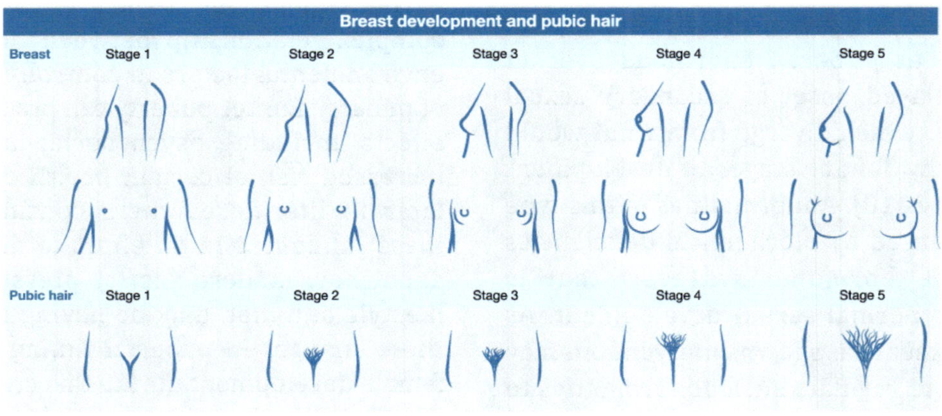

Figure 3.1. The tanner scale.

Source: https://www.seekpng.com/png/full/252-2520426_deepalu-png.png

Typically beginning at about 8 or 13 years of age, Tanner Stage 1 is prepuberty with minimal development, and Stage 5 is maturity with fully developed breasts and adult-pattern pubic hair. It is through awareness of these stages that normative development can be measured and abnormalities identified when growth advances deviantly from what is typical, a symptom perhaps of underlying health or endocrine disorders. Genetic and environmental influences have a major effect on the transition through Tanner stages, especially as regards hormonal effects. One study investigating the level of testosterone in children identified that there is a strong genetic influence on circulating testosterone as well as the timing of androgen-dependent pubertal development, with an estimated 50% heritability for both boys and girls (Archer *et al.*, 2005).

This suggests that while there is diversity in people, overall development via Tanner stages is over half determined by genetics. The study highlights the moderate correlation of testosterone levels with pubertal development and demonstrates that there are external components that go into moderating such a correlation at early and mid-puberty. Diseases such as P450 oxidoreductase deficiency (ORD) can significantly affect normal Tanner stage development, indicating the importance of clinical sensitivity during adolescence. In girls with ORD, cases have presented with incomplete development at puberty, enormous ovarian cysts, and delayed onset of secondary sexual features, all of which diverge from what would be predicted by Tanner stages of development (Adachi *et al.*, 2010). Abnormalities of this type are usually caused by biochemical deficiencies impairing the hormonal synthesis that is necessary for normal sexual development. As clinical assessment has shown, interventions may be necessary to regulate such abnormalities to allow normal development to occur. Monitoring deviations and abnormalities in Tanner stages by healthcare providers can effectively guarantee adolescent support during abnormal puberty, as the diagnosis and treatment of causative conditions at the right time.

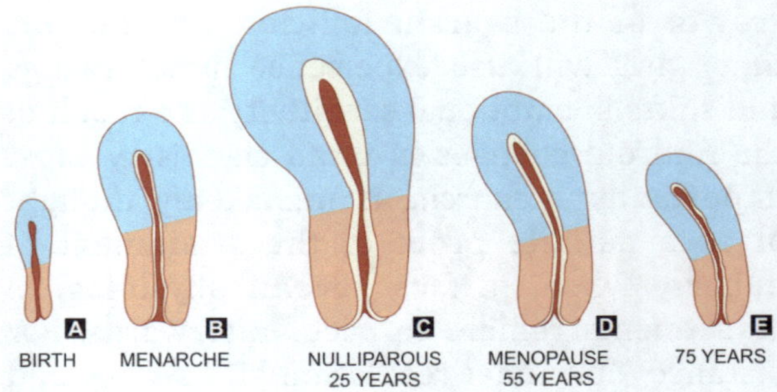

Figure 3.2. Changes in the size of the uterus from birth to 75 years of age.

Source: https://oshimu.com/wp-content/uploads/2021/07/Gynaecology-DC-Dutta.pdf

3.1.2. Average Age of Onset and Duration

The mean age of onset of puberty in females is the key developmental milestone that marks the transition from childhood to adulthood. Onset typically commences at the age of 8 and completes at 13, but it is influenced by genetic, environmental, and dietary conditions. For instance, studies have found that girls with increased body mass indices tend to experience earlier menarche, which encapsulates the complex relationship between biological and environmental factors in controlling the timing of puberty. Earlier puberty can produce different effects, including psychosocial issues and an increased risk of certain health complications later in life. Researchers continue to study these influences in an effort to discover more about how modern society pressures, such as lifestyle and diet, may be having an impact on these changes in pubertal timing and thus on female development during this critical phase of life. The duration of puberty, the several years that comprise assorted physical and emotional changes, is as important as the onset. Typically, the whole process of puberty lasts between approximately 2 and 4 years, during which girls grow secondary sex characteristics, experience growth spurts, and reach reproductive maturity.

Individual variations in length could account for variation in experience among individual girls, affecting their social life, self-image, and psychological well-being. Secondly, premature or delayed maturation may also be accompanied by challenges like differences in body image or levels of social acceptance.

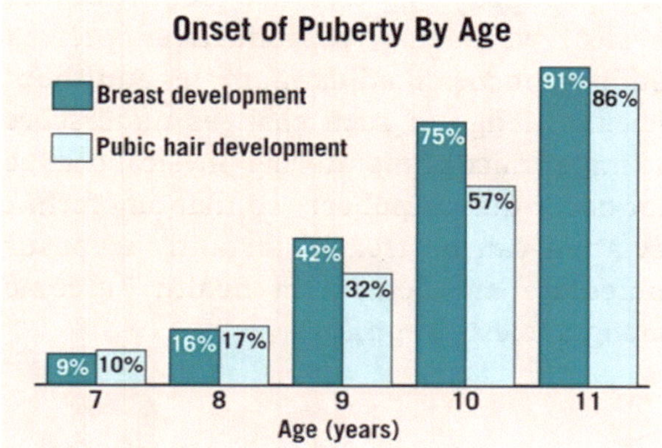

Figure 3.3. The average age of onset for female puberty.

Source: https://cdn.mdedge.com/files/s3fs-public/Image/September-2017/graph.JPG

Awareness of the average age and variability of puberty in females heightens sensitivity to the broader implications involving the timing of biological change onset and emphasizes the significance of education programs addressing the psychosocial effects of puberty. The implications of the mean age at onset and duration of puberty extend beyond individual experience to encompass broader public health issues. The increasing trend towards earlier puberty necessitates a multicomponent strategy to educate parents, educators, and providers regarding its possible health outcomes. For example, evidence indicates that early puberty could be connected with higher risks of future anxiety, depression, and even cardiovascular disease. Due to this, practitioners in such specialty areas as pediatrics and mental health must stay current with the latest trends in acknowledging the biological and psychological processes of puberty—a field that continues to evolve as studies continue to shed light on these complex processes. As discussed in several studies, early intervention and education are able to reduce adverse outcomes linked with abnormal timing in puberty, with particular importance placed on maintaining a continued research focus to monitor trends and develop effective support systems for girls undergoing this pivotal developmental stage.

3.1.3. Physical Changes During Puberty

Puberty is a pivotal stage of female development, characterized by an array of physical changes that signal the onset of reproductive maturation. Typically occurring anywhere from 8 to 13 years old, this development phase initiates the process of transforming a girl's body as it begins to produce greater levels of hormones, most notably estrogen. The first noticeable change, quite frequently, consists of the emergence of breast tissue, a physiological indicator of the maturing mammary glands. Accordingly, menarche, or the onset of menstruation, generally happens two to three years following breast development, heralding that ovulation has begun. They are needed not only for reproductive purposes but also for the psychological aspects of identity and self-concept during adolescence, supporting the intricate interrelationship between bodily growth and emotional well-being in adolescent girls. With ongoing puberty, a number of other physical changes take place that are essential for sexual differentiation and maturity. Growth spurts typically occur, leading to a surge in height and body size, with most girls peaking in growth at ages 11 and 12. Growth is regulated mostly by the activity of growth hormone and sex steroids, which cause changes in body composition, such as fat deposition in the hips and thighs.

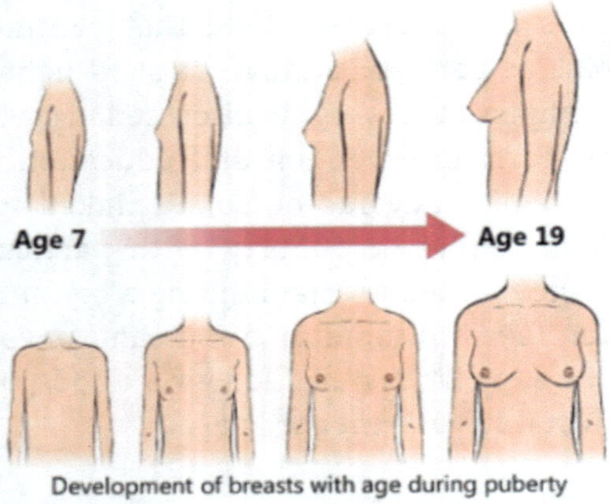

Figure 3.4. Between the ages of 8–13 years, girls start developing breasts.

Source: https://www.menstrupedia.com/articles/girls/physical-changes-girls

Moreover, the alteration of skin texture and development of body hair also occur significantly at this stage, coinciding with a rise in androgen levels. The alteration not only shapes the physical appearance of young women but also affects social and cultural definitions of femininity and body image to an extent of even increasing awareness of individual and societal standards of beauty. However, deviation from the usual sequence of physical change in puberty can be a sign of underlying health issues or hormonal issues. As an illustration, delayed puberty, which is the failure to develop breasts in puberty at the age of 13, can be an indication of hypogonadism or chronic diseases that disrupt the production of hormones. In contrast, precocious puberty before the age of eight can also be an issue, most frequently necessitating a medical evaluation to rule out pathological causes such as central nervous system dysfunction or exposure to exogenous hormones. Identification and therapy of these abnormal progressions are significant since they produce long-term consequences for physical well-being, reproductive potential, and psychosocial adjustment in adulthood. The knowledge of such changes underscores the importance of monitoring physical changes that occur during puberty so that any form of deviation can be treated instantly to ensure immediate and long-term health outcomes among adolescent girls.

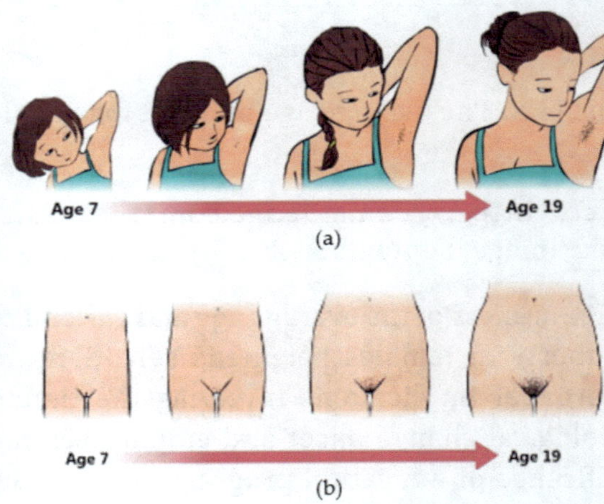

Figure 3.5. (a) Hair begins to grow in your armpits. (b) Hair in the genital region is known as pubic hair.

Source: https://www.menstrupedia.com/assets/quickguide/puberty/puberty-armpit.jpg

Test Your Knowledge

1. What are the Tanner Stages of Development, and what do they describe?
2. At what average age does puberty typically begin, and how long does it usually last?

3.2. Hormonal Changes during Puberty

Learning Outcome

1. Role of Estrogen and Progesterone
2. Impact of hormones on physical and emotional health
3. Hormonal fluctuations and their effects

The onset of puberty represents a hallmark milestone in the maturation of females, solidly rooted in hormonal changes specifically orchestrated by the endocrine system. Puberty is initiated when the hypothalamus begins to release gonadotropin-releasing hormone (GnRH), which stimulates the anterior pituitary gland to release luteinizing hormone (LH) and follicle-stimulating hormone (FSH). These hormones play central roles in ovarian function, such as the regulation of estrogen and progesterone secretion. The high levels of estrogen are particularly significant because they cause the development of secondary sexual characteristics such as the enlargement of breasts and hips. Furthermore, the interaction of these hormonal alterations not only regulates body change but also initiates biochemical reactions that influence growth spurts and sex organ maturation, setting the foundation for ultimate fertility. Prenatal research suggests that gestational circumstances influence the neuroendocrine machinery governing reproductive hormones in adult life. Developmental windows are essential, and exposure to many factors such as maternal diet, stress, and exogenous hormones during these windows can lead to reproductive dysfunction. For instance, exposure to androgens and estrogens at windows of development can lead to prenatal programming of the GnRH neurosecretory system and to variability in the development of normal reproductive function. This idea of prenatal programming highlights the significance of early hormonal environments in setting the reproductive health course of an individual. Hence, disruptions at this turning point can lead to adverse reproductive outcomes that persist during adolescent and adult life, pointing to the complexity of hormonal regulation during puberty as outlined in Bellingham *et al.* (2016).

Other than estrogen, the role of testosterone emerges as important during puberty, particularly with regard to personality traits such as dominance. These investigations indicate that there is a direct relationship between free testosterone levels and dominance behaviors in adolescent girls, but with the relationship being moderated by same-sex peer group membership. The testosterone-dominance link for boys is made more precise by masculine ideology, which holds that hormone changes not only orchestrate growth but also converge on social dynamics and identity during adolescence. These findings indicate the complexity of the effect of hormonal changes, demonstrating that the hormonal profile of adolescence involves physiological changes along with psychological implications, thus reflecting a holistic picture of female puberty both in a biological and socio-cultural context as presented in Kaufman *et al.* (2010).

3.2.1. Role of Estrogen and Progesterone

Adolescence is the defining transition in female growth since it is marked by the onset of the hypothalamic-pituitary-gonadal (HPG) axis. The basis of this growth rests on hormones progesterone and estrogen, which regulate physiological development necessary for fertility. Not only does estrogen facilitate physical growth, but it also contributes significantly towards the formation of secondary sexual characteristics, such as breast enlargement and sexual organ growth. Besides, it plays a significant function in regulating the initiation of menstrual cycles that are vital for future fertility. The interval and balance of estrogen secretion can also significantly affect not just reproductive but overall physical and psychological well-being during adolescence. Fluctuations of estrogen levels during this critical period may lead to abnormalities such as precocious puberty or delayed menarche, indicative of estrogens' vital role in normal pubertal development. Progesterone also plays a significant role at the age of puberty, although largely in preparation for potential pregnancy following ovulation. Progesterone rises following ovulation as the body gains reproductive capability, causing the endometrium to grow and facilitate pregnancy if it occurs. However, fluctuations in progesterone cause irregularities in the menstrual cycle, including frequency and hormonal balance. Alterations in progesterone levels in puberty can result in menstrual irregularities, which are a common complaint among adolescent girls. These irregularities can appear as polycystic ovary syndrome (PCOS) or other endocrine disorders, which can have reproductive implications in the long term. Understanding the dual role of estrogen and progesterone not only highlights their essential function in facilitating normal puberty but also sheds light on potential interferences that may result in abnormal development and associated health issues. The intricate role of estrogen and progesterone highlights the orchestral function of hormones necessary for healthy sexual development. Of major interest is the neuroendocrine basis of the process, which illustrates the sensitivity of the gonadotropin-releasing hormone (GnRH) system to various internal and external stimuli, which can, in turn, considerably influence reproductive function as well as consequent health. Prenatal exposure has been found to reprogram sexual development on an epigenetic level by several factors like steroids, diet, and environmental aspects, thereby influencing generations to come (Bellingham *et al.*, 2016).

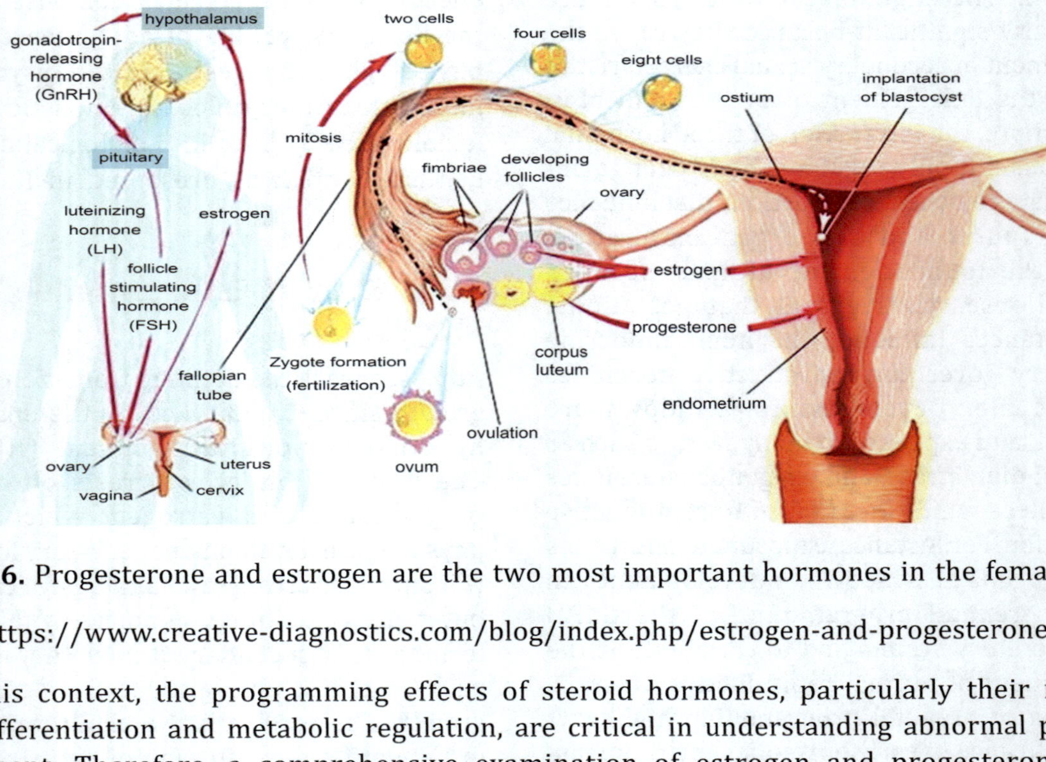

Figure 3.6. Progesterone and estrogen are the two most important hormones in the female body.

Source: https://www.creative-diagnostics.com/blog/index.php/estrogen-and-progesterone/

In this context, the programming effects of steroid hormones, particularly their roles in sexual differentiation and metabolic regulation, are critical in understanding abnormal pubertal development. Therefore, a comprehensive examination of estrogen and progesterone must consider these multifaceted interactions and their potential long-term consequences on a female's reproductive health and overall well-being (Deniselle *et al.*, 2016).

3.2.2. Impact of Hormones on Physical and Emotional Health

During female puberty, the intricate interplay of hormones plays a crucial role in both physical and psychological development. Bloom of sex hormones, primarily estrogen and progesterone, synchronizes the growth of reproductive organs, encourages the development of secondary sexual characteristics such as breast growth, and monitors menstrual cycle regularity. This biological transformation is often preceded by radical emotional changes, since hormonal changes have been linked with mood swings, anxiety, and heightened sensitivity. The impact of these hormones is notable in that not only do they produce physical maturity, but they also are involved in the developing adolescent brain, which implies that the hormonal profile of puberty extends far beyond biological repercussions into emotional health as well. As they experience puberty, their understanding and awareness of these developments are crucial to emotional health. It has been proven through research that teenagers, especially in the city, have little understanding of the hormonal shifts of puberty and how these affect their moods. For instance, research reveals that only 45.4% of private school boys and 36% of public school boys in Karachi demonstrated knowledge regarding the nuances of puberty changes. This disparity highlights the importance of tailored educational programs addressing both the biological and affective themes of puberty. Such interventions can make individuals younger, more attuned to what they are going through, and less worried and self-conscious about such natural processes, thus improving overall well-being at this early point in life (Nazim *et al.*, 2023).

Also, the changes in the endocrine system experienced during puberty can result in a series of emotional and mental challenges, which also must be recognized. Regulation of the neuroendocrine system at this time can be highly vulnerable, particularly in adolescents who have existing mental illness or neurodevelopmental disorders. Studies indicate that there is a vast overlap between disordered puberty and neurodevelopmental issues, a fact that forces healthcare providers to keep reproductive and mental health closely monitored. Identification of the connection between the two conditions can encourage early intervention strategies, which may mitigate potential long-term emotional and health effects. Through fostering an overall understanding of the impact that hormonal development has upon physical and emotional maturation, therapeutic aid and intervention can be created anew, ultimately ensuring a healthier transition through puberty (Howard *et al.*, 2024).

3.2.3. Hormonal Fluctuations and Their Effects

Hormonal fluctuations play a key role during puberty in female adolescents, as levels of progesterone and estrogen influence both physical and emotional development. Estradiol, a type of estrogen that promotes the growth and development of secondary sexual characteristics, starts being secreted by the ovaries during puberty. The elevation of estrogen levels is particularly pronounced in females going through puberty, causing breast enlargement, widening of the hips, and the onset of menstruation. Intriguingly, studies indicate that these hormonal fluctuations are not singular events but are interconnected with changes in gonadal morphology. Specifically, studies have shown that estrogen levels in the ovaries correspond sensitively with ovarian weight and the number of ovarian follicles, emphasizing the facet of hormonal fluctuations in fostering the physiological development typical of normal puberty (Bidlingmaier *et al.*, 1987).

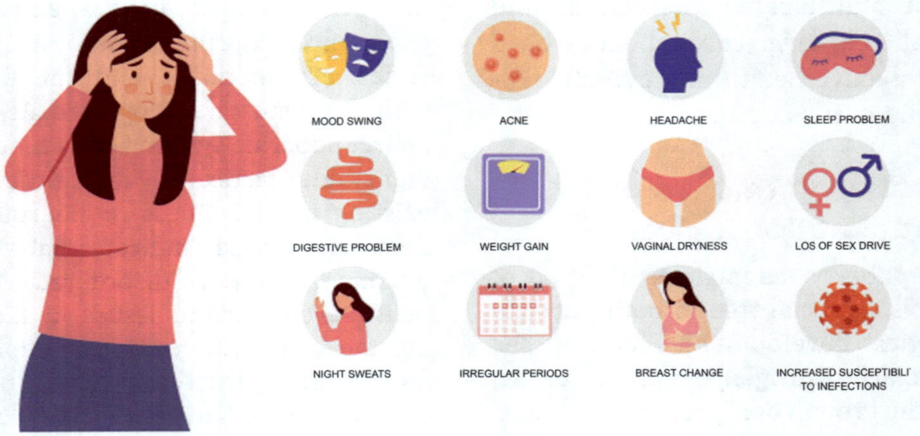
MOOD SWING
ACNE
HEADACHE
SLEEP PROBLEM
DIGESTIVE PROBLEM
WEIGHT GAIN
VAGINAL DRYNESS
LOS OF SEX DRIVE
NIGHT SWEATS
IRREGULAR PERIODS
BREAST CHANGE
INCREASED SUSCEPTIBILI
TO INEFECTIONS

Figure 3.7. Symptoms of hormonal imbalance.

Source: https://www.manipalhospitals.com/jaipur/blog/hormonal-imbalance-causes-symptoms-treatment/

Also, hormonal interactions at puberty may produce many abnormal conditions that disrupt normal development. Fluctuations of hormone levels may lead to irregular menstruation, endometriosis, or polycystic ovary syndrome (PCOS), which may all impact emotional and physical well-being. For example, overproduction of androgens may disrupt normal ovarian function, leading to irregular cycles and other signs of PCOS. In addition, as Linson *et al.* (2013) quote, hormonal imbalance can manifest in the form of gastrointestinal symptoms mimicking the syndrome of disorders like Irritable Bowel Syndrome. This interplay suggests that hormonal readjustments in puberty are multi-dimensional and would have far-reaching implications for physical well-being as well as psychological health, and hence require holistic plans for management and treatment. The effect of hormonal change extends beyond physical symptomatology, profoundly influencing emotional well-being throughout the tumultuous years of puberty. Moodiness, increased anxiety, and depression are apt to emerge as a direct effect of hormonal change. The bio-psychological model identifies hormones such as estrogen and progesterone, which affect neurotransmitter systems and can exacerbate mood disorders during this critical developmental period. Specifically, increases in progesterone have been linked with symptoms of anxiety and depression-like states. Knowledge of the endocrine underpinnings of these mood swings can be used to assist in the development of targeted therapeutic interventions that address causes, not just symptoms, ultimately establishing a healthier climate for adolescent girls to struggle through the challenges of puberty (Linson *et al.*, 2013).

Test Your Knowledge

1. What roles do estrogen and progesterone play in the female reproductive system?
2. How do estrogen and progesterone impact physical and emotional health?

3.3. Psychological and Emotional Development

Learning Outcome

1. Discuss the changes in self-esteem and body image
2. Define social interactions and peer relationships
3. Understand the coping with emotional challenges

Puberty marks the onset of an important development period that profoundly influences psychological and emotional development in females. The onset of teenage years in girls means the experience of an explosion of endocrine fluctuations, not only influencing physical appearance but also emotional state and mental illness. Such development can result in increased vulnerability to affective symptoms, which are frequently manifested in the form of mood changes, fearfulness, and depression. Research has indicated that premature maturation in females is likely to be a cause for concern with regard to the risk of developing such symptoms, but evidence indicates that late menarche may perhaps lead to lower adult-onset affective symptom risk, displaying a complex relationship between biological timing and emotional impact (Gaysina *et al.*, 2015).

Understanding of these results has the potential to inform the development of targeted interventions promoting psychological resilience at this phase of life. In addition, the affective terrain of the adolescent girl is often modulated by her social experience and self-concept development. Puberty brings with it a vast transformation, both biologically and socially, in that relationships with peers become more intense and societal demands accrue. It is in this time that impulsivity and emotional functioning difficulties can arise, probably leading to maladaptive eating behaviors or eating disorders, such as Binge Eating Disorder (BeD). In a study, the mediating role of alexithymia—difficulty in recognizing and expressing emotions—on impulsivity and emotional functioning in adolescents with BeD is found, and emotional awareness is found to be primarily involved in good psychological development (Ballarotto *et al.*, 2017).

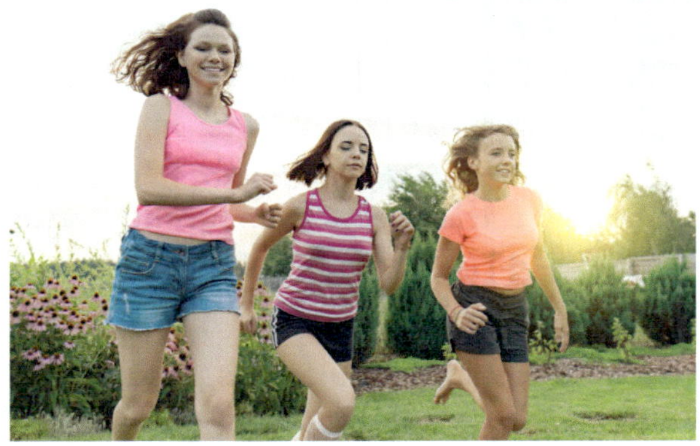

Source: https://images.ctfassets.net/aqfuj2z95p5p/3Dme2egtIJ2EkYhDr8RXhp/404bb64d500fb8b70f4e7c1bd40d6512/Always_EN_UK_Articles_A073-Emotional-Changes-During-Puberty_02-Emotional_changes_during_puberty.jpg?fm=webp&q=75

Thus, emotional literacy and coping strategies education for young girls can be a comfort point in diffusing these threats posed by these challenges of growth. Culturally and contextually, female puberty experiences can vary, further preventing psychological and emotional growth. Some of the variables that determine how girls cope with emotional adversity during this period include family dynamics, peer relationships, and social pressures. For instance, girls with adverse socio-environmental exposures may exhibit greater anxiety and depressive symptoms, which are carried forward into adulthood. Conversely, positive environments might forge resilience and improved emotional outcomes. Therefore, it is essential to recognize these dynamics in developing effective prevention strategies and treatment policies to support emotional well-being during puberty. By addressing the convergence of pubertal development and emotional well-being, teachers and physicians can craft interventions that enable adolescent girls to thrive through this developmental process and mitigate possible psychological costs of non-typical puberty progressions.

3.3.1. Changes in Self-Esteem and Body Image

By puberty in women, dominant physiological and psychological processes frequently result in changes in self-esteem and body image attitudes. When young people transition from adolescence to adulthood, they become increasingly attuned to societal expectations for beauty and attractiveness, further exacerbating feelings of inadequacy. Studies have shown that early adolescence is a critical stage, with a sudden increase in girls' body dissatisfaction that has a negative influence on self-esteem. These emotions are amplified by the effects of media representation, self-comparison to peers, and cultural ideals, making them more susceptible to forming unhealthy body images. This environment also contributes to the dynamic that self-esteem is made contingent upon conforming to these ideals, which then generates distress that is most often linked with body image issues. Understanding the psychological mechanisms of pubertal body image involves understanding the interplay between sociocultural ideals and self-esteem. Evidence suggests that body-dissatisfied females internalize sociocultural ideals of beauty and have decreased self-esteem. Comparing themselves to unattainable representations in the media, the adolescent girl may feel inadequate, and hence begins a vicious cycle in which low self-esteem begets body dissatisfaction, and body dissatisfaction begets low self-esteem. This cycle is particularly common in environments that lack supportive interventions; thus, the importance of educational programs that address self-esteem and positive body image before and during puberty. By teaching resilience against negative messages from society, it is possible to reverse the negative effect on psychological well-being that most teenagers undergo during this critical period. Treatment of body image concerns through intervention and education is one of the principles in helping adolescent girls build healthier self-esteem and overall well-being. Having school interventions that target enhancing body image and self-esteem has been a worthy alternative. The interventions help to counter the adverse correlates of self-esteem and body dissatisfaction, evidenced by research that finds robust relationships between the two concepts. Through healthier body image and countering of cultural expectations by means of extensive educational initiatives, equipping young girls with the resources to overcome the tribulations of puberty is achievable. Early engagement in self-esteem development tasks has a critical impact on changing the course of body image beliefs, leading to a generation of young women being able to resist destructive societal norms while gaining a more favorable sense of self.

3.3.2. Social Interactions and Peer Relationships

During female puberty, the processes of change that occur can have a significant impact on peer relationships and social relationships. As girls mature physically and emotionally, they will perhaps undergo alterations in their relationships with their peers. This is characterized by even greater concern with social approval and a tendency to become more sensitive to peer rejection and acceptance. Significantly, the nature of these relationships can influence self-esteem and emotional well-being. The peer relationship dynamics are further complicated by the onset of adolescence because girls are potentially working on such concerns as competition, body dissatisfaction, and social conformity pressure. These concerns can precipitate a crucial need for supportive friendships, which can serve as a buffer against some of the adverse effects of transitional stressors of puberty. Also, the beginning of puberty may be a significant influence on social relationships and peer interaction. Pubertal timing has been observed to expose girls to diverse social environments from their peers that can increase their risk for befriending deviant peer groups. This association is perhaps related to the development of conduct problems, where early maturing girls tend to associate with older peers who encourage the development of risk-taking behavior.

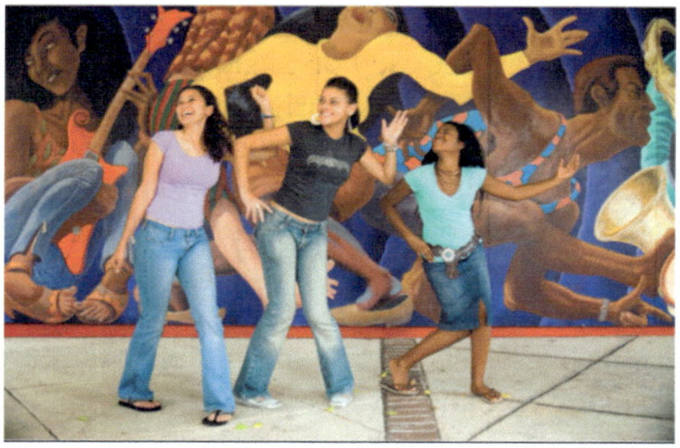

Figure 3.8. Adolescents develop strong friendships with peers who share similar interests and values.

Source: https://nerd.wwnorton.com/ebooks/epub/psychlife2/OEBPS/img/images/Fig4-27.jpg

By contrast, delayed menarchal girls are likely to have more conventional friendships and can benefit from positive peer relationships that enhance emotional stability. The interplay between pubertal timing and peer relations underscores the importance of information on gender-specific pathways to social development. Identification of such dynamics can assist practice to foster healthy relationships within a critical developmental phase. Also, social relationships during puberty are regulated both by developmental changes and by predisposing emotional problems. The development of affective symptoms, which in the case of females seem more intense, can drive girls' social behavior and peer relationships. Facts show that while early puberty is not the etiology of long-term affective symptoms, those who show very late menarche can be assisted with less susceptibility to adult-onset affective disorder. Emotional regulation is a key element of peer relationships because girls who struggle to communicate their feelings may struggle to maintain healthy relationships. The literature on conduct problems indicates that adolescent social experience will often interact with trouble regulating emotions to place girls at risk for unhealthy peer interaction. Recognizing these influences can be crucial in developing targeted interventions to support healthy social relationships for girls navigating the complexities of puberty (Gaysina *et al.*, 2015; Donnell *et al.*, 2007).

3.3.3. Coping With Emotional Challenges

It is particularly difficult to navigate the emotional rollercoaster of puberty in girls because puberty is a time of enormous physical, psychological, and social change. The emotional landscape changes abruptly during puberty, with a tendency to increase anxiety, uncertainty, and questioning about one's body image. Embarrassment and confusion are also likely to develop following the sudden appearance of puberty, and so it becomes necessary for young girls to acquire healthy coping strategies. Parents, teachers, and peers all have an important role to play in minimizing these emotional turbulences, as a supportive environment fosters good communication and facilitates adolescents' freedom of expression. Hence, emotional resilience must be enhanced;

girls can be assisted by the acquisition of stress management techniques, such as mindfulness and open communication, welcoming their developmental experiences constructively and positively. Social support networks become a critical factor in adolescent girls as they confront such emotional problems.

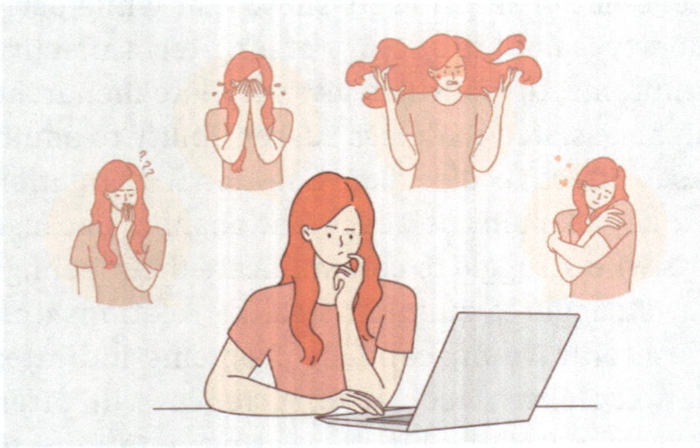

Figure 3.9. Emotional changes during puberty.

Source: https://images.ctfassets.net/6mz6gnctx58g/5y5WqNZlQb2rTyTt9Wx36B/bb9a3602739caa9c70ccdbe44211824f/TB_Callout_-1.png

The recognition of the value of friendships and family relationships may be able to eliminate isolation or terror. As reflected by emotional assessments in many studies, such as the one summarized in the Adolescent Idiopathic Scoliosis case (Wihak *et al.*, 2016), emotional responses to bodily change may significantly influence overall functioning. By involvement of these shifts in a comforting environment, females can learn not only how to embrace their developing selves but also learn to overcome pressures from society. Curriculum programs specifically designed to promote learning on puberty and the variations it creates can educate teenagers, as reported through revelations on knowledge gaps among young people (Nazim *et al.*, 2023). These programs foster coping and resilience behavior, yet again complementing emotional well-being at this stage of crisis. In addition, the psychological implications of puberty are not only the short-term emotional challenges but also result in long-term repercussions if not managed properly. During this vulnerable age, girls are exposed to external pressures from media presentations of ideal body images that once more mean a rise in feelings of inadequacy or anxiety. It is crucial to establish a body-positive culture of self-esteem and acceptance, which can avert adverse emotional responses. Interventions aiming to raise awareness of body changes and self-esteem can help establish an environment in which young girls can feel more secure in themselves. As girls learn constructive coping skills, they are most able to manage these problems, laying the groundwork for resilience later in life. Lastly, handling the emotional chaos of puberty with comprehension and vigilant environmental assistance can significantly enhance the quality of life for young adolescent females who are undergoing this natural but formidable process.

Test Your Knowledge

1. What impact do changes during puberty have on social interactions and peer relationships?
2. What are effective coping strategies for managing emotional challenges during puberty?

3.4. Signs of Normal Puberty

Learning Outcome

1. Define menarche and menstrual cycle regulation
2. Understand the development of secondary sexual characteristics
3. Explain the growth spurts and changes in body composition

Puberty onset is a significant developmental milestone in women, defined by a cascade of physiological changes signaling maturation. One of the earliest signs of normal puberty is the development of breast buds, which usually happens at 8 to 13 years. The development of breasts is triggered by increased levels of estrogen, signaling the initiation of secondary sexual characteristics. Apart from breast growth, the spurt in growth typically occurs, resulting in abrupt height increments that tend to occur between the ages of 9 and 14. During this phase, females may also experience changes in body composition, such as the buildup of increased fat primarily in the hips and thighs, which prepares their bodies for subsequent reproductive tasks.

These bodily changes are not merely biological; they play a vital role in the psychological maturation of adolescents, as they undergo the complicated aspects of identity and societal expectations of femininity. Menstruation or menarche is a definite marker of normal female puberty, marking the onset of reproductive potential. Menarche usually occurs at around age 12.5, but between 9 and 16 years is also within the realm of what is considered normal. The beginning of menses is a sign of preparedness for potential fertility, as it indicates that the ovaries are secreting mature eggs, as well as the endocrine regulation provided by the hypothalamic-pituitary-gonadal axis. Menstrual cycles will be unregulated at first, which is also usual since an adolescent's body is adapting to new hormone patterns. The understanding of the subtleties of this development can help parents and educators to recognize the signs of deviation that may indicate underlying conditions. Therefore, proper education regarding these signs has to be provided to create awareness and seek medical attention when any aberration takes place at this life stage. Furthermore, the development of pubic and axillary hair is a clear indicator of normal puberty, due to the androgens secreted by the adrenal glands. This hair growth typically begins shortly after breast development, typically at the age of between 9 to 14. The pattern and speed of hair growth can vary greatly from individual to individual and can be influenced by genetics, ethnicity, and environment. These body hair developments not only reflect the physical transformation of the body but also contribute to the development of sexual identity. Girls can be subjected to body pressures from society during puberty, highlighting the importance of establishing an environment where positive self-image and acceptance are permitted. Teachers and parents need to ensure open dialogue about the changes, directing young women through both the body and the emotional complexities of this pivotal development phase (Adachi *et al.*, 2010; Corsello *et al.*, 2016).

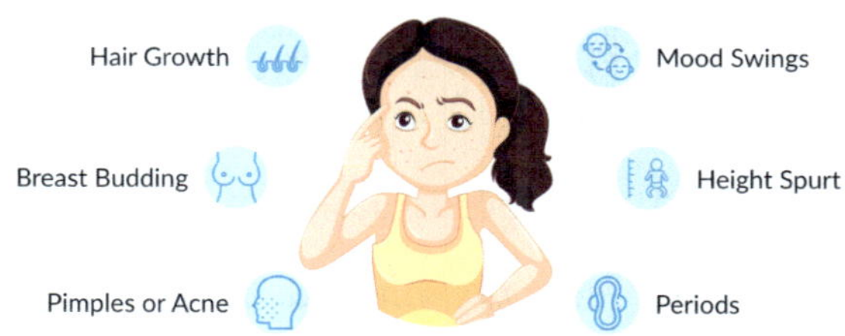
Hair Growth
Mood Swings
Breast Budding
Height Spurt
Pimples or Acne
Periods

Figure 3.10. Signs of puberty in girls.

Source: https://drsmitaramachandran.com/wp-content/uploads/2022/08/Signs-of-Puberty-in-Girls.png

3.4.1. Menarche and menstrual cycle regulation

Menarche, the onset of menstruation, is a significant event of female puberty and is governed by a multifaceted set of biological and environmental factors. Typically between 9 to 16 years of age, the timing of menarche can provide excellent insight into reproductive health and overall health. Research suggests that several factors, including genetics, diet, and physical activity, have a profound influence on when a girl will have her first menstruation. Moreover, premature or delayed menarche has been linked to different health outcomes, such as increased vulnerability to emotional disorders and long-term conditions like cardiovascular disease in adulthood. Understanding these correlations not only justifies following the menarche but also underscores its function as an initial indicator of impending future health conditions that require remediation and intervention (Chavarro *et al.*, 2024).

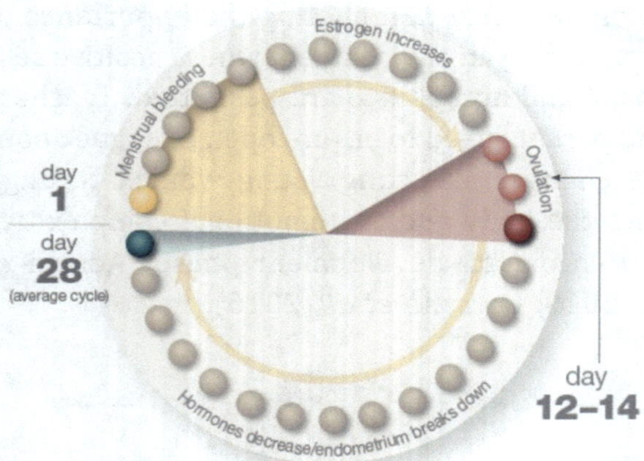

Figure 3.11. The menstrual cycle.

Source: https://www.nichd.nih.gov/sites/default/files/health/topics/menstruation/conditioninfo/PublishingImages/menstruation_02.jpg

Control of the menstrual cycle is an intricate hormonal interaction between the hypothalamus, pituitary gland, and ovaries. The interaction is intricate and regulates the phases of the menstrual cycle: the follicular phase, ovulation, and the luteal phase, with specific hormone changes regulating ovulation and preparing the endometrium for an eventual pregnancy. Disruption in this delicate balance may lead to menstrual irregularities, which are significant markers of health, particularly during adolescence, as the cycle is only just becoming regular. Disordered cycles or amenorrhea may represent underlying metabolic derangement or stress-related illnesses, thus serving as significant landmarks for clinicians to assess an adolescent woman's overall health and hopefully ward off reproductive diseases (Welp *et al.*, 1999). The significance of menstrual cycle control extends much beyond the realm of reproductive function, co-morally with metabolic health and problems typical of the female athlete triad. This triad is defined as disordered eating, amenorrhea, and osteoporosis, noting the adverse impact that high-level exercise may play on menstrual control. It is paramount that health professionals, particularly within the arena of athletics, are familiar with these disorders at early points in development to utilize appropriate interventions. By addressing menstrual irregularities at an early stage, physical therapists and health care providers can decrease long-term health consequences such as decreased bone mineral density and increased risk of fractures. Further, by exploring the interrelation of such conditions, therapeutic interventions that support healthy menstrual cycles as well as increased athletic performance and general health (Welp *et al.*, 1999).

3.4.2. Development of secondary sexual characteristics

The development of secondary sexual characteristics in women is a significant aspect of puberty, the period between childhood and adulthood. It typically happens between the ages of 8 and 13 and is controlled by a chain of hormonal and physical changes. Estrogen, which is mainly produced by the ovaries, also plays a role in developing these changes, which include breast expansion, redistribution of body fat, and the establishment of menstruation. As secondary sexual characteristics emerge, they not only signal biological maturation but also interact with psychosocial factors, including identity and self-concept regarding gender. Understanding the normal development of these characteristics is valuable, as deviations may lead to what will be deemed abnormal puberty and need to be further investigated and possibly treated. Irregular development of secondary sexual characteristics can take a variety of forms, leading to conditions such as delayed puberty or precocious puberty.

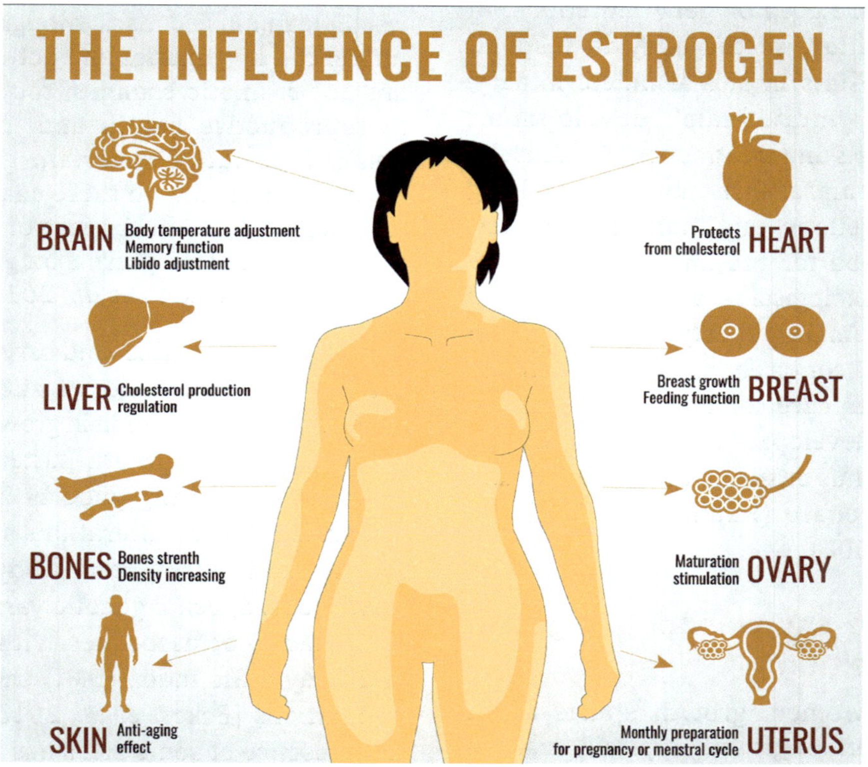

Figure 3.12. Secondary sexual characteristics.

Source: https://www.yaclass.in/p/science-state-board/class-8/reaching-the-age-of-adolescence-14830/adolescence-and-reproductive-health-5622/re-d8078aab-0c21-4a21-9bba-abd7046a212f

Delayed puberty, which is otherwise defined as failure to develop breasts by the age of 13 years, can be caused by underlying endocrine disturbances, genetics, or chronic illness. Precocious puberty, defined as the premature appearance of secondary sexual characteristics before the age of 8 years, could be due to premature activation of the hypothalamic-pituitary-gonadal axis. The implications of these disorders are important since they will affect physical health as well as emotional status. For instance, girls who exhibit precocious puberty can experience additional social pressure and psychological issues with their maturity level, while those with a delayed start can have issues regarding body image and self-esteem by comparing themselves to other people. Also, hormonal disorders can affect the expression of secondary sexual characteristics, like in Androgen Insensitivity Syndrome (AIS) cases. AIS provides a unique scenario in which individuals with an XY chromosome pattern acquire female secondary sexual characteristics despite the presence of male hormones, mainly due to Androgen Receptor gene mutations. In this case, the failure of the body to respond to androgens results in sexual indeterminacy, rendering the individuals' development complex. Diagnosis and treatment of AIS must be conducted in a comprehensive manner, involving hormonal, cytogenetic, and molecular studies, stressing the need for the medical staff to be conscious of the biological as well as psychosocial dimensions of female puberty. Providing such problems with a comprehensive approach can guarantee proper care for adolescent females with abnormal developments of secondary sex characteristics, thus ensuring their physical and psychological welfare (Kaufman *et al.*, 2010; Tonang *et al.*, 2006).

3.4.3. Growth spurts and changes in body composition

At puberty in women, growth spurts are a critical component of growth, typically marked by a sudden increase in height and a dramatic shift in body composition. It typically begins at 9 to 14 years of age, at which time girls may undergo a growth spurt one to two years preceding menarche. Height increase is dominated by hormonal changes, particularly in relation to estrogen, that cause the growth plates of bones to close after reaching maximum expansion. The timing and degree of these changes can vary significantly between individuals and lead to an enormous range of body shapes and development directions. Accordingly, understanding the variability in the onset and growth rate of growth spurts is necessary to distinguish between normal and abnormal pubertal development in girls. Throughout puberty in girls, body composition significantly changes, with variation in fat and muscle content becoming proportionally greater. Most typically, girls will experience an elevation in body fat percentage, particularly in regions such as the hips and breasts, that is tied to hormonal changes experienced during puberty. Concurrently, there is a more variable rise in lean muscle mass, though this too can be influenced by genetics and activity level. These are not cosmetic changes; they are important in reproductive health and in general well-being. Fascinatingly, certain genetic variants have been linked with these changes, according to research into the impact of specific single-nucleotide polymorphisms on growth and body composition (Eckert *et al.*, 2015).

Complexity of this kind serves to emphasize the multidimensionality of puberty as well as inter-individual variation in growth patterns. The interplay among growth patterns and genetic determinants during puberty is central to the understanding of alterations in development timing and associated body composition alterations. Specific genetic variants have been identified to be associated with weight change and body mass index (BMI) change in various populations (Eckert *et al.*, 2015). For instance, the presence of some SNPs has been associated with measures of growth in various ethnic groups and demonstrated the importance of considering race and gender in the assessment of normal pubertal maturation. Because these genetic differences may underlie more rapid weight and BMI gains, they may influence the pattern in which body composition alters during this developmental period. Identification of such variations not only contributes to a better understanding of female puberty but also assists in the detection of abnormalities that may need further medical evaluation and treatment.

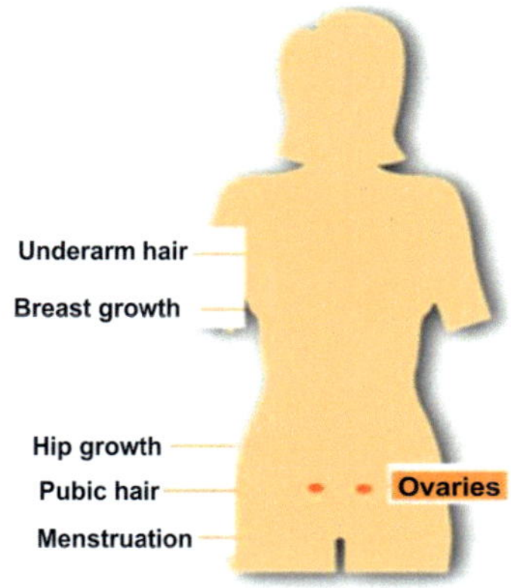

Figure 3.13. Growth spurt in puberty.

Source: https://study.com/cimages/multimages/16/hnet.com-image_41830378549692142797.png

Test Your Knowledge

1. Which secondary sexual characteristics develop during puberty?
2. How do growth spurts and body composition change during puberty?

3.5. Indicators of Abnormal Puberty

Learning Outcome

1. Define precocious puberty: causes and implications
2. Explain the delayed puberty: signs and potential issues
3. Discuss the disorders of sexual development

Female puberty is a complex biological process composed of many hormonal changes, marking the termination of adolescence and initiation of reproductive maturity. Puberty in most individuals typically begins between the ages of 8 and 13, marked by thelarche, breast growth. Abnormal pubertal signs can be in different ways, including precocious puberty, where there is the attainment of secondary sexual characteristics at an earlier age than 8, or delayed puberty, where menarche does not occur before the age of 15. This abnormality of growth pattern can have psychological and physiological implications. It is therefore necessary to identify these abnormal signs early, as early intervention may do a great deal to prevent future health issues resulting from abnormal growth patterns and hormonal imbalance. Through close observation of developmental milestones, medical practitioners can effectively identify abnormalities during puberty and provide the requisite support and therapy. Puberty is not only defined by physical changes; psychological and emotional factors are just as crucial in defining abnormal puberty. Girls with precocious onset, for instance, might face special social challenges, such as stigmatization or teasing, that impact their psychological well-being and self-esteem. Furthermore, delayed puberty girls can also experience anxiety due to their physical difference from their peers, leading to social withdrawal or depression. Endocrine system imbalance, such as in conditions like polycystic ovary syndrome (PCOS), can also be indicators of abnormal puberty. Data indicate that conditions affecting the endocrine system can disrupt the occurrence and progress of puberty, making it more difficult for the physiologic changes to occur. Identifying these emotional and psychological cues is very important in obtaining a well-rounded understanding of abnormal puberty in females. Another element of challenge in identifying abnormal puberty relates to the genetic and metabolic impacts on sexual development. Turner syndrome, for instance, is a chromosomal abnormality resulting from the absence of all or a portion of one X chromosome and can lead to short stature and delayed puberty. Likewise, metabolic states such as hypothyroidism may dramatically alter the rate and characteristics of puberty. Interacting relationships among environmental influences and genetic states make it difficult to make assessments of normal and abnormal puberty. As can be seen in studies that examine chromosomal segregation in oogenesis, genetic material abnormalities can set off an avalanche of problems involving women's reproductive status and development (Dyban *et al.*, 2010). Continued research and combined reviews of these numerous factors are required for understanding and addressing the numerous indicators of abnormal puberty (Gebre *et al.*, 2007).

3.5.1. Precocious puberty: causes and implications

Precocious puberty, defined as sexual development prior to nine years in males and eight years in females, is increasingly becoming a critical issue in public health. A wide range of factors has been invoked, including genetic predisposition to obesity, as well as environmental factors. Studies have focused on the role of endocrine disruptors in the environment to influence hormonal pathways. Researchers posit that the normalization of precocious puberty is part of a larger societal pattern in which conventional ideas of childhood are disrupted (Cozzi *et al.*, 2015). Not only does such premature maturation change the physical growth of girls, but it also causes one to question the psychosocial effects, as these individuals could experience emotional and behavioral issues related to premature adult-like behavior. In examining the effects of precocious puberty, there is a need to consider the psychosocial forces at play. Early growth typically harbors undesired attention and pressure, leading to issues like increased risk of sexualization and exploitation. Studies indicate that females who experience precocious puberty are likely to engage in risky behaviors at a greater percentage than their peers, an indicator that points to the psychological effects of early growth (Davies *et al.*, 2022). Additionally, this advancement can result in serious emotional distress since such individuals will be isolated from other children who are going through more typical pubertal stages. This difference in emotional well-being can negatively impact self-esteem and interpersonal relations, leading to cyclical anxiety and misfits within their formative environment. The applications of precocious puberty to the general population are health policy and education systems. Health professionals are now calling for generalized educational interventions to address the complexities inherent in early puberty. These interventions would most appropriately combine sensitivity to bodily changes with guidance on emotional and social adaptation (Cozzi *et al.*, 2015). Pediatric professionals must also possess the capacity to manage the intricacies inherent in children going through precocious puberty. This encompasses developing favorable environments that engage the children and parents in discussions about body changes and societal expectations. With the debate over precocious puberty maturing, it is still necessary to balance medical knowledge with experiences of involved subjects for the enhancement of a multi-faceted framework for knowledge on this developmental process.

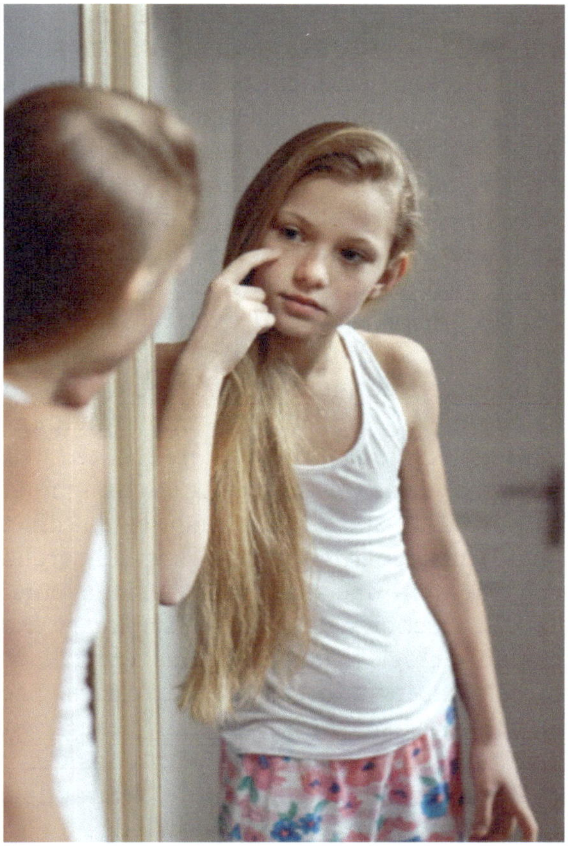

Figure 3.14. Precocious Puberty.

Source: https://cdn-memphismomsnew.b-cdn.net/wp-content/uploads/2018/08/precocious-puberty-3.jpeg

3.5.2. Delayed puberty: signs and potential issues

The onset of puberty is a crucial developmental milestone in female teenagers, which typically manifests between the ages of 8 and 13. Certain girls, however, might experience delayed puberty, which refers to the inability to develop breasts at the age of 13 or the inability to reach menarche at the age of 15. Clinically, it may be presented with a blend of characteristics, which include inadequate breast growth, lack of menstruation, and below-average growth rates. While it is necessary to consider environmental and genetic determinants of puberty onset, there are definite impacts that can be imparted by underlying medical conditions. Proper clinical evaluations to diagnose early delayed puberty can lead to interventions at the right time and mitigate potential impacts on self-esteem and psychosocial development in the patients. Delayed puberty may have several complications beyond the apparent physical signs. For instance, adolescents with delayed pubertal growth over a prolonged period of time might face psychological problems like anxiety, withdrawal, and a sense of inadequacy compared to peers. The psychological and social environment is critical in managing the consequences of delayed puberty. The physician should utilize a multidimensional approach, offering psychological support and determining whether medical interventions like hormone therapy are required to initiate puberty. In addition, careful monitoring of growth cycles and psychosocial well-being of such adolescents is crucial for emotional stability and healthy development into adulthood. Management protocols are successful if they are based on an understanding of why the pubertal delay occurred. Genetic causes, nutritional status, and certain disorders have implications on the timing of the onset of puberty. For example, the presence of conditions such as Turner syndrome or any other chromosomal abnormality can lead to sexual abnormalities. As mentioned, "children born with sex chromosomal mosaicism, including material derived from the Y chromosome, may present with a broad phenotypical spectrum," which can further mislead the clinical picture (Cools *et al.*, 2021). Secondly, the psychosocial implications of these conditions add to the challenges of delayed puberty, and clinicians must work in a multidisciplinary environment to attend to both the physical and the emotional aspects of care. Through collaboration between specialists, more effective and suitable management plans can be implemented in the affected adolescents (Ahmed *et al.*, 2017).

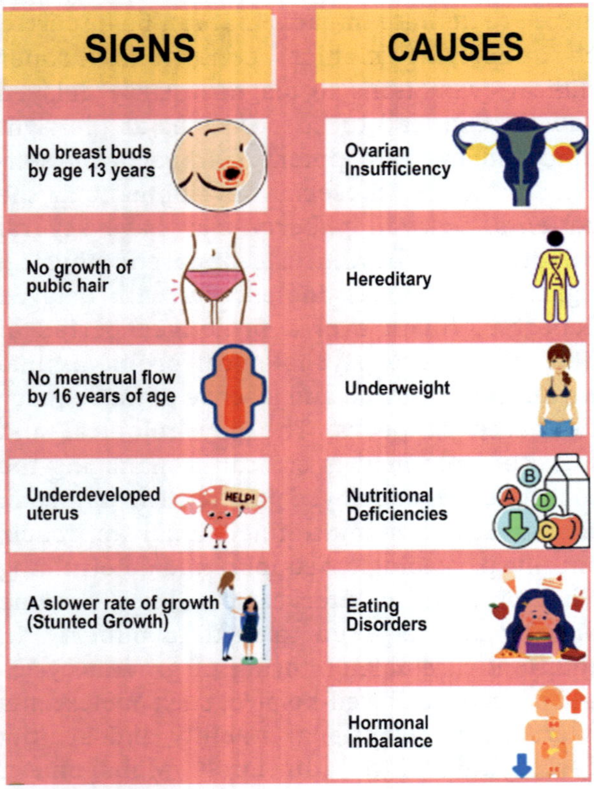

Figure 3.15. Signs and causes of delayed puberty.

Source: https://medhyaherbals.com/wp-content/uploads/2022/06/Signs-Causes-of-Delayed-Puberty-in-Girls-min-683x1024.png

3.5.3. Disorders of sexual development

Disorders of sexual development (DSDs) refer to a variety of medical conditions where atypical chromosomal, gonadal, or anatomic sex development occurs. DSDs usually manifest during different stages of puberty, affecting the physical and psychological growth of the afflicted subjects profoundly. DSDs may be caused by genetic abnormalities during embryonic growth or by hormonal disturbances. As contemporary medicine learns more about DSDs, the intricacy of female puberty becomes better understood. Particularly, presentation of DSDs during this early stage may pose challenges with sex assignment and the extent of psychosocial implications for adolescents seeking to establish themselves in a sex-gender system that the majority of societies maintain as binary. Consistently, treatment of the multivariable requirements of DSD individuals necessitates a multidisciplinary team to ensure care in this tumultuous phase of development (Ahmed *et al.*, 2017). The clinical care of DSD individuals includes not just medical treatment but psychological care and counseling addressing the individual's situation. Families are often presented with challenging decisions regarding sex assignment and potential surgery at diagnosis, raising ethical issues regarding child rights and parental involvement in decision-making. Management entails interaction with an interdisciplinary team of endocrinologists, geneticists, and psychiatric professionals to address the intricacies. Each case presents a need for a carefully thought-out individualized management plan considering the patient's needs and family interactions, in addition to improving knowledge of the population's attitude towards gender and sex diversity. As perceptions change, clinicians will have to remain sensitive to various perceptions in society in order for not just practices and suggestions to be medically fitting, but also culturally attuned (Ahmed *et al.*, 2017).

Scientific inquiry has begun revealing the neurologic implications of DSDs, particularly regarding the ways in which they may be related to gender identity. Studies have indicated that individuals with early-onset gender identity disorder (EO-GID) are structurally different in the brain compared to biological peers. Structural magnetic resonance imaging studies have reported regional brain volume and hormone level differences, suggesting a connection between the lack of hormonal deficiency and neurodevelopmental patterns. These findings not only contribute to an understanding of DSDs but also render standard models of gender identity development questionable. As more is learned about the biological foundations of gender development and identity, it is necessary to translate this into practice so that DSD patients can be better treated and discoveries inform future therapies, as well as the social rules guiding gender differences.

Test Your Knowledge

1. What are the signs of delayed puberty, and what potential health issues can it indicate?
2. How are disorders of sexual development identified, and what challenges do they present?

3.6. Health Implications of Abnormal Puberty

Learning Outcome

1. Define long-term physical health effects
2. Identify the psychological impact and mental health concerns
3. Discuss the importance of early intervention and treatment

The onset of abnormal puberty in females can lead to a range of health effects that extend past the immediate physiological changes. For instance, precocious puberty—girls gaining the secondary sexual characteristics prior to nine years of age—has been associated with increased risks of psychological and emotional problems. Studies indicate that early development can raise anxiety, depression, and body image problems because early sexual maturity may be hard to deal with for young girls. Moreover, irregular pubertal timing is likely to disrupt normal hormonal equilibrium, which in turn will lead to long-term reproductive problems such as polycystic ovary syndrome (PCOS) and infertility. It is necessary to recognize these psychological and physical effects in an effort to create interventions that can tackle the physical and mental health issues of the affected individuals. Besides psychological issues, precocious puberty can also cause drastic metabolic alterations that are potentially long-term health hazards. Researchers have found that early pregnancy in girls carries higher risks of overweight and obesity owing to alterations in the composition of the body as well as in metabolic rate. This, in turn, raises the risk of developing chronic diseases such as type 2 diabetes and cardiovascular disease at advanced ages. Hormonal disturbances resulting from abnormal puberty can also impair insulin sensitivity and raise the accumulation of visceral fat, aggravating health issues. As these metabolic effects arise from early hormonal disturbances, they underscore the need for healthcare providers to monitor growth patterns and metabolic health in girls with abnormal puberty in an effort not to suffer from long-term consequences. Abnormal puberty can also have health impacts across generations, which underscores the importance of understanding maternal effects on reproductive health. Maternal conditions such as obesity, stress, and exposure to endocrine-disrupting chemicals during pregnancy can pre-program daughters to enter puberty at an earlier age and lead to complications, typically initiating a cycle of health risk across generations. The concept of prenatal programming shines light on the process through which the prenatally affected environment organizes neuroendocrine mechanisms regulating reproductive mechanisms, which are bound to be extremely vulnerable to impacts from outside. As future generations' health will be based on conditions experienced in utero, it is imperative to address these foundational factors if one is to avoid the transgenerational inheritance of reproductive health issues, compounded by abnormal puberty. Knowledge regarding the interplay of environmental exposures and gene expression is vital to the effective deployment of public health interventions aimed at improving the reproductive outcomes of girls and their offspring.

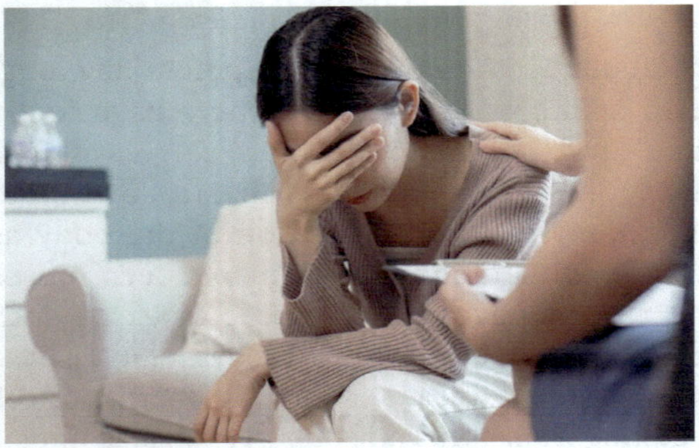

Source: https://www.bellybelly.com.au/wp-content/uploads/2016/06/puberty-more-common.jpg

3.6.1. Long-term physical health effects

Onset of puberty is a significant landmark in the development of girls, influencing not just reproductive capabilities but also long-term health consequences within the physiological system. One of the areas of health touched by puberty is the establishment and regulation of the neuroendocrine systems that serve reproductive purposes. Research has proven that prenatally induced exposure to stress and exogenous hormones, among other environmental factors, is capable of disrupting changes in the neuroendocrine system at this developmental point. These prenatal programming effects can predispose the female to reproductive dysfunction in later life, highlighting the significance of a healthy gestational environment. The consequences of these early hormonal effects reach far beyond the immediate reproductive health and could have implications for global health and well-being extending into generations, with changes in the neuroendocrine systems being epigenetically inherited (Bellingham *et al.*, 2016). Additionally, the age of puberty can have long-term, significant physical and mental health consequences for women. Studies have shown that adolescents who experience later menarche, i.e., those who start their periods at 15 years or older, may have a reduced risk of reporting affective symptoms in adulthood. Such a finding suggests that the age of reproductive events can modify the trajectory of psychological health. Notably, while early puberty has been linked to numerous negative health consequences, late development has been found to play a protective role against certain adult-onset affective disorders.

These findings suggest the complex interworkings between pubertal hormonal development and long-term psychological and physical health processes, with advice for an integrated understanding of these pubertal milestones (Gaysina *et al.*, 2015). Besides, the interface between physical health and puberty also extends to other long-term effects, with a particular emphasis on metabolic processes and cardiovascular health. Puberty is a time of physiological alterations that incline females towards the development of conditions such as obesity, insulin resistance, and cardiovascular disease later in life. As an example, nutritional considerations and lifestyle patterns during this critical growth phase have significant effects on metabolic processes and body composition. The health effects of poor lifestyle habits in puberty are likely to be disseminated into adulthood as chronic diseases. Such a multidisciplinary intervention involving health education, dietary counseling, and psychological guidance during puberty may facilitate healthier outcomes and reduce risks associated with abnormal growth patterns for subsequent generations.

3.6.2. Psychological impact and mental health concerns

When girls transition into puberty, they experience a range of physical and emotional changes that may drastically impact their mental health. Most females experience mood swings, self-esteem issues, and body image concerns during puberty, which are primarily brought about by sociocultural demands and hormonal fluctuations. Evidence indicates that the onset of affective symptoms is most likely to peak during adolescence, particularly among women, but the effects of the timing of puberty are complex. For instance, Gaysina *et al.*, 2015 discuss how subtle differences in the timing of puberty can affect long-term psychological well-being. Early development may amplify peer pressure and lead to psychological distress, while those with a late onset may encounter certain social challenges that give rise to anxiety or depression. A consideration of these aspects is paramount in understanding the mental health profile of adolescent girls. Furthermore, the psycho-emotional effect of abnormalities in puberty, such as delayed or premature development, can have a tremendous impact on the emotional life of a girl. Delayed menarche girls are found to be poorly prepared to deal with self-esteem problems or loneliness issues when comparing themselves with peers who have previously experienced the onset of puberty. In contrast, precocious pubertal girls undergo a heightened process of socialization that could lead to early sexualization and emotional disturbance. Research has demonstrated that such early or late onset experiences may have the potential to influence self-perception and coping, hence complicating a young girl's adolescent experience.

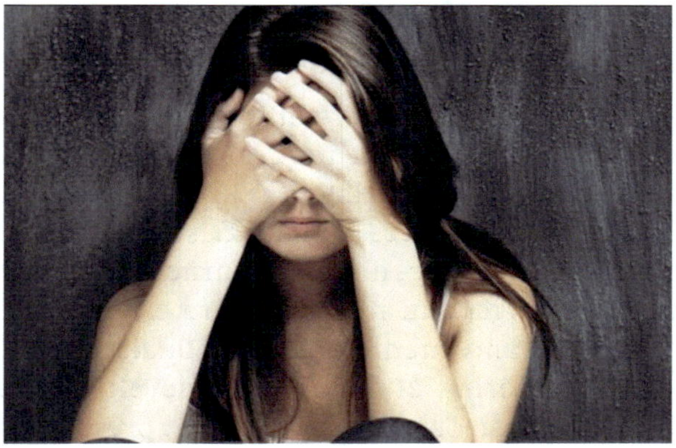

Source: https://parashospitals-web.s3.ap-south-1.amazonaws.com/uploads/2019/06/Mental-health.jpg

According to Gaysina *et al.* (2015), pubertal timing's influence on mental health may also depend substantially on sex, thereby suggesting that interventions aimed at girls and boys are individually needed in order to help them appropriately during adolescence. Besides this, family and parental relations are responsible for a girl's mental state during adolescence. As mentioned in research in adolescent idiopathic scoliosis, the experiences of the child and parent can be influenced by the interventions in medical care (e.g., bracing or surgery) that interrupt the regular process of puberty. indicates that parents of children receiving intensive medical treatments will often report higher levels of concern with their child's coping and pain, further complicating the adolescent's emotional life. The psychological burden of parental over-protectiveness and the atmosphere of stress surrounding medical procedures can unknowingly impact the way a girl thinks about herself and copes with problems. For this reason, it is critical to understand the multi-dimensional nature of such influences to devise pragmatic support systems that assist in bringing about positive psychological well-being during normal or abnormal female puberty.

3.6.3. Importance of early intervention and treatment

The significance of intervention and treatment in female puberty cannot be overstressed, particularly in preventing the psychological and physical consequences of abnormal development patterns. Adolescence is characterized by radical change, and it is therefore critical that caregivers and medical professionals ensure close monitoring of growth and development. Early detection of conditions such as precocious puberty or delayed maturation allows for early medical intervention, which can decrease the emotional stress and burden that typically accompany these conditions. Furthermore, sensitivity to the numerous differences in response to stressors throughout development allows more personalized treatment mechanisms (Karagiannis *et al.*, 2014), giving each young woman what she needs to ride out this difficult phase of her life. Moreover, the management of puberty-related issues at an early phase is most important in preventing long-term health consequences. For instance, puberty-related experiences of abnormal weight gain in women make them susceptible to obesity, a problem that has been identified by the World Health Organization as an epidemic globally among children and adults (Kyrou *et al.*, 2010). Early intervention methods that promote healthy lifestyle patterns—physical activity and nutrition—have the capacity to make a huge impact on the trajectory of a young woman's health. Focusing on these prevention mechanisms, healthcare providers can reduce the risks of obesity, ensuring young women not only navigate puberty in good health but also set themselves up for a lifetime of well-being. In addition to the physical and health benefits, intervention at an early age is essential to developing emotional resilience among adolescent girls. Puberty in women may be a time of upheaval characterized by self-doubt and anxiety, and with the inclusion of abnormal development experiences, these emotions can turn into more serious mental issues. Providing supportive environments that are centered on coping mechanisms can assist young women in managing stress and anxiety regarding their development. Such frameworks not only enhance their awareness of emotional challenges during puberty, but they also equip them with relevant life skills to manage future adversity effectively (Karagiannis *et al.*, 2014). Ultimately, an investment in early treatment and intervention at this critical point can lead to confident young women who can face adulthood's challenges with confidence.

Test Your Knowledge

1. How can abnormal puberty affect psychological well-being and mental health?
2. Why is early intervention and treatment important in cases of abnormal puberty?

SUMMARY

By and large, understanding female puberty as both an abnormal and normal process is crucial for the development of healthy outcomes. The intricacies of this stage of growth transcend the physical level, involving psychological, social, and environmental factors. Research highlights the fact that variations in the timing and duration of puberty can be influenced by a range of factors, including genetics, diet, and environmental toxin exposure. The importance of attention to such factors cannot be overestimated because they have the potential to cause abnormal developments that must be addressed clinically. For instance, maternal well-being in pregnancy can be important because studies have found that prenatal factors have the potential to permanently modify neuroendocrine functions. With this in mind, a multidisciplinary strategy needs to be employed to address the multiplicity of female puberty if it is to be more effectively predicted, prevented, and treated within clinical settings. The public health implications of atypical puberty cannot be ignored, particularly in those societies where cultural practice is inextricably bound up with health. Female genital mutilation (FGM) provides one key example, demonstrating how cultural practices can have adverse consequences on reproductive health and puberty. Case reports indicate that FGM may lead to delayed puberty or other anomalies of development, rendering diagnosis and treatment in subjects complicated. The convergence of medical understanding and culture dictates the necessity for culturally sensitive practice in healthcare. Eradication of practices like FGM must be supplemented by education programs aimed at building awareness concerning female health. These social conditions need to be resolved to enable young girls to navigate puberty free from the shackles of harmful practices, giving healthier generations and nondiscriminatory medicine. Research advances continue to illuminate the connection between female puberty and long-term health effects, justifying further research and education. With interdisciplinary cooperation between policymakers, teachers, and health professionals, steps can be taken to address the physiological and psychological issues of abnormal puberty. Adolescent women have to be given settings where they may receive proper guidance and support during the transitional phase. Taking note of recent studies that identify the impact of prenatal well-being and environmental exposure on reproductive development (Bellingham *et al.*, 2016) and the impact of FGM on intersex individuals (Elagib *et al.*, 2006), provisions for prevention education and care can be invigorated. Ultimately, increased awareness and education of female puberty will empower people and groups to advocate for healthier standards for generations to come.

Understanding normal female pubertal development is crucial in the recognition of normal developmental milestones and potential abnormalities. Puberty is a complicated process involving physical as well as hormonal development and typically occurs between the ages of 8 and 13. Breast development, known as thelarche, is one of the earliest signs to develop, and is followed by the onset of menstruation, known as menarche. It is regulated primarily by the hypothalamic-pituitary-gonadal axis, and gonadotropin-releasing hormone (GnRH) is the prime mover to elicit maximum release of luteinizing hormone (LH) and follicle-stimulating hormone (FSH) from the pituitary gland. LH and FSH, in their turn, regulate ovarian functions, which result in the production of estrogen and progesterone that cause the development of secondary sexual characteristics. A clear understanding of this typical pattern assists in the diagnosis of disorders of precocious or delayed puberty. Identification of abnormal puberty, as in disorders of precocious or delayed maturation, is essential for successful healthcare management. Precocious puberty, which involves the development of secondary sexual characteristics prior to age 8, has many psychosocial and physiological consequences for the involved individuals. This premature, abnormal maturation can result from genetic factors, environmental issues, or exposure to endocrine-disrupting chemicals, which are increasingly being attributed with the capability of altering hormonal balances and developmental pathways. Delayed puberty, however, typically presents itself when secondary sexual characteristics do not develop until the age of 13 and can be an indicator of illness such as hormonal imbalances or genetic disorders. Treatment involves careful evaluation and consideration of medical history as well as environmental exposures that can potentially impact development, such as the impact of toxicants according to Hitchcock *et al.* (2011). The intricate relationship between fertility and puberty emphasizes the importance of investigating the biological basis of this developmental phase. Gonadotropin-releasing hormone (GnRH) neurons, which regulate fertility, trigger differentiation and migration in fetal life, thereby influencing female reproductive capacity at adulthood. The new evidence emphasizes the role of some transcription factors, such as Vax1, in the maturation of GnRH neurons and in exhibiting genetic regulation of the initiation of puberty and subsequent fertility. Failure of properly functioning GnRH neurons could have severe reproductive consequences, including delayed puberty and fertility, results that deserve close follow-up in girls with atypical patterns of development. Understanding the gene and hormone mechanisms that control puberty not only guides improved clinical approaches to assessment and therapy but also encourages an educated appreciation for the subtleties of female reproductive health, as noted by (Hoffmann *et al.*, 2016).

KEY TERMS FROM THIS CHAPTER

- Thelarche
- Growth spurt
- Hypothalamic-pituitary-gonadal (HPG) axis
- Follicle-stimulating hormone (FSH)
- Secondary sexual characteristics
- Delayed puberty
- Turner syndrome
- Menarche
- Tanner stages
- Luteinizing hormone (LH)
- Estradiol
- Precocious puberty
- Hypogonadism

CRITICAL THINKING QUESTIONS

1. At what age range does normal puberty typically begin in females?

a. 5-7 years
b. 8-13 years
c. 14-16 years
d. 16-18 years

2. Precocious puberty in girls is defined as the onset of secondary sexual characteristics before the age of:

a. 6 years
b. 8 years
c. 10 years
d. 12 years

3. Which hormone primarily initiates the physical changes seen in puberty?

a. Progesterone
b. Follicle-stimulating hormone (FSH)
c. Luteinizing hormone (LH)
d. Gonadotropin-releasing hormone (GnRH)

4. Delayed puberty is generally diagnosed if there are no signs of breast development by age:

a. 10 years
b. 12 years
c. 13 years
d. 15 years

5. Which of the following can cause delayed puberty?

a. Hypogonadotropic hypogonadism
b. Precocious puberty
c. Early menarche
d. Hyperthyroidism

Short Answer Questions

1. What are the main stages of normal puberty in adolescents?
2. Which key hormones regulate the changes during puberty?
3. How does psychological and emotional development typically change during puberty?
4. What are common physical signs of normal puberty?
5. What are some indicators that puberty might be abnormal?
6. What are potential health implications of abnormal puberty?

Answer to Critical Thinking Questions

1. (b) 2. (b) 3. (d) 4. (c) 5. (a)

REFERENCES

1. Aagaard, A., Baggish, A., Ackerman, M., Anderson, J., La Gerche, A., Pelliccia, A., Antzelevitch, C., *et al.* (2017). International criteria for electrocardiographic interpretation in athletes: Consensus statement. https://core.ac.uk/download/287649657.pdf (accessed on 14th June 2025).
2. Adachi, M., Antley, R., Arlt, W., Auchus, R., Belgorosky, A., Köhler, B., Bulun, S., *et al.* (2010). Pubertal presentation in seven patients with congenital adrenal hyperplasia due to P450 Oxidoreductase deficiency. https://core.ac.uk/download/pdf/19023.pdf (accessed on 14th June 2025).
3. Ahmed, S. F., & Markosyan, R. (2017). Sex assignment in conditions affecting sex development. https://core.ac.uk/download/150597685.pdf (accessed on 14th June 2025).
4. Archer, J., Boomsma, D. I., Marshall, W. A., Marshall, W. A., Bartels, M., Meikle, A. W., Rogol, A. D., *et al.* (2005). Heritability of testosterone levels in 12-year-old twins and its relation to pubertal development. https://core.ac.uk/download/2355.pdf (accessed on 14th June 2025).
5. Ballarotto, G., Cerniglia, L., Cimino, S., Erriu, M., Porreca, A., Ronconi, L., & Tambelli, R. (2017). Does alexithymia have a mediating effect between impulsivity and emotional-behavioral functioning in adolescents with binge eating disorder? https://core.ac.uk/download/141694750.pdf (accessed on 14th June 2025).
6. Bellingham, M., Evans, N. P., & Robinson, J. E. (2016). Prenatal programming of neuroendocrine reproductive function. https://core.ac.uk/download/42371121.pdf (accessed on 14th June 2025).
7. Bidlingmaier, F., Dorr, H. G., Eisenmenger, W., Knorr, D., *et al.* (1987). Estrone and estradiol concentrations in human ovaries, testes, and adrenals during the first two years of life. https://core.ac.uk/download/12167712.pdf (accessed on 14th June 2025).
8. Bruchhage, M. M. K. (2013). Morphological differences in adolescent female to male transsexuals before cross-hormone treatment. https://core.ac.uk/download/30892640.pdf (accessed on 14th June 2025).
9. Chavarro, J., Nichols, A., & Oken, E. (2024). Reproductive risk factors across the female life course and later metabolic health. https://core.ac.uk/download/643236611.pdf (accessed on 14th June 2025).
10. Christian, M. (2020). Biological, cultural, and psychological factors that may predispose young adults to anorexia nervosa, bulimia nervosa, and binge eating disorders. https://core.ac.uk/download/480813589.pdf (accessed on 14th June 2025).
11. Cools, M., De Groote, K., De Leenheer, E., Debo, M., *et al.* (2021). Multidisciplinary approach to the child with sex chromosomal mosaicism including a Y-containing cell line. https://core.ac.uk/download/395604908.pdf (accessed on 14th June 2025).
12. Corsello, G., Falsaperla, R., Pavone, P., Pavone, V., Praticò, A. D., Ruggieri, M., Savasta, S., *et al.* (2016). Total hemi-overgrowth in pigmentary mosaicism of the (hypo melanosis of) Ito type: Eight case reports. https://core.ac.uk/download/286528715.pdf (accessed on 14th June 2025).
13. Cozzi, D., & Vinel, V. (2015). Risky, early, controversial. Puberty in medical discourses. https://core.ac.uk/download/53358420.pdf (accessed on 14th June 2025).

14. Davies, K., & Davies, K. (2022). An introduction to central precocious puberty. https://core.ac.uk/download/613729423.pdf (accessed on 14th June 2025).
15. Dimeglio, L. A., Geffner, M. E., Gerschenson, M., Hazra, R., *et al.* (2018). Changes in insulin sensitivity over time and associated factors in HIV-infected adolescents. https://core.ac.uk/download/227054243.pdf (accessed on 14th June 2025).
16. Dyban, A., Kuliev, A., Kuliev, A., Mantzouratou, A., Pujol, A., Barlow, A. L., Gutierrez-Mateo, C., *et al.* (2010). Errors in chromosome segregation during oogenesis and early embryogenesis. https://core.ac.uk/download/45628.pdf (accessed on 14th June 2025).
17. Eckert, G. J., Hannon, T., He, C., Pratt, J., *et al.* (2015). Associations between menarche-related genetic variants and pubertal growth in male and female adolescents. https://core.ac.uk/download/46963336.pdf (accessed on 14th June 2025).
18. Elagib, A., Gisselsson, D., Mitelman, F., Eltigani, H., Fadl-Elmula, I., Almroth, L., Almroth, L., *et al.* (2006). Female genital mutilation of a karyotypic male presenting as a female with delayed puberty. https://core.ac.uk/download/pdf/3936772.pdf (accessed on 14th June 2025).
19. Fike, K. E., & Miller, N. A. (2014). Exposure of prepubertal beef bulls to cycling females does not enhance sexual development. https://core.ac.uk/download/33355560.pdf (accessed on 14th June 2025).
20. Frankle, R. E. (2003). Does a marriage really need sex? A critical analysis of the gender restriction on marriage. https://core.ac.uk/download/144228409.pdf (accessed on 14th June 2025).
21. Frodella, C. M. (2015). The role of sex steroids and puberty on respiratory function. https://core.ac.uk/download/142061768.pdf (accessed on 14th June 2025).
22. Gaysina, D., Kuh, D., Hayward, H., Herva, A., Huerta, C., Li, L., Richards, M., *et al.* (2015). Pubertal maturation and affective symptoms in adolescence and adulthood: Evidence from a prospective birth cohort. https://core.ac.uk/download/30608851.pdf (accessed on 14th June 2025).
23. Gebre, M. Y. (2007). Reproductive traits in Ethiopian male goats. https://core.ac.uk/download/11695178.pdf (accessed on 14th June 2025).
24. Deniselle Gonzalez , M. C., Lara, H. E., Recabarren, S. E., Roselli, C. E., *et al.* (2016). Developmental and functional effects of steroid hormones on the neuroendocrine axis and spinal cord. https://core.ac.uk/download/159294623.pdf (accessed on 14th June 2025).
25. Hitchcock, E., & Madsen, T. (2011). Growing up toxic: Chemical exposures and increases in developmental disease. https://core.ac.uk/download/71358334.pdf (accessed on 14th June 2025).
26. Hoffmann, H. M., & Mellon, P. L. (2016). A small population of hypothalamic neurons govern fertility: The critical role of VAX1 in GnRH neuron development and fertility maintenance. https://core.ac.uk/download/323065271.pdf (accessed on 14th June 2025).
27. Howard, S. R., Lorente, M. J., Newsome, A., Pavón, J., *et al.* (2024). Disorders of puberty and neurodevelopment: A shared etiology? https://core.ac.uk/download/644554489.docx (accessed on 14th June 2025).
28. Karagiannis, C., Mills, D., & Zulch, H. (2014). Stress–its effects on health and behavior: A guide for practitioners. https://core.ac.uk/download/20320967.pdf (accessed on 14th June 2025).

29. Kaufman, J., T'Sjoen, G., Van Houtte, M., Vermeersch, H., *et al.* (2010). Gender ideology, same-sex peer group affiliation and the relationship between testosterone and dominance in adolescent boys and girls. https://core.ac.uk/download/55842905.pdf (accessed on 14th June 2025).
30. Kivastik, J. (2000). Lung function in Estonian schoolchildren: Relationship with anthropometric indices and respiratory symptoms, reference values for dynamic spirometry. https://core.ac.uk/download/79106802.pdf (accessed on 14th June 2025).
31. Kyrou, I., & Weickert, M. O. (2010). Clinical problems caused by obesity. https://core.ac.uk/download/46324.pdf (accessed on 14th June 2025).
32. Linson, E. A. (2013). The interplay between hormones and irritable bowel disease. https://open.bu.edu/bitstream/2144/12149/6/Linson_Elyse_2013_nosig_nocv.pdf (accessed on 14th June 2025).
33. MacDonald, T. M. (2010). School-based program to promote healthy body image and self-esteem in boys and girls. https://core.ac.uk/download/354477650.pdf (accessed on 14th June 2025).
34. Nazim, S. M. (2023). The knowledge and attitude regarding pubertal changes among adolescent males in urban Karachi, Pakistan. https://core.ac.uk/download/603659478.pdf (accessed on 14th June 2025).
35. O'Donnell, C. W. (2007). Development of conduct problems in girls: Testing theoretical models and examining the role of puberty. https://core.ac.uk/download/216836200.pdf (accessed on 14th June 2025).
36. Tonang, A. (2006). Clinical, hormonal and genetics features in patients with Androgen Insensitivity Syndrome in cytogenetic laboratories in Semarang. https://core.ac.uk/download/11720967.pdf (accessed on 14th June 2025).
37. Welp, R. (1999). Diet and exercise-induced menstrual dysfunction in the female athlete. https://core.ac.uk/download/235074084.pdf (accessed on 14th June 2025).
38. Wihak, A. A. (2016). Preliminary study comparing parent and child functioning by intervention for adolescent idiopathic scoliosis. https://open.bu.edu/bitstream/2144/16112/1/Wihak_bu_0017N_11107.pdf (accessed on 14th June 2025).

MENOPAUSE

4

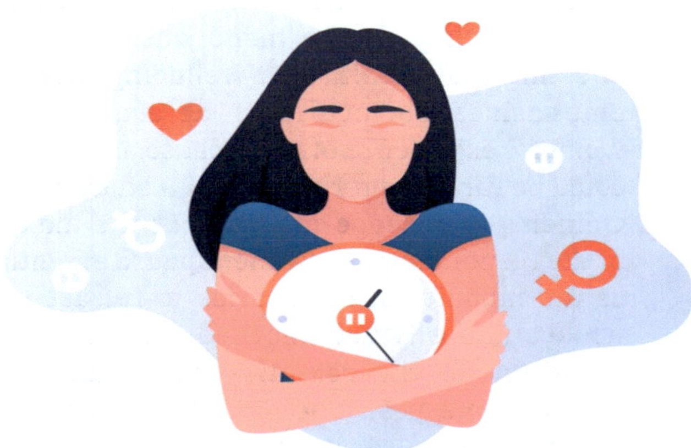

Introduction

Menopause is the start of a turning point in a woman's life, typically signaled by the cessation of menstrual periods and diminished levels of reproductive hormones. It typically occurs between the ages of 45 and 55, but can vary significantly in individuals. Menopause's radical hormone shifts bring about divergent physical and psychological symptoms that can immensely influence the quality of a woman's life. While many women would find menopause a normal part of life with no serious consequences for one's well-being, it takes the form of several complications in the shape of hot flashes, night sweats, and mood shifts. Understanding the nuances of menopause not only helps tolerate them but also indicates the necessity of applying management strategies applicable to this significant phase of life. These menopausal effects are not merely physiological but also mental and emotional health conditions. Women experience extreme levels of anxiety and depression at menopause, an affliction related to hormonal changes as well as cultural attitudes toward aging. Survivors of

LEARNING OBJECTIVES

After studying this chapter, you will be able to:

1. Explain the biological process of menopause
2. Analyze the psychological effects of menopause
3. Identify health risks associated with menopause
4. Evaluate lifestyle changes during menopause
5. Describe treatment options for menopause symptoms

breast cancer may have additional challenges in that menopause can cause specific health issues that are unique from those of women without such medical histories. Studies indicate that the roughly 9.3 million breast cancer survivors globally have certain menopausal symptoms due to the depletion of estrogen, hence complicating their transition. Recommendations usually discourage the application of traditional hormone replacement therapy and instead place greater emphasis on maximizing lifestyle and non-hormonal treatment (Davis *et al.*, 2017). This complex image serves as the foundation for defining the integrated experience of menopause, particularly among individuals with pre-existing health conditions. Menopause is more than a physical transition; it generally necessitates a recasting of personal identity, relationships, and long-range goals. Women feel loss—as they leave behind their reproductive years, many must confront the reality of aging as well as shifting roles in society. This phase may also initiate tough decisions relating to health care, including inquiry into preventive measures for age-related diseases like osteoporosis and cardiovascular disease. Statistics indicate that women with a history of genetic susceptibilities, such as BRCA mutations, may have additional considerations to navigate during their menopause experience (Breen *et al.*, 2016). This confirms the significance of customized approaches in menopause management to provide women with personalized care that accords with physical welfare and emotional well-being. In discussing menopause, it is important to appreciate the complexity of menopause and encourage women to embrace this period with confidence and strength.

Definition of Menopause

Menopause is a significant biological transition in a woman's life that leads to the permanent cessation of menstruation. Clinically, menopause refers to 12 consecutive months without menstrual periods. It is a sign of the reproductive capacity and typically takes place between ages 45 and 55. The menopause period is characterized by the decline in ovarian function, hence the decreased secretion of hormones such as estrogen and progesterone. The process may be gradual in nature, being more commonly identified with symptoms in the years around the perimenopausal period leading up to the final menstrual period. More awareness of the process is essential because the majority of women are not aware of the physiological, psychological, and emotional transformations that take place during menopause, ultimately affecting their health and wellbeing. Research emphasizes sociocultural determinants of women's experience of menopause, in that there could be various interpretations. A study of Saudi women's knowledge proved that the majority of the respondents knew menopause essentially as the inability of the ovaries to release eggs, while a minority had knowledge of the clinical definition of the cessation of menstruation for over one year. Such a lack of knowledge about menopause can lead to confusion and anxiety, particularly among common symptoms such as hot flashes and mood swings. Also, ignorance of proper knowledge can exacerbate the alienation and suffering women experience during this natural process. These gaps in knowledge must be met by health education interventions to empower women and improve their quality of life during this life transition (Alamer *et al.*, 2018). The intersection of menopause and health remains of continued interest, particularly in vulnerable populations, such as HIV-infected women. Research indicates that these women may experience premature menopause and bear a heavier symptom burden than their counterparts. A newly published literature review reported inconsistent methods in ascertaining menopause status, explaining that most studies use the World Health Organization's definition of menopause. Nevertheless, there are no universal measures for quantifying menopausal symptoms in HIV-positive women, which renders studies difficult to compare. Standardization of measurements and definitions is necessary to enhance the quality of research and align clinical treatments accordingly. As greater understanding becomes available, the emphasis on personalized health solutions will be able to significantly enhance outcomes for women, and therefore, it is crucial to continue research on this topic (Graham *et al.*, 2023).

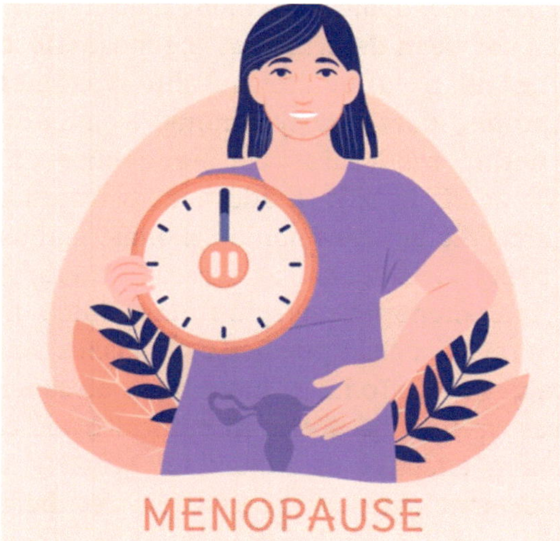

Source: https://images.herzindagi.info/image/2024/May/menopause-side-effects.jpg

Importance of Understanding Menopause

Awareness of menopause is imperative not just for women experiencing this life-changing period but also for healthcare systems managing their unique needs. During menopause, women experience a variety of symptoms ranging from physiological changes to emotional differences. Menopause awareness and education can help women in their right to efficient medical consultation and treatment. Moreover, a detailed understanding of menopause allows healthcare practitioners to provide tailored interventions, which ultimately enhance the quality of care. It is further essential to recognize that menopausal experiences are extremely varied, and hence, healthcare practitioners must incorporate an advanced perception of sex and gender into their actions. Gender medicine's emphasis on interdependence of biological and psychosocial concerns has a significant role to play in the determination of patient-specific needs across menopause, offering a more personalized healthcare experience (Bellini *et al.*, 2019).

In addition, social attitudes toward menopause often remain engulfed in stigma and misconception, and these have adverse effects on women's health outcomes. The context of menopause extends beyond individual experiences to encompass public health policy aimed at improving healthcare delivery. In contemporary discourse, it is urgent to break down myths surrounding menopause and relabel it as a natural life stage rather than a disease requiring treatment. Through an open culture of conversation about menopause, mental health professionals can better assist women experiencing menopausal symptoms, hence mitigating feelings of isolation and distress. Educating is a driving force behind this transformation, equipping women with the information and skills to manage menopausal challenges effectively, thus enhancing their quality of life and general health (Felice *et al.*, 2018).

Finally, having a solid understanding of menopause has immense implications for pushing research and policy further in women's health. By moving menopause to the center of the spectrum of gender medicine, researchers can identify distinctive markers of health and pathways that affect women's lives during this period of life. Centering menopause may result in the development of targeted therapeutic interventions and preventive strategies, ultimately filling knowledge gaps in women's healthcare. With advances in the area of gender medicine, the particular needs of postmenopausal women must be taken into consideration in health programs so that they are not left behind. The interface between research and practice can give rise to improved health policies focused on women's health at all stages of life, ultimately leading to improved health outcomes and patient satisfaction within the healthcare system (Bellini *et al.*, 2019).

4.1. The Biological Process of Menopause

Learning Outcome

1. Describe the hormonal changes during menopause
2. Discuss the stages of menopause: perimenopause, menopause, postmenopause
3. Identify the physical symptoms associated with menopause

Menopause is a significant biological milestone in a woman's life that indicates the cessation of her reproductive life. Menopause is caused by a slow decline in the ovaries' production of estrogen and progesterone, which in the majority of cases is followed by a set of physiological as well as psychological symptoms. When women age, typically between 45 and 55 years, ovarian reserve diminishes, and menstrual cycle irregularity develops that can last for years until menstruation ceases. This climacteric phase is not merely a physiological process; there are profound changes involved that might influence the quality of life of women. Understanding this biological context helps us better appreciate the diversity of symptoms women might encounter and the significance of individualized interventions during this phase of life.

Hot flashes, night sweats, and changes in mood are among the most prominent symptoms of menopause that owe much to unstable hormone levels. Vasomotor symptoms can interfere with daily functioning and sleep, inducing fatigue and emotional distress. Hormonal dysregulation in menopause affects neurotransmitter activity in the brain, leading to cognitive and mood changes. The heterogeneity of experiences highlights the need for individualized treatment strategies. The majority of women turn to obtaining a physician's advice during this period of transition, where health professionals have to weigh various forms of therapy, some of which are menopausal hormone therapy (MHT), which has been described as the most effective treatment to alleviate notable vasomotor symptoms, particularly among women who are within ten years post-menopause onset (Davis *et al.*, 2015). In addition to traditional hormone therapy, new non-hormonal treatments are being investigated as a rescue therapy to alleviate menopausal symptoms. Some new alternatives, such as purified cytoplasmic pollen extract, PureCyTonin®, have been discovered by research to be useful in clinical trials as a safe and effective treatment for women who are hormone-averse. This estrogen-free therapy works through mechanisms close to those of selective serotonin reuptake inhibitors (SSRIs), alleviating symptoms of hot flashes without the risks of hormone therapies (Biglia *et al.*, 2020). As research continues to progress, tailored treatment plans become increasingly vital on a daily basis. Clinicians need to consider a woman's medical history and preferences when developing a best-possible management plan for her during this biologically complex phase of life.

4.1.1. Hormonal Changes During Menopause

Menopause is the transitional stage of transformation in a woman's life that is marked by a series of hormonal adjustments that include the loss of estrogen and progesterone, the two hormones that have essential tasks to undertake to regulate several body functions, including menstrual cycles and reproductive activity. When a woman ages, typically between 45 and 55 years of age, the ovaries gradually reduce the levels of these hormones, and perimenopause starts, the stage of unpredictable menstrual cycles and shifting levels of hormones. These irregular hormone levels may lead to a range of symptoms, including hot flashes, night sweats, and mood swings. Having knowledge of the biological basis of these changes is crucial for women experiencing this life-altering transition because it can help them reduce symptoms and make informed decisions about potential therapies and lifestyle modifications. The loss of estrogen during menopause might also bear significant influence on women's general health. Estrogen is cardio-protective, and its deprivation could put women at increased risk for heart disease. Additionally, estrogen deficiency can lead to bone density loss, contributing to the development of osteoporosis. This increases their vulnerability to fractures and other skeletal disorders in later years. Consequently, in preparation for such vulnerabilities, the majority of women demand the application of hormonal therapy or a life change in a bid to reverse these effects. Hormonal treatments, either in the form of estrogen replacement or bioidentical hormones, aim to restore equilibrium and control symptoms experienced during menopause. However, it is important for women to weigh the benefits against potential risks, particularly in relation to long-term health implications, before they consider taking such treatments (Tharpe *et al.*, 2020).

Non-hormonal options have gained popularity as women increasingly look for non-invasive treatment options for menopausal symptoms. One of the hopeful alternatives is purified cytoplasmic pollen extract, PureCyTonin®. According to research, this non-estrogenic option might be able to reduce symptoms such as hot flashes safely without the dangers associated with hormone therapy. Clinical trials indicated that PureCyTonin® acts similarly to selective serotonin reuptake inhibitors (SSRIs), providing relief from symptoms through unique mechanisms not affecting hormonal equilibrium. This is of special significance for women with hormone therapy contraindications, such as women who are breast cancer survivors. The search for alternatives to hormones is a reflection of the growing body of evidence in favor of individualized treatment strategies for menopause (Biglia *et al.*, 2020). Through the consideration of more diverse alternatives, women are empowered in the self-management of symptoms while remaining aware of overall health and well-being.

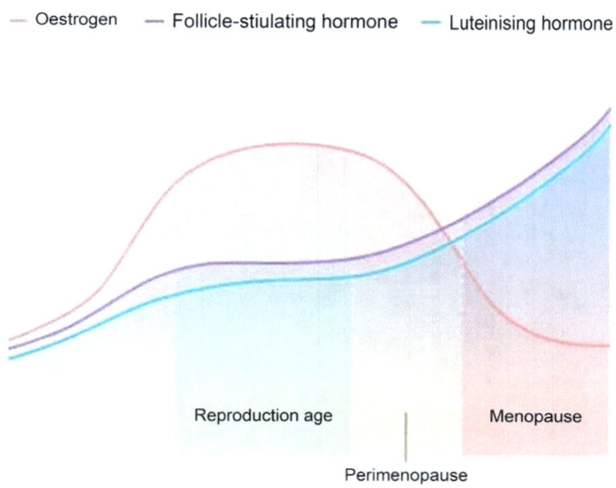

Figure 4.1. The main hormones are estrogen, progesterone, and testosterone, but others such as the control hormones follicle-stimulating hormone (FSH) and luteinizing hormone (LH) also play a part.

Source: https://www.forthwithlife.co.uk/blog/menopause-hormones/

4.1.2. Stages of Menopause: Perimenopause, Menopause, Postmenopause

Phases of menopause—perimenopause, menopause, and postmenopause—are a sudden change in a woman's life, characterized by hormonal fluctuations and many physical and emotional symptoms. Perimenopause, the initial phase of this transition, usually occurs in women in their 40s, lasting for a few years until menopause. During this phase, levels of estrogen and progesterone begin to decline periodically, leading to irregular menses, hot flashes, and mood swings. The majority of women during perimenopause undergo changes in cognition, including issues with memory and concentration, as reported recently (Bates *et al.*, 2019). These indicate the importance of understanding one's symptoms and the need for further research into their impact and management strategies at this critical time. Once women have gone through menopause, being free from a menstrual period for twelve consecutive months, there may be a whole new set of challenges.

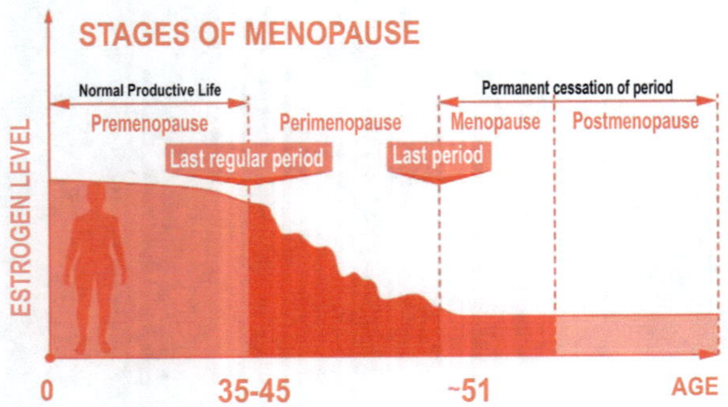

Figure 4.2. The stages of menopause—perimenopause, menopause, and postmenopause—represent a significant transition in a woman's life.

Source: https://cdn.responsumhealth.com/wp-content/uploads/2022/03/Stages-of-Menopause.png.webp

This phase is marked with a more precipitous fall in hormone levels, leading to a myriad of physiological changes, including increased risk for a number of health issues such as osteoporosis and cardiovascular disease. Postmenopausal women usually present with chronic perimenopausal symptoms initiated in perimenopause, and they severely affect their quality of life. For instance, research indicates that cognitive impairment may persist or even increase in postmenopausal women, especially those with other diseases such as diabetes, to the extent that they have greater cognitive impairment compared to similar counterparts who are premenopausal or in perimenopause (Bates *et al.*, 2019).

During the postmenopausal phase, from the past menstrual cycle to date, women must contend with a variety of long-term health effects. Research indicates that at this point, the majority of women have compromised overall cognitive performance and poor sleep quality, linked with increased menopausal symptoms of depression and anxiety (Hari *et al.*, 2024). Also, understanding menopause hormonal changes can bring sexual function alterations, causing effects on intimacy and relationships. It is critical that healthcare providers overcome these challenges through education and support for an enhanced quality of life during these times. Understanding and appreciating menopause complexities allow more targeted interventions and empower women to reclaim their health during these times.

4.1.3. Physical Symptoms Associated With Menopause

Menopause is typically heralded by an abundance of physical symptoms that can quite literally take women's quality of life. Vasomotor symptoms like hot flashes and night sweats are among the most prevalent. They can disrupt daily functioning and sleep. These unpleasant sensations are caused by changes in hormones, notably the drop in estrogen levels during this transitional period. Research has confirmed that the experience of symptoms varies widely between individuals, with some evidence in favor of a multiplicative model of biological, psychological, and environmental causative influences on symptom severity. While women may find little distress, others may view these symptoms as crippling, leading to increased use of healthcare and a lower overall health-related quality of life. Recognition of the range of physical symptoms that accompany menopause is significant in addressing the needs of women at this phase of transition and improving their healthcare outcomes (Eost-Telling *et al.*). In addition to vasomotor symptoms, women in menopause commonly experience urogenital disturbances, including vaginal dryness and urinary incontinence, that can destabilize intimate relationships and general well-being. These are the effects of the atrophic process in the vaginal and pelvic tissues due to declining estrogen levels, leading to reduced lubrication and elasticity. Most women also experience changes in their menstrual cycle, leading to irregular cycles or amenorrhea before menopause. The psychological impact of such physical symptoms can also lead to psychological distress, and depression and anxiety are prevalent in women who experience high menopausal symptoms. The interdependence of these concerns should be noted and holistic support taken, taking into account both the physical and psychological aspects of menopause, to enable women to navigate this stage of life with dignity and assistance (Gollschewski *et al.*, 2006). Physical exercise has been suggested as a potential intervention to combat some menopausal symptoms. Some evidence suggests that exercise, as a habitual activity, can result in the reduction of physical, urogenital, and psychological menopausal symptoms, particularly through structured programs like aerobic exercise and yoga. Systematic review offered some evidence that women engaging in these types of physical activity are more likely to improve total symptoms, and it suggests a positive role that exercise plays in symptom control. However, although the evidence is rather limited regarding what types of exercise are most effective to alleviate vasomotor symptoms, there is a necessity for further research in the form of specific guidance and taking into account individual choice and lifestyle factors. Exercise empowers women not only for physical health but also acknowledges their autonomy in controlling menopause complications (Eost-Telling *et al.*).

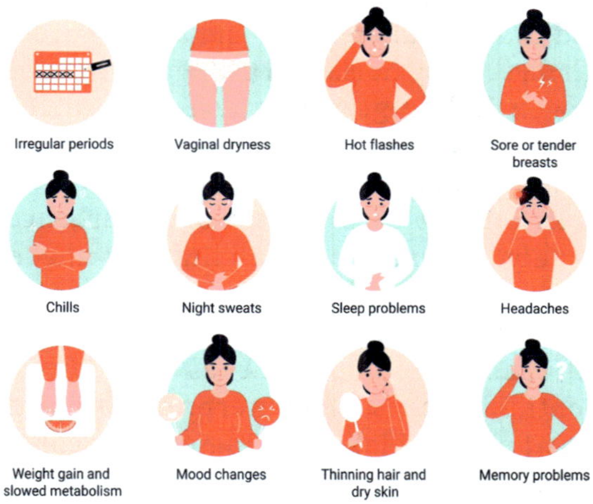

Figure 4.3. Symptoms of Menopause.

Source: https://propelphysiotherapy.com/wp-content/uploads/2022/11/symptoms-of-menopause-exercise-and-menopause-propel-physiotherapy.png

Test Your Knowledge

1. What are the main stages of menopause and how do they differ?
2. What are common physical symptoms experienced during menopause?

4.2. Psychological Effects of Menopause

Learning Outcome

1. Explain the emotional changes and mood swings
2. Analyze the impact on mental health: anxiety and depression
3. Identify effective coping mechanisms for psychological symptoms

The psychological menopause symptoms can appear in a number of ways and directly impact women's emotional and mental state. Menopause in most women is preceded by mood changes, depression, and anxiety brought forth directly by hormonal changes. Decrease in estrogen and progesterone levels can alter the functioning of neurotransmitters in the brain, leading to heightened emotional sensitivity and irritability. This emotional disturbance is not only common but debilitating, affecting interpersonal relationships, job performance, and overall quality of life. An awareness of such changes is important, as they have the potential to cause misinterpretation within social and familial environments, escalating loneliness at this period of transition. Moreover, the psychological effect of menopause extends beyond disruption in mood, often impacting women's self-esteem and body image. The majority of women are troubled with the physical alterations associated with menopause, such as weight gain, decreased elasticity of the skin, and alterations in hair patterning, causing negative self-concepts. The physical change lowers self-confidence, and they feel inadequate or unattractive. Research indicates that social standards of beauty contribute significantly to these attitudes that render women less powerful or valued at a point where they must embrace their identity and experiences. Therefore, the intersection of psychological and sociocultural factors brings into perspective the complexity of women's mental health during menopause, which needs an environment that is more empathetic and supportive. Finally, management of the psychological impact of menopause needs to be approached in a multi-dimensional manner, incorporating medical, psychological, and social support networks. Mental health needs promotion during this change and may include counseling or psychotherapy to allow women to express themselves and develop coping mechanisms. Furthermore, participation in community support groups is likely to bring women with similar difficulties together, minimizing feelings of loneliness and enhancing mental health. It is vital for medical professionals to recognize these psychological factors as major components of menopausal care. Abbott *et al.* (1986) identify differences in health experiences along age and gender dimensions, it is clear that differential interventions based on the particular psychological processes of menopausal women are required for supporting appropriate health and empowerment at this important juncture of life.

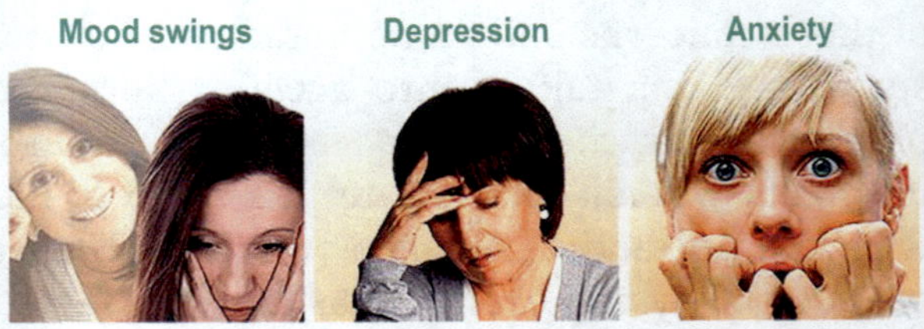

Figure 4.4. Emotional çhanges during menopause.

Source: https://www.menopausenow.com/pics/why-menopause-makes-you-mean.png

4.2.1. Emotional Changes and Mood Swings

When women pass menopause, they typically suffer extreme emotional changes and mood swings that greatly impact their general well-being. Most of these are caused by changes in the hormone levels in the body, primarily the decline in estrogen levels. Most women describe feeling extremely emotional in terms of irritation, worry, and depression at this time. Such emotional upheaval has the potential to interfere with everyday life, impacting interpersonal relationships, job performance, and self-esteem. Studies show that about 20% of women report having extreme emotional symptoms throughout this period, which underscores the need for exposure and knowledge surrounding these important changes. Menopausal affective profile is complex because women must deal not only with these immediate feelings but also with societal age-related and womanhood expectations that lie outside of them, which can both amplify their affective upheaval and feeling of isolation at this threshold time (Gavranich *et al.*, 2011). Menopausal mood swings' impact does not just unfold in the form of internal struggle, but also tends to carry over into the workplace. Women's leadership, in particular, may find such emotional transformations particularly challenging, as they strive to fulfill their professional responsibilities while experiencing high levels of emotional distress. Empirical data show that distraction and unease resulting from these symptoms may lead to loss of confidence and work performance, leading to feelings of isolation and loneliness among women who are at the peak of their professional careers (Gavranich *et al.*, 2011). The handling of personal and professional problems in the midst of these mood swings is overwhelming, so most seek assistance but find it insufficient or wanting. This indicates a stark imbalance in identifying and addressing the individualities of women experiencing menopause, particularly when augmented by the burden of career and hormonal disruption. Addressing the emotional needs of menopausal women requires a sensitive response both to individual experience and to the broader social context. The majority of women report that they employ a range of coping strategies, from alterations in lifestyle to workplace therapy, to reduce the emotional disruption of menopause. One of the important findings is that the support systems in place often break down, heightening the feeling of distress. In exploring the unique challenges menopausal women face, particularly in the workplace, researchers seek to encourage more targeted interventions that may foster better emotional health during this pivotal life stage. By emphasizing education and community as priorities, women can more effectively share information and advice with one another, thereby eradicating the shame that so readily attaches to this natural yet interruptive phase of life.

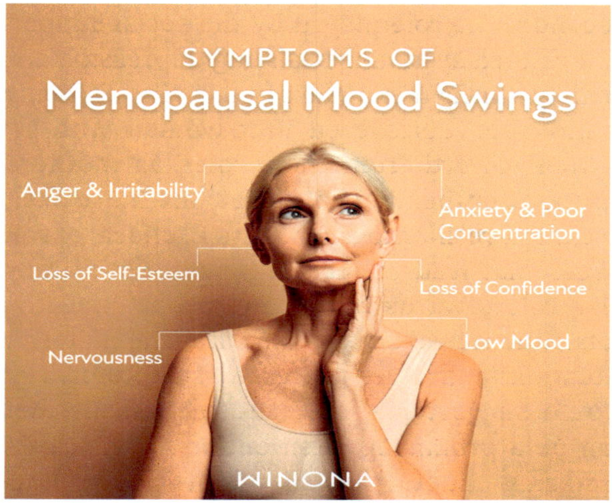
SYMPTOMS OF
Menopausal Mood Swings
Anger & Irritability
Anxiety & Poor Concentration
Loss of Self-Esteem
Loss of Confidence
Low Mood
Nervousness
WINONA

Figure 4.5. Symptoms of menopausal mood swings.

Source: https://images.ctfassets.net/lyqt8dkk29ch/1TggIaTyqxK9ZnSqDu1vDd/f83767ce076c917d947265db30f4c067/menopausal_mood_swings_symptoms.jpg

4.2.2. Impact on Mental Health: Anxiety and Depression

The menopause onset is also accompanied by numerous physiological changes that have the potential to significantly impact women's mental health, particularly anxiety and depression. Mood changes and emotional instability also feature at this point, and most women develop heightened symptoms of depression and anxiety. As also described in current studies, negative self-concept developed during menopause correlates highly with increased levels of stress, anxiety, and depression among postmenopausal women. For instance, research has noted that individuals whose sexual self-concept had a more negative skew were the women who exhibited high scores of these mental illnesses. The interdependence of self-perception and emotional health underscores the need to treat menopause as a physical stage but also as a critical period to heal and access care for emotional health (Ghodusi *et al.*, 2017). Secondly, the role played by the social support and reward system in resisting depression and anxiety during menopause is also vital. Recently, it has been discovered that women who get a high reward from their roles as mothers, partners, or members of society are more likely to exhibit resilience against the ill effects of role stress that lead to mental illness. Specifically, high role rewards can counteract the negative consequences of stress in marital and maternal situations and lower depressive symptoms. This would suggest that role satisfaction increase can be a promising intervention approach for fostering mental health results throughout menopause. Different ethnic groups of women respond differently to the stress of the role, and this again signifies that there is a necessity for specific support measures in addressing the mental health challenges of this stage of life (EM *et al.*, 2012). Mental health issues during menopause require multidimensional intervention measures that involve psychological support as well as encouraging positive self-concept. Psychosocial therapies aimed at enhancing sexual self-concept and neutralizing negative attitudes may be essential in lowering anxiety and depression levels. Collaboration among healthcare professionals is likely to yield more effective interventions that are responsive to the unique women's experiences during menopause. By establishing environments that promote positive role rewards and reduce stress, health care systems are better positioned to support women's mental health during this critical phase of their lives. Incorporating solutions that deal with the multidimensionality of mental health, including psychological, social, and physiological aspects, is at the core of a holistic approach to dealing with menopause issues (Ghodusi *et al.*, 2017).

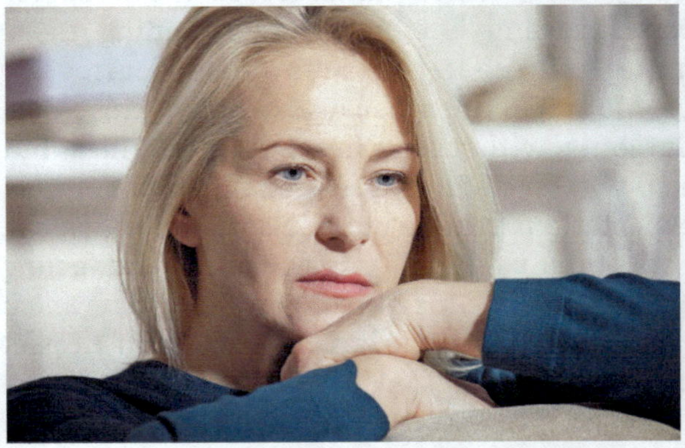

Source: https://domf5oio6qrcr.cloudfront.net/medialibrary/5953/18809866-bf58-4309-8715-cc5fc270c972.jpg

4.2.3. Coping Mechanisms For Psychological Symptoms

Working through the psychological symptoms of menopause can powerfully impact a woman's quality of life, and coping strategies are therefore important. Since these symptoms, such as anxiety, depression, and mood swings, are largely heightened by catastrophic thinking, knowing cognitive appraisal is essential. Women who have negative thoughts towards their menopausal experiences report more distress and less perceived control over their symptoms. The undesirable impact of catastrophic thinking, as evidenced, suggests that the acquisition of a thinking style that resists such negative interpretations would be to the advantage of psychological resilience as well as general tolerance for menopausal symptoms. Hence, incorporation of cognitive-behavioral methods aimed at reframing such thoughts would be a valuable intervention, allowing women to cope more effectively with this phase of life (Reynolds *et al.*, 2000). Moreover, the significance of varied coping mechanisms cannot be overstated, particularly in light of the varied psychological symptoms women undergo during menopause. It has been recently proven that Jordanian women employed intricate coping mechanisms, yet in most cases, they employed maladaptive mechanisms as well, such as increased consumption of tobacco and caffeine.

Employment of such maladaptive mechanisms primarily comes as a result of inadequate knowledge of healthier alternatives. Consequently, training programs that address both effective psychological coping skills and the risks of negative behaviors are needed. Through education and promotion of healthy coping skills, women would be in a better position to handle the psychological distress surrounding menopause, an outcome that enhances mental health results. An integrated approach in this manner would diminish the occurrence of menopausal symptoms as well as enhance women's overall wellbeing throughout the life-altering process (Alazawa *et al.*, 2023).

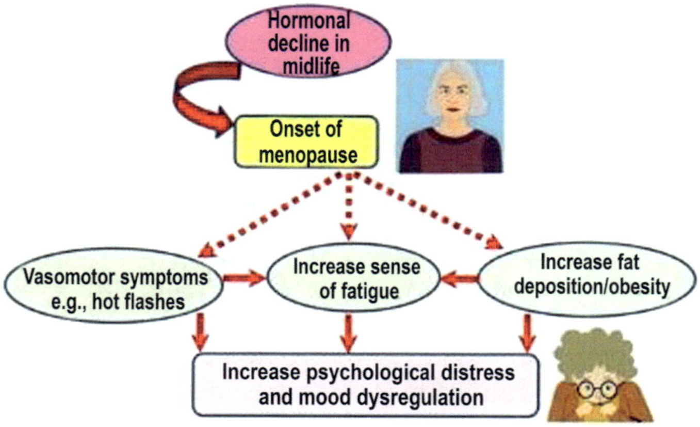

Figure 4.6. Psychological climacteric symptoms and attitudes toward menopause among Emirati Women.

Source: https://www.mdpi.com/1660-4601/17/14/5028

Lastly, the development of specialized interventions addressing the unique psychological needs of menopausal women is critical in the establishment of a supportive environment. Evidence suggests that interventions that combine cognitive-behavioral therapy (CBT) with psychoeducation might be especially beneficial in alleviating psychological distress. In educating women to recognize and modify maladaptive cognitions as well as equipping them with coping skills, such interventions give a sense of mastery over menopausal symptoms. Additionally, the integration of group counseling and support has the potential to offer the arenas in which to exchange experiences, reducing the feeling of isolation and enabling women to belong to a community with identical problems. Generally, an integrative treatment fusing individual coping strategies with support groups is essential in menopause psychological resilience enhancement, ultimately facilitating a less problematic transition and improved quality of life (Reynolds *et al.*, 2000; Alazawa *et al.*, 2023).

Test Your Knowledge

1. How can menopause impact mental health, particularly regarding anxiety and depression?
2. What are some effective coping mechanisms for managing psychological symptoms during menopause?

4.3. Health Risks Associated with Menopause

Learning Outcome

1. Describe osteoporosis and bone health
2. Assess cardiovascular health risks associated with menopause
3. Explain the increased risk of certain cancers

As women experience menopause, many health risks become more visible due to the hormonal changes in various body systems. Of concern is increased vulnerability to cardiovascular disease, which has been linked to an earlier age at menopause. It has been found in research that women who experience premature menopause are at higher risk for conditions such as heart disease and osteoporosis, which have been primarily attributed to widespread estrogen deprivation. Such estrogen deprivation, with its function of cardiovascular and bone health, presents even more motivation for the identification of effective interventions as a way of mitigating these risks. Lifestyle interventions, including diet and exercise, and hormonal and non-hormonal therapies, can be helpful strategies to promote health within this crucial transition period. Thus, knowledge of the timing and treatment of menopause is crucial in reducing long-term health consequences of this phase of life (Al-Wattar *et al.*, 2022). Besides cardiovascular disease, menopause has been associated with dramatic changes in bone mineral density, thereby potentially increasing the risk of osteoporosis and fractures. When estrogen decreases, bone resorption exceeds new bone formation, resulting in a net loss of bone. This is very much so in women experiencing premature ovarian failure or premature menopause. To their disadvantage, most women lack information on such risks and preventive measures. A study conducted among Caribbean women indicated a frightening trend: the vast majority of respondents had limited knowledge about menopause and its medical implications, and hence, insufficient healthcare-seeking behavior. Therefore, this knowledge gap demands specially formulated health education programs that suit the specific needs of diverse populations and promote practices leading to efficient prevention and control of bone health during and after menopause (Thomas *et al.*, 2005). Additionally, the multifaceted problems presented by menopause demand an aggressive approach toward health screening and preventive treatment. With the widespread lack of knowledge regarding menopause risk factors, medical practitioners have to give utmost importance to the sensitization of the patients regarding the cardiovascular and osteal dangers involved. Screening of cardiovascular ailments and assessment of bone mass needs to berendered the norm of women's treatment at this stage in life. Precisely, national and international guidelines recommend active surveillance in women who have undergone menopause at an age greater than the average because they are still at high risk despite not qualifying for hormone therapy for prevention of such complications. Coordinated health promotion and research efforts are essential in order to equip women with comprehensive care that addresses their unique needs at this juncture of life and thus halts the adverse health consequences of menopause (Al-Wattar *et al.*, 2022).

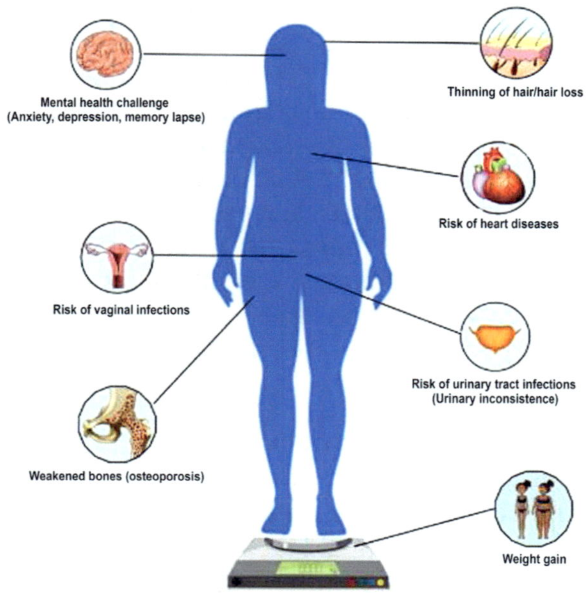

Figure 4.7. Health risks of menopause.

Source: https://www.datelinehealthafrica.org/ckfinder/userfiles/files/Menopause-health-risks.jpg

4.3.1. Osteoporosis and Bone Health

Menopause is a period of transformative crisis in a woman's life, first and foremost characterized by cessation of ovarian function and, as an aftermath, decreasing levels of estrogen. Such a hormonal shift is intimately related to bone density because estrogen plays a key role in bone mass conservation. Decreased levels of estrogen render women susceptible to losing bone mineral density (BMD) and to diseases like osteopenia and osteoporosis. Evidence indicates that surgical menopause, especially oophorectomy, is associated with quicker bone loss compared to naturally menopausal women. Specifically, evidence indicates that the incidence of osteoporosis is significantly higher among subjects with a history of hysterectomy and oophorectomy, and this is particularly higher with increasing numbers of years after surgery, indicating a necessity for very cautious follow-up of the bone status at this very crucial phase of life (Dhanalakshmi *et al.*, 2021). At the same time, the impact of menopause on osteoporosis transcends hormonal shifts, laying bare the multidimensional intersection of individual awareness, health behavior, and healthcare access. Studies investigating Korean American women's awareness of their bone health revealed significant disparities in osteoporosis risk awareness and prevention behaviors between stages of menopause. Notably, peri-menopausal explained a higher degree of awareness about their risk of osteoporosis compared to both the pre- and post-menopause groups. Though this awareness was not reliably predictive of pro-healthy actions nor in agreement with advice provided by healthcare professionals, it implies an immediate need for targeted education and improved communication concerning bone health, particularly for those post-menopausal women who are at higher risk of osteoporosis (Lee *et al.*, 2017). In the management of osteoporosis and bone health during menopause, holistic management strategies incorporating preventive in addition to therapeutic interventions are needed. Periodic BMD screening becomes important in identifying those who are at higher risk and treating them with interventions such as hormone therapy or dietary modification. Further, the application of lifestyle modifications such as weight-bearing exercises and adequate calcium and Vitamin D ingestion can fortify bone density. With regard to the unique challenges women face postmenopause, especially those who have had to deal with surgical interventions, specially formatted education plans and coordinated care by healthcare professionals are essential to the preservation and support of bone health. The additional research into alternative treatments and management further speaks to the growing need for healthcare practices to adapt to meet the changing needs of this group, making them aware and empowered regarding their bone health.

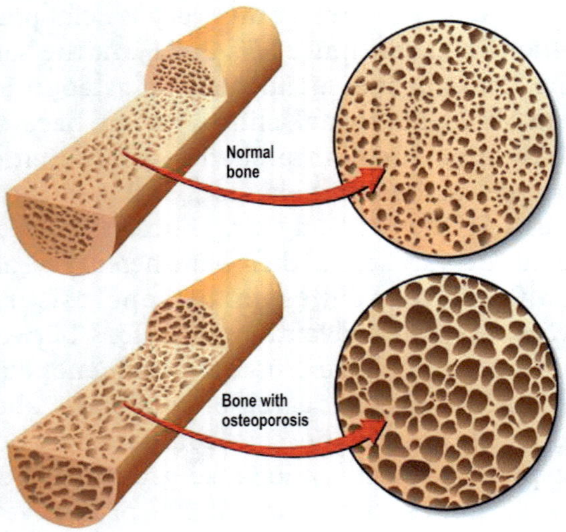

Figure 4.8. Low hormone levels and bone loss have been linked together for a long-time.

Source: https://drmagaziner.com/hormones/menopause-hormone-therapy-may-prevent-bone-loss/

4.3.2. Cardiovascular Health Risks

Menopause transition is a highly pivotal phase in a woman's life with far-reaching biological changes that are bound to have an impact on general health, particularly cardiovascular health. Near the top of the list of problems underscored is the increasing risk of cardiovascular disease (CVD) caused by the decline in estrogen levels after menopause. Estrogen also helps in the maintenance of vascular function and lipid profiles, and thus hormonal loss can encourage unwelcome changes such as increased cholesterol levels and arterial stiffness. Furthermore, the average age of menopause, which typically happens at 51 years, is a landmark at which most women may already be experiencing other cardiovascular risk factors such as high blood pressure or obesity. Knowledge of and exposure to these risks become essential for empowering women to adopt preventative health practices during this time of transition in life. Research has found an association between menopausal age and other health outcomes, such as cardiovascular risks. Women who experience menopause earlier in life, particularly those with conditions such as premature ovarian insufficiency (POI), have a higher risk of developing cardiovascular diseases, osteoporosis, and other complications during their later years (Al-Wattar *et al.*, 2022). This mostly occurs as a result of prolonged estrogen deprivation time, which emphasizes the importance of cardiovascular monitoring in these subjects.

Active interventions, including lifestyle modifications such as diet and physical exercise, have been shown to reduce these risks. Physicians should identify such conditions and discuss the implementation of proper management procedures with their patients that will enhance cardiovascular and general well-being following menopause. Hormone Replacement Therapy (HRT) remains a point of controversy in menopause management debate, particularly for cardiovascular well-being. In women with premature menopause or POI, HRT may be prescribed to counterbalance the adverse effects of low estrogen levels (Al-Shboul *et al.*, 2017). The application of HRT is not widely recommended for every menopausal woman, especially those above the mean age of menopause, where the risk might reduce the benefit for heart protection. Current guidelines suggest that advanced cardiovascular health screening and prevention, in accordance with the unique health profiles of women, should be highly prioritized for all post-menopausal women. Integration of such health interventions into routine healthcare practice ensures that women are able to effectively respond to cardiovascular risk factors as they transition through menopause.

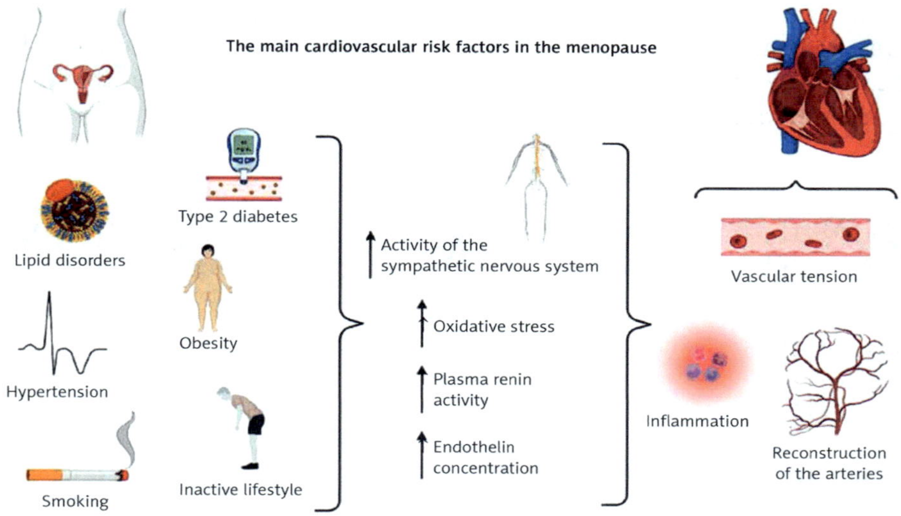

Figure 4.9. Menopause and cardiovascular disease.

Source: https://www.archivesofmedicalscience.com/Menopause-and-women-s-cardiovascular-health-is-it-really-an-obvious-relationship,157308,0,2.html#gallery-3

4.3.3. Increased Risk of Certain Cancers

Menopause is a life-defining process characterized by a core hormonal shift that not only affects reproductive function but also influences long-term health outcomes, including the emergence of certain cancers. Declines in estrogen levels during menopause have been identified as a critical process capable of redirecting susceptibility to cancer. For instance, estrogen plays a central role in regulating cell growth and differentiation within breast and endometrial tissues. When the levels of the hormone decrease, women can experience tissue changes that increase their likelihood of developing malignancies, predominantly breast and endometrial cancer. The scenario between cancer susceptibility and menopause exemplifies how important it is to understand the mechanisms through which hormonal changes impact cellular processes and the weaknesses already inherent in women's health. Recent research has highlighted the fact that women who undergo assisted reproductive technologies (ART), typically required due to infertility, are subjected to certain risks regarding cancer. Of specific interest is the impact of ovarian stimulation with hormone treatment, to the extent that such treatments can complicate cancer risk factors for certain cancers. An important component in determining this risk is discerning the impact of hormonal treatment from that of infertility itself. Interestingly, conception time for infertile history has been recognized in the literature (Codacci-Pisanelli *et al.*, 2018) as a risk factor for cancers of the ovary, endometrium, and breast. This multifaceted interaction calls for women receiving ART to be well-educated on the long-term cancer risks surrounding their menopause and reproductive choices. Apart from this, social and lifestyle dimensions related to menopause and cancer risk should also be investigated in the broader context of economic development and modernization. Industrialized nations have higher rates of cancer because of improved detection of cancer, as well as increased exposure to various carcinogens. Moreover, lifestyle modification such as nutrition enriched with growth factors and delaying childbearing can also result in raising cancer susceptibility among these populations (Yashin *et al.*). During transition to menopause, it is important to realize the variety of factors ,including genetic influence, environment, and lifestyle, that are affecting them. In general, the confluence of these variables necessitates a holistic approach to women's health premised upon proactive intervention in the menopausal transition as a means to stem cancer risks effectively.

Test Your Knowledge

1. What cardiovascular health risks are associated with osteoporosis or related conditions?
2. Which types of cancers have an increased risk linked to osteoporosis or its risk factors?

4.4. Lifestyle Changes during Menopause

Learning Outcome

1. Explain the importance of nutrition and diet
2. Describe exercise and physical activity recommendations
3. Analyze the role of sleep hygiene and its impact on menopause

The menopausal transition, on the other hand, introduces drastic changes in a woman's lifestyle, having the tendency of necessitating adjustments in everyday life and healthcare behaviors. Because estrogen levels decrease during menopause, many women experience symptoms such as hot flashes, night sweats, and mood changes, tending impacting their overall quality of life.

These symptoms tend to be highly inconvenient, leading many women to adopt lifestyle modifications to alleviate discomfort and promote well-being. Regular exercise, for example, has been shown to reverse some of the symptoms of menopause and improve mood. Exercise also plays a critical role in managing weight gain, which accompanies this stage with the shift in metabolism. Being physically active, in short, not only addresses issues with body health but also produces a sense of empowerment amidst hormonal fluxes that characterize this phase in life. Dietary modifications are yet another essential life change routinely adopted at the time of menopause. While women cope with the complexities of hormonal shift, they are ever more observant of their diet and have a well-balanced nutrition comprising high phytestrogens, fiber, and essential vitamins and minerals. Food intake of soy foods, whole grains, fruits, and vegetables has been shown to alleviate some of the menopausal symptoms and preserve bone health, countering increased osteoporosis risk following menopause. Cutting down on alcohol and caffeine intake is also advisable to lower the severity and frequency of hot flashes and insomnia.

Therefore. Diet can have a beneficial effect on various aspects of health and quality of life, as the significance of nutrition in overcoming menopause difficulties is asserted. Moreover, psychological adjustment in menopause is as significant a factor in enhancing quality of life. Women tend to use mindfulness exercises and stress management techniques to cope with mood swings and psychological stresses due to menopausal symptoms. Activities such as yoga, meditation, and relaxation techniques not only yield avenues for relief but also augment mental health effects. Possessing or maintaining a good support system among friends, family, or support groups may also render the necessary emotional support and validation in this process of transition.

Overall, these lifestyle changes result in an integrated approach to coping with menopause, with emphasis on interaction between the physical, emotional, and social domains. This global perspective is fundamental in helping postmenopausal women's quality of life be improved and contribute to establishing that lifestyle modifications at this stage are essential and beneficial interventions, particularly given the multifaceted nature of symptoms experienced (Bhalerao *et al.*, 2024; Anderson *et al.*, 2011).

4.4.1. Importance of Nutrition and Diet

The role of diet and nutrition during menopause simply cannot be overstated, as they play a very significant role in the management of symptoms and overall well-being. The hormonal changes of menopause are likely to promote weight gain and metabolic issues, and hence, an ideal dietary intake is necessary. A healthy diet high in fruits, vegetables, whole grain foods, and healthy fats is beneficial in minimizing the impacts of menopausal symptoms such as hot flushes and mood swings. Also, there are specific nutrients like calcium and vitamin D that are important in maintaining bone density during this phase. By following a healthy diet, women not only ease some of the symptoms of menopause but also take active measures towards long-term health gain, lowering their risk of chronic disease as they get older.

Nutrition is also important for cancer prevention, especially in women with a history of breast cancer. Evidence suggests that diet accounts for a majority of cancer risks in developed countries, indicating a high correlation between intake of food and health status. Although the evidence regarding diet and recurrent breast cancer remains indefinite, recent guidelines prioritize nutritional intake relative to certain needs. Recommendations for women with risk factors involve avoiding alcohol use, preventing weight gain following menopause, and adhering to a well-planned dietary regimen. This highlights the importance of making suitably informed dietary choices to maintain health during menopause, further underscoring the significance of personalized nutrition programs in alignment with international recommendations and evidence (Alexander *et al.*, 2011).

Lastly, the interplay between nutrition and social determinants is a key consideration in relation to women's health, notably menopause. Socioeconomic status and access to better food quality have a significant influence on food patterns and health conditions. The majority of women reside under stress caused by various social determinants that could lead to ill-suited food intake, thereby aggravating menopausal symptoms. The application of preventive care focusing on improvement in nutritional habits and stress management can offer the foundation for long-term, prolonged benefits to health. For instance, nutrition interventions that educate individuals about healthy eating can enable women to make informed lifestyle choices that, in the long run, lower their risk for cardiovascular diseases and enhance their overall well-being (Bucciarelli *et al.*, 2024). Identification and intervention on such interrelated factors are essential for optimizing nutritional responses and supporting women along the menopausal transition.

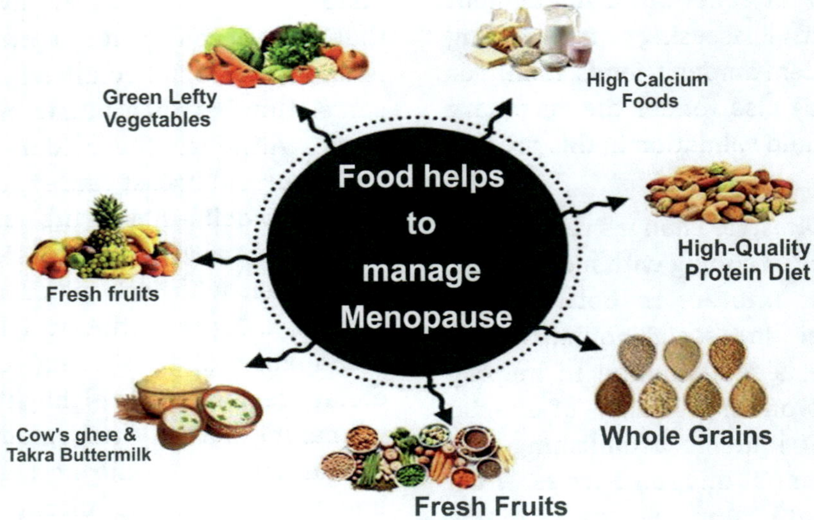

Figure 4.10. Diet to Manage Menopause.

Source: https://cdn.shopify.com/s/files/1/0586/8234/3501/files/food-to-manage-menopause.jpg?v=1716276646

4.4.2. Exercise and Physical Activity Recommendations

The initiation of menopause is accompanied by a significant life transition in a woman, which often arrives with many physical and emotional symptoms such as hot flushes, mood swings, and insomnia. Engagement with regular exercise emerges as a primary intervention to reduce these symptoms and improve quality of life. Research lays stress on the importance of exercise, which not only aids in weight management but also enhances cardiac function, reduces the risk of osteoporosis, and enhances the mood through the release of endorphins. All these benefits are especially important at menopause, when women already carry an added risk of heart disease and bone mineral density reduction. Hence, the inclusion of aerobic exercises, strength training, and flexibility exercises in daily life can serve to neutralize the negative effects of menopause, leading to a more balanced and healthier lifestyle. Moreover, scientific studies suggest that exercise could have a significant impact on menopausal symptoms. In a randomized trial, those who exercised regularly demonstrated a 24% improvement in symptom rates of menopausal symptoms and a 6% improvement in quality of life scores, demarcating the effectiveness of exercise as a non-pharmacological treatment. Additive effects of regular exercise not only yield relief from some symptoms like hot flashes and mood swings but also yield a generalized feeling of being well. By prioritizing physical exercise, women can take charge of their health, empowering themselves during this phase of transformation. These findings underscore the value of incorporating formal exercise programs specifically designed to counteract the particular difficulties of menopause, with an emphasis on transitioning toward lifestyle modification toward sustained well-being. As part of managing menopause, it is imperative to emphasize the inclusion of changes in diet as a component within the exercise regimes. The convergence of a healthy diet and physical exercise has been demonstrated to create synergistic effects in symptom relief in menopause and overall well-being. Diet plays an important part in symptom relief as well as leading to better health results through the provision of essential nutrients that sustain bone density and heart health. With the typically ensuing weight gain and increased vulnerability to disease during menopause, an intense emphasis on nutrient-rich foods can be extremely beneficial. Physically active programs, in conjunction with individualized dietary recommendations, can provide women with the knowledge to better navigate this stage of life, motivating optimal health and vitality. As recently documented, such lifestyle interventions show promise for enhancing the quality of life at menopause and are thus integral components of the holistic treatment of women at this time of transition.

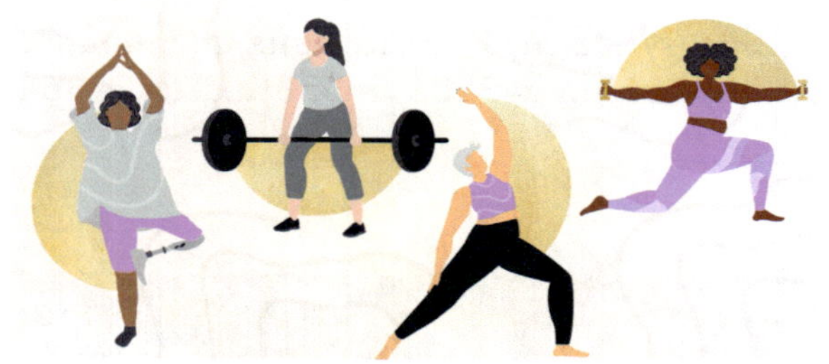

Source: https://news.cuanschutz.edu/hubfs/2024-12-02_Menopause_%26_Exercise.png

4.4.3. Sleep Hygiene and Its Impact on Menopause

Menopausal transition presents a number of physiological and psychological changes that can significantly affect the quality of sleep. Sleep disorders are commonly reported by women at this stage, typically as a result of vasomotor symptoms such as hot flashes and night sweats. These symptoms are the causes of the disruption in sleep and insomnia, and result in disturbed rest. Poor sleep during menopause has been found to exacerbate mood disorders, increase the risk of cardiovascular diseases, and reduce the overall quality of life. It is thus essential to manage women undergoing this phase to healthy sleep hygiene practices. Sleep hygiene refers to creating a sleep setting, adopting a standard sleeping schedule, and avoiding stimulating factors at night. By implementing these strategies, women can alleviate some of the sleep disturbances associated with menopause and improve overall health. The relationship between menopause and sleep hygiene underscores the importance of lifestyle modification at this time of life. Studies show that sleep pattern alterations during menopause can significantly impact mental health, leading to increased anxiety and depression. These psychiatric issues, along with insomnia, create a vicious cycle that again disrupts sleep. The latest evidence suggests that cognitive behavior modification (CBT) has been found effective in enhancing the sleep quality of postmenopausal women by adjusting the cognitive and behavioral mechanisms that impede restful sleep. Further, including aerobic exercise as part of one's lifestyle can influence sleep hygiene to allow menopausal symptoms to be better controlled. Therefore, medical personnel need to emphasize healthy sleeping practices to improve mental health and minimize the challenges menopause symptoms pose. When developing treatment plans, hormone replacement therapy (HRT) can be useful for women experiencing menopausal sleep problems. Research indicates that HRT alleviates vasomotor symptoms and improves sleep quality, reducing insomnia as well as overall health. Additionally, antidepressants have been established as a plausible treatment option, being found effective in the treatment of menopausal sleep disturbances. Certain SSRIs and SNRIs have been discovered to provide relief from insomnia when used with HRT, highlighting the importance of the use of a comprehensive approach to management at this age. Additionally, non-pharmacologic interventions, such as relaxation techniques and mindfulness, can also be used to improve sleep hygiene and minimize the heightened anxiety associated with menopause. As a woman goes through this transition, management and sleep hygiene with a multi-dimensional approach can improve sleep and general health outcomes and quality of life during a time of significant change (Hakim *et al.*, 2012; Arico *et al.*, 2019).

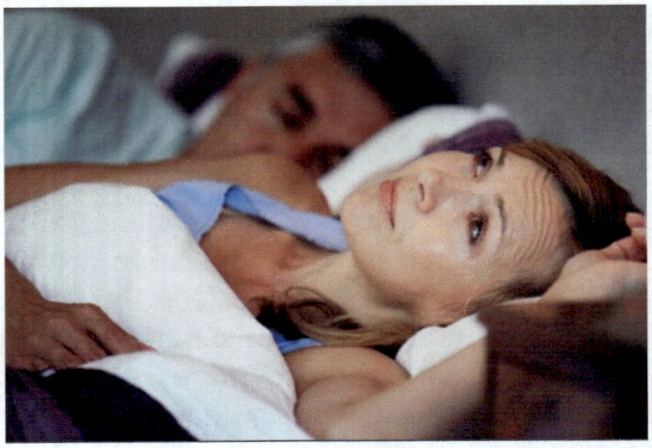

Figure 4.11. Poor sleep quality and sleep disturbance are lesser-known changes during this phase of life.

Source: https://www.hopkinsmedicine.org/-/media/images/health/1_-conditions/menopause/womaninsomnia640440_3_pyramid.jpg?h=357&iar=0&mh=360&mw=520&w=520&hash=B4F64CC5BF1F58798A0B4098F21A3C5E

Test Your Knowledge

1. Why is nutrition and diet important during menopause?
2. What types of exercise are recommended for women experiencing menopause?

4.5. Treatment Options for Menopause Symptoms

Learning Outcome

1. Describe the principles of hormone replacement therapy (HRT)
2. Identify non-hormonal medications and alternatives
3. Evaluate natural remedies and lifestyle adjustments

Treatment for symptoms of menopause is now much better, and women are offered a multitude of choices according to their requirements. Menopausal hormone therapy (MHT) has been found to be the best choice to manage vasomotor symptoms such as night sweats and hot flashes. In alignment with new guidelines from The Endocrine Society, the advantages of MHT generally outweigh the risks for most postmenopausal women under age 60 or within ten years after menopause begins. Striving for individualized care, taking into account such things as common medical conditions and patient desires, guidelines suggest therapy. Furthermore, before initiating MHT, doctors are advised to assess cardiovascular disease risk and breast cancer risk so that the treatments employed will be in consonance with each patient's unique health profile (Davis *et al.*, 2015).

Other treatments are available for women who do not want to take MHT or who may have contraindications. Nonhormonal therapies have gained wider use, offering effective means of managing vasomotor symptoms without the danger of hormone replacement. Low-dose vaginal estrogen and ospemifene are among those alternatives that have been shown to effectively treat the genitourinary syndrome of menopause, including vaginal dryness and pain. The use of vaginal moisturizers and lubricants can also be an additional symptomatic relief for those choosing aside from hormonal therapies. By considering these, medical practitioners can tackle the polyvalent needs of women during menopause so that quality of life is not disrupted even with the discomfort that may be associated with this natural process (Besong *et al.*, 2024).

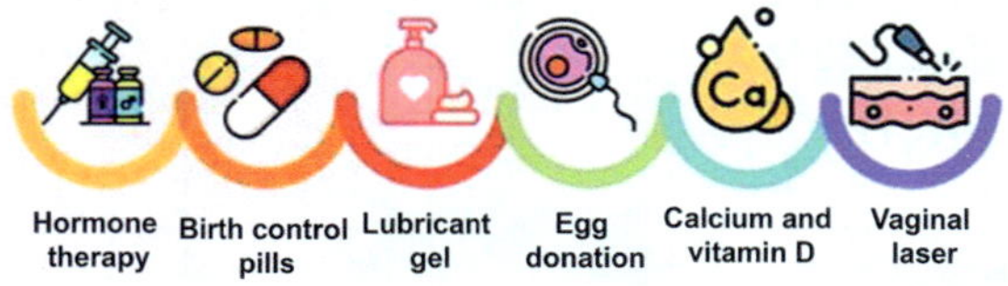

Figure 4.12. Early menopause treatment methods.

Source: https://raadinahealth.com/en/blog/premature-menopause-treatment

Apart from pharmacological management, lifestyle modifications also play a role in managing menopausal symptoms. A normal, regular diet rich in calcium and vitamin D, combined with regular exercise and stress management, can bring significant relief from some menopausal symptoms. Research indicates that women who lead active lives may experience alleviated frequency and severity of hot flashes, improved mood, and improved overall health conditions. Cognitive-behavioral therapy and mindfulness can also alleviate the psycho-emotional symptoms of menopause, such as anxiety and mood swings. With the addition of these lifestyle changes coupled with appropriate medical treatments, women can develop resistance to menopause problems so that they can glide through this phase of life with greater ease (Davis *et al.*, 2015).

4.5.1. Hormone Replacement Therapy (HRT)

Hormone Replacement Therapy (HRT) is now a landmark therapeutic option for the relief of the majority of menopausal symptoms, including hot flashes, night sweats, and mood swings. By both estrogen and, in some cases, progesterone replacement, HRT attempts to reverse the hormonal dyscrasias that define menopausal onset. Whether or not to initiate HRT is a factor of individual patients' health profiles and symptom gravities as well as lifestyle factors. Current evidence suggests that for most women, HRT can have a significant beneficial effect on quality of life, but it is not for all people, particularly in those with a history of hormone-sensitive cancer or cardiovascular disease. Thus, a knowledgeable understanding of the risks and benefits of HRT should inform treatment decisions at this complex time of life (Davison *et al.*, 2012).

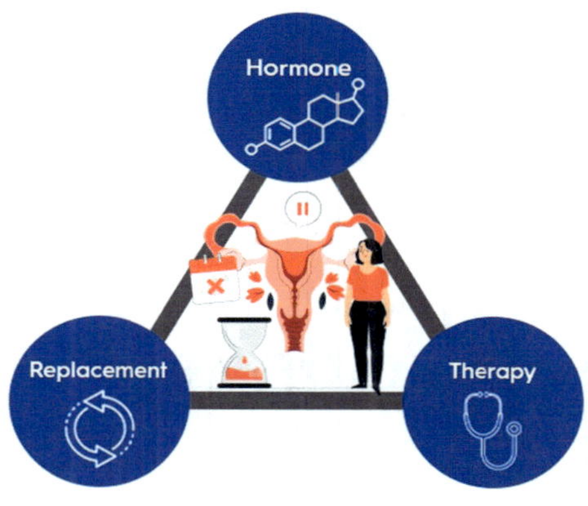

Figure 4.13. Hormone Replacement Therapy (HRT).

Source: https://progenesisivf.com/blog/hrt-relief-menopause/

Menopausal HRT has also sparked controversy about its long-term health implications. Data indicate that although HRT is effective in alleviating acute menopausal symptoms, its use may be associated with an increase in the risk of some diseases, such as breast cancer, venous thromboembolism, and stroke, especially when taken over an extended period of time. Therefore, healthcare providers must weigh such a risk against possible advantages on an individualized basis. Careful observation and reassessment during the course of treatment become essential to ensure that the therapy remains suitable for the evolving needs of the patients.

Above all, educating women on potential side effects and encouraging decision-making with healthcare professionals can lead to more personalized and effective care during the menopausal transition (Hakim *et al.*, 2012). Furthermore, the evolving situation of HRT brings to light the importance of individualized medicine with regard to genetic, environmental, and lifestyle determinants on women's health. Recent studies show that tailored approaches to HRT can optimize benefit while minimizing risk because different women metabolize hormones differently.

This paradigm change towards customization calls for further study of other therapies, such as phytestrogens or changes in lifestyle, that could be adjuncts or alternatives to traditional HRT. While controversy over menopause and HRT continues, it becomes more imperative that patients and physicians alike engage in frank discussion of the latest evidence and therapeutic possibilities. This collaborative approach can, in the long term, lead to healthier outcomes and a quality of life for women experiencing menopause (Davison *et al.*, 2012).

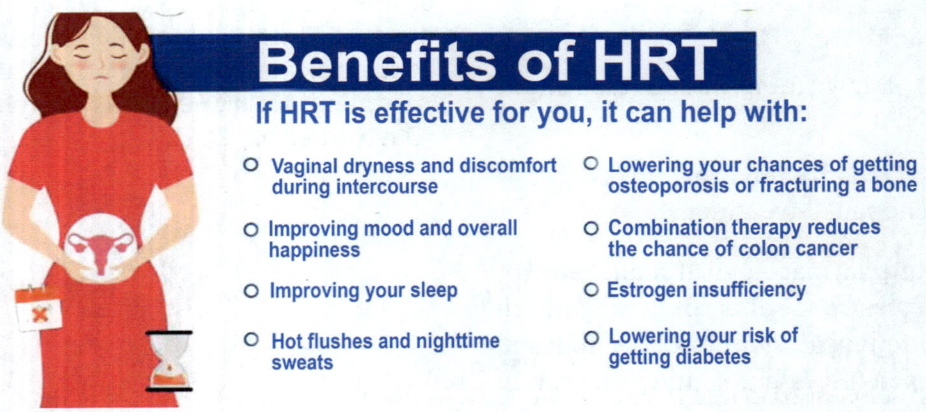

Source: https://progenesisivf.com/blog/hrt-relief-menopause/

4.5.2. Non-Hormonal Medications and Alternatives

In menopause management, non-hormonal medications and alternatives have also been received as a good option for women not willing to undergo hormone replacement therapy (HRT) or for women with contraindications for HRT. The clinical guidelines and systematic reviews developed by health organizations are stressing the provision of alternatives that act on the symptoms of menopause without the danger of hormonal therapy. Non-hormonal treatments like selective serotonin reuptake inhibitors (SSRIs) show promise, especially for symptom relief of vasomotor symptoms like hot flashes and night sweats. Lifestyle modifications like regular exercise, healthy eating, and stress-reducing exercises are also advised as the cornerstone ways of controlling menopausal symptoms effectively. As treatment becomes a consideration by health care professionals, knowledge of available treatment allows women to receive tailored care respecting their preferences and medical needs (Davis *et al.*, 2015). Aside from pharmacologic therapies, there are a number of non-hormonal therapies that have become increasingly adopted on the basis of their efficacy and safety profiles. For example, the use of gabapentin, originally designed to treat seizure disorders, has proved effective in suppressing hot flashes. Similarly, herbal remedies such as black cohosh have also been researched for their potential benefits, even with a complicated scientific community consensus regarding efficacy and safety. Added to the emotional well-being of menopause are cognitive behavior therapy and mindfulness, alleviating anxieties and mood swings, among others. The incorporation of these therapeutic modalities provides a multi-sided solution towards treating menopause that addresses women's diverse health needs amidst strong hormone changes. A patient-centered education and informed decision-making approach is critical in such a case, leading to better health outcomes as well as quality of life during menopause (Skotnes *et al.*, 2019). Non-hormonal treatment focuses eventually reveals a greater understanding of women's health and also the complexity involved in coping with menopausal symptoms. Evidence-based policy highlights the fact that while menopausal hormone therapy (MHT) is highly effective for some, alternatives must be equally accessible to those with specific health risks or individualistic preferences. This paradigm shift encourages the implementation of integrative care models that include both therapeutic and lifestyle interventions so that women are empowered to make some prudent decisions about their health. Thorough education about accessible options and routine communication with healthcare providers can provide a supportive environment, enabling women to combat menopause difficulties confidently and forcefully. As research evolves, producing an open culture of discussion about these alternatives can lead to improved identification of problems in women's health and enhanced knowledge about menopause care (Davis *et al.*, 2015).

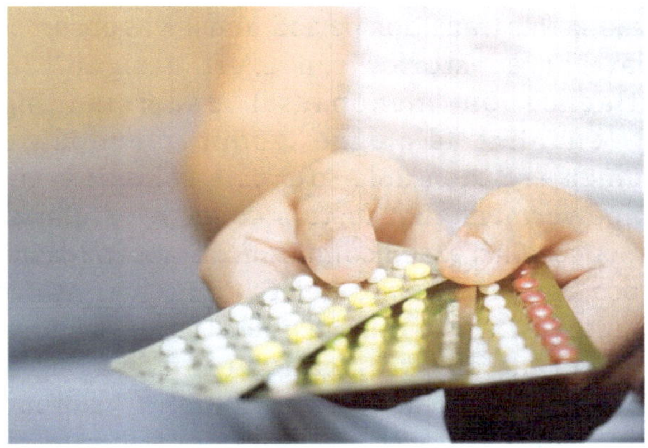

Source: https://www.pharmaceutical-technology.com/wp-content/uploads/sites/24/2019/10/menopause.jpg

4.5.3. Natural Remedies and Lifestyle Adjustments

During women's transition through menopause, natural therapies and lifestyle adjustments have gained popularity as good alternatives to standard hormone replacement therapy. The treatments are more likely to emphasize nutritional alterations, exercise, and stress management techniques that decrease the symptoms of hot flashes and mood swings during menopause. For instance, including soy foods or flaxseeds in the diet has been linked to the reduction of hot flashes because they contain phytoestrogens that may balance hormones naturally. Besides, routine physical exercises, particularly those of an aerobic nature and strengthening exercises, are required for weight control and enhancing psychological well-being. Through active involvement in these lifestyle modifications, women can positively influence their general quality of life and contribute to alleviating some of the debilitating menopausal symptoms, showing a growing preference for more integrated styles of management. The effects of these natural therapies extend far beyond merely symptom alleviation; they also serve to foster a support network among women experiencing menopause. A qualitative study observed the narratives of sedentary women making this transition period, and it was observed that shared stories can exert a significant influence on menopausal understanding. By enabling dialogue about menopause, women are then able to create solidarity and empowerment that fosters collective wellness practices. Increased communication can lead to more effective public health initiatives aimed at addressing the unique needs of menopausal women, thereby promoting healthier aging in general. This is a call to community support that is an overarching movement aiming to positively enhance menopause experience and empower women with the information and resources necessary for successful management of this life stage, therefore fighting menopause stigma. Additionally, growing interest in non-pharmacologic approaches to managing menopause necessitates massive research and determination of efficacy for such natural interventions. While many women report positive experiences with lifestyle modification, empirical data to support these findings are needed in order to establish evidence-based guidelines that can be trusted by women. The subtlety of menopause, including the range of symptoms and responses to therapy, emphasizes the need for ongoing investigation into individualized interventions. Interventions that educate women about these options would enhance women's agency during menopause, enabling healthier decision-making and fostering resilience through conscious choice. Ultimately, with more women seeking alternatives to traditional therapies, the integration of scientifically established natural therapies as integral care for the routine treatment could be adding value to quality of life in menopause by providing safe, efficient, and well-tolerated ways of controlling the symptoms, as has been suggested in current research literature (Utian *et al.*, 2005; Rietdyk *et al.*, 2011).

Test Your Knowledge

1. What is the purpose of Hormone Replacement Therapy (HRT) during menopause?
2. Name some non-hormonal medications used as alternatives to HRT.

SUMMARY

In summary, menopause is a multifaceted process that is largely influenced by both biological and culture-based factors. The heterogeneity of menopausal symptoms across various ethnic groups testifies to the complexity of the process. As cross-cultural research in the recent past has shown, women experiencing menopause are likely to experience vasomotor, psychological, somatic, and sexual symptoms that not only vary in prevalence but also severity and impact on quality of life. This highlights the importance of healthcare providers being culturally sensitive to respond to the needs of menopausal women, knowing that symptom expression and coping strategies can be deeply rooted in culture. Knowledge of the variables determining menopausal experiences is therefore central in developing successful support systems and interventions. Methodological concerns highlighted in recent research are an example of the importance of systematic and rigorous approaches to menopause research. As attested, significant differences in methodological processes, such as different age ranges, symptom checklists, and data collection mechanisms, make it challenging to juxtapose outcomes across studies. Particularly, the reviews outlined in the literature reveal that all but a few studies fail to account for significant determinants, i.e., psychosocial and lifestyle, that might enhance or diminish menopausal symptoms. Such divergence in methodology necessitates an official effort to standardize criteria for measuring menopausal symptoms that would then facilitate a better understanding and enhancement of women's health during this transitional period. Lastly, the implications of these findings suggest the need for a comprehensive and holistic research strategy for the future. There is a need for consistency of measurement of menopausal symptoms and attention to the interaction between dynamic cultural factors and experience. Cross-cultural comparison of data not only advances knowledge of menopause but also requires more localized interventions that address the diverse experiences of women globally. Closing the gaps in the methodology of existing research, specifically on the influence of acculturation and lifestyle, can go a long way in moving the menopause discourse forward. Overall, promoting inter-disciplinary study that seeks to place cross-cultural perspectives at the forefront will ultimately enable women to cope with menopause with more information, assistance, and determination.

Menopause is a significant life transition for most women, intertwined with a range of health-related problems that have a tendency to impact their careers. Women, Work and the Menopause: Releasing the Potential of Older Professional Women is a report that reveals complex intersections of menopausal symptoms and workplace experiences. The results reveal that sleep disturbance, anxiety, and memory loss can decrease job satisfaction and increase turnover intentions among working women. Significantly, while physical health declines with age, mental health improves, suggesting a multifaceted experience of aging that complicates menopause in the workplace. Such dualism indicates the necessity for organizations understand the forces operating on women of advanced ages, whose steady contribution lies at the core of the workforce yet routinely overlooked and misrepresented by employers and policymakers (Bariola *et al.*). The relationship between organizational support and the experiences of menopausal women is also an important aspect to be noted by the study. The study emphasized that negative organizational messages exacerbate the challenges faced by these women, leading to feelings of disconnection and marginalization. Women stated that gendered ageism and the unavailability of menopause information are to be blamed for the environment in which their needs are not addressed. Interestingly, organizational culture in some instances disregards menopause as a legitimate issue, and hence, women do not approach the issue or even talk about it to others. This lack of support lowers morale and may damage productivity, thus creating a need for change in workplaces to facilitate supportive environments where such issues can be addressed open-mindedly and compassionately (Bariola *et al.*). In addition, the study found work-related factors that can ameliorate or worsen menopausal symptoms. Small changes, such as offering temperature control and flexibility in working arrangements, have been seen to have positive outcomes for women experiencing menopause. Inactive workplace settings, on the other hand, tend to worsen symptoms, whereby organizations must carefully look into workplace ergonomics. The report suggests more formalized approaches to offering menopause-specific assistance and training, so that employees and employers can most effectively navigate this transition. While women said they did not desire formal intervention, they did describe a desire for education and organizational recognition of menopause, which is an increasing recognition of the essential contribution of older women in the workforce.

KEY TERMS FROM THIS CHAPTER

- Climacteric
- Postmenopause
- Hot flashes
- Osteoporosis
- Mood swings
- Menopausal transition
- Surgical menopause
- Phytoestrogens
- Perimenopause
- Ovarian reserve
- Night sweats
- Cardiovascular risk
- Sleep disturbances
- Premature ovarian insufficiency
- Hormone replacement therapy (HRT)
- Bone density loss

CRITICAL THINKING QUESTIONS

1. **Menopause is defined as the permanent cessation of:**
   a. Ovulation
   b. Menstruation
   c. Fertilization
   d. Hormone production
2. **At approximately what age does natural menopause typically occur in women?**
   a. 30-35 years
   b. 40-45 years
   c. 45-55 years
   d. 60-65 years
3. **Which hormone significantly decreases during menopause leading to symptoms such as hot flashes?**
   a. Progesterone
   b. Estrogen
   c. Testosterone
   d. Luteinizing hormone (LH)
4. **Which of the following is NOT a common symptom associated with menopause?**
   a. Hot flashes
   b. Vaginal dryness
   c. Increased fertility
   d. Mood swings
5. **Menopause can lead to an increased risk of which condition due to decreased estrogen levels?**
   a. Osteoporosis
   b. Hyperthyroidism
   c. Hypertension
   d. Diabetes mellitus

Short Answer Questions

1. What marks the official onset of menopause in women?
2. Name one common psychological effect experienced during menopause.
3. What is one increased health risk linked to menopause due to hormonal changes?
4. Give one lifestyle change that can help manage menopause symptoms.
5. What type of therapy is commonly used to relieve menopausal hot flashes?
6. Name one natural or alternative treatment option often considered for menopause symptoms.

Answer to Critical Thinking Questions

1. (b) 2. (c) 3. (b) 4. (c) 5. (a)

REFERENCES

1. Abbott, L. M. C. (1986). Female power, ethnicity, and aging. https://core.ac.uk/download/130355112.pdf (accessed on 14th June 2025).
2. Al-Shboul, Q., Jassim, G., & Smail, L. (2017). Emirati women's knowledge and attitudes towards menopause and hormone replacement therapy: Implications for health-care policy. https://core.ac.uk/download/480761666.pdf (accessed on 14th June 2025).
3. Al-Wattar, B. H., Davies, M., & Nash, Z. (2022). Bone and heart health in menopause. https://core.ac.uk/download/599585954.pdf (accessed on 14th June 2025).
4. Alamer, H., Alamri, M., Alhashem, H., Alkhursan, A., *et al.* (2018). Awareness and perceptions towards menopause among Saudi women. https://core.ac.uk/download/327077959.pdf (accessed on 14th June 2025).
5. Alazawa, Z. F. R., Ayassrah, N. E. S., Barrouq, D. M. S., Irshaidat, N., *et al.* (2023). A cross-sectional study for assessment of menopausal symptoms and coping strategies among Jordanian women of 40–60 years age group. https://core.ac.uk/download/599811377.pdf (accessed on 14th June 2025).
6. Alexander, A., Anderson, B., Beckjord, E., Bergman, H., Blackburn, J., Boyd, M., Boyd, R., *et al.* (2011). Dietary modification for women after breast cancer treatment: A narrative review. https://core.ac.uk/download/10906882.pdf (accessed on 14th June 2025).
7. Anderson, D., Sievert, L., Obermeyer, C. M., Melby, M. E., *et al.* (2011). Methods used in cross-cultural comparisons of vasomotor symptoms and their determinants. https://core.ac.uk/download/10908178.pdf (accessed on 14th June 2025).
8. Anderson, D., Sievert, L., Obermeyer, C. M., Melby, M. E., *et al.* (2011). Overview of methods used in cross-cultural comparisons of menopausal symptoms and their determinants: Guidelines for Strengthening the Reporting of Menopause and Aging (STROMA) studies. https://core.ac.uk/download/10908179.pdf (accessed on 14th June 2025).
9. Arico, I., Bonanni, E., Bonsignore, M., Caretto, M., Caruso, D., Di Perri, M. C., Galletta, S., *et al.* (2019). Italian Association of Sleep Medicine (AIMS) position statement and guideline on the treatment of menopausal sleep disorders. https://core.ac.uk/download/237172618.pdf (accessed on 14th June 2025).
10. Bariola, E., Jack, G., Schapper, J., Riach, K., Pitts, M., & Sarrel, P. (2025). Women, work and the menopause: Releasing the potential of older professional women. https://core.ac.uk/download/pdf/30673673.pdf (accessed on 14th June 2025).
11. Bates, K. A. (2019). The interaction of type II diabetes and gonadal steroids on cognition in middle-aged women. https://core.ac.uk/download/223071460.pdf (accessed on 14th June 2025).
12. Bellini, T., Bonaccorsi, G., Bramanti, B., Carè, A., *et al.* (2019). "Bridging the gap": Everything that could have been avoided if we had applied gender medicine, pharmacogenetics and personalized medicine in the gender-omics and sex-omics era. https://core.ac.uk/download/286075866.pdf (accessed on 14th June 2025).
13. Besong, C., Bham, A., Burroughs, C. R., Castine, M., *et al.* (2024). Managing menopause: The evolving role of estrogens, selective serotonin reuptake inhibitors, and phytoestrogens in balancing hormonal fluctuations. https://core.ac.uk/download/640946359.pdf (accessed on 14th June 2025).

14. Bhalerao, A., Kawthalkar, A., & Yemde, A. (2024). Determinants impacting the quality of life in postmenopausal women: An in-depth narrative review. https://core.ac.uk/download/620836146.pdf (accessed on 14th June 2025).

15. Biglia, N., Birkhaeuser, M., Brincat, M., Celis-Gonzales, C., *et al.* (2020). Purified and specific cytoplasmic pollen extract: A non-hormonal alternative for the treatment of menopausal symptoms. https://core.ac.uk/download/287622052.pdf (accessed on 14th June 2025).

16. Breen, V. E. (2016). Factors influencing uptake of risk-reducing salpingo-oophorectomy by BRCA1 and BRCA2 mutation carriers. https://core.ac.uk/download/46720399.pdf (accessed on 14th June 2025).

17. Brody, E. M., Brown, C., Cohen, J., Bromberger, J. T., Matthews, K. A., McKinlay, S. M., Avis, N. E., *et al.* (2012). Role stress, role reward, and mental health in a multiethnic sample of midlife women: Results from the Study of Women's Health Across the Nation (SWAN). http://deepblue.lib.umich.edu/bitstream/2027.42/98462/1/jwh%252E2011%252E3180.pdf (accessed on 14th June 2025).

18. Bucciarelli, V., Coppi, F., Gallina, S., Mattioli, A. V., Nasi, M., Nodari, S., Pinti, M., *et al.* (2024). The impact of stress and social determinants on diet in cardiovascular prevention in young women. https://core.ac.uk/download/614162600.pdf (accessed on 14th June 2025).

19. Codacci-Pisanelli, G., Del Pup, L., Levi-Setti, P. E., Patrizio, P., *et al.* (2018). Risk of cancer after assisted reproduction: A review of the available evidences and guidance to fertility counselors. https://core.ac.uk/download/188830441.pdf (accessed on 14th June 2025).

20. Davis, S. R., Gompel, A., Lumsden, M. A., Murad, M. H., *et al.* (2015). Treatment of symptoms of the menopause: An endocrine society clinical practice guideline. https://core.ac.uk/download/42367511.pdf (accessed on 14th June 2025).

21. Davis, S. R., Gompel, A., Lumsden, M. A., Pinkerton, J. V., *et al.* (2017). Managing menopausal symptoms and associated clinical issues in breast cancer survivors. https://core.ac.uk/download/96884955.pdf (accessed on 14th June 2025).

22. Davison, S., Elliott, C., & Hickey, M. (2012). Hormone replacement therapy. https://core.ac.uk/download/12793861.pdf (accessed on 14th June 2025).

23. Felice De , F., Di Pinto, A., Marchetti, C., Musella, A., *et al.* (2018). Fertility preservation in gynecologic cancers. https://core.ac.uk/download/154948073.pdf (accessed on 14th June 2025).

24. Dhanalakshmi, M. G., Ganesan, A., Lakshmanan, K., Myneni, R., *et al.* (2021). Bone health after menopause: Effect of surgical menopause on bone mineral density and osteoporosis. https://core.ac.uk/download/539899523.pdf (accessed on 14th June 2025).

25. Eost-Telling, C., Harris, D., MacKenzie, A., McDermott, J., Money, A., Norman, G., & Todd, C. (2025). The impact of physical activity and exercise interventions on symptoms for women experiencing menopause: Overview of reviews. https://core.ac.uk/download/637043369.pdf (accessed on 14th June 2025).

26. Ford, M. (2015). A descriptive study of menopausal woman's life experiences, stressors and their occupational meanings. https://core.ac.uk/download/232638258.pdf (accessed on 14th June 2025).

27. Gavranich, P. (2011). Perspectives of women in leadership roles: Working through "the change." https://core.ac.uk/download/61305625.pdf (accessed on 14th June 2025).

28. Ghodusi, M., Heidari, M., & Rafiei, H. (2017). Sexual self-concept and its relationship to depression, stress and anxiety in postmenopausal women. https://core.ac.uk/download/143840308.pdf (accessed on 14th June 2025).

29. Gollschewski, S. E. (2006). The use of complementary and alternative medications by menopausal women living in South East Queensland. https://core.ac.uk/download/10885129.pdf (accessed on 14th June 2025).

30. Graham, E. E., Hatchfeld, A., Michala, L., Moseholm, E., *et al.* (2023). Collection of menopause data in studies of women living with HIV: A systematic literature review. https://core.ac.uk/download/590330478.pdf (accessed on 14th June 2025).

31. Hakim, J., Ross, D. A., South, A., Weller, I., *et al.* (2012). Evidence for action on HIV treatment and care systems in low and middle-income countries: Background and introduction.

32. Hari, G., Kalyan, P. N., Manaswi, P., *et al.* (2024). A study on the symptoms, sleep quality and cognitive function of the women during menopause. https://core.ac.uk/download/603896338.pdf (accessed on 14th June 2025).

33. Hayman, M. (2024). Breaking the silence: Exploring the impact of supervisor vulnerability on menstrual disclosures at work. https://core.ac.uk/download/619597331.pdf (accessed on 14th June 2025).

34. Hutted, I., Padmadas, S. S., & Willekens, F. (2004). On the compression of reproductive spans: The case of Andhra Pradesh in India.

35. Kang, A. R. (2023). Managing menopausal symptoms through exercise and dietary changes. https://core.ac.uk/download/571288513.pdf (accessed on 14th June 2025).

36. Kelsey, T. W., & Wallace, W. H. B. (2010). Machine science in biomedicine: Practicalities, pitfalls and potential. http://arxiv.org/abs/1008.3795 (accessed on 14th June 2025).

37. Lee, Y. S. (2017). Care coordination in bone health screening between individual behaviors and health care services among Korean-American women across three age groups. https://digitalscholarship.unlv.edu/cgi/viewcontent.cgi?article=1029&context=apin (accessed on 14th June 2025).

38. Mavroeidi, A., & Skelton, D. A. (2018). How do muscle and bone strengthening and balance activities (MBSBA) vary across the life course, and are there particular ages where MBSBA are most important? https://core.ac.uk/download/293863667.pdf (accessed on 14th June 2025).

39. Mohamad Diah, N. (2009). "What's wrong with mak?": Understanding menopause among young Malay adults. https://core.ac.uk/download/300389694.pdf (accessed on 14th June 2025).

40. N/A. (2025). Not just an older woman's disease: Breast cancer in your 20s and 30s. https://core.ac.uk/download/pdf/30673830.pdf (accessed on 14th June 2025).

41. Nieroda, M., Posso, D., & Seckam, A. (2024). Women's expectations for system support for a healthy menopausal transition: A pilot study. https://core.ac.uk/download/621694561.pdf (accessed on 14th June 2025).

42. Reynolds, F. (1999). Distress and coping with hot flushes at work: Implications for counsellors in occupational settings. https://core.ac.uk/download/334730.pdf (accessed on 14th June 2025).

43. Reynolds, F. (2000). Relationships between catastrophic thoughts, perceived control and distress during menopausal hot flushes: Exploring the correlates of a questionnaire measure. https://core.ac.uk/download/334729.pdf (accessed on 14th June 2025).

44. Rietdyk, A. E. A. (2011). The experience of menopause as reported by sedentary women. https://core.ac.uk/download/147832381.pdf (accessed on 14th June 2025).

45. Skotnes, L. L. H. (2019). An exploratory view of female reproductive health issues: A case study in Norway. https://core.ac.uk/download/542326928.pdf (accessed on 14th June 2025).

46. Tharpe, M., & Wessells, M. (2020). Are hormone therapies more effective in treating the manifestations/symptoms of menopause than lifestyle, exercise, and diet changes? https://core.ac.uk/download/534774730.pdf (accessed on 14th June 2025).

47. Thomas, S. E. (2005). Menopause knowledge and attitudes of English-speaking Caribbean women: Implications for health education. https://core.ac.uk/download/267865166.pdf (accessed on 14th June 2025).

48. Utian, W. H. (2005). Psychosocial and socioeconomic burden of vasomotor symptoms in menopause: A comprehensive review. https://core.ac.uk/download/pdf/3717431.pdf (accessed on 14th June 2025).

49. Wharton, C. Y. (2020). Middle-aged women negotiating the ageing process through participation in outdoor adventure activities. https://core.ac.uk/download/228178497.pdf (accessed on 14th June 2025).

50. Yashin, A. I., & Ukraintseva, S. V. (2025). Economic progress as cancer risk factor. II: Why is overall cancer risk higher in more developed countries? https://core.ac.uk/download/pdf/7127514.pdf (accessed on 14th June 2025).

MENSTRUATION

5

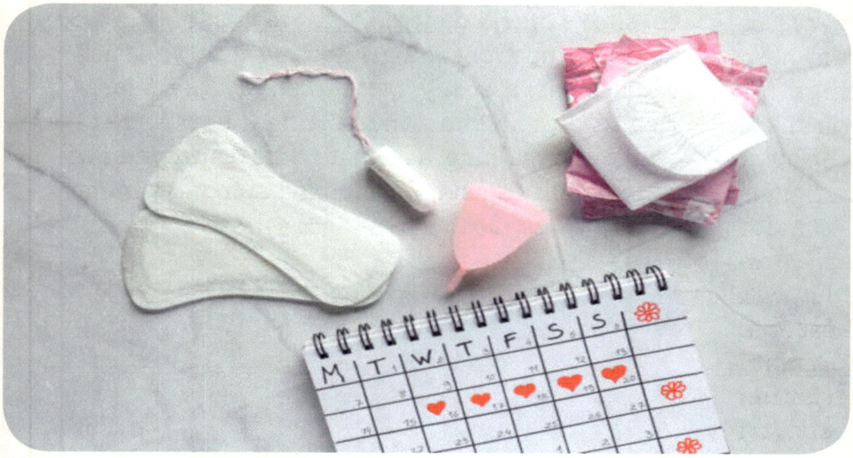

Introduction

There is a need to comprehend menstruation both biologically as a process and socially as a phenomenon that directly affects the lives of menstruating people. The natural process has historically been stigmatized, and the resulting cultural discourse has been inclined to exclude the talk on it. In most societies, menstruation is viewed as a taboo that not only stifles open conversation but also creates a culture where menstruating individuals can be isolated in their private lives and in the workplace. Ignorance and denial of menstruation have the potential to cause isolation, ultimately affecting mental health. This chapter aims to explore the multifaceted aspects of menstruation, questioning its social backdrop, subjective understanding of menstruators, and the necessity of an extended dialogue in educational institutions and workplaces as well. Menstruation has organizational implications, most prominently concerning organizational dynamics. Recent studies have identified a notable disparity in management scholarship; menstruation has been nearly invisible compared to other bodily functions, such as pregnancy

LEARNING OBJECTIVES

After studying this chapter, you will be able to:

1. Explain the biological aspects of menstruation
2. Analyze various cultural perspectives on menstruation
3. Examine the psychological effects of menstruation
4. Demonstrate understanding of menstrual health and hygiene
5. Define menstruation and reproductive health
6. Evaluate the societal implications of menstruation

and lactation, which have been brought into focus (Hayman *et al.*, 2024). The invisibility invites a conclusive misinterpretation of the unique issues that menstruating employees face in the workplace. Menstrual invisibility could discourage managers from being in a position to assist their workers appropriately, denying them necessary adjustments. A core process in building a comprehensive workplace environment is the driver behind menstruating workers reporting symptoms and accessing support. Deconstruction of the dynamics provides useful information that can help organizations develop effective settings for employees. Disclosure motivation awareness for menstruation also illuminates significant organizational body work and hidden stigmas at the workplace (Hayman *et al.*, 2024). With organizations looking to make it inclusive, an understanding of menstruation subtleties will lead to better practices and policies. Research has also put forward supervisors' vulnerability and organizational culture for menstruation as the key to programs' success. Based on qualitative and quantitative research into the menstruating workforce experience, the chapter tries to present a feeling of urgency regarding filling knowledge and support gaps. Ultimately, a complete understanding of menstruation and its impact is not merely one of health, but of dignity and well-being for each and every worker within any organizational setting.

Definition of Menstruation

Menstruation, or the period, is a recurring biological process that generally occurs on a monthly basis in someone with a uterus from the age of puberty until menopause. Menstruation is the sloughing off of the lining of the endometrium when there is no fertilized egg produced during the time of ovulation. This is regulated by a delicate balance of hormones, such as estrogen and progesterone, which regulate the thickening and eventual shedding of the uterine lining. The typical menstrual cycle lasts 28 days, but cycles can differ widely from woman to woman in length, from 21 to 35 days. The bodily presence of menstruation is not only biological in intent but also embodies numerous cultural, social, and psychological significances that impact women's health and experiences all over the world. Defining menstruation is not only an affair of the biological machinery but also encompasses the sociocultural contexts and experiences of menstruators. Menstrual hygiene products and facilities are utilized extensively to show stark contrasts in terms of public health, education, and gender equality. One such example is a study conducted by the World Health Organization, illustrating the struggle of women in gaining access to safe and hygienic toilet facilities used for menstrual management (Berry *et al.*, 2019).

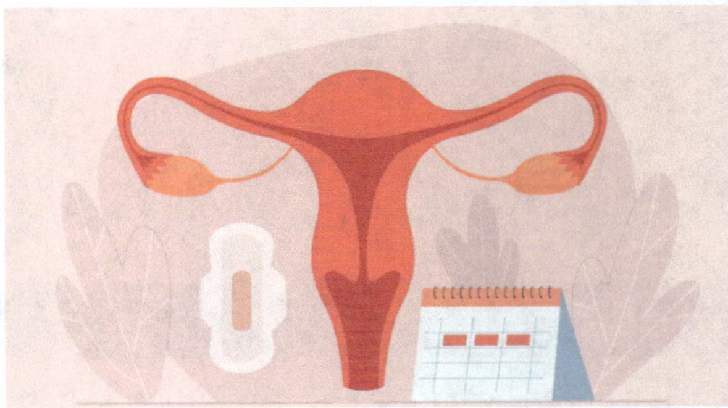

Source: https://images.healthshots.com/healthshots/en/uploads/2022/06/15093731/menstrual-hygiene-management.jpg

This brings into focus the necessity to acknowledge menstruation as not just a biological process but also as a significant social problem that intersects with education, economic participation, and health rights. Stigmatization of menstruation also contributes to these challenges, which have a tendency to lead to social exclusion, shame, and inadequate health responses, thus exacerbating the problems most women experience when attempting to manage their periods. Moreover, primary dysmenorrhea, which is pathological pain-free menstrual cramps, is evident as a prevalent condition in menstruators. Based on research, a vast majority of high school students have reported this painful symptom, which can be caused by decreased concentration and participation in learning settings (Fantaw *et al.*, 2024). The prevalence of primary dysmenorrhea is a sign that demands proper menstrual health education and the provision of the right resources, particularly to the younger population. Understanding of menstruation, therefore, must involve its effects on day-to-day living, psychosocial health, and the necessity for medical and social care planning for the sufferers. Providing universal health resource access and creating enabling environments can allow individuals to successfully manage the complexities of menstruation.

Historical Context of Menstruation

Menstruation has been welcomed in various cultural understanding and practice across history, which have all influenced women's experience of the natural biological process. Society has regulated both the understanding and regulation of menstruation in most cultures, which has been accomplished through introducing controlling practices that impact women's health and well-being. For instance, Elizabeth Gumbaket's research indicates the challenge faced by adolescent girls during menarche in Papua New Guinea, which reveals an immense inhibition against pre-menarche preparation in socio-cultural attitudes towards menstruation. This lack of preparation of adolescent girls can negatively affect young women's menstrual well-being and thereby the overall quality of their lives. These cultural contexts illustrate how ancient attitudes toward menstruation can build systemic barriers, and why more communication and education regarding adolescent menstrual health is needed. In Jewish culture, the history of menstruation is intertwined with religious practice, mainly through the practice of niddah. Niddah or menstrual purity observance has evolved within Jewish law and culture and builds challenging issues regarding women's agency. Scholarship of niddah practice attests to an advanced interaction of tradition and contemporary interpretations of the women's roles in the ritual context. While traditionally regarded as a symbol of patriarchal thought, the practice may also work to empower and enable women to define themselves. Academics propose that the evolution of the rituals of niddah follows broader societal evolution, most notably with regard to the ideas of purity and sexuality in religious contexts. This dynamic also points towards menstruation's past record as more than simply a biological reality, but shifting cultural tides and beliefs too. With menstruation still being studied in various academic and social contexts, its richness of history beyond mere biology must be realized. Cultural practice during menstruation is found to exhibit ongoing power negotiation and identity formation throughout societies. Both Gumbaketi's writings and niddah research prove the far-reaching impact that cultural ideals have on the menstruation experience and upkeep. Additionally, the evolution of these practices proves a mirror image of what's occurred in society at large, such as with changes in gender roles and increased pressure toward female rights in health education. Lastly, understanding the history of menstruation informs us of the ways in which women have managed their reality, and reveals to us the challenges that remain in having balanced health resources and support to menstruators throughout the world.

Importance of Discussing Menstruation

Talking about the significance of menstruation brings some key issues regarding how social taboo and stigmatization could limit open discussion of what is a biological, natural process. Lack of communication typically equates to false information and the absence of knowledge regarding women's health needs. In many cultures, particularly in nations like India, menstruation remains a secret subject that significantly impacts women's health decision-making. The Reproductive and Child Health Programme brings to light that stigma and communication barriers have a critical influence on women's access to relevant healthcare resources and information. Therefore, promoting thorough discussions regarding menstruation is important to enable women to make well-informed decisions regarding their wellbeing, leading to enhanced community health. By talking, people can deconstruct harmful myths and ignorance myths that mandate silence over the monthly cycle undergone by menstruators and create a secure environment for learning and acceptance (Saha *et al.*, 2005). The workplace is yet another significant venue where menstruation is traditionally taken for granted, and the consequence is that there will be no accommodations required for working menstruators. This surveillance emphasizes the need to include menstruation health discourse in organizational policy, which can do much to promote workplace inclusivity. Research indicates that the invisibility of menstruation can constrain supervisors' understanding of employees' needs and, hence, poor support for afflicted employees. Stigmatizing menstruation as an inherent aspect of women's health is the key to the development of an inclusive workplace. Through the open conversation of menstruation, the organizations can create a culture where menstruators feel free to report symptoms, eventually leading to better management practices. This, in turn, can cut down potential stigmas and lead to more positive workplace policies with respect to the special needs of women, thereby increasing overall employee morale and productivity (Hayman *et al.*, 2024). Apart from this, schools also play a crucial role in making menstruation topics routine, especially among the underage who are undergoing their first menstrual periods. Offering whole-school sex education covering menstruation can more effectively equip students with the knowledge and support they need to navigate these transitions confidently. Menstruation in school can assist in dispelling myths, reducing stigma, and building a supportive environment for all young people. Menstruation discussions can also help create an understanding and empathy among peers, creating a culture in which young menstruators can feel welcome and understood. By prioritizing these discussions, schools prepare students not only for the physical realities of menstruation but also for the emotional and social aspects that accompany it. Thus, this creation of an open menstruation discourse framework in school is critical to producing informed, well-rounded citizens who are able to pass on this information to their communities (Saha *et al.*, 2005).

5.1. Biological Aspects of Menstruation

Learning Outcome

1. Define the menstrual cycle phases
2. Explain the hormonal regulation of menstruation
3. Identify common physiological symptoms

The body process of menstruation comes automatically linked to the reproductive cycle, which is managed through complex interactions between hormones specifically estrogen and progesterone. The 28-day menstrual cycle has several phases: the menstrual phase, the follicular phase, ovulation, and the luteal phase. During the menstrual phase, the endometrial lining is shed if it is not fertilized, resulting in the visible menstrual discharge. This shedding is an essential part of the female reproductive system's health, an expression of the body's cyclical readiness for potential pregnancy. In addition, hormonal fluctuations within the cycle influence other physiological and psychological conditions, not just the biological process but also the psychological responses that come with menstruation in women, as established in studies on the subject. Symptoms of menstruation are not solely issues of reproductive readiness; they have implications for women's health and well-being. Disruptions to the menstrual cycle may herald underlying illness, such as polycystic ovary syndrome (PCOS) or thyroid disease, and awareness of these biological markers is critical for early diagnosis and management. Secondarily, menstrual abnormalities such as dysmenorrhea and premenstrual syndrome (PMS) also present the same kinds of challenges to a high proportion of menstruators, impacting daily functioning and quality of life. These reinforce the necessity for balanced reproductive health education that not only rejects the biological realities of menstruation but also the social and medical reactions required to attend to individuals suffering from menstrual pain. Awareness and proactive management result in menstruators' well-being, which underscores the interconnectedness of biological events to daily life.

Regardless of biological relevance, socio-cultural realities always prevail and render their relevance invisible, thus leading to stigma and marginalization of menstruators. The economics of menstruation introduce the additional layer that states impose a sales tax on menstrual products but not on other health products, a policy that discriminates against society's values and gender equality. The tampon tax is a financial burden on menstruators as well as a public health issue regarding access and affordability of necessary products. Legal action and activism are increasingly being pursued against the discriminatory taxation of that sort, and an ever-growing awareness of menstrual equity as a fundamental principle of social justice. Simply put, biological, economic, and sociopolitical forces intersect to define the sphere in which menstruation is experienced and thus require a multifaceted approach to the complexity of the issue represented by this natural biological process.

5.1.1. The Menstrual Cycle Phases

The menstrual cycle, a physiological monthly process, can be broadly categorized into four individual phases: the menstrual phase, the follicular phase, the ovulation phase, and the luteal phase. Beginning with the menstrual phase, which lasts from approximately day one to day five, the period is marked by the shedding of the uterine lining in the event that fertilization fails to occur. During menstruation, levels of progesterone and estrogen decrease, leading to breakdown of this lining and causing bleeding from the menstrual system. Curiously, there are physiological alterations at this point, and research has determined alterations in blood viscosity and hematocrit levels. In one study, relative blood viscosity decreases significantly during menstruation compared with values obtained during the premenstrual phase, which could reduce the risk of cardiovascular complications among women (Agoreyo *et al.*, 2017). The follicular phase then ensues, running from day six to day fourteen of the cycle. During this phase, the pituitary gland releases follicle-stimulating hormone (FSH) that stimulates the growth of the ovarian follicles and estrogen secretion. As the estrogen levels increase, the uterine lining thickens in anticipation of possible implantation. This phase is highly critical in regulating the menstrual cycle, as it facilitates the process leading up to ovulation. This is the phase when women are able to sense more energy and an improved mood due to hormonal changes. Women with heightened risk-taking during their menstrual and premenstrual phases are characterized by variations in bidding behaviour in experimental settings, as expressed by how intrinsic hormonal conditions will shape behaviour based on the phase of the menstrual cycle (Pearson *et al.*).

Ovulation occurs around day fourteen, when the mature egg is released from the ovary. This phase is highly critical to reproduction as the egg must meet the sperm so that the egg can be fertilized. Ovulation is triggered by the luteinizing hormone surge, resulting in the egg being available for fertilization for a brief window of time, about 24 hours. Once ovulation has occurred, the cycle enters the luteal phase, which is between day fifteen and the start of menstruation. During this time, the anovulatory follicle is converted to a corpus luteum that produces progesterone in order to prepare the lining of the uterus even more for potential implantation of a fertilized ovum. Upon failure of fertilization, the progesterone level drops, which causes menstruation and the beginning of a new cycle. Familiarity with all these stages is essential in learning the complex interplay between the hormones and their consequences on women's health throughout the menstrual cycle.

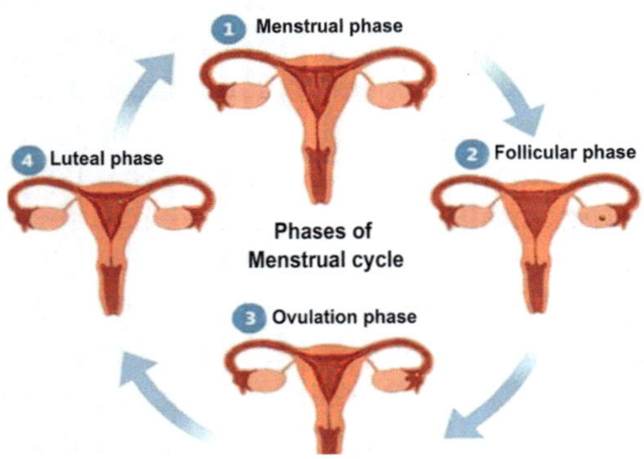

Figure 5.1. Phases of menstrual cycle.

Source: https://www.menstrupedia.com/assets/quickguide/physiology/pysiology-menstrual-phases.jpg

5.1.2. Hormonal Regulation of Menstruation

The hormonal regulation of menstruation is a complex interplay of several hormones that governs the menstrual cycle phases. It is at the core of this regulation that the ovaries, pituitary gland, and hypothalamus synergize to regulate levels of estrogen and progesterone. The hypothalamus first secretes gonadotropin-releasing hormone (GnRH), which stimulates the anterior pituitary to release follicle-stimulating hormone (FSH) and luteinizing hormone (LH). FSH stimulates the growth of ovarian follicles, while LH stimulates ovulation, which results in the expulsion of an egg at maturity. Fluctuations in estrogen during the follicular phase play a key role in thickening the uterine lining in readiness for possible implantation. This intricate hormonal exchange not only regulates the menstrual cycle but also has considerable implications on most health conditions, as indicated by evidence that the frequency of migraines in women is concomitant with alterations in estrogen levels throughout their reproductive lives, as cited in Terrin *et al.* (2018).

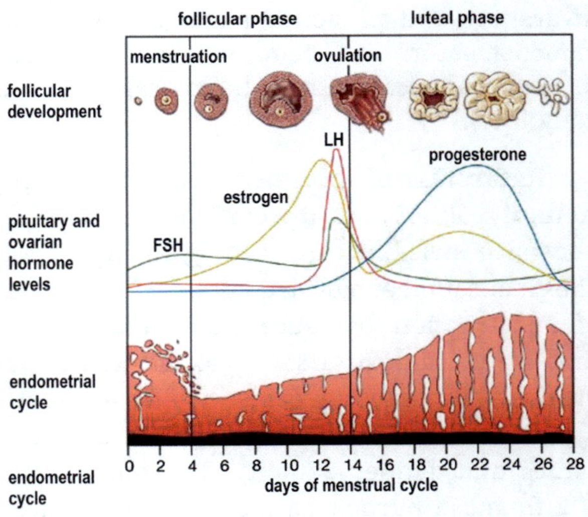

Figure 5.2. Cyclical changes during a woman's normal ovulatory menstrual cycle.

Source: https://cdn.britannica.com/07/55707-050-5927EDFB/changes-woman-cycle.jpg

Following ovulation, the corpus luteum is formed and secretes progesterone, which is the luteal phase of the menstrual cycle.

Progesterone functions to maintain the uterine lining intact and ready for implantation in case it gets pregnant. If pregnancy does not occur, the corpus luteum degenerates, and there's a drop in progesterone and estrogen. This drop in hormones results in the shedding of the uterine lining—menstruation. Surprisingly, the timing of this cascade of hormones can create various physical and emotional symptoms, according to self-reported data collected by menstrual tracking apps.

Recent research based on Clue app longitudinal data indicates that variability in cycle length is highly correlated with users' qualitative symptoms, which indicate the interaction between levels of hormones and feelings of menstrual well-being, as highlighted in Druet *et al.* (2020). Regulation of hormones is more than just monitoring menstrual periods; it gives feedback on women's health conditions such as endometriosis and polycystic ovary syndrome (PCOS).

The detection of hormonal changes will be able to detect symptoms and manage conditions that profoundly impact quality of life. For instance, research shows that women who have cycle variability extremes present certain patterns of symptoms, which underline the need for individualized healthcare interventions. With the use of technology and patient-provided information, clinicians can modify their treatment and symptom management protocols, thus enabling a more personalized care experience. Continuous research into the hormonal regulation of menstruation not only demystifies cycles but also adds to the general pool of knowledge around women's health, paving the way for innovation in medical practice and research..

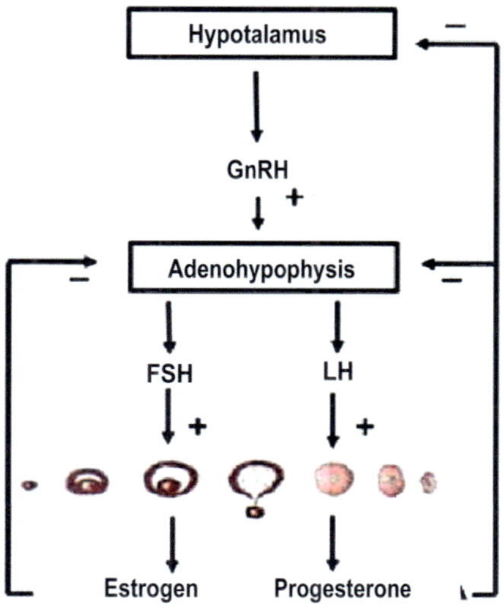

Figure 5.3. Hormonal control of the menstrual cycle.

Source: https://www.researchgate.net/figure/Hormonal-control-of-the-menstrual-cycle_fig2_330663356

5.1.3. Common Physiological Symptoms

It is necessary to know the normal physiological symptoms occurring with menstruation, so that female health and well-being can be promoted. Women can have variable symptoms during the menstrual cycle that interfere with their daily lives. These may involve abdominal cramps, bloating, breast tenderness, and mood change. These are considered to be normal physiological responses to hormonal changes—primarily estrogen and progesterone—while individual experiences may be very varied. Stress and lifestyle may exacerbate these signs, affecting the physical as well as the mental state of women during menstruation. An overall understanding of the physiological symptoms helps to make women's experiences ordinary, and it also facilitates empathy towards the subject matter of menstrual health, which remains significant in various cultures. Aside from the widely recognized symptoms of menstruation, there are some women who have more severe symptoms in the form of premenstrual syndrome (PMS) or premenstrual dysphoric disorder (PMDD). These conditions greatly affect emotional and mental health, and symptoms of such include violent irritability, depression, anxiety, and fatigue. Recognizing the distinction between typical symptoms and those typical of PMS or PMDD is critical, as it can lead to appropriate intervention and treatment. In addition, examining further socio-cultural determinants of the experience of these symptoms can inform barriers to optimal management. Experiments prove that enhancing menstrual hygiene and management through education can maximize the quality of life in the majority of women, enabling them to have greater control over their physiologic symptoms during menstruation (N/A, 2011).

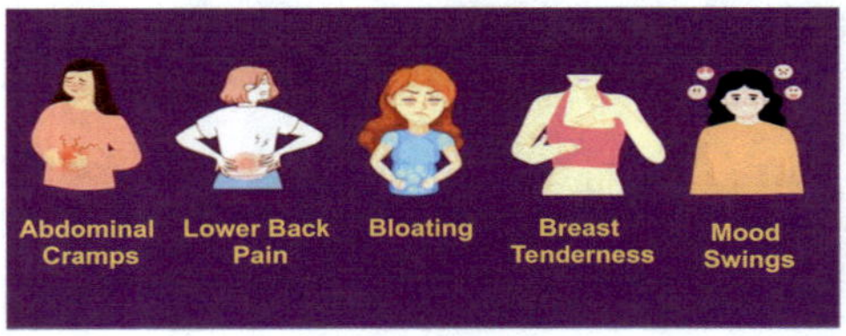

Figure 5.4. Symptoms of premenstrual syndrome.

Source: https://nimaaya.com/wp-content/uploads/2024/05/Common-Periods-Symptoms.png

Another common physiological symptom of menstruation is the onset of migraines, in this instance, due to changes in hormones. Episodic migraines have been found to occur at their highest levels during the premenstrual phase due to changes in levels of estrogen. The majority of individuals experience that they have synchronous symptoms with the menstrual cycle and worsening headaches with or preceding menstruation. The correlation emphasizes the complexity of physiological responses that take place during menstruation, illustrating how both hormonal control and neurological state perhaps impact one another. Clinical data suggest that lifestyle management, diet, and stress can minimize symptoms for these events (Marmura *et al.*, 2018). By acknowledging the variations of physiological presentation that manifest as a consequence of menstruation, healthcare practitioners can create personalized plans of treatment, improving quality of life in menorrhagic patients.

Test Your Knowledge

1. Which hormones are primarily responsible for regulating the menstrual cycle?
2. What are some common physiological symptoms experienced during menstruation?

5.2. Cultural Perspectives on Menstruation

Learning Outcome

1. Discuss menstruation in different cultures
2. Define taboos and stigmas surrounding menstruation
3. Identify the impact of culture on menstrual health

Menstrual culture is heavily determined by time-tested beliefs, taboos, and myths, which vary significantly across cultures. Menstruation in the majority of cultures is surrounded by a stigma expressed in prohibitions on women's activity and contact during menstruation. Women, for instance, are forbidden to cook, go to religious places, or take part in social gatherings in most of India, which all express deeply ingrained beliefs linking menstruation with dirt and pollution. These cultural beliefs not only influence individuals' perceptions of menstruation but also have an impact on access to menstrual health education and management. Where menstruation taboos do exist, the stigma attached to menstruation can lead to a deficiency of information concerning proper hygiene practices, again exacerbating women's issues with the proper management of their menstrual hygiene. All these cultural barriers must be addressed by solutions to improve menstrual hygiene and provide a favorable condition for women's health. The problem of period poverty also overlaps well with cultural perspectives on menstruation, as one observes in most cultures around the world. Period poverty is the lack of access to menstrual hygiene products due to poverty, and this can be overlaid by cultural attitudes that devalue menstrual health. It has been found that, for example, in Kerala, 25.5% of young girls experience period poverty, particularly those with lower socioeconomic status (*et al.*, 2024). These cultural attitudes not only illustrate what options women have when it comes to menstruation products but also themselves and their self-confidence and dignity when discussing menstruation. As the study illustrates, inadequate attitudes toward menstruation and low socioeconomic status are closely associated with a high prevalence of period poverty, highlighting the need for interventions towards financial as well as cultural obstacles. Providing free menstrual products and enhanced education around menstruation can be an important consideration for reducing these issues. Discovering how different groups view menstruation also shows that there are cultural nuances that surround this natural process. For example, the knowledge of menstruation among male medical students in Tamil Nadu was found to be highly mediated by media rather than formal education. This shows that traditional beliefs continue to prevail even among educated individuals, leading to variations regarding empathy and sympathy towards women's experience during menstruation (*et al.*, 2024). The struggle between shifting educational perspectives and traditional, long-held beliefs signifies the necessity of whole-body sex education that includes honest discussions of menstruation. Through filling in the gaps in education, myths can be debunked, misconceptions reduced, and a more informed and supportive environment fostered for women. Through the inclusion of men and women in this dialogue, society could advance towards dismantling harmful cultural expectations and creating a healthier discourse of menstruation.

5.2.1. Menstruation in Different Cultures

Menstruation is a sociocultural sign in most cultures, as it changes the way humans perceive and conceptualize this biological event. The onset of menstruation, in most cultures, is a time of festival to mark the girl's transition to womanhood. Menstruation may be preceded or followed by ceremonies or rituals that indicate the significance a society attaches to gender and reproduction. For instance, in some Indigenous societies, menstruation is considered to be a sacred occurrence, validating women's roles within their communities. This cultural respect is evident in the way menarche is often celebrated with specific festivities, which validate social bonds and transfer knowledge among women. Cultural practices cross over into stereotypes that affect knowledge on women's roles within society, as highlighted through the work of Plains Indian cultures. This study shows how the records of the past may overlook women's experiences and hence the necessity for more subtle insights into their cultural relevance (Mello *et al.*, 2004).

Other cultures, on the other hand, may have restrictions or prohibitions about menstruation affecting women's health and well-being. Socio-cultural norms and how the interaction of such norms influences how young women experience the time leading up to menarche. As seen in the case of Papua New Guinea, these norms can limit pre-menarche preparation and education, adversely affecting menstrual health. Young women's lives will be marked by misinformation and shame, which can bring about shame and fear over the natural process. These findings emphasize putting menstrual education into education and health systems for enhancing young women's knowledge and confidence in their bodies. By removing such cultural barriers, sexual and reproductive health among adolescent girls across different cultural contexts can be enhanced (Maulingin-Gumbaketi *et al.*, 2021). The study of menstruation across cultures is a rich ethnographic tapestry of perspectives, beliefs, and practices, which can have a dramatic impact on women's lives. Understanding these cultural orientations, it is possible to see better how menstruation can be both a physiological phenomenon and a marker of cultural identity. It provides the incentive for programs that respect cultural diversity but promote education regarding menstruation on the basis of fact. Programs that synthesize traditional beliefs and factual health knowledge can empower women and girls, providing an environment that appreciates their cultural identities. Realization of the different interpretations of menstruation that have been related to different societies is one of getting rid of stigma and making menstrual education and health accessible to and beneficial for all, thereby bringing about social change and gender equality on a mass scale.

5.2.2. Taboos and Stigmas Surrounding Menstruation

The social stigmas and taboos generated during menstruation give rise to a culture of silence and shame that inhibits open talk about this natural biological phenomenon.

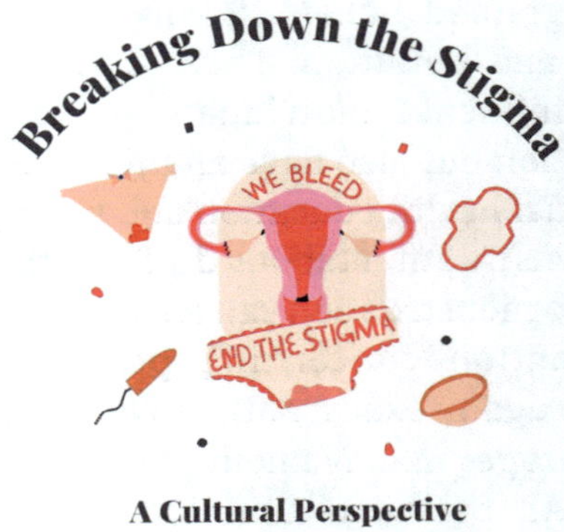

Source: https://www.ujaas.in/uploads/images/Menstrual-Taboo-Breaking-Down-the-Stigma-A-Cultural-Perspective.jpg

Menstruation is concealed in secrecy in most societies, where it is understood as a cause of pollution or frailty. Such a general attitude not only makes those who menstruate outcasts but also keeps them outside the sphere of knowledge and health services. For example, research has established that it is hard for women to make knowledgeable choices regarding menstrual health and hygiene due to such deeply rooted stigmas, highlighting overall public opinion that regards menstruation as taboo. Such taboos need to be countered so women can be enabled, health equity can be promoted, and it can be made possible to live in a society where menstrual health is made normal rather than hidden or neglected (Saha *et al.*, 2005).

Stigma's impact is also compounded by menstrual product advertising, which is usually rooted in ambiguous communication, recycling societal discomfort with menstruation. Advertising messages prefer the use of euphemisms and circumlocutions rather than making an open reference to the topic in question, which has the effect of reinforcing consumer embarrassment. This sort of evasiveness can lead to a lack of understanding and confusion about the available methods of menstrual hygiene management. Women require explicit, informative, and validating messaging when selecting hygiene products, but the prevailing marketing approach is constructing a feeling of need to conceal menstruation rather than embracing or normalizing it. The female hygiene product advertising space must thus be reoriented in such a manner that creativity becomes balanced with transparency regarding menstrual health and its implications for women (Schulte *et al.*, 2019). In addition, menstruation stigma has severe implications for women's access to healthcare and decision-making. The majority of women are ashamed to seek medical assistance or discuss menstruation issues with physicians for fear of being judged or misunderstood. Such reluctance can lead to undiagnosed menstrual disease and overall reproductive health abandonment. For instance, in rural communities, the intersection of traditional practices and modern health care is often a cause of imbalance where women's choices for their health are more and more controlled by stigma and lack of support. Health communication campaigns will need to address the sociocultural context of menstruation, emphasizing dialogue and education, in order to be successful in counteracting such obstacles. By developing a learning culture instead of a culture of stigma, society can support better overall health outcomes for menstruating individuals (Saha *et al.*, 2005).

5.2.3. The Impact of Culture on Menstrual Health

Menstrual perceptions have a profound cultural influence on menstrual health, particularly in the third world context. Menstruation tends to be tainted by cultural taboo and stigma in most cultures, so that menstruating individuals are ostracized. Stigma discourages open debate of menstrual health, and ignorance and misinformation ensue. In countries like India, where traditional beliefs are likely to have a strong bearing on practice, adolescent girls may be conditioned to view menstruation as shameful rather than a biological process. This cultural construct, in turn, influences their belief regarding menstrual hygiene management (MHM) and leads to unsafe practices harming physical and psychological health. These cultural beliefs need to be addressed because they are directly linked to the health and self-esteem of girls and are a hindrance to appropriate health education and access (Anne *et al.*, 2024). Finally, cultural norms control the availability and use of menstrual hygiene products, and this has a significant influence on the overall health outcome for menstruators. In urban areas of India, while information and access to medical care may be higher than in rural areas, many girls are still hindered from accessing sanitary products under current cultural beliefs. These are further compounded by poor facilities, e.g., no access to sanitation facilities within schools that discourage the attendance of girls at school during menstruation. As noted in different research articles, where culture limits the efficient management of menstruation, the consequent physical distress and social exclusion impair girls' school achievement and mental health (N/A, 2010). Therefore, reversing these deeply ingrained cultural customs is required so that a situation can be established where menstruating men and women can operate efficiently. Lastly, the connection between culture and menstrual health emphasizes the importance of locally relevant education and intervention measures. Cultural change must take place to break down stigma around menstruation and promote healthier behavior. Menstrual health education that works must be culturally sensitive and aim to involve communities, building understanding and accepting menstruation as part of normal life. Enhanced access to menstrual products, as well as education capable of deconstructing harmful cultural presumptions, must be included in programs. These programs have the potential to empower adolescent girls to manage their menstruation with dignity and confidence, and ultimately lead to the achievement of broader Sustainable Development Goals in gender equality and health (Anne *et al.*, 2024). Breaking down cultural barriers through community engagement has the potential to transform perceptions and practices regarding menstrual health at its very foundation, ushering in a more just world.

Test Your Knowledge

1. What are some common taboos and stigmas associated with menstruation?
2. How can cultural beliefs impact menstrual health and access to hygiene products?

5.3. Psychological Effects of Menstruation

Learning Outcome

1. Discuss the emotional changes during the menstrual cycle
2. Analyze the relationship between menstruation and mental health
3. Identify effective coping strategies for menstrual-related mood swings

The psychological effect of menstruation can be felt in many forms, having a significant effect on women's emotional and psychological status. Most women complain of mood swings, increased irritability, and heightened anxiety during menstruation. All these psychological changes can be attributed to hormonal changes, particularly the change in estrogen and progesterone levels. This hormonally cyclical process often co-occurs with changes in neurotransmitter functioning, and emotional stability and mood can be directly impacted. Also, social stigma surrounding menstruation may increase distress or anxiety further, leading the woman to internalize her experience in a negative way. Thus, understanding the psychosomatic correlation between the hormonal changes and emotional responses is essential in order to address the psychological effects associated with menstruation. In addition to mood swings, the psychological impact of menstruation is intensified by other significant contributing factors such as stress, sleep, and body image. Evidence confirms that a direct connection between states of stress and disturbances of the menstrual cycle is prevalent, reflecting that women who are subjected to increased stress are more susceptible to psychological disturbances during menstruation. In addition, the sleep quality is also critical; women who do not sleep well report more emotional distress, including depression and anxiety, in the time frame of their menstrual cycle. Observational research has determined that women with irregular body mass indices also suffer psychologically with regard to their menstrual cycles. Such findings draw attention to the importance of recognition of contextual effects on emotional well-being in menstruation and indicate the necessity for an integrated health approach towards women's health that involves psychological support.

The convergence between psychological implications and menstruation draws a call towards raising awareness and education around such an experience. Placing the heightened conversation surrounding menstruation within the context of society can minimize stigma and establish enabling environments for women. School and community-based educational programs can orient individuals to learn about the psychological effects of menstruation as well as coping mechanisms to manage distress. Peer support groups and counseling can also provide women with a safe space to discuss their experiences openly. As studies on menstrual well-being point out, it is important to address the psychological effect of menstruation not just for the person but also to improve understanding of women's health issues at a broader level (Fitriani *et al.*, 2019; Gharravi *et al.*, 2009).

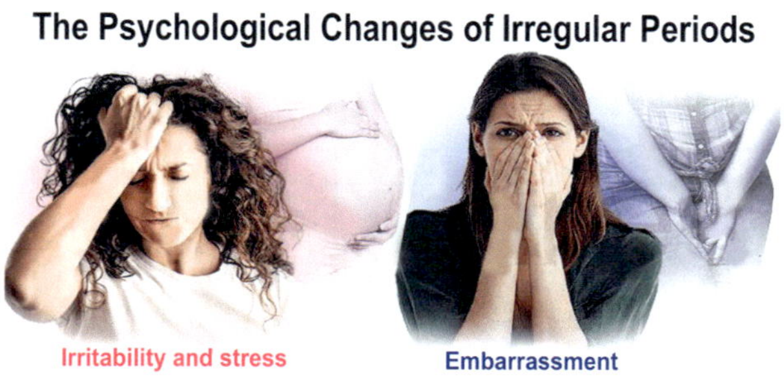

Figure 5.5. The Psychological changes of irregular period.

Source: https://www.shecares.com/imgs/e/9/8/911270/the-effects-of-irregular-periods-psychological-and-physical.png

5.3.1. Emotional Changes During the Menstrual Cycle

The affective profile women experience during their menstrual cycle is a complex mixture of hormonal fluctuations and psychosocial factors. Every phase of the cycle, and particularly the luteal phase, is marked by changing states of mood. This period is typically also marked by heightened irritability, anxiety, and mood swings, commonly debated within the context of premenstrual syndrome (PMS). PMS provides a range of affective symptoms that can go a long way in diminishing the productivity and overall quality of life for women, illustrating the great impact hormonal changes have on emotional well-being. Incorporating the knowledge of how these cycles affect daily activities, especially for teenagers, is important in raising knowledge and facilitating better coping mechanisms for those who experience such changes (Fitriani *et al.*, 2019). Studies accentuate that emotional variation during the menstrual cycle can be brought about by factors external to the body, such as body mass index (BMI), sleep quality, and stress. Interaction among these factors and menstrual cycle disorders is well established; women with high levels of stress are most vulnerable to emotional disturbances. For example, studies indicate that adolescents with a poor quality of sleep are at a higher risk of irregularities in menstrual cycles, which can lead to the associated emotional changes during this phase (Fitriani *et al.*, 2019). Additionally, maintaining a healthy BMI can eliminate some of the deleterious impacts on emotional stability, thereby validating the necessity for overall wellness in managing menstrual-related emotional symptoms. The widespread occurrence of PMS among young females, particularly in learning institutions, raises profound implications on educational performance and overall mental health. Almost 60.8% of nursing students reported having endured PMS, a symptom associated with lowered quality of life in most domains like physical wellbeing, psychological state, and social functioning. As research indicates, the psychological effects of PMS can disrupt learning outcomes, reducing concentration and class attendance. Management of these emotional changes requires a holistic approach blending health education, mental health interventions, and lifestyle intervention, thereby enhancing resilience and the quality of life for those undergoing the emotional alterations caused by the menstrual cycle (Kustriyanti *et al.*, 2020).

5.3.2. The Relationship Between Menstruation and Mental Health

The intricate interaction between menstruation and psychiatry is evident in the case of the majority of women who are PMS victims. PMS is characterized by a range of physical, behavioral, and emotional symptoms seen during the luteal phase of the menstrual cycle. The evidence indicates that PMS not only affects quality of life but also academic and workplace performance. Especially, in a study of nursing female students, an impressive 60.8% prevalence rate of PMS has been found. Symptoms such as reduced concentration and absence can further increase the level of stress and anxiety, ultimately leading to a compromised mental health setting for those individuals (Kustriyanti *et al.*, 2020). Due to these reasons, understanding the implications of PMS on mental health is crucial in addressing the bigger issues of women's health and well-being. Aside from PMS, the menstrual cycle in general can influence emotional mood throughout different periods. Mood swings and cognitive function have been linked to endogenous variations of estrogen and progesterone. It has been suggested that females would experience increased symptoms of depression or anxiety at certain times of their menstrual cycle, particularly the premenstrual and menstrual periods. This emotional instability can interfere with day-to-day functioning and interpersonal relationships, and the recognition of menstruation as a significant influencer on mental health becomes more and more vital. Moreover, the social stress with respect to menstruation can augment stigma and anxiety regarding these normal physiological events, which ultimately impact the mental health condition of women (Chapman *et al.*, 2015).

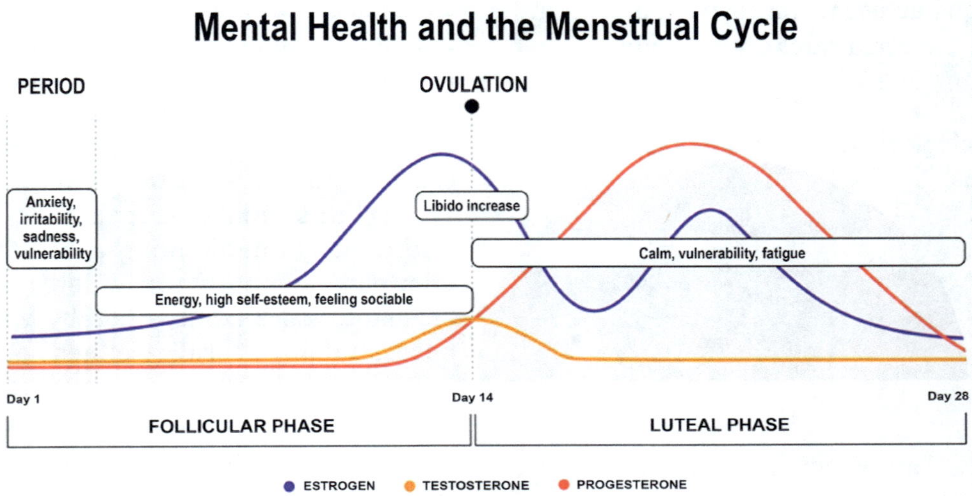

Figure 5.6. The menstrual cycle affect mental health.

Source: https://images.prismic.io/tuune-blog/21a1d29c-f035-4b97-9f7d-fd40d9c0d057_Mental+Health+%26+the+Menstrual+Cycle.png?auto=compress%2Cformat&fit=max&q=100&w=900&h=490

The intersection of menstruation, mood, and social attitudes is worthy of complete consideration for better treating women's emotional and psychological needs. Managing the mental health issues of menstruation is vital in the development of effective care practices. Increased knowledge and sensitivity in the clinical and educational settings can assist in providing comforting environments to the women who experience PMS and other related mental health issues.

Psychological therapies, such as counseling and lifestyle changes, may also benefit the sufferers. In addition, education of women about the menstrual cycle and its likely impact on mental wellbeing can help them approach resources when they need them. This kind of awareness may also push researchers and healthcare professionals to devise targeted interventions that consider the psychological impact of menstruation. In this manner, they can significantly enhance the health of women who undergo the complex interplay of menstruation and mental well-being (Kustriyanti *et al.*, 2020; Chapman *et al.*, 2015).

5.3.3. Coping Strategies For Menstrual-Related Mood Swings

Menstrual mood swings are a common occurrence for most individuals experiencing menstruation, which primarily brings about significant emotional distress. Awareness of effective coping strategies is essential in dealing with such changes. A study conducted among female students revealed that 77.7% of the subjects reported experiencing mood swings, an indication of the commonality of the experience among university students. Resting and sleeping were two of the most common coping activities, and they were effective mechanisms to reduce distress brought about by mood swings. By putting the importance of adequate sleep and taking breaks throughout their menstrual cycle first, individuals can de-intensify the emotional pain of such fluctuations. Stating that accepting menstruation as a natural process may help ease the psychological load and hence facilitate a healthier attitude towards one's menstrual cycle could also be effective. In addition to the mere coping strategies, more official means of coping may enhance emotional health during menstruation. Aerobic exercise and exercise of muscle strength have been proposed as effective coping strategies.

Engaging in such exercise not only causes the release of endorphins, which can spontaneously improve mood, but also leads to improved physical health. The inclusion of light to moderate exercise in lifestyle can be an anticipatory strategy for coping with mood swings. Moreover, support for stress management behaviors, such as yoga or mindfulness, can help individuals develop emotional resilience in their most challenging menstrual cycles. These changes in lifestyle are essential in creating a supportive environment for menstruators, promoting physical and emotional welfare.

Lastly, the value of social support cannot be overestimated in managing menstrual mood fluctuations. Peer groups have the potential to serve as a great source of friendship and support in difficult situations. Menstrual education programs that demystify menstruation and its related symptoms are needed to build an educated community. Such programs may facilitate open discussion about menstruation, de-stigmatize it, and provide a peer support network. The insight based on research is that learners often exhibit poor health-seeking behavior, suggesting the need for improved awareness and availability. Universities can improve overall mental health during menstruation for students by implementing environments that involve healthy coping as well as proper understanding (Akpoigho *et al.*, 2022; Matsuura *et al.*, 2024).

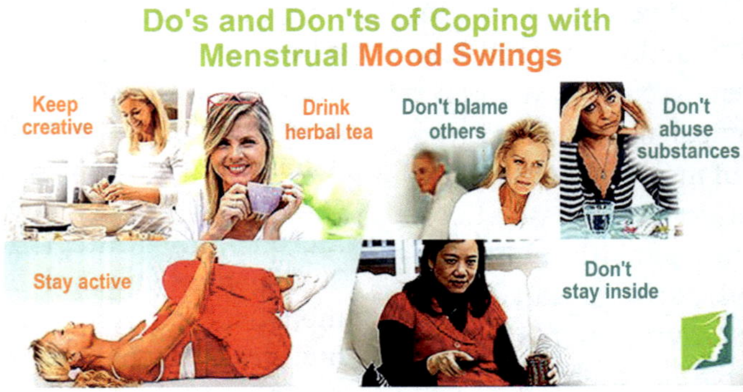
Do's and Don'ts of Coping with
Menstrual Mood Swings
Keep creative
Drink herbal tea
Don't blame others
Don't abuse substances
Stay active
Don't stay inside

Figure 5.7. Do's and Don'ts of Coping with Menstrual Mood Swings

Source: https://www.menopausenow.com/mood-swings/articles/dos-and-donts-of-coping-with-menstrual-mood-swings

Test Your Knowledge

1. How can menstruation affect mental health conditions such as anxiety or depression?
2. What are some effective coping strategies for managing mood swings related to the menstrual cycle?

5.4. Menstrual Health and Hygiene

Learning Outcome

1. Explain the importance of menstrual hygiene management
2. Evaluate the impact of access to menstrual products
3. Demonstrate an understanding of effective education on menstrual health

Menstrual hygiene and health (MHM) are key components of health education that touch the lives of adolescent girls in a profound manner. Menstruation is still a cause of stigma and myths in most parts of the globe, particularly in developing countries. As such, sanitary products and proper information regarding menstrual care are not easily accessible to most girls. MHM is not just important for physical health; dignity, privacy, and emotional well-being are also involved. The solution to menstruation problems is central to girls' and women's empowerment so that they can manage their menstruation free from any hindrance. Deconstructing education against the cultural taboo of menstruation not only builds a more enlightened society but also drives policy changes towards improving resources for women and girls, which eventually contributes to their health outcomes and the global goals. Studies have established that knowledge and information about menstrual hygiene differ markedly between adolescent populations. A study among urban adolescent girls in India found that although the participants had some basic knowledge about menstruation, they lacked hygiene practices related to its management and received different social stigmas. Specifically, girls reported difficulty accessing good hygiene facilities within homes as well as schools. These obstacles are not only practical but deeply embedded in cultural beliefs that view menstruation as unattractive or something to be ashamed of. The consequences of inadequate menstrual education can have manifestations in higher risks of infection, pain, and psychological discomfort during menstruation, and therefore the demand for extensive outreach programs that offer girls the information and resources to maintain proper menstrual health, thus enabling them to cope with this natural process of life adequately and without fear (Anne *et al.*, 2024). Moreover, the impact of poor menstrual hygiene is not only personal; it also affects education and gender equality. Poor facilities and the lack of ongoing education create a culture that dissuades girls' school attendance during menstruation. Proper menstrual hygiene facilities are indispensable to the power to concentrate and may lead to absenteeism, harming grades. Studies have shown that focused intervention to improve access to menstrual products and facilities in schools can lead to a considerable positive impact on the learning experience of adolescent girls. As reported, there exists an urgent need for comprehensive menstrual health education in schools alongside a public campaign to help change society's perceptions of menstruation (Aluma *et al.*, 2021). By addressing these linked challenges, we can establish a society where girls are confident and dignified in their ability to manage their menstruation, thereby achieving sustainable development outcomes.

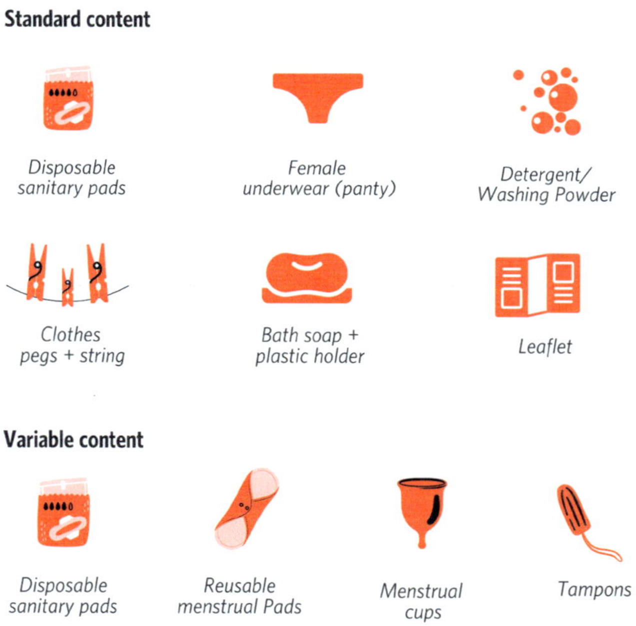
Standard content
Disposable sanitary pads
Female underwear (panty)
Detergent/ Washing Powder
Clothes pegs + string
Bath soap + plastic holder
Leaflet
Variable content
Disposable sanitary pads
Reusable menstrual Pads
Menstrual cups
Tampons

Figure 5.8. Menstrual Hygiene Management.

Source: https://www.unfpa.org/sites/default/files/styles/common_style/public/resource-cover-image/MHM%20kit%20-%20infographic.png?itok=bQJ_q1fZ

5.4.1. Importance of Menstrual Hygiene Management

Menstrual hygiene management (MHM) is an important element of gender equality and public health, particularly for menstruators. Essentially, MHM refers to a collection of practices enabling menstruators to maintain cleanliness and good dignity during their menstrual cycles. Provision of appropriate menstrual products, sanitation facilities, and education empowers menstruators with information to manage their menstruation well, reducing infections and ensuring well-being. Besides individual health, the value of MHM extends beyond societal institutions; it has a significant role within broader societal institutions, exerting impacts on education and economic progress. If individuals are secure and not bothered during menstruation, they will be actively participating in school and at the workplace, thus leading to a more just society.

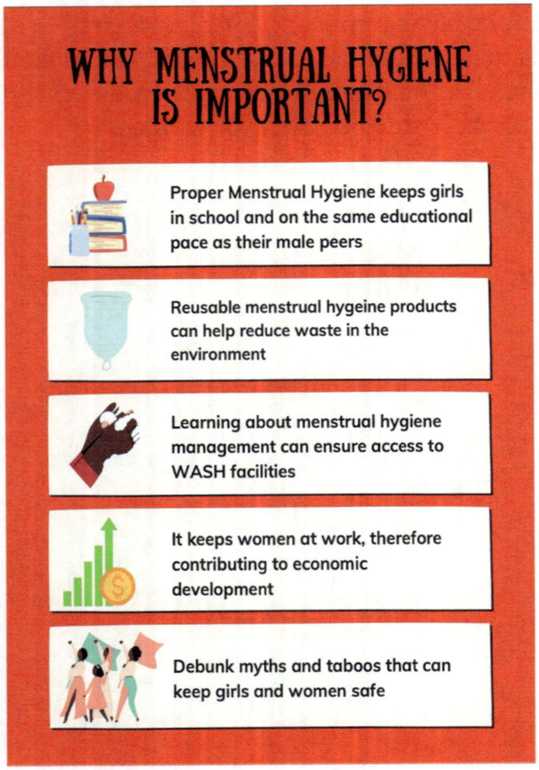

Source: https://external-content.duckduckgo.com/iu/?u=https%3A%2F%2Fpbs.twimg.com%2Fmedia%2FE5AllD3WEAMtRmQ.jpg%3Alarge&f=1&nofb=1&ipt=533fb00cfd72ef87bacfcb01e3ee8fff3945529e420c487c6900f14740583024

Menstrual hygiene can thus be enhanced through public policies that are embraced holistically. The recognition of MHM as a key part of human rights puts the realization of gender equality at its center. Legal regimes have been prone to ignoring the significance of menstrual hygiene, with menstruators both denied access to products and burdened by egregious taxes that characterize hygiene products as non-essential luxury items. Campaigns to end the tampon tax highlight the gender stereotypes deeply embedded in legal regimes around menstruation. By acknowledging menstrual hygiene products as necessities, and not luxuries, societies can begin to tackle inequalities embedded in the system. Legal reforms can be potent tools in the endeavor, demanding a shift in society that recognizes MHM as a fundamental right essential to gender equality and human dignity. Activists are increasingly resisting punitive policies in court cases and campaigns, a sign of a growing awareness of the need for legal recognition of menstrual equity in human rights agendas.

Educating individuals is also imperative in helping to instill menstrual hygiene management. Organized public health programs that raise awareness and knowledge of menstrual health can potentially break down deep-rooted stigmas and cultural taboos surrounding menstruation. Education allows menstruators to make sound-informed choices on product usage, hygiene routine, and self-care during menstruation. In particular, incorporating menstrual hygiene education in school curricula can introduce proper discourse among young people, establishing a culture of openness and comprehension. As social norms shift to embrace menstruation as an open-to-discuss issue, the long-term impact on health outcomes as well as on gender equity grows increasingly significant. By promoting inclusive education focusing on MHM, societies can provide future generations with the information and confidence to take care of their menstrual health without any difficulties, eventually building a more equitable society at large.

5.4.2. Access To Menstrual Products

Availability of menstrual products is a significant part of human menstruation that transcends individuals' experience and into the broader public health and social justice discourse. There are many individuals with significant barriers to using these essential products due to financial concerns, stigma, or unavailability in their area. Exclusion from access can lead to negative health effects, including increased vulnerability to disease and psychological distress, which are added features to what is already a natural physiological process. It's of particular concern in marginalized communities where economic constraints could prevent individuals from accessing menstrual products. Abolitionists would argue that efforts towards menstrual equity must prioritize policies dismantling such barriers so that all people can access such products without stigma or shame (Crawford *et al.*, 2020). In addition, the terms of menstrual product access are wrapped up in broader societal perceptions of menstruation itself. Several commercials and the general public conversation regarding menstrual products have been inclined to avoid the realities of menstruation by being euphemistic in their language, thus having a tendency to maintain an air of embarrassment towards this natural biological function. The ambiguity of the majority of female hygiene commercials can not only lead to the lack of extensive awareness of the options available but also diminished interest in menstrual health (Schulte *et al.*, 2019). This gap serves to sustain stereotypes and stigma around menstruation, ultimately eroding the strides towards increasing access to menstrual products. Advocacy groups and policymakers should thus move to bridge this gap by promoting free conversation and lobbying for widespread education on menstruation that covers information on products accessed and their value. Addressing access to menstrual products has significant implications on gender justice and human rights. Menstrual equity involves not only access to products but also ensuring the promotion of the acceptance of menstruation as a vital aspect of health that merits recognition in legal structures and public policy. The present trend of menstrual equity has brought into perspective the importance of integrating this discussion in gender justice debates, where women, particularly low-income women and marginalized women, are disproportionately affected by a lack of access to menstrual items (Crawford *et al.*, 2020).

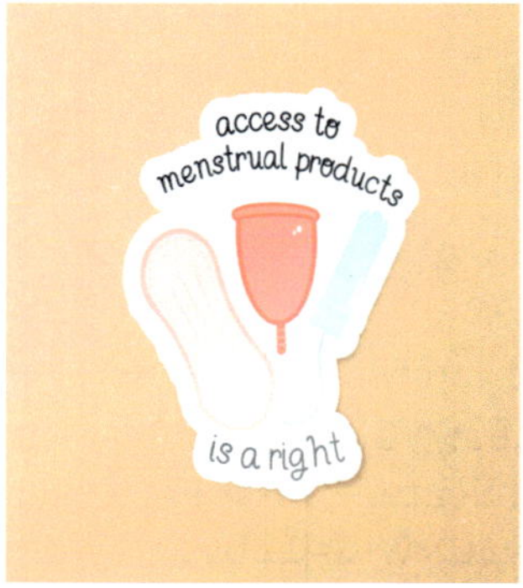

Figure 5.9. Access to menstrual hygiene products.

Source: https://i.etsystatic.com/22457845/r/il/dfbd42/3786300226/il_fullxfull.3786300226_9h6m.jpg

Future initiatives must not only focus on the distribution of menstrual products but also recognize the complex interplay of social factors that contribute to inequalities in access. Efforts geared toward promoting menstrual equity can facilitate broader discussions about health equity and the need for inclusive policies that acknowledge and address the diverse experiences of menstruators.

5.4.3. Education on Menstrual Health

Menstrual health education is crucial in the process of dispelling social taboos and stigma around menstruation. The majority of adolescent girls, especially in developing countries, have severe menstrual hygiene management constraints based on prevalent cultural assumptions stigmatizing open discussion on menstruation. Such silence may lead to myths and fear regarding body transformation, thus complicating menstruation management among young people.

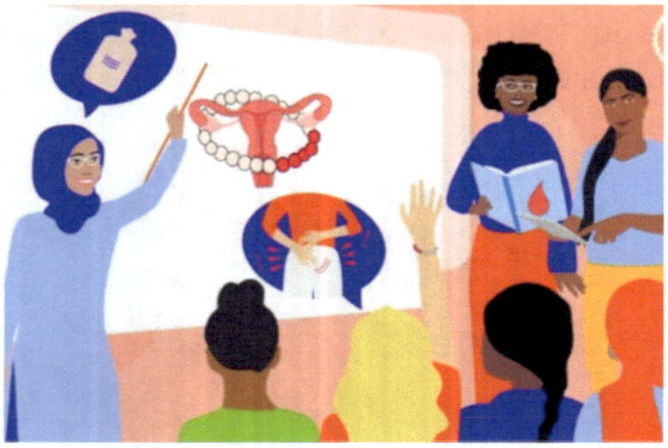

Source: https://s7d1.scene7.com/is/image/wbcollab/Education_fb-standard-fb-shared1?qlt=90&hei=630&wid=1200&fit=hfit

As has been observed in research on urban Indian adolescent girls, even where access to education has been relatively enhanced, there continues to exist a substantive knowledge deficiency in menstrual management and its hygiene habits (Anne *et al.*, 2024). This is a testimony to the urgent necessity for comprehensive education programs that not only impart factual knowledge but also facilitate easy communication so as to create an enabling environment for girls undergoing these biological transformations in life. Additionally, the impact of effective education programs in molding menstrual health cannot be overstated. Recent conferences, such as the Second Annual Virtual MHM in WinS Conference, emphasize the necessity of strategies that are uniquely tailored to identify barriers and quantify the efficacy of those strategies implemented (Vasquez *et al.*, 2014).

By recognizing the unique challenges encountered in varying environments, school programs can be designed to suit specific needs. Such interventions must involve community and cultural elements, resulting in a program attractive to the target group. Improved access to sanitary products, along with hygiene etiquette education, can profoundly enhance the health and welfare of menstruating individuals beyond merely academic knowledge to give them confidence and dignity at the time of menstruation. In expanding the discourse around menstrual health education, it is of utmost importance to engage various stakeholders, including parents, teachers, and healthcare providers. These group dynamics may provide a better understanding of menstrual change and adolescents' support needs. Education programs can be given in schools, communities, and home settings, where discussion may normalize and desensitize menstruation, thus reducing stigma. Moreover, establishing open communication lines may allow girls to seek required medical assistance in situations of menstrual health issues. This comprehensive response is aligned with global education goals and underscores the interconnections among education, health, and gender equity. The vision is a world in which menstruation is freely discussed, well-managed, and without stigma (Anne *et al.*, 2024).

Test Your Knowledge

1. What are the consequences of limited access to menstrual products on girls and women?
2. How does education on menstrual health contribute to breaking stigma and improving hygiene practices?

5.5. Menstruation and Reproductive Health

Learning Outcome

1. Describe menstruation as an indicator of reproductive health
2. Identify common menstrual disorders
3. Explain the role of menstruation in fertility

Menstruation is a critical reproductive health indicator, having a direct relation to the health and daily lives of menstruating people. Menstruation is not only a biological phenomenon but also a complex web of cultural, social, and personal influences. Adequate information on menstrual hygiene management (MHM) is required, as inadequate information can lead to stigmatization, health issues, and loss of education. For instance, studies on Nepali schoolgirls' experience and knowledge found severe gaps in knowledge about proper menstrual hygiene practice and suggested that there is a need for educational intervention to improve reproductive health outcomes. The findings are particularly significant in emphasizing the need for specially focused educational campaigns that start addressing the obstacles to effective MHM and attempt to dismantle myths surrounding menstruation (N/A, 2011). The reproductive health and menstruation implications are most forcefully felt in the developing world, where cultural biases tend to undermine optimal practices. Conferences like the MHM in WinS Conference offer a forum to discuss research and methodology that address these issues directly. The process of dialogue at conferences like the MHM in WinS Conference underscores the importance of empirical research instruments that can test MHM interventions in varied settings. This is essential in establishing local menstrual hygiene barriers, which can have a significant influence on school attendance and general health among menstruators. Through the use of scientifically sound study techniques, stakeholders can formulate locally responsive interventions that address particular communities, ultimately resulting in better reproductive health service quality and supporting broader development goals (Vasquez *et al.*, 2014). Furthermore, the intersection of menstruation and reproductive health is key to promoting gender equality and empowerment. Menstrual stigma can dramatically lower girls' confidence and limit their participation in education and public life. Addressing such issues will require coordinated action by policymakers, educators, and health professionals to create facilitative environments. Interventions that focus on the education of parents and teachers on menstrual health can contribute to a culture of openness and compassion, an imperative move towards de-stigmatizing menstruation. By promoting menstrual health, therefore, not only does it improve the well-being of individuals, but it also sparks social change, with ripple effects towards the empowerment of women and girls in various facets of society. Understanding the intricate dynamics of menstruation in reproductive health is therefore important to an integrated approach in health care and education.

5.5.1. Menstruation As An Indicator of Reproductive Health

Menstruation is a significant marker of female reproductive well-being, an expression of a multifaceted array of physiological and psychological states that affect women. The menstrual cycle is controlled by various factors, including body mass index (BMI), quality of sleep, and levels of stress. Research has found that changes in menstrual cycles can act as markers of pathology; e.g., women with abnormal BMI have almost a twofold likelihood of experiencing menstrual disorders. Moreover, the study highlights that low-quality sleep and elevated levels of stress have an integral role to play in menstrual disturbances, highlighting the interrelationship between physical and psychological health. The awareness of these interactions allows medical practitioners to enhance patient assessment of a woman's reproductive health and implement proper intervention with customized strategies, resulting in greater overall well-being and, in turn, potentially preventing further severe health complications (Fitriani *et al.*, 2019). The advent of technology has rewired our capacity to monitor and understand menstruation as an indicator of health. The growth of menstrual monitoring apps such as Clue has accumulated massive user data, showing trends that were previously difficult to quantify using traditional survey tools. Research of over 378,000 users established that irregularities in cycle length and predictability are predictors of larger-scale health conditions, such as endometriosis. By reaching self-reported qualitative symptoms alongside statistical data, health workers can gain better insight into individual menstrual health. It is this blending of technology and medicine that makes for better insight into characteristics within usual cycles, allowing for more accurate health assessments and the ability to implement early interventions (Druet *et al.*, 2020).

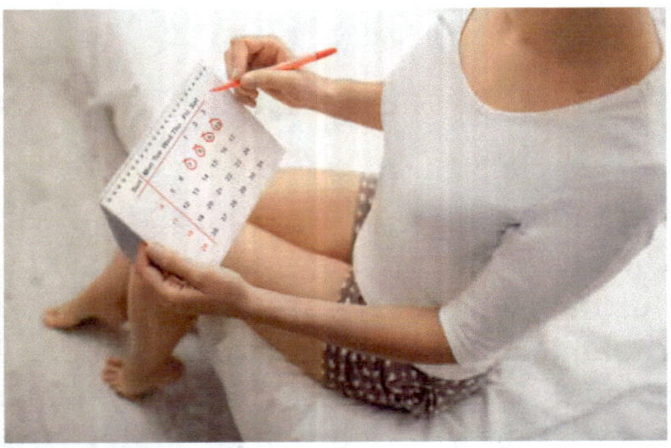

Figure 5.10. Menstrual cycle is a vital sign and important indicator of reproductive health.

Source: https://images.theconversation.com/files/610635/original/file-20240731-17-vbqgfd.jpg?ixlib=rb-4.1.0&rect=0%2C0%2C5484%2C3840&q=20&auto=format&w=320&fit=clip&dpr=2&usm=12&cs=strip

Additionally, menstrual health is not just evidenced by the biological processes of menstruation, but also by the psychological consequences that accompany menstrual disorders. The majority of women acquire serious emotional disturbances from irregular menstruation or disabling symptoms like dysmenorrhea, which then compromises overall well-being. An understanding of the psychological and emotional dimensions of menstruation is critical in the holistic conceptualization of reproductive health. As research grows, qualitative data by way of menstrual monitoring can be incorporated to identify symptomatic trends in experience, ultimately guiding clinicians to forecast menstrual irregularities. On this premise, a whole-person approach towards accounting for physical as well as psychological dimensions of menstruation can lead to improved health outcomes and well-being for women at various stages in life (Fitriani *et al.*, 2019; Druet *et al.*, 2020).

5.5.2. Common Menstrual Disorders

Menstruation is always accompanied by some disorders that have a significant impact on a woman's quality of life. The most prevalent disorders include dysmenorrhea, amenorrhea, and oligomenorrhea. Dysmenorrhea refers to the aching menstrual cramps experienced by most women during their periods, interfering with their daily routine and general health. Dysmenorrhea can be classified as primary dysmenorrhea, which is brought about by hormonal disturbances, and secondary dysmenorrhea, which is related to conditions such as fibroids or endometriosis. The impact of dysmenorrhea is far greater than mere physical discomfort and, in most instances, reaches psychological morbidity and loss of productivity. Therefore, the knowledge and management of these menstrual disorders are significant towards the promotion of women's well-being and health as they are key indicators of women's general health that may be dependent on the body mass index (BMI), sleep quality, and stress level (Fitriani *et al.*, 2019).

Amenorrhea, or the lack of menses, can occur in different manners due to various etiologies such as lifestyle habits, hormonal imbalance, and disease conditions. Primary amenorrhea happens in teenagers who have not yet begun menstruation at the age of 16 years, while secondary amenorrhea is the failure to experience menstruation for three months or more in females who have previously menstruated (Gharravi *et al.*, 2009). These disturbances are highly disruptive, and they are largely reflective of underlying ailments such as polycystic ovary syndrome (PCOS), thyroid diseases, or undue exercise and stress. This highlights the importance of increased awareness and monitoring of menstrual cycles, especially among adolescent girls and young women, as they may be indicators of general health problems. Menstrual abnormalities can then not only be rectified by treating amenorrhea, but also the general health of the individual can be improved. Oligomenorrhea, or infrequent periods that are typically characterized as cycles over 35 days, is another common menstrual abnormality with significant impacts on health. It is typically an indication of underlying hormonal disturbances, such as in PCOS, which may lead to infertility if untreated. Aside from its physiological impacts, oligomenorrhea is most commonly linked with mental illnesses due to the anxiety and pressure of not knowing when menstrual cycles might return. Evidence suggests a basic interplay between variables such as BMI, degree of stress, and sleep quality on menstrual cycle regularity, which suggests that integral treatment is required for such conditions (Fitriani *et al.*, 2019). Having an understanding of the complex etiology of oligomenorrhea can allow women to receive appropriate care and treatment, which can improve their reproductive health and overall well-being.

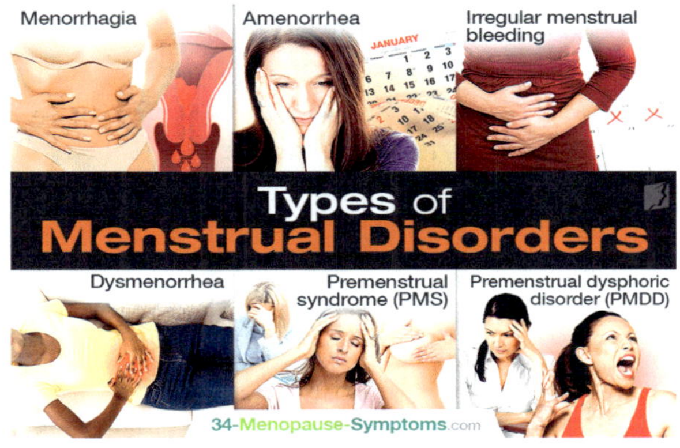
Menorrhagia
Amenorrhea
Irregular menstrual bleeding
Types of
Menstrual Disorders
Dysmenorrhea
Premenstrual syndrome (PMS)
Premenstrual dysphoric disorder (PMDD)
34-Menopause-Symptoms.com

Figure 5.11. Common menstrual disorders.

Source: https://www.menopausenow.com/pics/6/b/2/738832/menstrual-disorders.png

5.5.3. The Role of Menstruation in Fertility

Menstruation plays a central role in the complex menstrual cycle of women's fertility, acting as a significant sign of reproductive well-being. Menstruation is part of several distinct hormonal changes that prepare the body for potential conception. During each month, the ovaries release an egg during the process of ovulation, which generally occurs at the midpoint of the cycle. In the event of a breakdown in fertilization, the endometrial lining that had been thickened in anticipation of implantation is shed off during menstruation. This repetitive process is required to restore hormonal balance as well as prepare the female body for future pregnancy. Abnormalities during this cycle may be an indicator of other underlying conditions and thus point to menstruation as a predictive factor for reproductive capability and health, such as is emphasized in studies of natural family planning methods (Fehring *et al.*, 2010).

In addition, the relationship between menstruation and fertility has particular applicability when addressing disorders such as polycystic ovary syndrome (PCOS), which affects a noteworthy percentage of the reproductive-age female population. PCOS disrupts regular hormonal balance, leading to irregular or even absent menstruation that consequently impacts ovulation and fertility. Understanding this relationship is essential; treatment of PCOS with success typically involves lifestyle modification and hormone regulation to attain a regular menstrual cycle and, hence, enhance fertility possibilities. Studies highlight how, by addressing hormonal imbalances common with PCOS, women can overcome most of the fertility problems and aid a healthier reproductive system (Bernier *et al.*, 2012). This illustrates the need for general public education and awareness regarding the significance of the menstrual cycle to fertility.

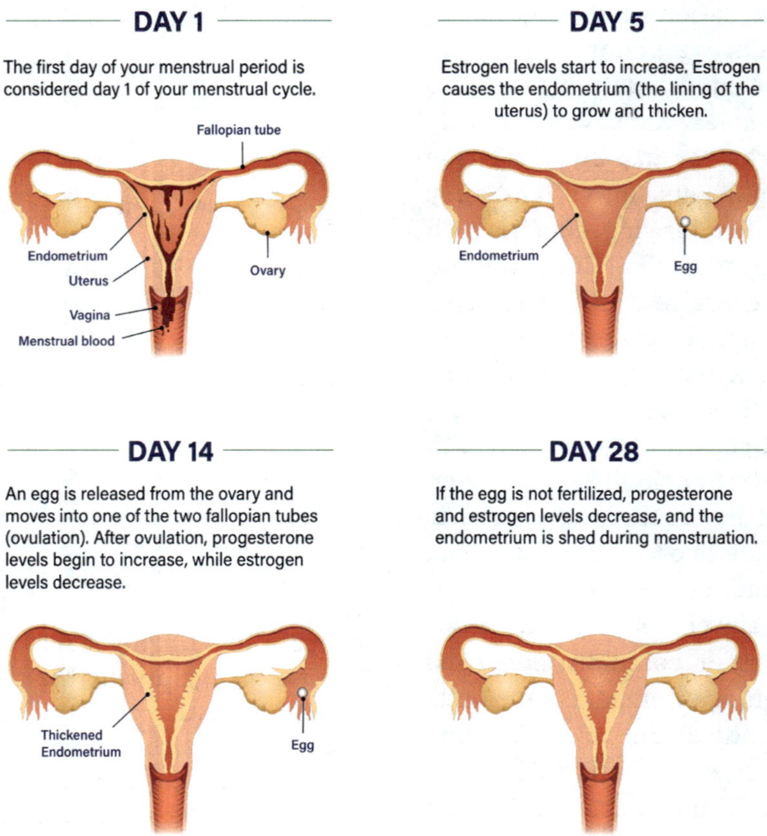

Figure 5.12. Menstrual cycle is one of the most powerful tools for understanding your fertility.

Source: https://positivestepsfertility.com/blog/menstrual-cycle-and-fertility/

Menstruation also has implications beyond the individual's health, influencing society's understanding of female reproduction and healthcare strategies. Menstrual cycle knowledge is vital for women and health care providers alike since it guides family planning and reproductive health management choices. The ability to track and understand one's menstrual cycle allows women to control their reproductive health, facilitating quick medical action in the event of anomalies. Culturally, increased understanding of menstruation will assist in dismantling stigmas and taboos regarding women's health issues, allowing for improved access to reproductive health information and more honest discourse. Ultimately, having knowledge that menstruation is a very important aspect of fertility not only provides individuals with improved health outcomes but also assists in developing a more educated, more supportive community for women's reproductive rights and health (Fehring *et al.*, 2010).

Test Your Knowledge

1. How does menstruation serve as an indicator of reproductive health?
2. What are some common menstrual disorders and their symptoms?

5.6. Societal Implications of Menstruation

Learning Outcome

1. Define menstruation in the workplace
2. Evaluate the importance of advocacy for menstrual equity
3. Explain the role of policy in menstrual health

The social impact of menstruation extends to public lives, generally shaping cultural discourse and public health policy. Menstruation is generally devalued in most societies by stigma, producing overall silence around the topic. Silence may perpetuate misinformation and introduce feelings of shame in menstruators. Incidentally, this cultural taboo keeps women back from confidence and participation in numerous fields of society, for example, education and work. To push past such adversity, effective awareness campaigns are key. These campaigns can provide clear information on menstrual health and remove the secrecy around the process itself to make way for a salubrious discussion on menstruation. Notably, ads for menstrual hygiene products consistently have trouble with this vagueness, and require striking a touchy balance between creative advertising and actual education. By prioritizing informative approaches, the globe can empower menstruators and reduce the stigma surrounding this natural biological phenomenon (Schulte *et al.*, 2019).

Schools are also key battlegrounds for dealing with the social impacts of menstruation, particularly in the developing world. Where access to education varies substantially by gender, such as in countries like Ethiopia, menstruation is a primary determinant of girls' educational trajectories. Research shows that only 57% of Ethiopian girls attend primary school, and enrollment declines to a paltry 31% at secondary levels (Aman *et al.*, 2024). Menstruation combined with gender-positive cultural attitudes and the absence of enhanced sanitary facilities leads to absenteeism and increased drop-out rates among girls. Such disruption not only deepens gender inequality but also stifles economic and social development. Thus, it is necessary that steps for raising access to feminine hygiene and schooling are taken. Working with menstruation serves to end gender discrimination and enforce a culture of equality for education. Moreover, the significance of menstruation is deeply ingrained in public health programming. Access to menstrual products forms part of ensuring women's well-being and well-roundedness.

While in other societies, the lack of affordable sanitary materials opens a window of unsafe behavior where women resort to using unclean materials to control their menstrual flow, endangering infection and long-term health issues. Public campaigns must target making available safe, sanitary supplies and information about menstrual health. This entails advocating for policy change that ensures women's access to basic healthcare commodities. The demand for these programs is further heightened where girls are faced with additional barriers such as child marriage and discrimination based on gender. By promoting education and access to menstrual products, society can enhance women's health indicators significantly and consequently their wellbeing, hence leading to improved societal well-being (Aman *et al.*, 2024).

5.6.1. Menstruation in the Workplace

The problem of menstruation at work is typically shrouded in stigma and myths, hence a lack of realization in the adoption of supporting actions for menstruating staff. The majority of workplaces are not prepared to meet the physiological and psychological effects of menstruation, and this can bring significant problems to the involved staff. The cultural silence surrounding menstruation leaves the staff isolated and unwilling to expose their needs or grievances regarding their menstrual cycle. This invisibility not only impacts personal well-being but can also affect overall workplace productivity and morale. To overcome these barriers, a shift in workplace culture that encourages open communication and educational initiatives on menstrual health is necessary. By creating a conducive environment, organizations can avert the adverse impacts of menstruation on workers and foster an inclusive environment. Implementing large-scale health programs focused on menstruation is a significant move towards acknowledging and addressing the needs of menstruating employees. Research has indicated that businesses that pursue sensitization health programs are capable of constructing healthier employees in addition to enhancing worker engagement and retention. Organizations such as HERproject illustrate how it is possible to spur awareness as well as support through training sessions on menstrual health by taking employees and employers through such opportunities. By stimulating the business value of workplace menstruation-focused health programs, companies can step forward to become more inclusive and accommodating in their policies. Moreover, such initiatives can reduce the stigma associated with menstruation, enabling employees to access aid or concessions when necessary, with greater ease, thus promoting overall workplace well-being and satisfaction (N/A, 2010).

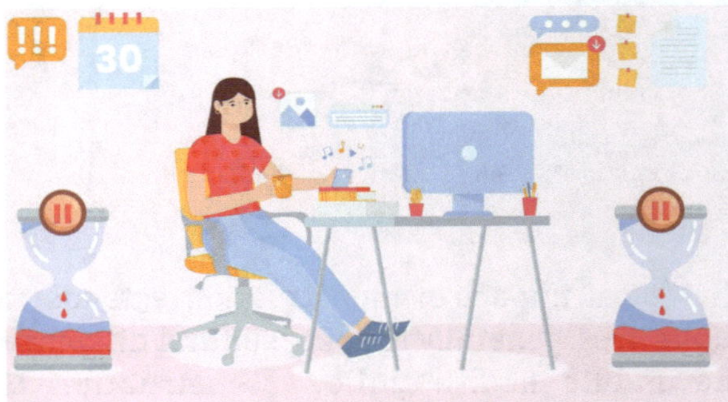

Figure 5.13. Menstrual health is a fundamental aspect of women's well-being that deserves attention and support in all aspects of life, including the workplace.

Source: https://safestree.com/blogs/period-tips/menstrual-health-in-the-workplace-supporting-women-in-every-environment

The complexity of menstrual difficulties is typically exacerbated by social stigma, which impinges on how employees manage their menstrual symptoms in the workplace. Disclosure dynamics of menstruation are a key area to understand in a secure setting that is a safe haven for addressing employee needs. A study identifies that supervisor vulnerability and employee willingness to disclose their needs as they perceive management support as a key area to observe. As noted, the failure to consider menstruation is contributing to employees' challenges in accessing proper accommodations. By fostering a culture that ensures open discussion and empathetic responses from managers, organizations can reduce barriers that discourage menstruating workers from seeking help. The shift not only improves retention and performance but also creates a more inclusive workplace, ultimately for all employees (Hayman *et al.*, 2024).

5.6.2. Advocacy For Menstrual Equity

Menstrual equity advocacy has gained momentum as an integral part of gender justice, which strives to address the social stigmas and barriers encompassing menstruation. Menstrual equity is an effort aimed at providing individuals with adequate access to menstrual products, education, and facilities without facing discrimination or financial hardship. This emergent issue overlaps with broader discussions regarding women's rights and public health and illustrates how policy far too frequently ignores the needs of menstruators, particularly those from marginalized populations. Analyzing previous advocacy efforts and litigation, it is evident that there has been progress, yet plenty of work remains to be undertaken. Activists emphasize the importance of intersectionality, where the deep experiences of menstruators are recognized and tackled in the larger agenda of menstrual justice (Crawford *et al.*, 2020). By advancing policies that ensure menstrual products are made available and inclusive, activists are building a future where menstruation is normalized and valued. The focus on menstrual equity is particularly significant in school environments, where access to menstrual products can directly impact attendance and academic performance. Schools often become sites of controversy around menstruation, with schools themselves failing to provide adequate support to students. As research done during conferences, such as the Second Annual Virtual MHM in WinS Conference, shows, menstrual health management issues usually lead to absenteeism as well as to disruption of learning activities (Vasquez *et al.*, 2014). These issues need to be overcome with multi-faceted interventions that include policy changes and education interventions that will facilitate the de-stigmatization of menstruation. By placing menstruators' needs at the forefront of institutions, activists can make an impact within institutionally grounded, educated, and empathetic policies, paving the way for a welcoming space for all learners. Moreover, the topic of menstrual equity shines a light on the economic reality of menstruation, where access to necessary products is disproportionately expensive for poor individuals. Availability and access to menstrual products vary extensively, sustaining poverty cycles as well as gender inequality. Campaigns of advocacy seek to implement legislative policies that not only reduce or eliminate taxes on menstrual products but also offer them in public institutions and facilities, particularly for poor individuals . Through partnering with broader social justice movements, menstrual equity activists are following common initiatives for economic justice while knowing that a response to menstruation is a piece of a broader pursuit of gender justice. In future work, there must be ongoing advocacy and commitment to developing cross-stakeholder partnerships to construct systemic change in the way menstruation is perceived and accounted for in society (Crawford *et al.*, 2020).

5.6.3. The Role of Policy in Menstrual Health

The policy function in menstrual health is central to shaping social attitudes and establishing norms of menstruation. Effective policies can deconstruct the stigma associated with menstruation and establish a culture of acceptance and openness. Policies address various fields such as education, access to healthcare services, and sanitation facilities for menstruating women. On that note, the integration of menstrual health management (MHM) into school curricula is essential. By educating students on menstruation in early life, policymakers can assist in reducing misinformation and fostering a more sympathetic context for individuals who go through menstruation. On top of this, sanitary product and facility guidelines within schools and workplaces can assist in ensuring that menstruation is treated with respect, thereby improving academic and professional attendance. Through such interventions, policy not only affects individual welfare but also creates a broader societal movement towards acceptance and openness regarding menstrual health. Menstrual hygiene management policies are also intrinsically connected with human rights. The ability to manage menstruation in a dignified manner has direct implications for a chain of rights, including health, education, and access to sanitation. When poorly written or non-existent policies prevail, they have the potential to greatly hinder women and girls' ability to participate in normal activities, in effect impacting their quality of life as well as human rights. There have been widespread accounts of insufficient menstrual health policies, such as the inability to be seen among refugee camps and marginalized communities where sanitary amenities are non-existent or non-functional. (N/A, 2017) indicates the adverse effects on women's and girls' rights when menstrual health is neglected. By aligning menstrual health policies with a human rights agenda, stakeholders are better positioned to address such inequalities and promote equitable access to the required resources, thus enhancing the dignity and autonomy of menstruating individuals. At the level of implementation, the success of menstrual health policies also largely relies on how effectively organizations and practitioners can put these plans into practice. The development of policy-informing tools, such as the practitioner's guide, is a key process to do so. These guides assist organizations in unraveling the complex intersections of dignity, human rights, and menstrual health, providing an actionable template for plugging described gaps in policy. (Vasquez *et al.*, 2014) emphasizes the importance of employing research tools in evaluating and enhancing MHM practices periodically. By providing improved training and education to the personnel who actually implement these policies, organizations can effectively maximize prioritization of menstrual health in environments as varied as schools and emergency response environments. Last but not least, with robust policies and informed practitioners, menstrual health can be positioned as a key component of holistic health and human rights strategies.

Test Your Knowledge

1. What challenges do menstruating individuals face in the workplace?
2. How does advocacy for menstrual equity aim to improve access and awareness?

SUMMARY

The discussion of menstruation is essential to understand the multifaceted implications that this biological process has on a lot of aspects of women's lives. From hygiene and health to social perceptions, menstruation is a very private yet very stigmatised issue. As some research has indicated, marketing of women's hygiene products is frequently untransparent, so women's identification of their requirements at menstruation becomes more complicated. The vagueness of advertising can create a culture of silence around menstruation, thus reinforcing the feeling of shame and embarrassment. It becomes crucial to spot these dynamics as it emphasizes the necessity for awareness campaigns empowering women rather than just offering products. These shifts in advertising can assist in the formation of an enlightened society with a high sense of respect towards natural cyclical phenomena found in women's biology (Schulte *et al.*, 2019). It is a timely reminder of such balance in advertising. Along with this, the link between menstruation and health has wider implications for the overall well-being of women. Research has shown that hormonal fluctuation in menstrual cycles can have direct impacts on physical and mental well-being. For example, the premenstrual phase is characterized by cyclical fluctuations in estrogen and progesterone levels, which can be a reason for mood swings and headache states like migraines. Recognizing these interrelations helps women not only to maintain control over their health but also to emphasize the importance of healthcare practitioners embracing a multidisciplinary perspective when describing menstrual health. As *et al.*Terrin *et al.* (2018) observe, there is an intricate interdependence between hormone levels and the development of certain diseases that affect women disproportionately. By prioritizing in-depth education on these dynamics, health practitioners can better serve women's needs throughout the course of their reproductive lives.

Ultimately, honoring menstruation's social nature is also integral to supporting a more inclusive conversation. It is necessary to break down and transcend stigma around this natural phenomenon so that frank conversation about menstruation can make it commonplace. In integrating menstruation education into broader public health schemes, societies are able to give women the freedom to report their experiences and challenges without fear of stigma. These programs would pave the way for policy reforms that ensure access to menstrual products and care, ultimately bringing about gender equality. The findings in all these studies, including those on the effects of menstruation on health and practices, emphasize a general need for change at the societal level. It is only through careful consideration of these questions that we can realistically reconceptualize cultural attitudes around menstruation and enable women to celebrate their natural rhythms.

Menstrual knowledge encompasses not only the physiological processes but also the influence of menstrual health on women's overall well-being. An integral component of managing menstruation is the treatment of disorders such as symptomatic uterine fibroids that can negatively impact quality of life. Existing studies have proven that drugs like ulipristal acetate (UPA) can control heavy menstrual bleeding from fibroids effectively, with a significant number of women experiencing amenorrhea after treatment. Specifically, research has proven that after a single course of UPA, 79% of the women experienced amenorrhea, which indicates the drug's efficacy in menstrual disorder management (Fauser *et al.*, 2014). Further, the average volume reduction of fibroids post-treatment demonstrates the capability of pharmacotherapy to minimize physical symptoms during menstruation, thus making an argument stronger for easily accessible treatments. Menstrual hygiene management (MHM) is another critical area of study with overlap in broader public health initiatives. Effective

MHM techniques are necessary for menstruating individuals to be able to maintain dignity, health, and hygiene throughout their menstrual cycles. This encompasses access to appropriate sanitary products, safe disposal facilities, and menstrual health education. Importantly, there is also the equally necessary need to mainstream water, sanitation, and hygiene (WASH) policies in schools, particularly among adolescent girls, in order to enable them to safely manage their menstrual cycles. With strengthened evidence generation on MHM, stakeholders are better placed to implement programs that reduce menstrual stigma and improve women's and girls' health (N/A, 2014). These developments not only impact individuals' health but also educational and societal advancement more broadly. Lastly, the menstruation discussion must include a comprehensive appreciation of its sociocultural consequences. Large percentages of individuals still encounter significant stigma with regard to menstruation, and this can erode their ability to function actively and fully in education and workplaces. By fostering open discussion of menstrual health and the necessity for proper management channels, societies can eliminate customary taboos. Education on the physiological as well as psychological consequences of menstruation facilitates individuals and fosters a culture of acceptance and support. Furthermore, the overlap between medical science and public health policy concerning the issue of menstruation underscores the necessity for a multidisciplinary approach to this natural biological process. Hence, condensing the above-mentioned facts points out that menstruation is not only a biological phenomenon but a very complex phenomenon which is deeply interwoven with medical, social, and cultural paradigms.

KEY TERMS FROM THIS CHAPTER

- Menstrual cycle
- Follicular phase
- Ovulation
- Progesterone
- Gonadotropin-releasing hormone (GnRH)
- Menarche
- Dysmenorrhea
- Oligomenorrhea
- Endometrium
- Luteal phase
- Corpus luteum
- Estrogen
- Luteinizing hormone (LH)
- Menstrual flow
- Amenorrhea
- Premenstrual syndrome (PMS)

CRITICAL THINKING QUESTIONS

1. **Which of the following is considered the most accurate diagnostic test for confirming menopause?**
   a. Ultrasound
   b. Estrogen level
   c. Follicle-stimulating hormone (FSH) level
   d. Progesterone level
2. **The transitional phase before menopause, characterized by irregular periods and hormonal changes, is called:**
   a. Postmenopause
   b. Perimenopause
   c. Premenstrual syndrome
   d. Menarche
3. **Hormone replacement therapy (HRT) is primarily used to:**
   a. Prevent pregnancy
   b. Enhance fertility
   c. Relieve menopausal symptoms
   d. Induce menopause
4. **Which of the following is a long-term health risk associated with menopause?**
   a. Acne
   b. Hypotension
   c. Osteoporosis
   d. Glaucoma
5. **A woman is considered to be in menopause after she has had no menstrual periods for:**
   a. 3 consecutive months
   b. 6 consecutive months
   c. 9 consecutive months
   d. 12 consecutive months

Short Answer Questions

1. Which two main hormones regulate the menstrual cycle?
2. Name one cultural belief or practice associated with menstruation.
3. What is a common emotional or psychological symptom experienced during menstruation?
4. Why is proper menstrual hygiene important for overall health?
5. How can irregular menstruation affect a person's reproductive health?
6. What is one social barrier that can prevent access to menstrual hygiene products?

Answer to Critical Thinking Questions

1. (c) 2. (b) 3. (c) 4. (c) 5. (d)

REFERENCES

1. Agoreyo, F. O., & Okorie, C. (2017). Evaluation of relative blood viscosity during menstruation in reproductive females. https://core.ac.uk/download/478427484.pdf (accessed on 14th June 2025).
2. Akpoigho, E. C., & Nwankwo, C. U. (2022). Assessment of premenstrual syndrome and coping strategies among female students of the School of Basic Medical Sciences, University of Benin, Benin City, Nigeria. https://core.ac.uk/download/544242419.pdf (accessed on 14th June 2025).
3. Aluma, F., & Ongom, A. (2021). Challenges faced by girl child aged between 9–18 years in menstrual hygiene in schools: A cross-sectional study of Ogur Sub-County, Lira District, Uganda. https://core.ac.uk/download/489417548.pdf (accessed on 14th June 2025).
4. Aman, H. (2024). Women's right to education in Ethiopia. https://core.ac.uk/download/641670205.pdf (accessed on 14th June 2025).
5. Anne, S. K., & Vijayalakshmi. (2024). Menstrual hygiene and its awareness among adolescent girls: A study from an urban area. https://core.ac.uk/download/620836191.pdf (accessed on 14th June 2025).
6. Bernier, D. (2012). Polycystic ovary syndrome: Pathogenesis, health consequences, and treatment of PCOS in relation to insulin resistance. https://core.ac.uk/download/72048051.pdf (accessed on 14th June 2025).
7. Berry, A., Brady, S. S., Burgio, K., Camenga, D., *et al.* (2019). U.S. adolescent and adult women's experiences accessing and using toilets in schools, workplaces, and public spaces: A multi-site focus group study to inform future research in bladder health. https://core.ac.uk/download/231816798.pdf (accessed on 14th June 2025).
8. Chapman, R., Earle, S., Ledger, S., Townson, L., *et al.* (2015). Contraceptive choices for women with learning disabilities. https://core.ac.uk/download/30475368.pdf (accessed on 14th June 2025).
9. Crawford, B. J. (2017). Tampon taxes, discrimination, and human rights. https://core.ac.uk/download/84502085.pdf (accessed on 14th June 2025).
10. Crawford, B. J., & Waldman, E. G. (2019). The unconstitutional tampon tax. https://core.ac.uk/download/212892736.pdf (accessed on 14th June 2025).
11. Crawford, B. J., Johnson, M. E., Karin, M. L., Strausfeld, R., *et al.* (2020). The ground on which we all stand: A conversation about menstrual equity law and activism. https://core.ac.uk/download/322808787.pdf (accessed on 14th June 2025).
12. Druet, A., Elhadad, N., Li, K., Shea, A., *et al.* (2020). Characterizing physiological and symptomatic variation in menstrual cycles using self-tracked mobile health data. http://arxiv.org/abs/1909.11211 (accessed on 14th June 2025).
13. Fantaw, S., Hassen, M., Hussen, M., Kayro, S., *et al.* (2024). Prevalence of primary dysmenorrhea and associated factors among high school students in Hawassa, Sidama Region, Ethiopia. https://core.ac.uk/download/629287348.pdf (accessed on 14th June 2025).
14. Fauser, B. C. J. M., Brown, A., Busfield, D., Barlow, D. H., Dolan, S., Donnez, J., Donnez, O., *et al.* (2014). Long-term treatment of uterine fibroids with ulipristal acetate. https://core.ac.uk/download/9367119.pdf (accessed on 14th June 2025).

15. Fehring, R. (2010). Current medical research: Summer–Fall 2009. https://core.ac.uk/download/213085473.pdf (accessed on 14th June 2025).
16. Fitriani, R. J., Probandari, A., & Wiboworini, B. (2019). Body mass index, sleep quality, stress conditions determine menstrual cycles among female adolescents. https://media.neliti.com/media/publications/300781-body-mass-index-sleep-quality-stress-con-0575c812.pdf (accessed on 14th June 2025).
17. Flaherty, E. M. (2008). Howling (and bleeding) at the moon: Menstruation, monstrosity and the double in the *Ginger Snaps* werewolf trilogy. https://core.ac.uk/download/46712680.pdf (accessed on 14th June 2025).
18. G. K., Mini, S. K., Godwin, U. C. U., Lakshmi, V. M., *et al.* (2024). Menstrual product choice and the extent of period poverty among young adult females: Findings from a cross-sectional study in Kerala, India. https://core.ac.uk/download/613230464.pdf (accessed on 14th June 2025).
19. Gharravi, A. M. (2009). Menstrual cycle patterns of college students in Gorgan–Northeast of Iran: Identify its association with sociodemographic factors. https://core.ac.uk/download/52204963.pdf (accessed on 14th June 2025).
20. Hayman, M. (2024). Breaking the silence: Exploring the impact of supervisor vulnerability on menstrual disclosures at work. https://core.ac.uk/download/619597331.pdf (accessed on 14th June 2025).
21. Kustriyanti, D., & Rahayu, H. (2020). Prevalence of premenstrual syndrome and quality of life among health science college student. https://core.ac.uk/download/480550077.pdf (accessed on 14th June 2025).
22. Marmura, M. J. (2018). Triggers, protectors, and predictors in episodic migraine. https://core.ac.uk/download/213444199.pdf (accessed on 14th June 2025).
23. Matsuura, Y., Nguyen, B. T., Nguyen, K. T., Phan, H. M., *et al.* (2024). Menstruation-related symptoms and associated factors among female university students in Vietnam. https://core.ac.uk/download/604491001.pdf (accessed on 14th June 2025).
24. Maulingin-Gumbaketi, E. S. (2021). "Making of a strong woman": A constructivist grounded theory on young women's experiences at menarche in Papua New Guinea. https://core.ac.uk/download/482707185.pdf (accessed on 14th June 2025).
25. Mello, C. G. (2004). Gender and empowerment: Contemporary Lakota women of Rosebud. https://core.ac.uk/download/10685503.pdf (accessed on 14th June 2025).
26. N/A. (2010). Investing in women for a better world. https://core.ac.uk/download/71352416.pdf (accessed on 14th June 2025).
27. N/A. (2010). Menstrual hygiene in South Asia: A neglected issue for WASH (Water, Sanitation and Hygiene) programmers. https://core.ac.uk/download/75783154.pdf (accessed on 14th June 2025).
28. N/A. (2011). Is menstrual hygiene and management an issue for adolescent school girls? https://core.ac.uk/download/71358560.pdf (accessed on 14th June 2025).
29. N/A. (2014). Maintaining the momentum: Advancing health, learning and equity through WASH in schools. https://core.ac.uk/download/75783080.pdf (accessed on 14th June 2025).
30. N/A. (2015). The history of Niddah in America as social drama: Genealogy of a ritual practice. https://core.ac.uk/download/79584418.pdf (accessed on 14th June 2025).

31. N/A. (2017). Understanding menstrual hygiene management and human rights. https://core.ac.uk/download/141922771.pdf (accessed on 14th June 2025).

32. Pearson, M., & Schipper, B. C. (2025). Menstrual cycle and competitive bidding. https://core.ac.uk/download/pdf/6470406.pdf (accessed on 14th June 2025).

33. Saha, S. (2005). Dynamics governing women's decision on reproductive health matters: Reflections from a qualitative study in Central India. https://core.ac.uk/download/pdf/86410.pdf (accessed on 14th June 2025).

34. Schulte, L. (2019). A critique of advertisements for female hygiene products: A silent crisis in America. https://core.ac.uk/download/213463717.pdf (accessed on 14th June 2025).

35. Terrin, A., Negro, A., Raffaelli, B., Mitsikostas, D. D., Ornello, R., Khan, S., *et al.* (2018). Male and female sex hormones in primary headaches. https://core.ac.uk/download/188830209.pdf (accessed on 14th June 2025).

36. Thirunaaukarasu, D., Karthikeyan, M., Geetha, K., Naidu, V., *et al.* (2024). Perceptions related to menstruation among male medical students in Chengalpattu, Tamil Nadu: A qualitative study. https://core.ac.uk/download/640070350.pdf (accessed on 14th June 2025).

37. Vasquez, E., Sommer, M., Sahin, M., Worthington, N., & Dooley, T. (2014). WASH in schools empowers girls' education: Proceedings of the Menstrual Hygiene Management in Schools Virtual Conference 2013. https://core.ac.uk/download/75783637.pdf (accessed on 14th June 2025).

AMENORRHEA

6

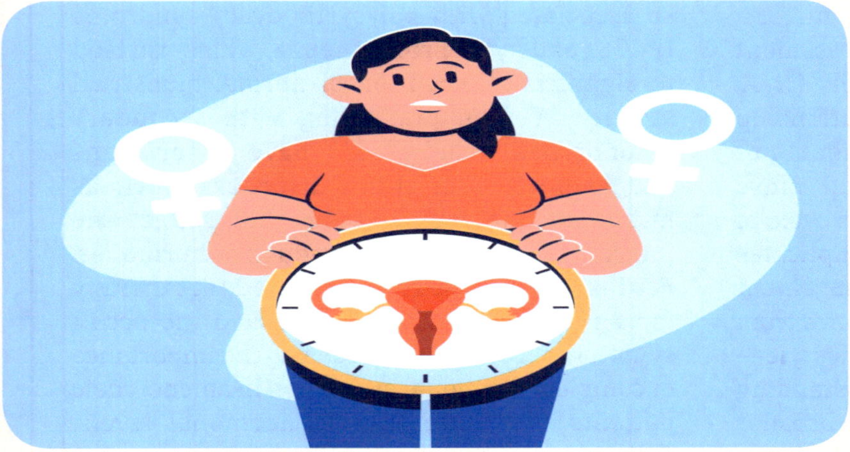

Introduction

Amenorrhea, or the absence of menstruation, is a significant indicator of numerous underlying health conditions, and hence its probing is a significant field of gynecological study. Broadly categorized into primary and secondary types of amenorrhea, amenorrhea can be brought about by numerous reasons such as hormonal disturbances, lifestyle factors, or clinical conditions. Primary amenorrhea is characterized by not having had the first menses by age 16, whereas secondary amenorrhea is the cessation of menses following a normal previous menstrual period. These distinctions are significant because they lead to appropriate avenues of diagnosis and treatment. In addition, amenorrhea is not merely a physiological state; it has long-term consequences for a woman's overall well-being, impacting fertility and leading to concern regarding bone health and cardiovascular status, particularly since it can lead to a deficiency in estrogen (N/A, 2025). The etiology of amenorrhea needs extensive evaluation since it involves a broad variety of biological, environmental, and psychological

LEARNING OBJECTIVES

After studying this chapter, you will be able to:

1. Identify and classify the different types of amenorrhea.
2. Analyze the various causes contributing to amenorrhea.
3. Recognize the symptoms and diagnostic methods for amenorrhea.
4. Evaluate the impact of amenorrhea on overall health.
5. Assess available treatment options for managing amenorrhea.
6. Develop strategies for the prevention of amenorrhea.

influences. Hormonal imbalances may be secondary to disease such as polycystic ovary syndrome (PCOS) or thyroid disease, which disrupts the normal menstrual cycle. Lifestyle, in the guise of excessive exercise, starvation diet, or stress, is also a leading cause of amenorrhea. While some conditions, such as pregnancy or use of hormonal contraceptives, cause temporary amenorrhea, differentiation from more distressing causes is crucial in healthcare. Specifically, each cause is associated with its constellation of symptoms and risk factors, highlighting the need for medical assessment and individualized treatment protocols (N/A, 2025). In treating amenorrhea, the relationship between physical and mental health should not be ignored. Lack of menstruation can cause distress and anxiety, initiating a vicious cycle of psychological distress that further complicates the syndrome. Therefore, effective management involves both medical treatment—variance from hormone therapies to adjustment of lifestyle—and psychological management. Understanding amenorrhea promotes awareness of the broader implications this condition has on a woman's life, such as future fertility. Due to its long-term health consequences, early diagnosis and intervention are critical. With the evolution of medicine, continued research into the etiology of amenorrhea allows women to receive complete care that includes not only the symptoms but the emotional and psychological components of this illness (N/A, 2025).

Definition of Amenorrhea

Amenorrhea, or failure or absence of menstruation, can happen in primary and secondary forms. Primary amenorrhea is defined by the fact that a woman has never menstruated by age 15 or three years from the time secondary sexual characteristics begin. This can be an indication of underlying genetic or anatomical issues that need to be analyzed further. On the other hand, secondary amenorrhea refers to the cessation of menstruation for three months in women who previously experienced normal menstrual cycles. The incidence may be attributed to several physiological and pathological reasons, such as hormonal imbalance, stress, and gene mutations. Being aware of these definitions matters in terms of diagnosing and treating menstrual disorders because they are chief indicators of an individual's reproductive status and health. Among the usual reasons for secondary amenorrhea are hormonal imbalances, more so associated with polycystic ovary syndrome (PCOS) and hyperprolactinemia, which can lead to significant disruption of normal menstrual activity. Women presenting with secondary amenorrhea usually also have other signs and symptoms of these disorders, such as hirsutism and weight gain, that reflect the interconnectedness of reproductive hormones. For instance, a case report showed that therapy for a microprolactinoma unmasked the occult symptoms of PCOS, underscoring the importance of complete hormonal evaluation in amenorrheic patients. The difference in hormonal levels, particularly with higher prolactin and androgen, provides insight into the pathophysiology of such cases and also the value in diagnosing amenorrhea in the selection of effective treatment modalities (Erenler *et al.*, 2024). Other recent evidence indicates that amenorrhea may also be a manifestation of systemic diseases such as autoimmune disorders, wherein dysautonomia may be a significant factor to consider. In certain autoimmune conditions, amenorrhea may occur along with other systemic symptoms, such as dysautonomia, which involves more than one system of the body. This association is exemplified in autoimmune autonomic ganglionopathy, where dysautonomia occurs with amenorrhea, suggesting an interplay between the immune and reproductive systems. Clinicians should be aware of these associations when trying to unravel and treat amenorrhea in general. By taking on a broader understanding of amenorrhea, along with its potential connections to systemic disease processes, doctors are able to develop more beneficial treatment protocols that are mindful of the causes as well as symptoms (Kaida, 2021).

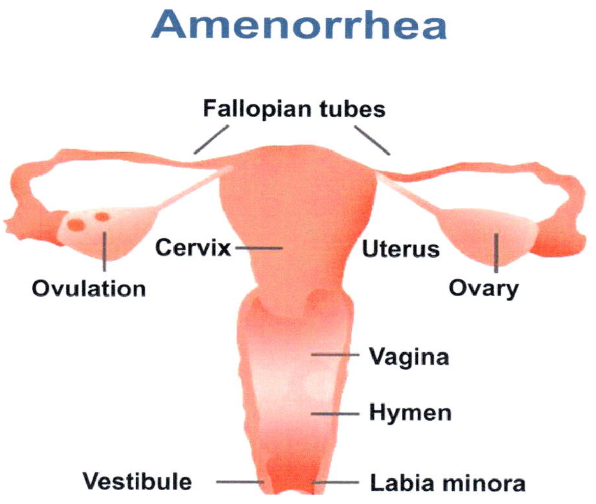

Figure 6.1. Amenorrhea.

Source: https://cdnrmi-19948.kxcdn.com/sites/default/files/Disease-2020-10/Amenorrhea-1024x1024.png

Importance of Understanding Amenorrhea

It is essential to know about amenorrhea not merely due to its immediate and direct effects on women's reproductive health but due to its potential long-term effects on overall well-being as well. Absence of menstruation can be a sign of underlying hormonal imbalances, dietary malnutrition, or more critical conditions such as polycystic ovary syndrome (PCOS). Proper knowledge about amenorrhea allows clinical practitioners to offer prompt assessment and intervention. For instance, adolescent females with disordered menstrual cycles may need special training and lifestyle modifications in order to prevent the progression of conditions like PCOS, which affects a high proportion of reproductive-aged women. Early detection and proper management can prevent amenorrhea-associated risks, ensuring healthier development and reproductive health outcomes. The psychological impacts of amenorrhea also cannot be downplayed, particularly within specific groups of elite athletes. Studies have indicated that mental disorders and mental illness symptoms are prevalent in this group, typically exacerbated by medical conditions presenting as amenorrhea. The interaction between physical and mental health serves to highlight the need for an interdisciplinary response to treating amenorrhea. Understanding the psychosocial causes of this condition enables practitioners to develop comprehensive interventions dealing with both psychological and physical aspects of an athlete's health. Therefore, with the prioritization of amenorrhea, clinicians can ensure overall well-being, which aids in better performance and quality of life for both athletes and non-athletes, as evidenced by expert recommendations towards standardization in sport mental health care. Lastly, the treatment of amenorrhea contributes to an increase in awareness of the bigger picture for women's health. This status is a marker of a possible hormonal disorder that affects other systems of the body, apart from reproduction. Amenorrhea increases women's risk of osteoporosis, cardiovascular morbidities, and metabolic syndromes due to long-term estrogen deprivation. Thus, knowledge of amenorrhea encourages healthy behavior and preventive management. Follow-up visits and lifestyle modification may be key in maximizing long-term prognosis. Encouraging recognition of amenorrhea not only aids in the clinical management of the involved populace but also aids in encouraging a cultural understanding of women's health issues, spreading the word that menstruation disorders are stigmatized and that must be broken. In line with these observations, an integrated understanding of amenorrhea is needed to promote women's health results in today and tomorrow.

6.1. Types of Amenorrhea

Learning Outcome

1. Discuss the primary amenorrhea and secondary amenorrhea
2. Explain the functional amenorrhea

Amenorrhea, or absence of menstruation, can be categorized into two categories: primary amenorrhea and secondary amenorrhea. Primary amenorrhea is when an adolescent woman has not experienced her first menses by the age of 15 or five years following the initiation of breast development. This can be a manifestation of different underlying etiologies, like genetic disease, congenital malformation of the reproductive system, or abnormalities in puberty-related hormones. The challenge of diagnosing primary amenorrhea is that there are so many possible causes that a complete medical evaluation is required in an effort to decide on the proper treatment. This type of amenorrhea is important to treat not only for physical health but also for the emotional well-being of individuals affected by it, because the beginning of menstruation is a time period linked to greater social and developmental milestones. Conversely, secondary amenorrhea is diagnosed when a woman who once had regular menstrual cycles experiences a three-month or longer absence of menstruation. Secondary amenorrhea may be brought on by a variety of different factors, including hormonal imbalance, extreme weight fluctuation, intense exercise, and underlying health conditions such as polycystic ovary syndrome (PCOS) and hyperthyroidism. Diagnosis of secondary amenorrhea will usually involve meticulous history-taking and clinical examination, supplemented with laboratory tests to evaluate the hormonal status. In contrast to such expectations, international evidence-based guidelines for the diagnosis and treatment of diseases like PCOS stipulate the necessity of identifying secondary amenorrhea with precision, as it may lead to delayed treatment and finally cause chronic complications and adverse health results in women. This complexity also places more focus on the need for individualized care in such cases (Teede *et al.*, 2018*et al.*).

Another aspect of considerable importance in understanding amenorrhea is the distinction between functional and organic etiologies. Functional amenorrhea typically happens as a result of lifestyle factors such as exercise, diet, and stress, highlighting the role of psychosocial factors in menstrual well-being. Some athletes or those with eating disorders, for instance, will exhibit changes in their menstrual cycle due to energy deficit or psychological stressors. Organic amenorrhea, on the other hand, is comprised of definable anatomical or physiological abnormalities, such as anatomical defects, tumors, or chronic disease. The understanding of these distinctions is important to healthcare providers because it determines the management plan and the kind of interventions required. This dual consideration of functional versus organic causation also reflects the need for holistic care methods that combine medical treatment with lifestyle modification, thereby promoting overall reproductive health and well-being.

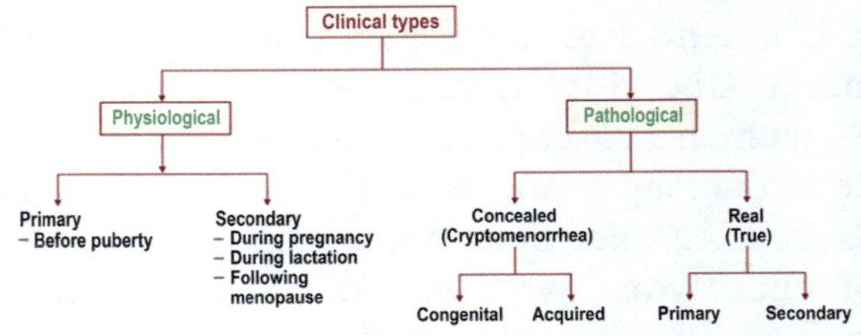

Figure 6.2. The following types are amenorrhea.

Source: https://oshimu.com/wp-content/uploads/2021/07/Gynaecology-DC-Dutta.pdf

6.1.1. Primary Amenorrhea

Primary amenorrhea, which is the absence of menarche at fifteen or thirteen years of age in the presence of secondary sexual characteristics, is a most critical topic in adolescent health. It is not only its physiologic implications but also its potential psychosocial impact on the involved population. The onset of menarche typically marks the passage from girlhood to womanhood, or more specifically, a milestone in the woman's development. Delays in doing so, particularly in combination with other abnormal growth or development factors, will necessitate a thorough medical work-up to uncover etiologies therefor. Indeed, suppose menarche has not been attained three years after thelarche or five years after the commencement of puberty. In that case, health professionals are compelled to investigate the etiology of this condition in order to establish appropriate intervention and management strategies (Seppä *et al.*, 2021).

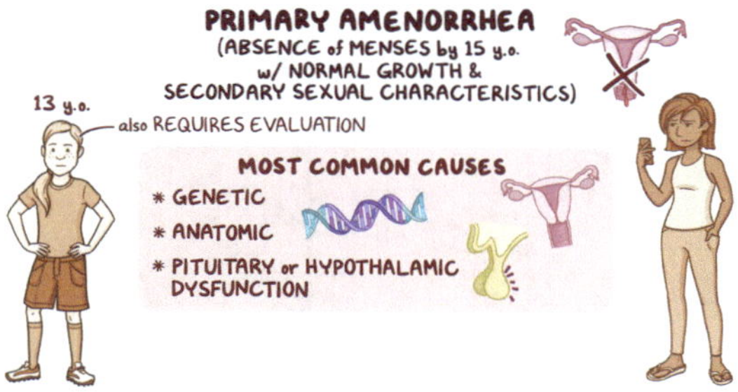

Figure 6.3. Primary amenorrhea.

Source: https://d16qt3wv6xm098.cloudfront.net/IIhx3yE9TO6_S7sgWtB9mOf0Rryyj33V/_.jpg

The etiology of primary amenorrhea is multifarious and complex and extends from disorders of the hypothalamic-pituitary-gonadal axis, anatomical defects, to a variety of endocrine disorders. Primary amenorrhea etiologies include such disorders as outflow tract obstructions and gonadal dysgenesis, emphasizing the heterogeneity of causes for primary amenorrhea. Hypothalamic-pituitary endocrine disorder could result in hypogonadotropic amenorrhea, and ovarian malformations could induce hypergonadotropic amenorrhea. Chronic illnesses and psychiatric illness are also implicated, complicating the clinical syndrome and necessitating an individualized diagnostic approach. An understanding of these underlying causes is vital for appropriate management and treatment because misdiagnosis can significantly affect reproductive health and well-being (Yoon *et al.*, 2019).

Primary amenorrhea treatment must be tailored according to the individual's particular diagnosis and needs, requiring a multidisciplinary approach by pediatric endocrinologists, gynecologists, and mental health professionals. Good-quality evaluation should include thorough clinical history-taking, physical examination, and appropriate laboratory investigations to assess levels of hormones and imaging studies to assess anatomical abnormalities. Management modalities range from hormone replacement to surgical intervention for anatomic issues, depending on the diagnosed condition. The management goals can include restoration of menstrual function, achievement of fertility, and elimination of any psychosocial consequences resulting from the condition. By presenting a comprehensive and anticipatory management plan, those who are affected can be guided by healthcare providers in overcoming the ordeal of primary amenorrhea with a better quality of life and health outcomes (Seppä *et al.*, 2021).

6.1.2. Secondary Amenorrhea

Secondary amenorrhea, or loss of menstruation for three cycles consecutively or six months in women who had regular menstrual cycles in the past, is of special interest in the field of women's health. The condition can be a warning sign of underlying physiological or psychological issues, and hence its understanding is important to enable early diagnosis and intervention. Stress, excessive physical exercise, drastic weight fluctuations, and hormonal imbalance are frequent etiologic factors for this phenomenon. The relationship between menstrual health and weight is of particular concern, in which both being fat and underweight can disrupt hormonal processes essential to ovulation. Furthermore, disorders like polycystic ovary syndrome (PCOS) and thyroid disease may also exacerbate this situation, with long-term fertility implications if not treated as outlined in N/A (2025). Comprehensive evaluation most often necessitates extensive diagnostics, including hormonal profiling and imaging modalities. Particular emphasis is placed on the identification of some hormonal abnormalities likely to be responsible for the absence of menstruation. For instance, elevated levels of luteinizing hormone (LH) and androgens are characteristic findings in diagnosing PCOS, a common cause of secondary amenorrhea. In cases like those of Ms. N, where the hormonal tests had revealed characteristic features of PCOS, it is particularly important to have a person-specific approach to treatment. In addition, lifestyle interventions such as exercise and weight management are most crucial in relieving this syndrome's symptoms along with enhancing general well-being. Adding medical therapy, like combined hormonal contraceptives, serves to not only regulate menstrual cycles but also relieve associated symptoms, enhancing the quality of life among the patients as demonstrated in Apriliana *et al.* (2022).

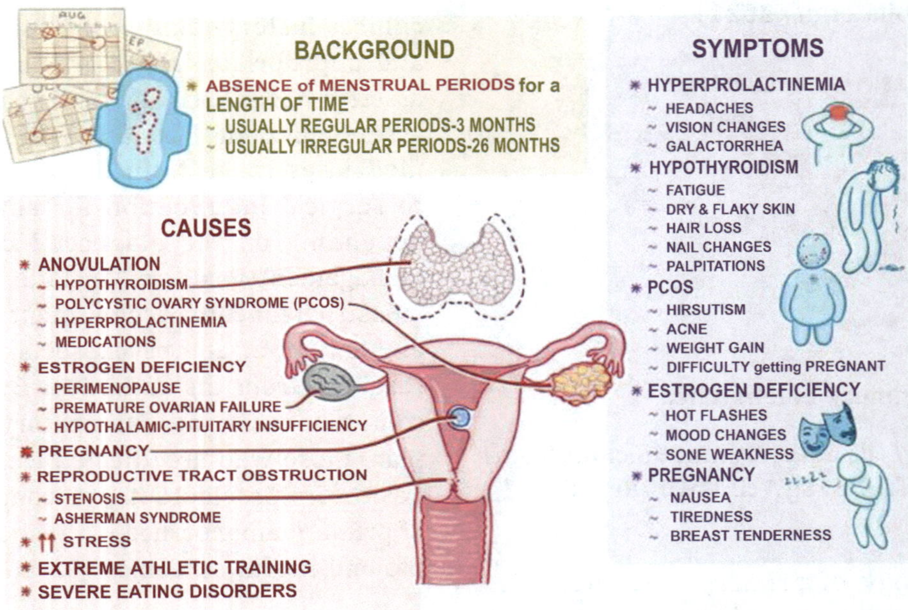

Figure 6.4. Secondary Amenorrhea.

Source: https://www.osmosis.org/answers/secondary-amenorrhea

The effects of secondary amenorrhea go beyond mere menstrual disturbances and comment on a number of aspects of a woman's overall health, including her fertility and bone mineral density. Absence of menstruation is normally accompanied by low estrogen levels, and these may lead to lower bone mineral density and encourage the occurrence of osteoporosis in advanced age. Long-term management of secondary amenorrhea is thus critical to cater for the prevention of systemic health complications. Treatment of underlying conditions, bringing about lifestyle modifications, and applying rightful medical interventions are all involved in the treatment. As research continues to expand our understanding of secondary amenorrhea, it is increasingly clear that early discovery and intervention can have a real impact on outcomes, enhancing reproductive well-being and general health for affected women, and hence underscoring the significance of bringing awareness and education regarding this condition as described in N/A (2025).

6.1.3. Functional Amenorrhea

Functional amenorrhea is a broad group of menstrual disturbances, best defined as the absence of menstrual flow on the basis of non-organic etiology. It is often the result of a complex interaction of physiological and psychological factors and is most frequently the result of stress. Often in these cases, significant life changes or chronic stressors lead to hypothalamic dysfunction, disrupting the hormonal communication necessary for the usual menstrual cycle. The condition affects women of all ages, primarily women in the reproductive age group, and is concerning due to its effects on fertility and overall well-being. Management of functional amenorrhea requires a multi-faceted approach, where not only is the biology addressed, but also the psychosocial conditions under which such women live. More recent texts highlight the incorporation of psychological counseling and non-hormonal therapy in the management of functional amenorrhea. Treatments such as psychological counseling combined with natural supplements such as *Vitex agnus-castus* extract have been proven effective in the restoration of regularity in menstrual periods. A study revealed that women who were being psychologically counseled in combination with some food supplements observed significant improvement, and hormonal balance was restored in a majority of patients (Tatarchuk *et al.*, 2024). This approach emphasizes the significance of personalized interventions that meet both mental and physical needs, and thus it is a key area for future research and clinical practice in women's health care. Functional amenorrhea can also be overlooked or misdiagnosed by the specialist community, who recognize that it can frequently appear somewhat ambiguously. Current recommendations highlight the necessity for comprehensive diagnostic tests to distinguish functional from organic etiology of amenorrhea. The controversy around the neurophysiological basis of mechanisms, such as the role of progesterone metabolites, is valuable in understanding the complexity of the conditions (N/A, 2024). By developing a better understanding of functional amenorrhea, clinicians can design improved individualized treatment plans that not only treat symptom suppression but also long-term reproductive well-being. With greater recognition of the disorder, an equal need exists for proper intervention and screening methods within the broader context of menstrual disorders.

Test Your Knowledge

1. What is the difference between primary and secondary amenorrhea?
2. What are common causes of functional amenorrhea?

6.2. Causes of Amenorrhea

Learning Outcome

1. Discuss the hormonal imbalances
2. Describe the lifestyle factors
3. Identify the medical conditions

Amenorrhea, or the absence of menstrual cycles, may be caused by a vast array of reasons that span physiological, psychological, and pathological settings. Hormonal imbalance is the most common cause of amenorrhea and usually arises from conditions such as polycystic ovary syndrome (PCOS). PCOS disrupts the usual growth of follicles in the ovaries, leading to irregular ovulation and menstruation. In addition, endocrine disorders such as hypothyroidism or hyperprolactinemia can adversely affect the hypothalamic-pituitary-ovarian (HPO) axis significantly and cause amenorrhea. The scenario demonstrates the significance of regular hormonal assessment among women with absent menstruation, as it informs proper therapeutic management using known resulting hormonal patterns.

The effect of lifestyle and psychological factors is also a significant factor in causing amenorrhea. For instance, acute weight loss, excessive exertion, or starvation may disrupt the energy balance necessary for regular ovulation, known as hypothalamic amenorrhea. Furthermore, emotional disorders and stress can activate the hypothalamus, inhibiting the release of gonadotropin-releasing hormone (GnRH), again disrupting menstrual function. The mutual relationship between mental health and normal menses demands that treatment be multifaceted, involving both psychological therapy and modification of lifestyle. By considering these factors along with hormonal evaluation, doctors can give a better treatment schedule to women who have amenorrhea. Structural abnormalities and chronic illnesses also cause amenorrhea. Conditions like Turner syndrome or androgen insensitivity syndrome lead to structural defects which may prevent normal menstrual function.

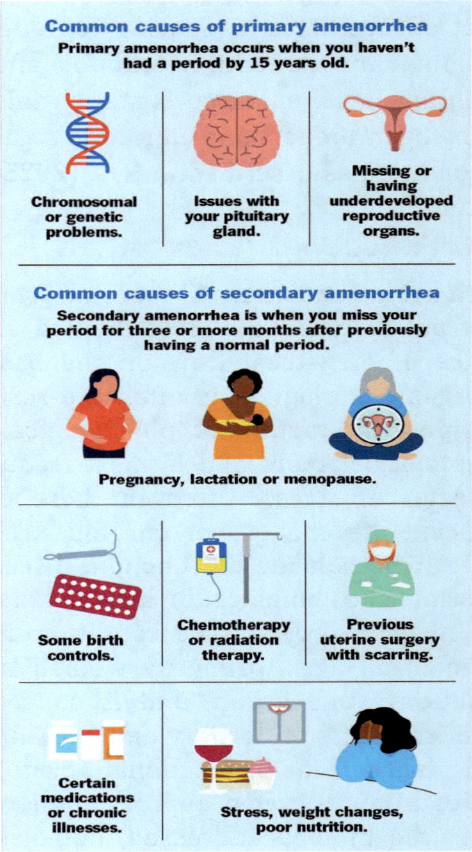

Figure 6.5. Common causes of amenorrhea.

Source: https://my.clevelandclinic.org/-/scassets/images/org/health/articles/3924-amenorrhea

Furthermore, prolonged illnesses such as diabetes or celiac disease may lead to hormonal derangement and consequent amenorrhea. These conditions underscore the necessity of thorough medical checks that consider both systemic and reproductive health in order to adequately diagnose and treat the pathologies underlying amenorrhea. New approaches to health education and delivery, such as electronic platforms targeting women's health, can potentially make diagnostic efforts more streamlined and beneficial for those affected, as described in recent studies identifying the prospect of integrated care improving conditions like secondary amenorrhea (Nelson *et al.*, 2023). Hence, correct management needs to be multi-faceted in nature, addressing both the physiological and psychosocial dimensions of this complex disorder (Teede *et al.*, 2018).

6.2.1. Hormonal Imbalances

The amenorrhea state, or the cessation of menstruation, is said to be closely linked to the hormonal imbalances in the body. They occur due to some underlying conditions like stress, sudden fluctuations in weight, or endocrine diseases. For instance, diabetic mellitus patients usually have abnormal menstrual cycles due to high levels of androgens that inhibit the normal mechanism of the menstrual cycle. Analogously, hypothalamic amenorrhea, which arises due to an aberrant hypothalamic response to stress or inadequate energy availability, indicates the delicate equilibrium between hormonal regulation and menstrual health. Lastly, certain medications, such as isotretinoin, most commonly used in the management of acne, have been reported to be causative agents of menstrual disturbance, which suggests one more avenue through which hormonal balance may be disrupted (Alhetheli *et al.*, 2022). Therefore, an understanding of these hormonal dynamics is critical in the diagnosis and management of amenorrhea. Nutrition is another critical component that is involved in amenorrhea's hormonal imbalances, i.e., diseases like celiac disease that disrupt the endocrine system via malabsorption of nutrients. The autoimmune nature of celiac disease has a tendency to create many physiological changes that not only affect gastrointestinal well-being but also hormonal regulation (Caio *et al.*, 2019).

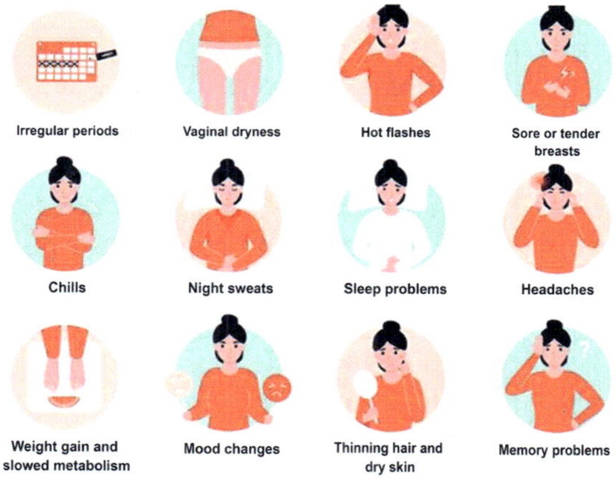

Figure 6.6. Signs of hormonal imbalances.

Source: https://www.womenshealthnetwork.com/wp-content/uploads/2022/11/Symptoms-of-Hormonal-Imbalance-1.jpg

When individuals suffering from celiac disease consume gluten, it can trigger an inflammatory response that exacerbates deficiency states, hence impacting hormonal pathways crucial to the sustenance of the menstrual cycle. This relationship between dietary intake and hormonal health illustrates how secondary medical conditions can have far-reaching implications on reproductive health. Hence, relief from these nutritional insufficiencies through dietary modification becomes essential to restoring hormonal balance and, in turn, potentially reducing symptoms of amenorrhea. Additionally, stress relief and lifestyle also need to be highly prominent in conversations regarding hormonal imbalance and amenorrhea. Ongoing stress will lead to alterations in cortisol levels, which will then suppress the functioning of reproductive hormones like luteinizing hormone (LH) and follicle-stimulating hormone (FSH). The ensuing hormonal dysregulation can suppress the development of ovarian follicles and disrupt the usual menstrual cycle. The understanding of this association has, in turn, led to heightened awareness of the need for treatment of amenorrhea as a whole-person process, incorporating stress reduction techniques and lifestyle adjustments as well as medical therapy. By encouraging holistic management strategies that cope with physical and emotional well-being, healthcare practitioners are in a better position to respond to the etiology of hormonal imbalance causing amenorrhea.

6.2.2. Lifestyle Factors

The interaction between lifestyle determinants and amenorrhea is an important research field in reproductive health. Several factors like diet, exercise, and stress have a critical impact on menstrual cycles. High levels of exercise, particularly among athletes, may cause energy depletion, which alters the hormonal balance and thus causes amenorrhea. Similarly, inadequate caloric consumption, as in the case of restrictive diets, is shown to have major effects on the hypothalamic-pituitary-ovarian axis and reduce ovulation. Education on such associations is critical for the recognition of vulnerable populations and the tailoring of interventions to restore menstrual function and, thus, the value of an integrative approach to the treatment of amenorrhea through lifestyle modification. In addition, psychological distress can reinforce amenorrhea prevalence by disturbing the physiological processes that underlie hormonal regulation. Stress activates the hypothalamic-pituitary-adrenal (HPA) axis, hence potentially disrupting menstrual cycles. Dietary alterations due to significant life events, like the Fukushima Daiichi Nuclear Power Plant accident, also illustrate how environmental pressures can lead to negative lifestyle habits, placing one under a higher risk for metabolic syndromes like amenorrhea (Takahashi *et al.*, 2024). Stress management and psychological well-being receive attention as they bear a direct relationship with the maintenance of hormone balance along with total reproductive well-being, highlighting the intricate relationship between menstruation and mental well-being. Educational interventions among lifestyle determinants offer a potential path towards the prevention of amenorrhea, particularly among adolescent women. For example, evidence has found that increasing awareness of healthy lifestyles can bring about dramatic change in menstrual health outcomes. Enhanced knowledge of lifestyle changes and hypertension among Indian adolescents showed the impact where psychological engagement resulted in enhanced health behavior (Semou *et al.*, 2024). Similarly, increasing awareness of nutrition, physical exercise, and stress reduction is essential in fostering an environment favorable to menstrual health. Early interventions can empower individuals to adopt healthier lifestyles, and in the process, they can even reverse or prevent the onset of amenorrhea, which underscores the necessity of including educational programs in public health programs.

6.2.3. Medical Conditions

Amenorrhea, or absence of menstruation, is a significant indicator of underlying medical conditions that may require additional testing. It is further classified into two: primary amenorrhea, which occurs when no initiation of menstruation has occurred by age 15, and secondary amenorrhea, which occurs when frequent menstrual periods previously present stop for at least three successive cycles. Such causes cover hormonal imbalance, lifestyle-related problems like stress or excessive exercise, as well as medical illnesses like thyroid disease or polycystic ovary syndrome (PCOS). Understanding the problems posed in amenorrhea is essential to avoid potential long-term complications of health issues such as infertility, osteoporosis, and cardiovascular disorders that may result from extended hormonal imbalance (N/A, 2025). The process of diagnosing amenorrhea consists of a meticulous clinical assessment, where doctors interview the patients about their history, lifestyle, and underlying psychological stressors that could be causing amenorrhea. Doctors employ a set of tests to diagnose the underlying cause of amenorrhea, such as blood tests to determine the levels of hormones and imaging scans, such as ultrasounds, to determine the presence of ovarian or uterine problems. Treatment of the potential causes, such as chronic stress or severe weight loss, is key to effective treatment. Significantly, amenorrhea has the potential to significantly affect women's mental health, since the social stigma and personal significance of menstruation have the potential to compound anxiety or depression. Therefore, integrative treatment incorporating psychological care alongside medical therapy is essential in the management of the extensive variety of influences that come with amenorrhea to ensure that treatment is all-encompassing for the victims (N/A, 2025).

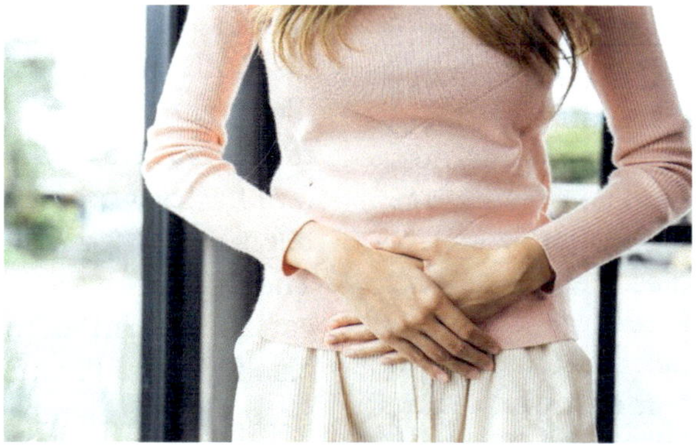

Source: https://insiderhealthytactics.com/wp-content/uploads/2024/01/Menstrual-Disorders-cause.jpg

The management of amenorrhea varies widely with its etiologic agent. In primary amenorrhea, drug therapy or anatomical interventions can be used, whereas secondary amenorrhea can include lifestyle modification or medication. In conditions such as PCOS, typically involving hormonal imbalance, medications to regulate menstrual cycles and improve fertility might be required. Where amenorrhea is caused by excessive stress or excess strain, changes in lifestyle, such as treatment programs for counseling and stress management, are vital. Due to the risk of amenorrhea being linked with other serious diseases, including chronic lymphocytic leukemia (CLL), the larger implications of amenorrhea must be taken into consideration. Amenorrhea patients must be closely monitored for associated health complications, hence cementing the importance of a thorough medical examination.

Test Your Knowledge

1. How can hormonal imbalances affect the menstrual cycle?
2. What medical conditions are known to disrupt normal hormonal function?

6.3. Symptoms and Diagnosis

Learning Outcome

1. Identify common symptoms associated with amenorrhea
2. Explain the diagnostic tests and procedures
3. Assess the importance of medical history in diagnosis

Amenorrhea diagnosis has a multi-dimensional approach that defines the probable reason for the cessation of normal menstrual cycles. Primary and secondary amenorrhea are differentiated by direct investigation. Primary amenorrhea, which is the absence of menstruation by age 15 with the development of secondary sexual traits, typically points toward congenital defects or chromosomal abnormalities. By contrast, secondary amenorrhea, i.e., lack of menstruation for three or more consecutive months following normal menstrual cycles, may have a plethora of causes. These include disturbances of the endocrine system due to dysfunction of the hypothalamus or ovarian failure and systemic disease, including extreme weight loss, stress, or chronic disease. Prompt diagnosis is crucial, as amenorrhea may be a warning sign of serious illness that needs to be treated early to prevent long-term effects such as infertility or decreased bone density. Diagnosis of amenorrhea begins with a complete clinical evaluation consisting of a detailed medical history and physical examination. Amenorrhea symptoms are often the prime clues for further diagnostic evaluation. A thorough analysis may reveal signs of hyperandrogenism—e.g., hirsutism or acne—that indicate incipient diseases like polycystic ovary syndrome (PCOS) or adrenal hyperplasia. In addition, evaluation of factors like lifestyle and stressors is significant because psychological or environmental influences can effectively control endocrine regulation. Blood tests to evaluate hormone levels like prolactin and thyroid-stimulating hormone give insight into incipient endocrine disturbances. It is particularly necessary to take into account hyperprolactinemia, as this is a common condition that is linked with secondary amenorrhea and may present with different clinical manifestations, as highlighted in explanations regarding the impact of pituitary tumors on reproductive health (Auriemma *et al.*, 2023).

The inclusion of imaging tests, such as ultrasound or MRI, can also help define structural causes of amenorrhea when physiological disruption is suspected. For example, conditions like primary ovarian insufficiency can lead to premature ovarian failure and necessitate familiarity with their multicausal etiologies—beginning with genetic to autoimmune causes. Their identification is critical not just for the establishment of amenorrhea diagnosis but also for the education of targeted management. Secondary amenorrhea can also reflect more widespread systemic conditions and, therefore, should be followed by investigation of the overall health of the patient, as systemic disorders can compromise reproductive function. As emphasized in amenorrhea literature, restoration of reproductive homeostasis is essential to the prevention of future fertility and long-term hormonal health, and necessitates a sensitive strategy for diagnosis and management in this population (Stuenkel *et al.*, 2021).

6.3.1. Common Symptoms Associated With Amenorrhea

Amenorrhea, or absence of menstruation, is typically accompanied by a range of other symptoms that may vary significantly depending on the causes. Some of these signs include alterations in bodily functions such as changes in libido, weight gain or loss, or expressions of endocrine diseases such as excessive hair growth, or hirsutism. The endocrine significance of amenorrhea can extend to more generalized issues, not only reproductive but also general health. The psychosocial impact is also to be considered, with usual emotional distress, worry, or depression, which exacerbate the symptomatology. These need to be determined since they could be vital signs of what may possibly be behind amenorrhea—be it lifestyle factors or more complex medical conditions, thereby making it imperative to have immediate medical evaluation when such phenomena are noticed (N/A, 2025). In some cases, amenorrhea may be a sign of more widespread endocrine abnormalities. In women with Cushing's syndrome, for instance, menstrual irregularities are seen in conjunction with other symptoms such as weight gain or a characteristic facial appearance. One report documented a 33-year-old woman diagnosed initially with polycystic ovarian syndrome who developed amenorrhea after stopping oral contraceptive treatment. Although she had exhibited depressive and anxious symptoms, her condition was ultimately caused by central hypogonadism and underlying Cushing's syndrome, revealing the complex interrelationships between hormonal disorder and menstrual health (Alhajeri *et al.*, 2024).

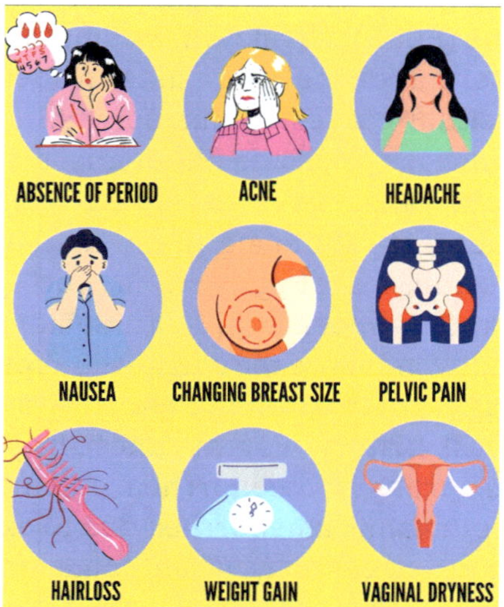

Figure 6.7. Amenorrhea symptoms.

Source: https://247homeopathy.com/wp-content/uploads/2022/10/amenorrhea-symptoms.jpeg

Understanding the way that these conditions overlap is necessary in order to enable clinicians to create effective treatment modalities that are specific to the symptomatology found in their patients. The other widespread symptom associated with amenorrhea is a decrease in estrogen level, which may give rise to other illness issues such as osteoporosis or cardiovascular disease. Amenorrhea is also typical of an interruption of regular hormonal patterns, which can give rise to lower bone density over a period of time. Women with amenorrhea must also watch out for other symptoms such as night sweats or hot flashes, which may indicate menopause-like alterations but at a younger age. Furthermore, amenorrhea can cause infertility and other reproductive problems in the long term. Thus, a comprehensive understanding of amenorrhea encompasses not only acute symptoms but also the broader picture of long-term health consequences, again reinforcing the necessity for early diagnosis and treatment in victims (N/A, 2025).

6.3.2. Diagnostic Tests and Procedures

Amenorrhea diagnosis needs an overall strategy involving several diagnostic tests and processes. A proper physical examination and medical history serve as the foundation of the evaluation process, enabling doctors to identify potential underlying etiologies. The age of the patient, menstrual history, and symptoms present are crucial in classifying amenorrhea as primary or secondary. Following the clinical examination, laboratory tests are usually conducted to determine the levels of hormones like follicle-stimulating hormone (FSH), luteinizing hormone (LH), estrogen, and prolactin, which are very important in diagnosing diseases like polycystic ovary syndrome (PCOS) or hypothalamic amenorrhea. The accuracy of these tests can be decisive in determining treatment because improper diagnosis will lead to inappropriate therapeutic interventions. Imaging tests could be called for in more complex situations to determine anatomical structures that could be responsible for amenorrhea. Transvaginal ultrasonography can be employed to screen the ovaries and lining of the uterus to provide information about such issues as ovarian cysts or uterine abnormalities. Moreover, magnetic resonance imaging (MRI) can also be employed to identify pituitary adenomas or hypothalamic dysfunctions that interfere with the hormonal regulation of menstruation.

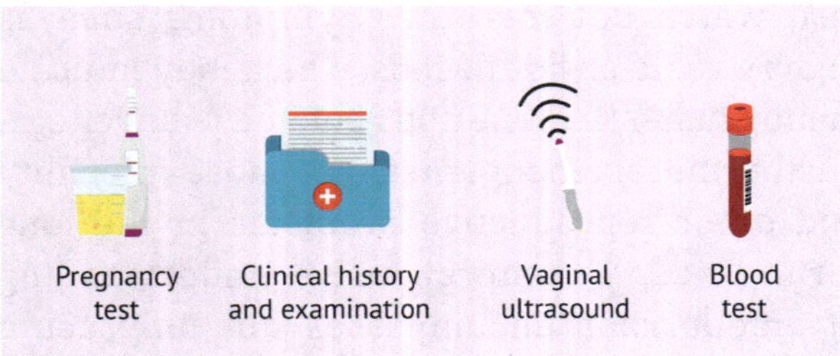

Figure 6.8. Diagnostic tests for amenorrhea.

Source: https://www.invitra.com/en/amenorrhea/diagnosis-amenorrhea/

All imaging modalities have their strengths and limitations, which makes it a must for healthcare professionals to select the appropriate test based on the presenting patient. Both laboratory and imaging results together provide more information for purposeful management plans based on the patient's particular condition. Also important in the diagnostic workup of amenorrhea is awareness of the patient's lifestyle and psychological component. Stress, malnutrition, and excessive exercise are all known variables that can alter menstrual function. Non-invasive procedures, such as the use of the non-invasive vaginal lavage technique, can be recommended by medical practitioners to gather more information regarding reproductive health, as illustrated through investigations on confirmation of mating in animal models like Wistar rats (Yugesh *et al.*, 2023). The incorporation of lifestyle assessment and laboratory testing into a comprehensive framework enhances the depth of diagnosis and treatment of amenorrhea. Furthermore, with developments in the technology of diagnosis, being cognizant of these developments—such as antigen rapid diagnostic tests—is important for healthcare workers to make correct and effective diagnoses in complex cases (Lippi *et al.*, 2022).

6.3.3. Importance of Medical History in Diagnosis

The significance of meticulous medical history taking in the diagnosis of amenorrhea cannot be overstated. Medical history serves as a foundation for understanding a patient's reproductive health, personal habits, and medical background, which are all critical factors influencing menstrual regularity. A comprehensive history includes relevant aspects such as the onset of menarche, the regularity of menstrual cycles, contraceptive use, and any previous gynecological issues. Additionally, it provides insight into broader health conditions such as thyroid disorders or polycystic ovary syndrome (PCOS) that may impact menstruation. This information not only aids in identifying the potential causes of amenorrhea but also helps clinicians prioritize differential diagnoses, which can range from hormonal imbalances to structural abnormalities that require intervention, as suggested in Yoo (2025). Furthermore, specific patient demographics significantly influence the diagnostic approach to amenorrhea, necessitating even more attention to medical history. For instance, in younger patients, primary amenorrhea or conditions like hypothalamic amenorrhea due to excessive exercise or stress may often come into play. In contrast, secondary amenorrhea frequently indicates underlying hormonal issues or lifestyle factors, especially among women of reproductive age. The importance of understanding these contextual nuances is emphasized in studies highlighting the diverse causes of amenorrhea, which require clinicians to be astute in recognizing patterns based on individual case histories. Comprehensive assessment of a patient's medical background, including previous treatments and psychosocial factors, is crucial for effective clinical management and tailored therapeutic interventions, as noted by Yoo (2025). Lastly, the integration of medical history with diagnostic tools enhances the overall patient assessment process. While laboratory tests and imaging studies play vital roles in confirming diagnoses, the initial medical history often reveals red flags that direct the course of testing and treatment. For example, a history of weight fluctuations or significant stressors may prompt a clinician to evaluate for conditions like hypothalamic amenorrhea or hyperprolactinemia more aggressively. The synergy between thorough history-taking and appropriate diagnostic testing has shown favorable outcomes in managing amenorrhea, as individualized treatment plans often lead to the resolution of symptoms. These interactions underline the necessity of a multidisciplinary approach in understanding and addressing the complexities of amenorrhea, ultimately leading to improved patient care and health outcomes as supported by findings in Behera *et al.* (2024).

Test Your Knowledge

1. Which diagnostic tests are typically used to evaluate amenorrhea?
2. Why is taking a detailed medical history important in diagnosing amenorrhea?

6.4. Impact on Health

Learning Outcome

1. Describe the physical health implications of amenorrhea
2. Explain the psychological effects associated with amenorrhea
3. Evaluate the long-term health risks linked to amenorrhea.

Amenorrhea, or absence of menstruation, can have a very significant effect on a woman's overall health, both physical and psychological. Beyond the apparent disruption of the menstrual cycle, the effects of this disorder extend to interfere with other body systems. For instance, the hormonal dysfunction typically present with amenorrhea can lead to such issues as osteoporosis, a condition of brittle bones, with a higher chance of fractures. Furthermore, the lack of regular menstrual cycles could be an indication of underlying diseases such as polycystic ovary syndrome (PCOS) or thyroid disease, both of which need to be medically screened and treated. The knowledge of these health implications is essential since it ensures responsible healthcare measures directed at lowering eventual health risks linked with amenorrhea. Beyond its physical health implications, amenorrhea also has profound psychological impacts on the individual. Women afflicted by this condition are apt to demonstrate inadequacy, anxiety, and depression due to the expectations and pressures exerted on femininity and reproduction from society. The psychological impairment of amenorrhea falls most forcefully on younger women who are searching for identity and body image. Further, stigmatization of menstrual disorders generates reduced disclosure of health problems, hence isolation and avoidance of professional help. Raising awareness regarding the psychological effects of amenorrhea is necessary in order to foster mental health care and educate women on their reproductive cycle processes.

Socioeconomic status also plays a significant role when it comes to the health effects of amenorrhea. Studies have revealed that women from low-income socioeconomic categories may experience higher levels of menstrual disorders due to the fact that they do not have easy access to health care services, education, and self-practice of health care resources (Islam *et al.*, 2024). This disparity tends to increase the severity of health results because such women may be ignorant of the health management needed. Additionally, the point at which cultural beliefs regarding menstruation intersect with socioeconomic status has the potential to further complicate health. These factors must be taken into consideration so that thorough healthcare plans can be established that give everyone the support and education required for treating amenorrhea and its larger implications for health (Jensen *et al.*, 2025).

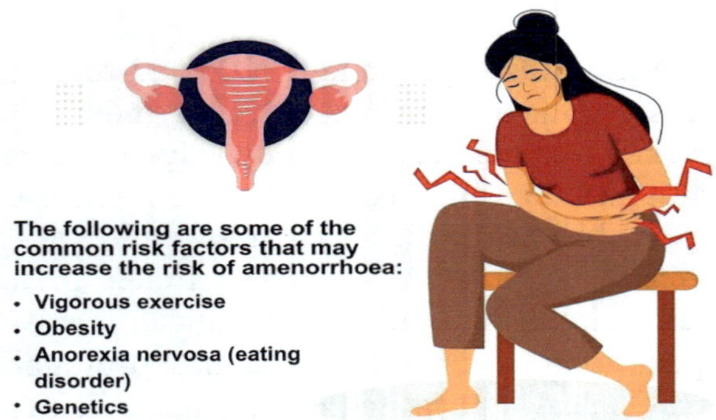

Figure 6.9. Risk factors of amenorrhea.

Source: https://lirp.cdn-website.com/69c0b277/dms3rep/multi/opt/Risk+factors+of+Amenorrhea+-+PACE+Hospitals-1920w.jpg

6.4.1. Physical Health Implications

Physical health effects of amenorrhea are profound, impacting varied biological processes in women. Amenorrhea is not only a symptom but may be a sign of possible health issues, such as the lack of menses. Lack of hormonal regulation, for instance, may lead to increased risk of osteoporosis due to low estrogen levels, which is crucial for maintaining bone density. Amenorrheic women may develop reduced bone mineral density, thereby promoting fractures and chronic skeletal disorders. Moreover, the psychological manifestations such as anxiety and depression that are part of the disorder tend to exacerbate physical health issues through the impact on diet and exercise levels, further creating a vicious circle of poor health. It is crucial to have management and treatment measures in place to reverse the implications of these conditions. Additionally, the physiological consequences of amenorrhea continue into metabolic health, further complicating its physical manifestations. When menstruation is lost, there tends to be a disruption in metabolic regulation that comes with it. This dysregulation may lead to weight fluctuation, which poses problems such as obesity or malnourishment, both of which carry their unique health consequences. Research has shown that metabolic derangement, which is caused by amenorrhea, also increases the risk of developing type 2 diabetes and insulin resistance. The interaction of amenorrhea and metabolic health points to the necessity of treatment approaches that address the multi-faceted condition. Therefore, reinstating not only the lack of menstruation but also the overall effect on metabolic status is critical in the formulation of sound intervention programs for patients suffering from the condition. Moreover, the psychosocial character of amenorrhea has far-reaching ramifications for body health, since chronic stress can fuel and worsen the condition. Described as "technostress," this phenomenon highlights the impact of modern work environments on employee health and well-being. When women experience difficulties in balancing family and career responsibilities, work-related stress can trigger or exacerbate amenorrhea, creating a lethal cycle of decline that impacts physical and mental health. The combination of technostress with amenorrhea illustrates the manner in which contemporary problems affect health beyond standard biological frameworks. Increased awareness and preventative measures are necessary when treating amenorrhea in a holistic sense, taking workplace dynamics and techno stressors into account that can aggravate outcomes for reducing health. More informed strategies like these can avoid long-term ramifications of this ailment, ultimately resulting in better health for women with amenorrhea.

6.4.2. Psychological Effects

Amenorrhea, or absence of menstruation, has extremely severe psychological impacts far greater than the physical impact of the condition. Individuals who experience amenorrhea typically face emotional distress in the form of depression, anxiety, and low self-esteem. The psychological distress may be due to body image and femininity pressures in society, which encourage feelings of failure or inadequacy once the body fails to live up to traditional ideals. Furthermore, the stress associated with the underlying conditions of amenorrhea, including disorders such as Polycystic Ovary Syndrome (PCOS), aggravates such emotional problems. The sense of health and fertility control generates an enhanced sense of vulnerability that challenges one's self-concept and mental health. Thus, psychological impact is significant in maintaining overall amenorrhea management because mental well-being is intrinsically linked to physical well-being outcomes. Research provides a very concerning interaction between psychological stressors and menstrual pathology, particularly in terms of significant life events or medical emergencies. For instance, with the COVID-19 pandemic, most women have reported menstrual cycle changes, including amenorrhea, with increased psychosocial stress. Social isolation, concern, and the overall anxiety related to health disturbances have been reported to dysregulate the hypothalamic-pituitary-adrenal axis, hence influencing hormonal balance and menstrual function. Research indicates that psychological distress caused by stress may also be physical, hence the need for addressing mental health when treating amenorrhea. Recognition of this intricate relationship underscores that psychological treatment has to be an integral part of care regimens for those suffering from amenorrhea since it can positively alter physiological outcomes. In addition to the immediate psychological impacts, long-term effects of amenorrhea can have cascading influences upon mental health and other aspects of health. Chronic amenorrhea, particularly when linked to disorders like PCOS, can lead to persistent feelings of frustration and distress that can produce chronic ailments like clinical depression or anxiety disorders. The persistent cycle of hope followed by disappointment regarding potential fertility or symptom relief can be disabling emotionally for the patient. Also, the embarrassment of reproductive health problems tends to compel the individual to internalize the issue, further excluding them and causing them to feel sad or worthless. Clinicians must, therefore, make sure that they cover both the psychological and physical sides of amenorrhea while promoting resilience and allowing the individual to successfully tackle their problems alongside controlling their reproductive health.

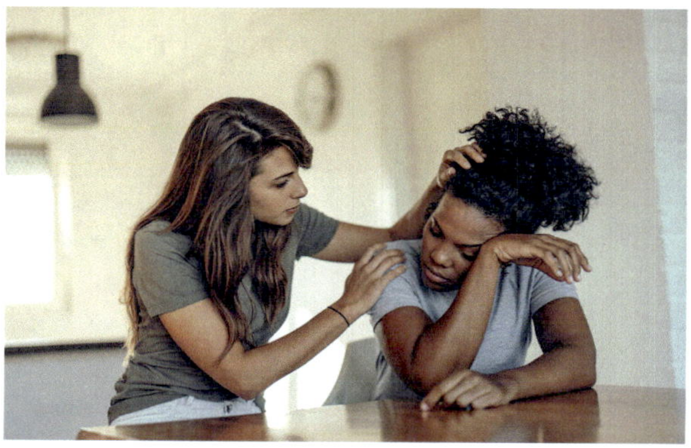

Source: https://www.my5palms.com/wp-content/uploads/2024/06/How-to-Help-Someone-With-Depression.png

6.4.3. Long-Term Health Risks

Amenorrhea would be a severe long-term health risk to those affected, particularly their reproductive health and well-being. One of the main concerns includes the impact of hormonal imbalance due to the absence of menstruation, which may result in complications such as infertility and decreased bone density. Women with long-standing amenorrhea may be unable to adapt to the physiological changes that follow estrogen deficiency, including an increased risk of osteoporosis. Such a condition can result in fractures and decreased quality of life, considering the key importance of menstrual health to the maintenance of skeletal strength over a lifespan. There has been evidence of a link between heavy metal exposure and long-standing amenorrhea. Particularly, research on the associations of blood concentrations of lead, cadmium, and mercury revealed elevated levels of lead to be related to prior infertility and chronic amenorrhea in women aged 20–49 years. More particularly, the research showed that lead exposure has a dose-dependent effect, which can possibly impair women's reproductive health and enhance the risks of infertility and amenorrhea. These findings illustrate the significance of environmental variables in women's health and the complex relationship between harmful exposures and reproductive function, further complicating the long-term medical hazards of amenorrhea. In addition to environmental variables, amenorrhea treatment, particularly if it is hypogonadism-induced, emphasizes the significance of long-term hormone replacement therapy (HRT). HRT aims to induce secondary sexual characteristics and guarantee psychosexual health in such involved adolescents. One should carefully note the risks and benefits provided by such therapy, as improper management can lead to amplified long-term diseases. Proper administration of estrogens and progesterones can also neutralize the adverse effects of amenorrhea, like potential fertility issues. Long-term effects of HRT require additional research to fully understand. Meanwhile, comprehensive management approaches must be developed to address the multifaceted health risks associated with amenorrhea, promoting a healthier future for those affected.

Test Your Knowledge

1. What are some physical health implications of amenorrhea?
- How can amenorrhea affect psychological well-being?

6.5. Treatment Options

Learning Outcome

1. Define hormonal therapies
2. Explain the lifestyle modifications
3. Discuss addressing underlying medical conditions

The treatment of amenorrhea is multifaceted, based on the cause of the condition. Proper clinical assessment is crucial in establishing the correct diagnosis, which in turn determines therapy. For patients with hypothalamic amenorrhea, lifestyle modifications such as weight gain and stress reduction have been found to be beneficial since these are most likely to disrupt hormonal equilibrium. Where amenorrhea occurs with polycystic ovary syndrome (PCOS), health practitioners can recommend pharmacologic treatment in the form of hormonal contraceptives to regulate menstrual cycles and to rectify associated symptoms. The comprehensive range approach emphasizes a treatment program to suit the individual subject, incorporating one that is compatible with the specific etiology of amenorrhea, thus ensuring maximum benefits for each subject. More severe forms of amenorrhea, such as those resulting from disorders like Asherman's syndrome, require more innovative treatments. Asherman's syndrome is characterized by the formation of scarring of the uterus, which can lead to reduced menstrual volume or complete amenorrhea. Treatments are commonly hysteroscopic surgery to remove adhesions and restore uterine function. This procedure is a pillar in the condition management due to the fact that it allows visualization and treatment of the uterine cavity directly. In addition, various restoration therapies, including hormone therapy and even recently explored stem cell therapies, are being developed in order to optimize recovery and fertility among the affected persons (Priya *et al.*, 2022). The evolving nature of the treatment modalities strives to improve the quality of life in these patients as well as address the subtleties of the condition. Also, some congenital abnormalities, such as Mullerian agenesis, offer particular challenges when amenorrhea is being treated. Diagnosed commonly in adolescence due to amenorrhea, the syndrome must be treated sensitively and individually.

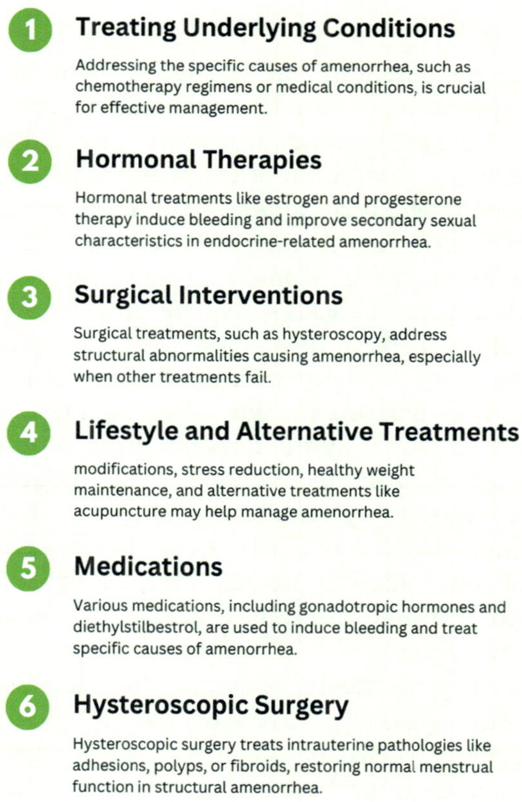
1
Treating Underlying Conditions
Addressing the specific causes of amenorrhea, such as chemotherapy regimens or medical conditions, is crucial for effective management.
2
Hormonal Therapies
Hormonal treatments like estrogen and progesterone therapy induce bleeding and improve secondary sexual characteristics in endocrine-related amenorrhea.
3
Surgical Interventions
Surgical treatments, such as hysteroscopy, address structural abnormalities causing amenorrhea, especially when other treatments fail.
4
Lifestyle and Alternative Treatments
modifications, stress reduction, healthy weight maintenance, and alternative treatments like acupuncture may help manage amenorrhea.
5
Medications
Various medications, including gonadotropic hormones and diethylstilbestrol, are used to induce bleeding and treat specific causes of amenorrhea.
6
Hysteroscopic Surgery
Hysteroscopic surgery treats intrauterine pathologies like adhesions, polyps, or fibroids, restoring normal menstrual function in structural amenorrhea.

Figure 6.10. Treatment option for amenorrhea.

Source: https://www.healthbenefitstimes.com/9/uploads/2024/06/Treatment-Options-for-Amenorrhea.png

Treatment can involve surgical procedures to form a functional vagina, allowing sexual function and psychosocial issues to be treated. Surgical and nonsurgical methods have been developed, recognizing the importance of patient education in the effective deployment of these treatments (Stanhiser *et al.*, 2016). Additionally, offering reproductive alternatives for patients with Mullerian agenesis is essential as it aids in a better understanding of their reproductive health and possible family planning. While treatment methods improve, individualized care stands as a point of emphasis in the solution to amenorrheas' varied etiologies.

6.5.1. Hormonal Therapies

The management of amenorrhea often involves the exploration of various hormonal treatments that restore menstrual cycles and adjust underlying hormonal disturbances. Among the significant techniques in the management of stress-induced amenorrhea, which is often prevalent in women undergoing severe psychological stresses, is the use of non-hormonal medications along with counseling of the patient's psychology. Recent studies show that treatments like *Vitex agnus-castus* extract may offer subtle dopaminergic support, thereby stabilizing endocrine homeostasis and restoring regular menstrual cycles. These findings underscore the need to integrate drugs with mental health care in order to obtain optimal treatment results, since the proper regulation of stressors is required in order to promote reproductive health among women, especially those who live in war-torn territories, such as Ukraine, where stress-induced amenorrhea has been increasingly observed (Tatarchuk *et al.*, 2024). In premature ovarian insufficiency (POI), hormonal therapy is key to bone density preservation and prevention of cardiovascular risk usually associated with premature menopause. Estrogen replacement is very significant in women under age 40 because it reverses the adverse effects of estrogen deficiency. Compared studies indicated that both menopausal hormone replacement therapy (HRT) and oral contraceptives (OCs) also have a positive impact on bone mineral density, significant in osteoporosis prevention. These therapies also have a normal lipid profile and liver function, showing reassuring evidence of their safety and efficacy. These observations indicate that the choice between OCs and HRT can be determined based on individual preference and need, emphasizing the importance of personalized healthcare in the management of amenorrhea in POI (Park, 2024).

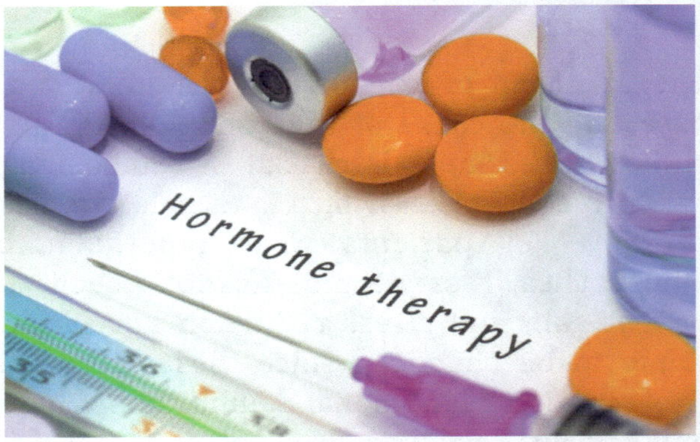

Source: https://thcobgyn.com/wp-content/uploads/2018/09/Texas-Health-Care-OBGYN-hormone-therapy.jpg

Though hormonal therapies are promising avenues for the treatment of both primary and secondary amenorrhea, it is important to consider thinking along the lines of a multi-faceted treatment plan that incorporates lifestyle modification and dietary surveillance. Taking the approach of combining psychological counseling, dietary intervention, and exercise conditioning can significantly enhance the effectiveness of hormonal treatments, offering a multidisciplinary treatment strategy to patients. Also, the long-term management of amenorrhea involves extensive assessment and follow-up to ascertain whether there are conditions underlying that may lead to menstrual irregularity. With a holistic model of care, health care practitioners are better positioned to help women with amenorrhea, not just restoring menstrual function but also general well-being. Thus, by embracing an array of treatment modalities, women are given the optimal care individualized to suit their specific situation for ultimate reproductive health outcomes.

6.5.2. Lifestyle Modifications

Effective management of amenorrhea often involves the addition of lifestyle modifications that have a significant influence on overall reproductive function. Of these adaptations, nutritional intake is most critical. A balanced diet made up of essential nutrients, particularly those with a role in hormonal balance, is crucial. Incorporating food sources high in omega-3 fatty acids, calcium, and iron is one type of food intake that could act to counteract some of the physiological stresses behind amenorrhea. These dietary modifications not only aim to restore menstrual cycles but also serve to enhance energy, regulate weight, and overall health. Moreover, the transition to a healthier diet can be empowering as one is able to become engaged with their own health. Therefore, understanding how diet affects hormonal regulation is important in the treatment of amenorrhea through lifestyle modifications specific to the condition, further indicating that a holistic approach can yield sustained health benefits. One other lifestyle modification that can positively impact individuals with amenorrhea is regular exercise. Moderate exercise helps with the regulation of body weight, stress, and metabolism improvement, all of which are essential in restoring menstrual cycles.

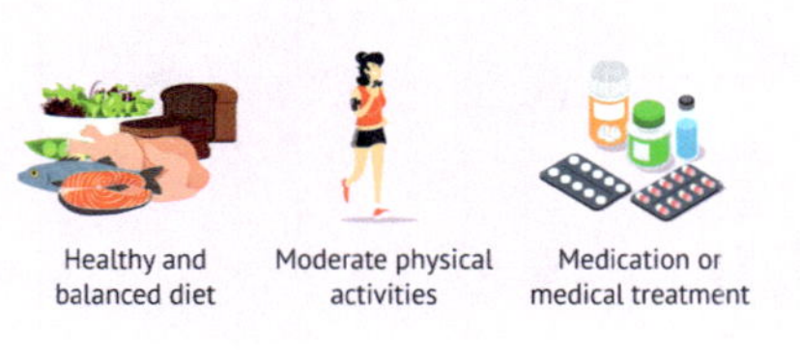

Source: https://www.invitra.com/en/amenorrhea/treatment-amenorrhea/

Research has indicated that both excessive and insufficient physical exercise can have a role to play in derailing hormone balance and leading to amenorrhea. Finding balance in the selection of low-impact exercises such as walking, yoga, or swimming can help alleviate some of the symptoms inflicted by the condition and also lead to general feelings of well-being. Physical exercise is also widely linked with improved mental health outcomes, hence solving the psychobehavioral issues that accompany amenorrhea. Thus, developing a particular fitness regimen can be a beneficial advantage for patients afflicted with this condition, not only keeping the body in general health but also mentally strong. Reduction of stress via mental health treatment is fundamental in the cure of amenorrhea. Chronic stress may have the ability to interfere with the hypothalamic-pituitary-ovarian axis and lead to irregular menses. Thus, the inclusion of such exercises as mindfulness, meditation, or cognitive-behavioral strategies can serve to counteract the stress and anxiety levels, thereby supporting an environment of hormonal balance. Psychological prioritization and the construction of coping mechanisms will enable one to effectively deal with the emotional burdens of amenorrhea. Moreover, such lifestyle modifications highlight the connection between mind and body, which makes it imperative that comprehensive treatment is required to recover. Addressing stress not only preserves hormonal health but also enhances overall quality of life, justifying the importance of incorporating mental well-being strategies into lifestyle change. Adopting a holistic approach guarantees individuals can construct lasting change that enhances amenorrhea treatment results as well as long-term well-being.

6.5.3. Addressing Underlying Medical Conditions

It is critical to treat and manage underlying medical conditions when managing amenorrhea since some conditions may be a significant contributing factor to abnormal menstrual cycles. For instance, polycystic ovary syndrome (PCOS), thyroid dysfunctions, and endocrinological disturbances often lead to abnormal menstrual cycles. The diagnosis of these disturbances is achieved through proper evaluation in the form of a complete history, physical examination, and applicable laboratory studies. Once such underlying conditions are diagnosed, treatment can be designed to address these, thereby enabling the control of amenorrhea. Addressing the root causes, medical professionals can devise treatment regimens that cure both amenorrhea itself and the underlying medical conditions, eventually enhancing the overall well-being and health of patients. In addition to the direct symptoms of amenorrhea, the effects of the underlying, untreated conditions may extend to quality of life as well. Medical diseases such as autoimmune diseases, metabolic syndromes, or even malignancies might be manifested in the form of menstrual abnormalities. Such medical diseases should be managed early, not only for normalization of menstruation but also for prevention of long-term sequelae. For example, early identification of thyroid dysfunction will avert weight gain, mood disorders, and cardiovascular disease risks, all of which may be secondary to chronic amenorrhea. Additionally, situations highlighted in recent studies, such as repeated pneumonia because of congenital heart disease, show how comorbid basic medical conditions can worsen the problems with amenorrhea. With the implementation of a strategy that treats these underlying complications, healthcare workers can significantly enhance patient results and quality of life (Sen *et al.*, 2024). Finally, holistic treatment of amenorrhea must entail a good understanding of potential underlying medical conditions and their impacts. This means not only direct symptoms of amenorrhea but also the general health implications that can arise from neglect of these conditions. Emphasis on the importance of holistic examinations and subsequent interventions will ensure that patients are given appropriate care and attention. This exchange will also encourage patients to seek care at an early stage, cultivating a proactive attitude toward their health. Lastly, the proper management of underlying medical conditions will not only restore menstrual function but will also enable individuals to maintain optimum health and prevent future complications, vindicating the importance of a holistic approach to amenorrhea management (Alayed, 2024).

Test Your Knowledge

1. What lifestyle modifications can support treatment outcomes?
2. Why is it important to address underlying medical conditions in treatment plans?

6.6. Prevention Strategies

Learning Outcome

1. Explain the importance of maintaining a healthy lifestyle
2. Discuss the role of regular medical check-ups for amenorrhea
3. Define how education and awareness contribute to the prevention and treatment of amenorrhea

Prevention of amenorrhea frequently requires a multi-component strategy based on lifestyle changes and preventive healthcare measures. Education about menstruation is crucial, especially among adolescents who are experiencing profound physiological shifts. Broader interventions that include topics of nutrition, physical exercise, and stress reduction can make young women more likely to keep their menstrual cycle healthy. Studies have shown that up to 67.8% of adolescent girls experience menstrual disorders, and thus, the need for the establishment of certain prevention methods through lifestyle choices is pressing. Exercise on a regular basis, along with a balanced diet, can lower the vulnerability to amenorrhea and other menstrual irregularities. Apart from that, the development of environments to ensure mental wellness is likely to de-stress, which has also been shown to play a part in menstrual disorders (Sappe ARK *et al.*, 2024).

Prevention, based on the function of hormonal influence, particularly for the young female population receiving treatments for breast cancer, becomes more complicated. Chemotherapy and some anti-cancer therapies induce amenorrhea and pose risks of premature ovarian failure (POI). Studies support the application of temporary ovarian suppression by gonadotropin-releasing hormone analogues (GnRHa) for chemotherapy as a very effective approach. The technique has been found to significantly reduce the likelihood of chemotherapeutic amenorrhea and preserve fertility in premenopausal women (Lei *et al.*, 2021). These procedures indicate the need for integrating preventive health care into settings in which young women are at risk of amenorrhea as a side effect of necessary treatments. Lastly, prevention of amenorrhea must include publicity and access to reproductive health care. Young women must become aware and be encouraged to request visits to health providers for individualized assessments and interventions addressing their own individual needs. Providing access to information on the effects of drugs, habits, and the management of stress can provide individuals with the capacity for decision-making. Also important is the availability of options for maintaining fertility, such as embryo or oocyte cryopreservation in individuals at risk of infertility due to treatment-induced amenorrhea. With improved education and support for menstrual health, health systems can improve the treatment and prevention of amenorrhea to yield improved reproductive outcomes in young women (Lei *et al.*, 2021). Ultimately, an integrated approach with lifestyle intervention, medical treatment, and comprehensive reproductive health education is likely the solution to addressing the complex problems of amenorrhea.

6.6.1. Maintaining A Healthy Lifestyle

The concept of following a healthy lifestyle has much to do with the overall well-being of the person, particularly in the context of amenorrhea, or the inability to menstruate. Adopting healthy lifestyle practices like regular exercise, a healthy diet, and sufficient water intake can significantly affect menstrual well-being. For instance, women who are physically active enough are less likely to experience hormonal disturbances that may cause amenorrhea. Research shows that problems related to lifestyle, like maintaining good body weight, can lead to better reproductive health and regular menstrual cycles. People can prevent the dangers of amenorrhea and enhance their reproductive health through an active lifestyle. Balancing hormonal function and menstrual health requires nutrition. The correct diet that involves fruits, vegetables, whole grains, and necessary nutrients supports proper body functions, including reproductive health. Some dietary styles, such as those based on a Mediterranean diet, have been associated with improved health, including normal menstruation. Individuals who implement these dietary habits into their lifestyle not only enhance their overall health but also decrease the risk of ailments like amenorrhea. Nutrition is claimed to result in better hormonal equilibrium and ultimately assist in regulating normal menstrual cycles. Nutrition thus becomes an essential element in a good lifestyle regimen for individuals who wish to maintain reproductive health and prevent amenorrhea.

Also, the emotional aspect of a balanced life cannot be left out in the case of amenorrhea. Stress and mental health management are equally crucial, as psychological factors can greatly impact hormonal balance and menstrual cycles. Stress-reducing therapies such as mindfulness, yoga, or meditation can help create emotional equilibrium and even reverse amenorrhea in the victim. This is crucial in light of the fact that excessive levels of stress directly correlate with disrupted hormonal pathways and thus menstrual cycle irregularities. Therefore, adopting an approach that encompasses physical health, diet, and mental well-being is vital for maintaining a healthy lifestyle as well as in the management of conditions like amenorrhea. Emphasizing the interconnectedness of the factors can give individuals a comprehensive framework for enhancing their reproductive health as well as overall well-being.

6.6.2. Regular Medical Check-Ups

Regular medical check-ups also play a core role in the early detection and treatment of amenorrhea, particularly among adolescents. These routine assessments provide a great platform for medical experts to assess and monitor reproductive health among young women. Because most individuals fear seeking help with menstrual ailments because of ignorance or stigma, regular check-ups can provide an open platform for discussing such concerns and demystifying the subject. By focusing on the early identification of conditions such as polycystic ovary syndrome or hypothalamic amenorrhea, healthcare practitioners are able to intervene at the appropriate time, facilitating optimal long-term outcomes. The significance of early detection is further underscored by findings that show that anticipatory use of healthcare significantly improves the reproductive health of adolescents, suppressing the risk of chronic conditions worsening over time (Agarwal *et al.*, 2024). In addition to remedying physical health problems, regular medical check-ups also provide psychological support for teenage girls who undergo the ordeal of adolescence. The care of their psychological problems in dealing with amenorrhea must not be dismissed, as teenage girls may be confronted with distress and feelings of self-esteem due to their menstruation. By means of these check-ups, clinicians are able to give recommendations and reassurance to adolescent girls so they can air their concerns in a non-judgmental environment. Also, issues of lifestyle factors—nutrition, physical activity, and stress—ordinarily become a discussion point, which can prove decisive in preventing amenorrhea. Pediatric gynecologic practice allows for a holistic approach to health in recognizing the interrelationship between physical and emotional well-being and thus supporting a more holistic approach to adolescent gynecologic issues (Bhavana V Waghmare *et al.*, 2024). Lastly, the value of regular check-ups is not just to individual health but ultimately results in more significant public health effects. Public awareness programs that encourage routine gynecological examinations can enhance amenorrhea and related disorder awareness, fostering a prevention culture. Education campaigns have the potential to play a central role in demystifying reproductive health complications and giving young women confidence to access care without anxiety. Furthermore, the integration of information from regular check-ups can inform healthcare policy and resource allocation so that healthcare systems can effectively treat adolescent gynecological demands. Medical check-ups are thus not only a tool for individual care but also a platform on which reproductive health can be optimized on a mass level to ensure wellness among subsequent generations (Agarwal *et al.*, 2024).

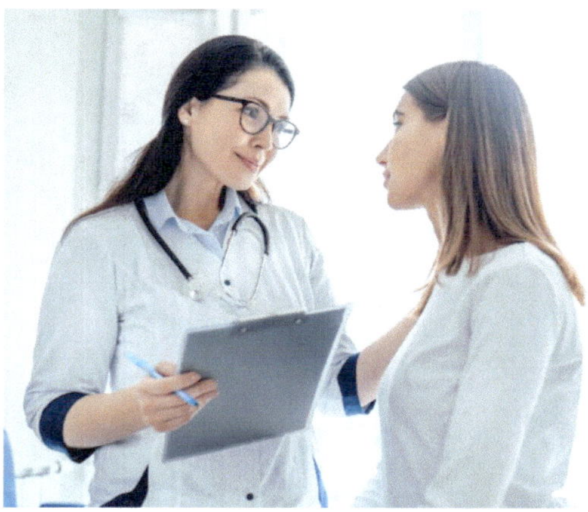

Source: https://htv.com.pk/wp-content/uploads/2195671.jpeg

6.6.3. Education and Awareness

Education and awareness form the cornerstone of the understanding and treatment of amenorrhea, particularly in groups with higher risk, i.e., athletes and those with polycystic ovary syndrome (PCOS). The multifactorial causation of amenorrhea makes it necessary that clients and healthcare professionals are well-informed about its physiological, psychological, and sociocultural dimensions. Comprehensive educational programs have the potential to enhance symptom awareness, empower women to seek early treatment, and provide an open setting for discussion of menstrual health. Greater awareness of the capacity of psychological stressors to induce amenorrhea is particularly important among elite athletes. As highlighted by recent policy statements, physical and mental health are inseparable, and a holistic education approach that addresses both in the debate of amenorrhea and the overall influence on general health and athletic performance is appropriate (Reardon *et al.*, 2019).

Also, guidelines outlined for PCOS management stress the importance of informed consent and active patient involvement in treatment planning. PCOS women normally present with more than just reproductive complications, such as psychological well-being and lifestyle management. Appropriate education on the symptoms, potential health impacts, and treatment of the syndromes assists women in empowering themselves in their own healthcare journey. More awareness of PCOS can mean appropriate diagnoses as well as individualized management based on women's personal experience with the condition. Global guidelines underscore the necessity of enhanced health education with the assistance of consumer feedback into educational material preparation to address both physical and mental well-being (Teede *et al.*, 2018). Such innovation can facilitate widespread awareness regarding amenorrhea in relation to PCOS. Finally, public health interventions and community outreach can further promote education and awareness about menstruation and work to correct myths and stigmatization related to menstrual disorders. They must be targeted towards various communities with culturally relevant information that will attract a variety of groups. Women can be educated by public health education about the significance of menstrual health as a component of good overall health and the warning signs that need to be seen. The formation of support groups, like peer discussions or forums, can also create a sense of community and sharedness among women. Focusing on education and awareness, health workers can facilitate ease of access to intervention and support in the initial stages, thus optimizing the outcome on health for those who have amenorrhea (Reardon *et al.*, 2019; Teede *et al.*, 2018).

Test Your Knowledge

1. Why are regular medical check-ups important for individuals with amenorrhea?
2. How can education and awareness improve outcomes for those affected by amenorrhea?

SUMMARY

Briefly put, amenorrhea, while a symptom rather than an independently existing condition, involves a wide comprehension of its underlying causes and effects on women's health. The intricate interplay between amenorrhea and ailments such as Polycystic Ovarian Syndrome (PCOS) and Non-Alcoholic Hepatic Steatosis Disease (NAHSD) illustrates the multidimensionality of reproductive health ailments. Evidence shows that women with PCOS are more at risk for liver conditions, and the interrelation calls for active surveillance of health and intervention against related risks. Seeing and reacting to these relationships matters not only as a method of avoiding long-term health complications but also as a method of improving the quality of life in women with amenorrhea and related conditions (Khan *et al.*, 2024). Aside from its significance for reproduction, amenorrhea also has a wide variety of impacts on other aspects of women's general health, such as sexual and psychological health. Similar to the situation with sexual dysfunction in patients with chronic illness, the psychological impact of such reproductive symptomatology cannot be overestimated. The majority of women with amenorrhea are usually upset and experience loss of sexual function, particularly if the amenorrhea per se is untreated or poorly managed in clinical practice. Healthcare providers must recognize the merits of addressing these sensitive topics under consideration and integrating sexual health examinations into routine assessment of amenorrheic individuals to facilitate a holistic approach in caregiving (Nørskov *et al.*, 2024).

Lastly, the need for multi-disciplinary treatment avenues for amenorrhea becomes all the more pronounced. As more intensively the interrelations among various health conditions are probed, one understands that interdisciplinary collaboration between medical specialists—like endocrinologists, gynecologists, and psychologists—is important. Treating the connection of physical and emotional welfare in women suffering from amenorrhea, healthcare providers are able to create efficient treatment plans that not only address the physiological aspects of the disease but also enhance emotional and sexual well-being. This integrative treatment is important to deliver comprehensive management strategies that enable women to regain their reproductive health and overall well-being (Khan *et al.*, 2024).

Amenorrhea, or non-menses, is a multifaceted disorder with numerous physiological, psychological, and lifestyle determinants. Identification of underlying etiology, from normal states such as pregnancy and lactation to more complex disorders of PCOS and hypothalamic amenorrhea, is necessary. The potential etiologies are so wide-ranging that a broad diagnostic approach must consider patient history, hormonal status, and lifestyle. Early diagnosis is imperative, as prolonged amenorrhea can lead to grave health issues, including bone loss and infertility, and therefore highlights the need for early treatment and control with a proper sense of the various causes of amenorrhea. The coincidence between endometriosis and amenorrhea also highlights another major area in the understanding of menstrual pathology. Endometriosis, affecting approximately 190 million women and individuals assigned female at birth worldwide, is characterized by the presence of endometrial-type tissue in locations outside the uterus, typically with consequent crippling pain as well as infertility. Because the condition is frequently heterogeneous in presentation, a persistent diagnostic delay remains a common feature, reflecting the need for greater familiarity among health professionals. Understanding how endometriosis can contribute to amenorrhea is critical for clinicians because patients presenting with these symptoms will usually require both reproductive and pain management interventions to treat their complex disease, ultimately being treated in a tailored, multidisciplinary manner (Horne *et al.*, 2022). Psychological components, such as stress and eating disorders, also have a broad influence on the prevalence of amenorrhea. Such disorders as anorexia nervosa have the consequence of inducing hormonal imbalance, and in reaction, the hypothalamus will be compelled to suppress menstruation. This calls for taking a biopsychosocial approach in treating amenorrhea, considering both physical health and psychological health in treatment programs. Studies have shown that by addressing these psychological factors, reproductive health outcomes can be optimized and the severity of related symptoms reduced. With advancing healthcare, a thorough understanding of all the cross-cutting determinants behind amenorrhea—multiple which vary from hormonal variations to psychological tension and debilitating diseases—will be required for proper patient management and improved overall health (Anand *et al.*, 2022).

KEY TERMS FROM THIS CHAPTER

- Primary amenorrhea
- Hypothalamic dysfunction
- Premature ovarian insufficiency
- Asherman's syndrome
- Thyroid dysfunction
- Eating disorders
- Medications
- Secondary amenorrhea
- Hyperprolactinemia
- Turner syndrome
- Androgen insensitivity syndrome
- Chronic illness
- Excessive exercise

CRITICAL THINKING QUESTIONS

1. **Amenorrhea is defined as the absence of:**
   a. Ovulation
   b. Menstruation
   c. Fertilization
   d. Pregnancy
2. **Primary amenorrhea is diagnosed when a girl has not had her first menstrual period by age:**
   a. 12 years
   b. 13 years
   c. 15 years
   d. 18 years
3. **Secondary amenorrhea refers to the absence of menstruation for how many months in a woman who previously had normal cycles?**
   a. 1 month
   b. 3 months
   c. 6 months
   d. 12 months
4. **Which of the following is NOT a common cause of amenorrhea?**
   a. Pregnancy
   b. Polycystic ovary syndrome (PCOS)
   c. Hypothyroidism
   d. Appendicitis
5. **Which hormone is typically low in cases of hypothalamic amenorrhea?**
   a. Prolactin
   b. Gonadotropin-releasing hormone (GnRH)
   c. Estrogen
   d. Progesterone

Short Answer Questions

1. What is the difference between primary and secondary amenorrhea?
2. Name one common cause of amenorrhea.
3. Besides the absence of menstruation, name one symptom that may accompany amenorrhea.
4. How can amenorrhea affect bone health?
5. What is one common treatment approach for amenorrhea caused by hormonal imbalance?
6. Name one lifestyle change that can help prevent amenorrhea.

Answer to Critical Thinking Questions

1. (b) 2. (c) 3. (b) 4. (d) 5. (b)

REFERENCES

1. Agarwal, M., Singh, S., Jyoti, C., Sinha, S., & Simran, S. (2024). Understanding adolescent gynecological issues: A cross-sectional study at a tertiary care center. *Cureus*. https://doi.org/10.7759/cureus.57713 (accessed on 14th June 2025).
2. Alayed, K. M. (2024). Multiple immune dysregulation conditions with a single underlying root cause of NRAS gene-positivity: A case report. *Middle East Journal of Medical Case Reports*. https://www.semanticscholar.org/paper/b536ef26d6dbf58bff02c98613eb13c76d5a8c18 (accessed on 14th June 2025).
3. Alhajeri, A., Hajji, S., & Aljenaee, K. (2024). Amenorrhea as a presentation of Cushing's syndrome. *Endocrinology, Diabetes & Metabolism Case Reports, 2024*. https://www.semanticscholar.org/paper/ec489dc664ca3d8247ed0416048c0f8af8185506 (accessed on 14th June 2025).
4. Alhetheli, G., Alhazmi, S., Almutairi, S. M., Alharbi, S., Alharbi, N., Alsweed, M., Al-Dhubaibi, M. S., *et al.* (2022). The effects of isotretinoin on the menstrual cycle: A cross-sectional study. *Clinics and Practice, 12*, 908–917. https://doi.org/10.3390/clinpract12060095 (accessed on 14th June 2025).
5. Anand, U., Dey, A., Singh Chandel, A. K., Sanyal, R., Mishra, A., Pandey, D. K., De Falco, V., *et al.* (2022). Cancer chemotherapy and beyond: Current status, drug candidates, associated risks and progress in targeted therapeutics. *Genes & Diseases, 10*, 1367–1401. https://doi.org/10.1016/j.gendis.2022.02.007 (accessed on 14th June 2025).
6. Apriliana, D. N., Restiana, R. P., Dalope, I. Y., Perdana, A. A., & Widiyasa, A. (2022). Irregular menstruation, acne, hirsutism, and the possibility with PCOS. *International Journal of Medical Science and Clinical Invention*. https://www.semanticscholar.org/paper/74ca98af6f60a8190 1239ef58f16776ebec3ff35 (accessed on 14th June 2025).
7. Auriemma, R. S., Pirchio, R., Pivonello, C., Garifalos, F., Colao, A., & Pivonello, R. (2023). Approach to the patient with prolactinoma. *The Journal of Clinical Endocrinology & Metabolism, 108*, 2400–2423. https://doi.org/10.1210/clinem/dgad174 (accessed on 14th June 2025).
8. Barot, S., Rantanen, P., Nordenvall, C., Lindforss, U., Hallqvist Everhov, Å., Larsson, S. C., Lindblom, A., *et al.* (2023). Combined associations of a healthy lifestyle and body mass index with colorectal cancer recurrence and survival: A cohort study. *Cancer Causes & Control, 35*, 367–376. https://www.semanticscholar.org/paper/c4888405480162a3821a8035a383dc2fdcff1600 (accessed on 14th June 2025).
9. Behera, A., Panda, S., Choudhary, A. K., & Sahu, M. (2024). Evaluation and management of secondary amenorrhea: A case series in a tertiary care center. *International Journal of Medical and Biomedical Studies*. https://www.semanticscholar.org/paper/35bf96f750bdc261b5a5f1 b2d6ac2a7e92fdddc9 (accessed on 14th June 2025).
10. Caio, G., Volta, U., Sapone, A., Leffler, D. A., De Giorgio, R., Catassi, C., & Fasano, A. (2019). Celiac disease: A comprehensive current review. *BMC Medicine, 17*. https://doi.org/10.1186/s12916-019-1380-z (accessed on 14th June 2025).
11. Costa, T. A., & Menezes, M. P. N. (2024). The biological and psychological impact of the Coronavirus disease-19 pandemic on the characteristics of the menstrual cycle. *Journal of the Turkish German Gynecological Association, 25*, 259–265. https://www.semanticscholar.org/paper/5e8caebddb0e3c096eebfd1ccfbcc39f06fcaef0 (accessed on 14th June 2025).

12. Elmakki, E. (2024). The role of lifestyle modifications in preventing and managing systemic hypertension: Current guidelines and future directions. *Annals of African Medicine, 24*, 1–8. https://www.semanticscholar.org/paper/c2f973899425b0386b929de448319684b212e9bf (accessed on 14th June 2025).

13. Erenler, F., & Mathyk, B. (2024). 7521 Unmasking of PCOS after macroprolactinoma treatment. *Journal of the Endocrine Society, 8*. https://www.semanticscholar.org/paper/c495366e005966ae6ebb0ac1e076203335d2c749 (accessed on 14th June 2025).

14. Goswami, Y., & Gaurkar, S. (2023). Ramsay Hunt syndrome: An introduction, signs and symptoms, and treatment. *Cureus, 15*. https://www.semanticscholar.org/paper/d1156ab20a108fe569a25ebe45da0fbcb5caf864 (accessed on 14th June 2025).

15. Horne, A. W., & Missmer, S. A. (2022). Pathophysiology, diagnosis, and management of endometriosis. *BMJ*. https://doi.org/10.1136/bmj-2022-070750 (accessed on 14th June 2025).

16. Islam, S., Afrin, W., & Khatun, K. (2024). Menstrual disorders and self-care practices: A study on prevalence among female undergraduate students. *Scholars International Journal of Obstetrics and Gynecology*. https://www.semanticscholar.org/paper/72a1c19e03f97769a32ade62f8e6ec9dbd4a8410 (accessed on 14th June 2025).

17. Jensen, A., Clarke, E. J., Nugent, Z., Paice, E., Gringel, I., Yamamoto, K., Rocchigiani, G., *et al.* (2025). Inflammation and response to bacterial infection as potential drivers of equine odontoclastic tooth resorption and hypercementosis: A proteomics insight. *Equine Veterinary Journal*. https://www.semanticscholar.org/paper/68b07eef1871fe31a8298042cf98cc6bfba8c714 (accessed on 14th June 2025).

18. Jeong, J., Kim, B. J., & Lee, J. (2024). Navigating AI transitions: How coaching leadership buffers against job stress and protects employee physical health. *Frontiers in Public Health, 12*. https://www.semanticscholar.org/paper/ab690837d81dc1118b253a6470da1a5315deb728 (accessed on 14th June 2025).

19. Kaida, K. (2021). Dysautonomia in immune-mediated neuropathies. *Neurology and Clinical Neuroscience, 10*, 124–129. https://www.semanticscholar.org/paper/182ed4d1e5681e150c4d7f60abde57a87f8cf62d (accessed on 14th June 2025).

20. Khan, S., Zubair, M., Rehman, A., Zahid, I., Gulali, S. S., Yousafzai, S. Y., & Khan, M. (2024). Sonographic association between hepatic steatosis disease and polycystic ovarian syndrome in Swabi women. *Journal of Health and Rehabilitation Research*. https://www.semanticscholar.org/paper/27a36f428d75a4f8f4881c1c3753edd40b330f23 (accessed on 14th June 2025).

21. Lei, Y., & Yeo, W. (2021). The risk of menopausal symptoms in premenopausal breast cancer patients and current pharmacological prevention strategies. *Expert Opinion on Drug Safety, 20*, 1163–1175. https://www.semanticscholar.org/paper/07d1744f60d7e8ba6a97133817e99e1477dcf376 (accessed on 14th June 2025).

22. Lippi, G., Henry, B., & Plebani, M. (2022). An overview of the most important preanalytical factors influencing the clinical performance of SARS-CoV-2 antigen rapid diagnostic tests (Ag-RDTs). *Clinical Chemistry and Laboratory Medicine (CCLM), 61*, 196–204. https://www.semanticscholar.org/paper/98297e7f3b0447b6077306c12a83efc18817ca21 (accessed on 14th June 2025).

23. Lo, W. C., Hu, T., Shih, C. Y., Lin, H. H., & Hwang, J. S. (2024). Impact of healthy lifestyle factors on life expectancy and lifetime health care expenditure: Nationwide cohort study. *JMIR Public*

Health and Surveillance, *10*. https://www.semanticscholar.org/paper/1696731194d00edde1b7e8279c1d1f2e1eed1adf (accessed on 14th June 2025).

24. McClam, M., Liu, J., Fan, Y., Zhan, T., Zhang, Q., Porter, D., Scott, G. I., *et al.* (2023). Associations between exposure to cadmium, lead, mercury and mixtures and women's infertility and long-term amenorrhea. *Archives of Public Health*, *81*. https://www.semanticscholar.org/paper/43afeee79c00887f78a00ca70375496115675c2e (accessed on 14th June 2025).
25. Mohd Shukri, M. F., Norhayati, M. N., Badrin, S., & Abdul Kadir, A. (2022). Effects of L-carnitine supplementation for women with polycystic ovary syndrome: A systematic review and meta-analysis. *PeerJ*, *10*. https://www.semanticscholar.org/paper/60ca60bc0ce410ccab1985c775fade93bb7d0dae (accessed on 14th June 2025).
26. Nelson, L. M., Spencer, H., Hijane, K., Thinuan, P., Nelson, C. W., Vincent, A., Gordon, C. M., *et al.* (2023). My 28 Days–A global digital women's health initiative for evaluation and management of secondary amenorrhea: Case report and literature review. *Frontiers in Endocrinology*, *14*. https://doi.org/10.3389/fendo.2023.1227253 (accessed on 14th June 2025).
27. Nørskov, K., Schjoedt, I., Tolver, A., & Jarden, M. (2024). Sexual health in patients with malignant hematological disease: A Danish cross-sectional study. *Sexual Medicine*, *12*. https://www.semanticscholar.org/paper/3c11fff7b2f82b3a6fc6fec84e056e33b9175028 (accessed on 14th June 2025).
28. Park, J. C. (2024). Comparison of the effectiveness of hormonal replacement therapy and oral contraceptive pills in women with premature ovarian insufficiency. *Journal of the Korea Academia-Industrial Cooperation Society*. https://www.semanticscholar.org/paper/ce275745ea10bbcb2ac3264d0cc0646d0c9c52e2 (accessed on 14th June 2025).
29. Priya, S., & M, U. (2022). Asherman's syndrome (intrauterine synechiae). *International Journal of Nursing Education and Research*. https://www.semanticscholar.org/paper/206fd84a0179f100daf9e90c505ec70b862958db (accessed on 14th June 2025).
30. Reardon, C. L., Hainline, B., Miller Aron, C., Baron, D., Baum, A., Bindra, A., Budgett, R., *et al.* (2019). Mental health in elite athletes: International Olympic Committee consensus statement (2019). *British Journal of Sports Medicine*, *53*, 667–699. https://doi.org/10.1136/bjsports-2019-100715 (accessed on 14th June 2025).
31. Sappe, A. R. K., Oktavia, A. T., Chairunnisa, A., & Undaryat, Y. M. (2024). Menstrual cycle disorders in adolescents. *Journal Multidiscipline Indonesia*. https://www.semanticscholar.org/paper/11c38858b07896e3ea69e8cf5b9a3dcc26009ca5 (accessed on 14th June 2025).
32. Semou, T., Monteiro, S., Hariharan, M., Padhy, M., & Chivukula, U. (2024). Impact of hypertension education on knowledge and healthy lifestyle practices among Indian adolescents: A quasi-experimental study. *Health Education Journal*, *84*, 33–44. https://www.semanticscholar.org/paper/7c2a5a23c7d891b0d0047051061262f9a94e732a (accessed on 14th June 2025).
33. Sen, T., Datta, G. C., Islam, M. M. Z., Islam, A., Iqbal, M. J., & Ahmed, A. S. M. N. U. (2024). Clinical profile and underlying causes of recurrent pneumonia in young children. *International Journal of Research in Medical Sciences*. https://www.semanticscholar.org/paper/2932d96fd30f510c9020a2cf3e46a3beb1125d93 (accessed on 14th June 2025).
34. Seppä, S., Kuiri-Hänninen, T., Holopainen, E., & Voutilainen, R. (2021). Management of endocrine disease: Diagnosis and management of primary amenorrhea and female delayed puberty. *European Journal of Endocrinology*, *184*, R225–R242. https://doi.org/10.1530/eje-20-1487 (accessed on 14th June 2025).

35. Shadman, M. (2023). Diagnosis and treatment of chronic lymphocytic leukemia: A review. *JAMA*, *329*(11), 918–932. https://www.semanticscholar.org/paper/57507ae473307f3cf9330 25aa7dda407fbd45aa9 (accessed on 14th June 2025).

36. Sitthiyod Samakkhiwitthayakhom, T. (2024). Advancements in Alzheimer's disease: Emerging therapies, lifestyle modifications, and early intervention strategies. *International Journal of Current Science Research and Review*. https://www.semanticscholar.org/paper/fbc7f2c9e77e6050205c24c35a24db9200893993 (accessed on 14th June 2025).

37. Sommovigo, V., Bernuzzi, C., Finstad, G. L., Setti, I., Gabanelli, P., Giorgi, G., & Fiabane, E. (2023). How and when may technostress impact workers' psycho-physical health and work-family interface? A study during the COVID-19 pandemic in Italy. *International Journal of Environmental Research and Public Health*, *20*. https://www.semanticscholar.org/paper/4bb 3d552026ea7d357f43d6c93c1cc10fafadd06 (accessed on 14th June 2025).

38. Stanhiser, J., & Attaran, M. (2016). Müllerian agenesis: Diagnosis, treatment, and future fertility. https://www.semanticscholar.org/paper/5c94c56d33988a739ae4d560da7f2753 cb381616 (accessed on 14th June 2025).

39. Stuenkel, C. A., Gompel, A., Davis, S. R., Pinkerton, J. V., Lumsden, M. A., & Santen, R. J. (2021). Approach to the patient with new-onset secondary amenorrhea: Is this primary ovarian insufficiency? *The Journal of Clinical Endocrinology & Metabolism*, *107*, 825–835. https://doi.org/10.1210/clinem/dgab766 (accessed on 14th June 2025).

40. Takahashi, A., Hayashi, F., Ohira, T., Shimabukuro, M., Sakai, A., Maeda, M., Hosoya, M., *et al.* (2024). Impact of changes in lifestyle and psychological factors on the incidence of metabolic syndrome after the Great East Japan Earthquake: Follow-up of the Fukushima Health Management Survey. *Journal of Atherosclerosis and Thrombosis*, *32*, 345–355. https://www.semanticscholar.org/paper/600248c6bc58e62cb151c825e487e4aa4d1f2275 (accessed on 14th June 2025).

41. Takahashi, T., Kosei, N. V., Yakimets, V. M., Plaksiieva, K., Regeda, S., & Pylypenko, A. (2024). Stress-induced amenorrhea–possibilities for non-hormonal correction. *Reproductive Endocrinology*. https://www.semanticscholar.org/paper/5ec5afdc2063a32c6a0432bb4718a 74a48265651 (accessed on 14th June 2025).

42. Teede, H., Misso, M., Costello, M., Dokras, A., Laven, J. S. E., Moran, L., Piltonen, T., *et al.* (2018). Recommendations from the international evidence-based guideline for the assessment and management of polycystic ovary syndrome. *Clinical Endocrinology*, *89*, 251–268. https://doi.org/10.1111/cen.13795 (accessed on 14th June 2025).

43. Voutsadaki, K., Matalliotakis, M., & Ladomenou, F. (2022). Hypogonadism in adolescent girls: Treatment and long-term effects. *Acta Bio Medica: Atenei Parmensis*, *93*. https://www.semanticscholar.org/paper/e784a761430e6565880a6dab084adbf678efff57 (accessed on 14th June 2025).

44. Waghmare, B. V., & Jajoo, S. (2024). Navigating the challenges: A comprehensive review of adolescent gynecological problems. *Cureus*. https://doi.org/10.7759/cureus.56200 (accessed on 14th June 2025).

45. Witchel, S. F., Oberfield, S. E., & Peña, A. S. (2019). Polycystic ovary syndrome: Pathophysiology, presentation, and treatment with emphasis on adolescent girls. *Journal of the Endocrine Society*, *3*, 1545–1573. https://doi.org/10.1210/js.2019-00078 (accessed on 14th June 2025).

46. Yoo, I. H. (2025). Pediatric abdominal pain: The need for a careful differential diagnosis according to age. *Journal of the Korean Medical Association*. https://www.semanticscholar.org/paper/fe4d1948af082209d8ef9d58b57a3cb696e5f1ee (accessed on 14th June 2025).

47. Yoon, J. Y., & Cheon, C. K. (2019). Evaluation and management of amenorrhea related to congenital sex hormonal disorders. *Annals of Pediatric Endocrinology & Metabolism, 24*, 149–157. https://doi.org/10.6065/apem.2019.24.3.149 (accessed on 14th June 2025).

48. Yugesh, K., Sampath Kumar, S. K., & Kalaivani, P. (2023). Diagnostic tests for confirmation of mating in adult female Wistar rats: An experimental study. *Journal of Clinical and Diagnostic Research*. https://www.semanticscholar.org/paper/5f8a2e74f90586b30e62fb470b42e46fea500703 (accessed on 14th June 2025).

ABNORMAL UTERINE BLEEDING

7

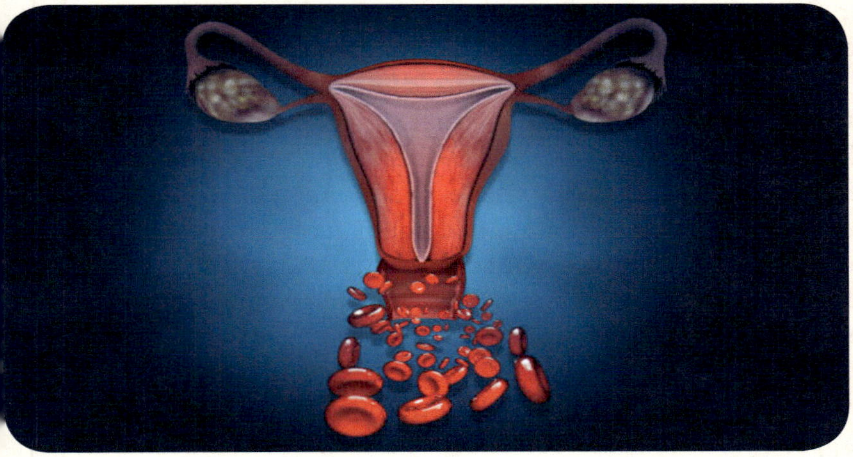

LEARNING OBJECTIVES

After studying this chapter, you will be able to:

1. Identify the different types of abnormal uterine bleeding
2. Explain the various causes of abnormal uterine bleeding
3. Recognize the symptoms associated with AUB
4. Describe the diagnosis of abnormal uterine bleeding
5. Evaluate treatment options for AUB

Introduction

Abnormal uterine bleeding (AUB) is a prevalent clinical challenge faced by a significant proportion of the female population. Bleeding from the uterus that is different from a woman's regular menstrual cycle, AUB may present as menorrhagia, oligomenorrhea, or intermenstrual bleeding. Its presentation affects approximately 10%–25% of women, hence posing an immediate need to comprehensively understand the condition (Cantarelli *et al.*, 2024). There are multiple etiologies of AUB, ranging from endocrine disturbances to structural lesions, such as polyps and fibroids. By examining the underlying etiology and an awareness of the clinical presentations of AUB, healthcare practitioners can initiate timely and appropriate interventions, thus enhancing the quality of life of individuals with AUB. The clinical importance of the diagnosis and treatment of AUB must not be overlooked, considering its influence on women's health and well-being. Doctors must conduct thorough evaluations, including an accurate history of menstruation and physical examinations, to effectively diagnose the condition.

Evolving technologies in diagnostic techniques, including imaging modalities like ultrasound and hysteroscopy, make it possible to identify underlying causes, facilitating an individualized treatment plan (Cantarelli *et al.*, 2024). The treatment choices for AUB range from hormone therapy to surgery, depending on severity and on what underlying issue, for instance, uterine fibroids or ovarian failure.

They not only eliminate the symptom but also address the root problem, reducing morbidity and enhancing overall health outcomes in women. Given the complexity of AUB, its subdivision into causes like polyp, adenomyosis, leiomyoma, and coagulopathy highlights the multifaceted nature of the disease (Arikarevula *et al.*, 2024). Knowing that presentations of AUB are varied, clinicians are challenged to embrace a systematic diagnosis and treatment approach. Use of a framework like the PALM-COEIN classification assists in understanding the individual etiologic factors of AUB so that care stratification is enhanced. The holistic approach ensures management plans are customized to an individual woman's unique medical history and personal belief systems. As research on AUB continues to progress, the continued creation of awareness and education becomes essential in providing women with reproductive health information, facilitating adherence to treatment regimens, and motivating better health outcomes.

Definition of Abnormal Uterine Bleeding

Abnormal Uterine Bleeding (AUB) has been defined as any deviation from the typical menstrual bleeding patterns, such as variations in duration, volume, frequency, and regularity. The effects of AUB extend beyond the true physical symptoms; it can indeed change the quality of life of a person, leading to psychological morbidity and social limitation. As up to one-third of women in the reproductive age group experience AUB, its treatment and diagnosis are crucial to maintain overall wellness. According to the International Federation of Gynecology and Obstetrics, the condition is categorized under structural and non-structural causes and is otherwise referred to as the PALM-COEIN classification.

This model not only makes sense of the diagnostic course but also forms the foundation of the therapeutic intervention specific to the cause, resulting in improved health status for the involved. The endometrial cycle is the pathophysiologic basis of AUB and is intricately connected with the circulating hormones and local tissue reactions, which regulate menstruation. Endometrium is an active tissue that undergoes cycles of breakdown and growth under the regulation of sex hormones, estrogen, and progesterone. This very balanced system can be disrupted to produce pathological states manifested as abnormal bleeding patterns. There is some evidence that even subtle imbalances in control factors of the endometrium can trigger symptoms of AUB, especially in patients who experience anovulatory cycles because of endocrine disturbances. This is most prominent among adolescents, where an immature hypothalamic-pituitary axis leads to a preponderance of anovulatory menstruation, and is a cause for the high incidence of AUB among them (Jain *et al.*, 2022).

Incidence in a significant number of adolescents, AUB requires a thorough understanding of the etiology and the management strategy. The consequences of AUB not being managed are not just physical, such as anemia due to repeated blood loss, but also long-term psychological and social consequences on a patient's life. These options for treatment are multifaceted, with both hormonal and non-hormonal modalities depending on the severity of bleeding, implications for anemia, and patient stability. The need for follow-up care once more supports the need for repetitive checking and adjustment of treatment regimens to guarantee comprehensive care. With greater knowledge of AUB and its subtleties, healthcare workers are able to provide appropriate and tailored management strategies, ultimately contributing to improved patient outcomes and quality of life (Jain *et al.*, 2022).

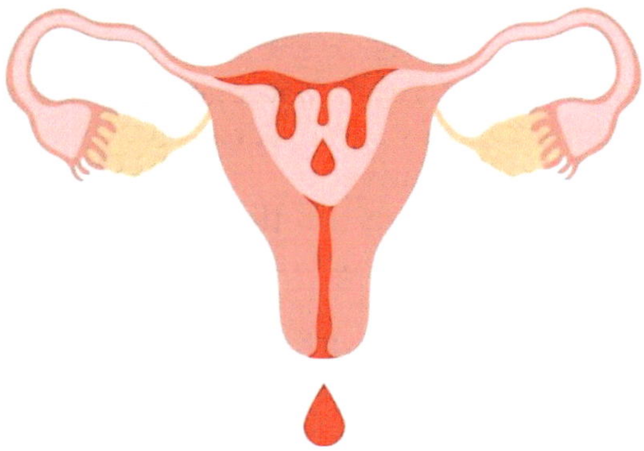

Figure 7.1. Abnormal uterine bleeding (AUB) is a common issue many women experience at some point in their lives.

Source: http://sukhipariwarclinic.com.np/abnormal-uterine-bleeding-a-simple-guide/

Importance of Understanding AUB

Understanding abnormal uterine bleeding (AUB) is important for many reasons, primarily because of its significant effect on women's quality of life and health. AUB encompasses many bleeding patterns that are not normal for menstruation, such as irregular volume, frequency, and duration. Abnormalities may have many etiologies, and therefore, proper diagnosis is necessary for effective management. As pointed out in research, AUB is a frequent disorder among different age groups, particularly the perimenopausal women, where it tends to signify concomitant physiological alterations or conditions. Confirmation of these patterns allows practitioners to implement appropriate interventions, enhancing women's overall outcome and reducing the likelihood of severe complications, e.g., anemia or even malignancy (Philip *et al.*, 2022). Furthermore, the psychological and emotional burden of AUB should not be overlooked. The majority of women with AUB report a significant level of distress, which secondarily influences the quality of life and results in social withdrawal. The interconnection between discomfort and concern about possible health effects is a multidimensional issue. Standardized terminology and unambiguous definitions of AUB, as discussed in the recent FIGO consensus statement, could facilitate better communication between patients and physicians.

This approach not only aids in the improvement of patient understanding but also establishes an environment in which women feel assured to seek out medical consultations and discuss their symptoms freely (Chodankar *et al.*, 2022). Raised awareness about AUB ensures early diagnosis and treatment, potentially alleviating a huge emotional burden. Lastly, the importance of knowledge on AUB extends to the clinical practice and research domains in highlighting requirements for education and awareness. Standardized classifications and definitions can help well-established research programs, thereby paving the way to improved epidemiological studies and trials.

This foundation enables practitioners not only to understand the intricacy of AUB but also to stay abreast with new therapeutic approaches. By integrating full education on AUB into medical training, health practitioners will be in a better position to meet the complicated demands of their patients. The ultimate, this information translates to pre-emptive management strategies that improve long-term health outcomes and empower women to maintain reproductive health and quality of life (Philip *et al.*, 2022).

7.1. Types of Abnormal Uterine Bleeding

Learning Outcome

1. Define heavy menstrual bleeding (Menorrhagia)
2. Explain the irregular menstrual bleeding
3. Describe intermenstrual bleeding

bnormal uterine bleeding (AUB) is a complex series of patterns of bleeding, including menorrhagia, metrorrhagia, and dysmenorrhea, all indicating underlying dysfunctions of the menstrual cycle. Menorrhagia, the abnormally heavy or prolonged menstrual bleeding, is most often encountered by women at the menopause period and can be triggered by a range of factors, including uterine fibroids and hormonal imbalance. Metrorrhagia is intermenstrual bleeding and is caused by polyps, submucosal fibroids, or congenital uterine malformations. It is reported that women with recurrent miscarriage may have an increased frequency of congenital uterine malformations, underlining the necessity of early diagnosis and treatment in this population (Cocksedge *et al.*, 2008). It is essential to recognize these differences as it aids healthcare practitioners in personalizing treatment regimens, focusing not only on the symptoms but also on the etiology of AUB. The PALM-COEIN classification system has a systematic methodology to categorize the various etiologies of AUB, and it is essential to do so in order to treat it effectively. This classification divides the potential causes into two categories: structural (PALM), including polyps, adenomyosis, leiomyomas, and malignancy; and non-structural (COEIN), including hormonal dysfunctions, coagulopathy, endometrial disorders, iatrogenic causes, and not yet classified mechanisms. According to a retrospective analysis at AIIMS Patna, the most common category of AUB presented in clinic was AUB-E due to endometrial causes and accounted for a significant number of cases (Bhadani *et al.*, 2018). Based on such classification, clinicians can prioritize diagnostic tests, such as hysteroscopy or imaging, aimed at specific types of AUB, allowing more accurate treatment protocols. In the study of prevalence and age distribution of the types of AUB, it can be seen that AUB occurs in varying ways at different stages of life. For example, it has been found that most frequently affected are women aged 40 to 49 years, an age group generally characterized by perimenopausal alterations (Bhadani *et al.*, 2018). In this, endocrine changes can manifest with various patterns of bleeding, making it imperative to perform thorough evaluation regimens in this crucial period of a woman's life. Furthermore, histological patterns identified among these patients yield valuable information, with most presenting with secretory patterns. These findings sustain the argument that age-targeted medical approaches to diagnosis and treatment of AUB are needed to improve women's health results and address the nuances of various bleeding conditions.

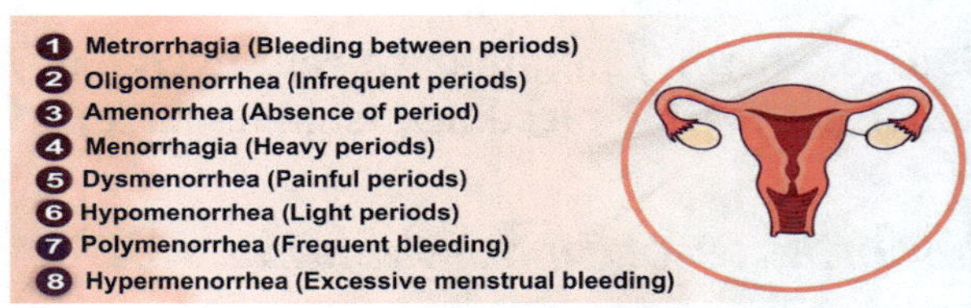

Figure 7.2. Different types of abnormal uterine bleeding (AUB).

Source: https://clinicone.com.np/wp-content/uploads/2025/02/Types-of-abnormal-periods.png

7.1.1. Heavy Menstrual Bleeding (Menorrhagia)

Menorrhagia, or excessive menstrual bleeding, is a frequent presentation of abnormal uterine bleeding (AUB) that has a major effect on women's quality of life and health. Defined by abnormally heavy or prolonged menstrual flow, menorrhagia produces considerable physical and emotional morbidity. Women with menorrhagia complain of weakness, fatigue, and decreased daily functioning due to the unpredictability of their cycles and the lack of ability to manage excessive blood loss. It is not only a nuisance; it can result in serious health consequences in the form of iron deficiency anemia that requires immediate medical care and treatment. Recognition of menorrhagia's complexity calls for an exploration of its etiology, from hormonal dysfunction to structural pathology of the uterus, to explain the heterogeneous presentation of AUB in reproductive-age women (Chodankar *et al.*, 2022).

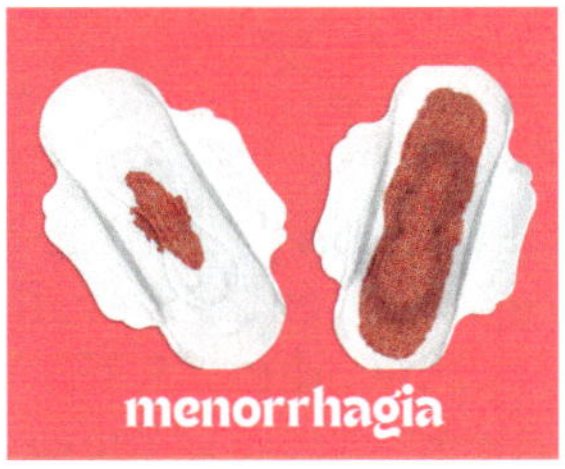

Source: https://assets.zyrosite.com/AoPPvkMw6vSrnvpn/classic-dWxbGX827WTgKl0e.png

Menorrhagia treatment remains an integral aspect of gynecological health care since it comprises not only medical interventions but also lifestyle modifications. It may present in a variety of forms, ranging from over-the-counter (OTC) medications such as non-steroidal anti-inflammatory drugs (NSAIDs) to moderate symptom control to hormonal therapies to normalize menstrual cycles and, most seriously, to surgical interventions such as endometrial ablation or hysterectomy. Recent studies point towards the application of selective estrogen receptor modulators like ormeloxifene, which have shown potential in the treatment of AUB by nullifying estrogen's action on the uterine lining (Singh *et al.*, 2024). These studies put forward the importance of customized treatment strategies with regard to the patient's needs, particularly for women who may be hesitant to accept surgery, thus making it simpler to treat menorrhagia's disabling symptoms. Furthermore, the psychosocial impact of menorrhagia should not be exaggerated since the disorder can extend beyond physiological presentations to impact women's emotional well-being and social behavior.

The majority of women report feeling embarrassed, anxious, and lacking in self-esteem concerning their experience of heavy bleeding, thus avoiding social contact or physical activity. The psychological burden reinforces the need for integrative therapy that aligns the medical and affective aspects of AUB. It is important that healthcare workers embrace a holistic model, encompassing counseling and support in conjunction with clinical treatment. By recognizing the multifaceted experience of women suffering from menorrhagia, the medical community can enhance compliance with treatments and overall prognosis, leading to a better quality of life for persons afflicted by this very common yet frequently overlooked disorder (Chodankar *et al.*, 2022).

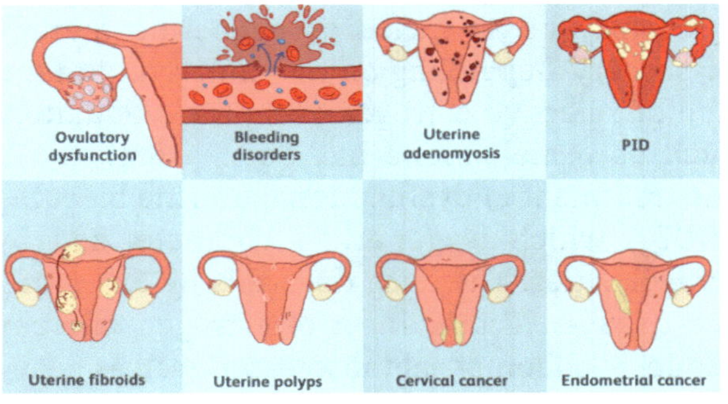

Figure 7.3. Common causes of heavy menstrual bleeding.

Source: https://www.verywellhealth.com/thmb/x8AuC-tERBa9JJ7krPra6m3DmGw=/1500x0/filters:no_upscale():max_bytes(150000):strip_icc()/op-causes-of-heavy-menstrual-bleeding-3522223-5c04a43346e0fb0001838004.png

7.1.2. Irregular Menstrual Bleeding

Irregular menstrual bleeding, being one of the most common symptoms of abnormal uterine bleeding (AUB), has a significant impact on the lives of women of all ages. AUB encompasses various abnormalities of cycle frequency, duration of the flow, and amount of blood. The PALM-COEIN classification system of AUB offers valuable information concerning its etiology by categorizing potential causes under nine categories. Notably, the latest research identifies heavy menstrual bleeding as the most prevalent presentation among women with AUB, in approximately 60% of women who are evaluated. Identification of causes is important for effective treatment and diagnosis, with irregular patterns of bleeding potentially anticipating benign or malignant processes that will necessitate unique therapeutic approaches (Banmeru *et al.*, 2025). Therefore, a need exists for ongoing research into clinical and histopathological correlations of abnormal menstrual bleeding to improve patient outcomes. Management of abnormal menstrual bleeding usually involves the exclusion of the various underlying causes, as this determines treatment. Measures for regulation of the cycle may be as varied as endocrine therapy or surgery, depending on the underlying cause. Use of selective estrogen receptor modulators such as ormeloxifene has been promising in the treatment of dysfunctional uterine bleeding (DUB), which is generally characterized by irregularities. The drug does this by exploiting the tissue-selective effect of estrogen, thereby reducing endometrial thickness as well as heavy bleeding episodes. A recent study showed that ormeloxifene therapy caused a marked rise in hemoglobin levels and decreased bleeding scores among women with DUB (Singh, 2024). This new treatment highlights the importance of personalized strategies in managing AUB, particularly regulating the abnormal bleeding that disrupts women's lives. In AUB in women, the complications are dramatic and can affect mental well-being and overall health. Uncertainty of the disease can lead to significant distress, with many consulting a healthcare professional. Awareness of this condition's potential to become serious complications like hyperplasia or endometrial cancer imposes an acute need for early intervention and diagnosis. Research validates that detailed treatment strategies aligned with a patient's background can be helpful, boosting physical and emotional health. As healthcare professionals struggle to treat abnormal menstrual bleeding, ongoing studies and new therapies will be crucial in developing more efficient management protocols. Therefore, diagnosis of the diverse manifestations of AUB will enable better-targeted treatment and better overall women's health (Banmeru *et al.*, 2025).

7.1.3. Intermenstrual Bleeding

Intermenstrual bleeding (IMB) is an important clinical concern in the overall context of abnormal uterine bleeding (AUB). It is bleeding that occurs between regular menstrual periods and can be a manifestation of a variety of underlying conditions, including hormonal disturbances, endometrial pathology, or structural abnormalities such as fibroids. Systematic diagnosis of the etiology of IMB is crucial since it guides treatment intervention that can significantly enhance a woman's quality of life. Utilization of the FIGO classification system, incorporating the widest range of possible etiological causes, allows for precise diagnosis of the underlying reasons for intermenstrual bleeding and planning of management strategies according to individual patient needs. The connection of IMB with conditions like fibroids also complicates diagnosis, emphasizing the need for strict evaluation and imaging processes like hysteroscopy to facilitate proper demarcation of the etiology of AUB (Whitaker *et al.*, 2015). The impact of intermenstrual bleeding extends beyond the physical to include women's psychological and emotional health. For the majority, IMB leads to more tension and anxiety due to the unpredictable nature of bleeding that may disrupt personal and professional life. Having recurrent bleeding evokes health fears regarding reproduction and lowers quality of life as women attempt to comprehend the potential consequences of their condition. Most significantly, studies have found that the presence of pelvic pain, most commonly in association with intermenstrual bleeding, exacerbates the symptoms and may lead to chronic pain conditions such as primary dysmenorrhea. The complex influence of IMB must be understood, since it impacts therapy options and the overall management of AUB. Addressing these psychosocial dimensions must be part of a comprehensive healthcare strategy to ensure that women receive holistic and empathetic care (Iacovides *et al.*, 2015). Management strategies for intermenstrual bleeding depend on the underlying causes established through thorough diagnostic evaluation. Depending upon the aetiology, treatment may range from conservative approaches such as hormonal therapy to invasive procedures such as endometrial ablation or surgery if fibroids or other structural abnormalities are identified as the etiology. With evolving medical therapies, women are living with fewer surgeries and better results, and so intermenstrual bleeding becomes easier to manage. Individualized treatment is necessary, taking into consideration a woman's age, her reproductive requirements, and her overall health. With ongoing advancements in knowledge regarding AUB and its manifestations like IMB, highlighting integral care will lead to improved treatment modalities and, ultimately, improve the quality of life in affected women (Whitaker *et al.*, 2015).

Test Your Knowledge

1. What are the common causes of heavy menstrual bleeding (menorrhagia)?
2. How does irregular menstrual bleeding differ from normal cycle variations?

7.2. Causes of Abnormal Uterine Bleeding

Learning Outcome

1. Identify the hormonal imbalances that contribute to abnormal uterine bleeding (AUB)
2. Describe structural abnormalities of the reproductive system associated with AUB
3. Explain how medical conditions and medications can lead to abnormal uterine bleeding

The etiology of abnormal uterine bleeding (AUB) is different and affects women of various ages. One of the primary systems utilized to classify the causes is the PALM-COEIN classification system, in which the etiologies are classified into structural and non-structural classes. According to this classification, the structural etiologies include polyps, adenomyosis, leiomyomas, and malignancies, and the non-structural etiologies include coagulopathies, ovulatory dysfunction, endometrial causes, iatrogenic, and classifications as yet undefined. This step-by-step approach not only assists in the proper diagnosis of the underlying conditions causing AUB but also in appropriate management strategies depending on the patient's condition. The complexity of such causes underscores the importance of optimal patient evaluation so that potentially curable conditions are not overlooked. A study of patients who come in with AUB is demonstrated through research to reveal ovulatory dysfunction as the leading etiology at about 28% of cases reported. This is then followed by leiomyomas, or fibroids, in about

24.67% of cases presented, and endometrial at 15.33% of the diagnosis. These findings highlight that women of childbearing age, particularly those aged perimenopause, usually experience heavy menstrual bleeding with functional menstrual cycle disorders or with structural lesions such as fibroids. In addition, abnormal uterine bleeding presents a risk for subsequent complications, which include anemia, thereby necessitating timely diagnosis and treatment even more (Soni *et al.*, 2024). Treating these causes not only alleviates the acute symptoms of AUB but also enhances global health and quality of life in impacted women. Beyond acute physical discomfort, AUB's impact can significantly affect emotional and psychological states as well. Although the physical causes are of paramount importance in terms of diagnosis and treatment, psychosocial impacts cannot be discounted. Females with AUB typically present with distress, anxiety, and compromised quality of life due to the unpredictability of their menstrual cycle and risk of embarrassment in social settings. The interconnection between physical and emotional health emphasizes the importance of comprehensive treatment with the combination of medical and psychological therapies (Soni *et al.*, 2024). By diagnosing and treating reversible causes of AUB, health care professionals can enhance women's health, leading to more comprehensive care that not only cures the symptoms but also relieves the significant emotional distress this condition can initiate.

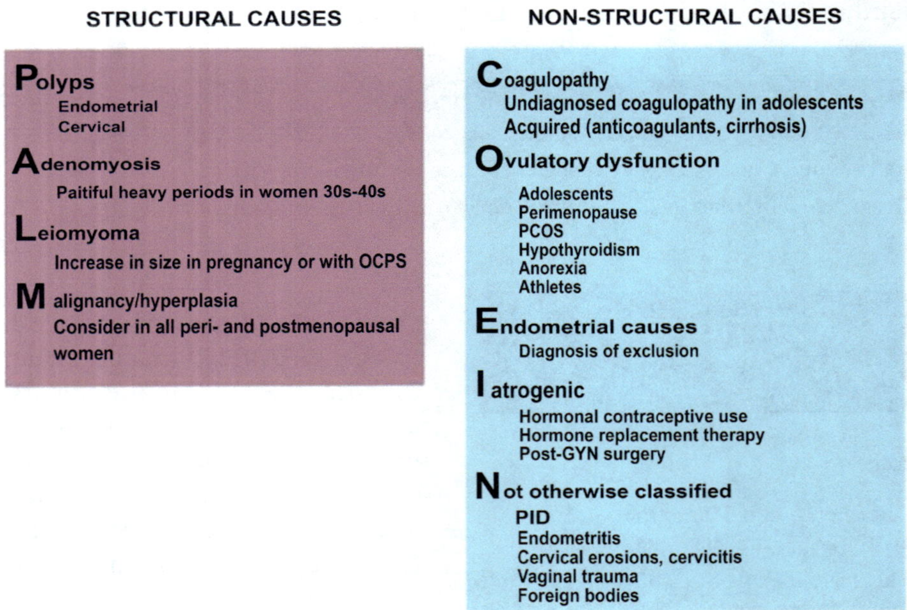

Figure 7.4. Causes of abnormal uterine bleeding.

Source: https://img.grepmed.com/uploads/3857/gynecology-palmcoein-mnemonic-abnormal-obstetrics-original.jpeg

7.2.1. Hormonal Imbalances

Hormonal disorders are the central cause of developing abnormal uterine bleeding (AUB), which affects the complex interaction of reproductive hormones that control menstrual cycles.

More specifically, disruptions in estrogen and progesterone levels can trigger alterations in endometrial lining, which result in variability in bleeding patterns. Thyroid disease and polycystic ovary syndrome are medical conditions that can exacerbate such hormonal disturbances to cause AUB. The role of thyroid hormones, in particular, has been found to have a tremendous impact on menstrual regularity. For example, hypothyroidism is associated with longer and more frequent menstrual cycles, mainly because the production of such hormones that play a critical role in maintaining the menstrual cycle and endometrial health is incomplete (Shree *et al.*, 2025). Therefore, it is paramount to identify and manage these hormonal imbalances to ensure proper intervention and treatment of women presenting with AUB. The importance of hormonal therapy in the treatment of AUB cannot be overemphasized. Upon diagnosing hormonal imbalance, doctors are known to prescribe a myriad of treatment options with the view of establishing balance. Combined oral contraceptive pills are some of the most commonly used hormonal contraceptives that can regulate menstrual flow by providing a constant dose of estrogen and progesterone. In addition, the levonorgestrel-releasing intrauterine device (LNG-IUD) has been shown to be effective in reducing menstrual blood loss with limited systemic effects (Shree *et al.*, 2025). Evidence indicates that a high percentage of women experience good outcomes with this intervention because it works on the endometrium rather than systemic levels of hormones and thus provides a focused intervention for women with AUB. The expanding understanding of hormonal therapy portends improved quality of life and reproductive health for women with these disorders. Greater study of the intricate interactions between hormonal imbalances and AUB is clinically important and relevant to patient care. For instance, careful evaluation of thyroid function has emerged as a crucial part of AUB management, particularly in light of observed correlations in most studies. Since 38% of AUB women also suffer from hypothyroidism, the screening of this condition during clinical evaluation has been advocated for greater efficacy in treating it (Pooja *et al.*, 2024). Fine-tuning of the procedures by healthcare professionals through the integration of hormonal testing in routine practice helps them enhance diagnostic accuracy and optimize the treatment process. By treating underlying hormonal imbalance, clinicians are not only able to correct symptoms, but also optimize overall reproductive health, and thereby enhance quality of life in women suffering from AUB. Continued investigations into these interrelated factors will open the way for innovative treatment options attuned to the individual patient's distinctive hormonal environment.

7.2.2. Structural Abnormalities

The search for structural abnormalities is a critical step in the understanding of abnormal uterine bleeding (AUB) since these abnormalities can have far-reaching implications for a woman's reproductive well-being. Structural abnormalities comprise a series of conditions like uterine polyps, fibroids, and adenomyosis that arise from altered uterine architecture. All of these abnormalities can disrupt normal menstrual function, leading to heavy or irregular bleeding. For instance, uterine fibroids, which are benign growths that develop from the uterine smooth muscle, can lead to severe menstrual disturbances, and referral for medical therapy and possible intervention becomes warranted. Structural abnormalities are identified using a step-by-step process, sometimes beginning with a careful history and physical examination. Medical imaging technologies, such as ultrasound, which is the initial test used to assess uterine shape, are used by medical practitioners to determine the presence of these abnormalities. In addition, hysteroscopy allows one to directly visualize and biopsy the endometrial lining, from which one can diagnose lesions that are implicated in AUB. These tests are effective with evidence provided in the context of the PALM-COEIN classification system, where causes of AUB are systematized into clear categories to facilitate accelerated diagnosis and treatment strategies (Viganò *et al.*, 2024).

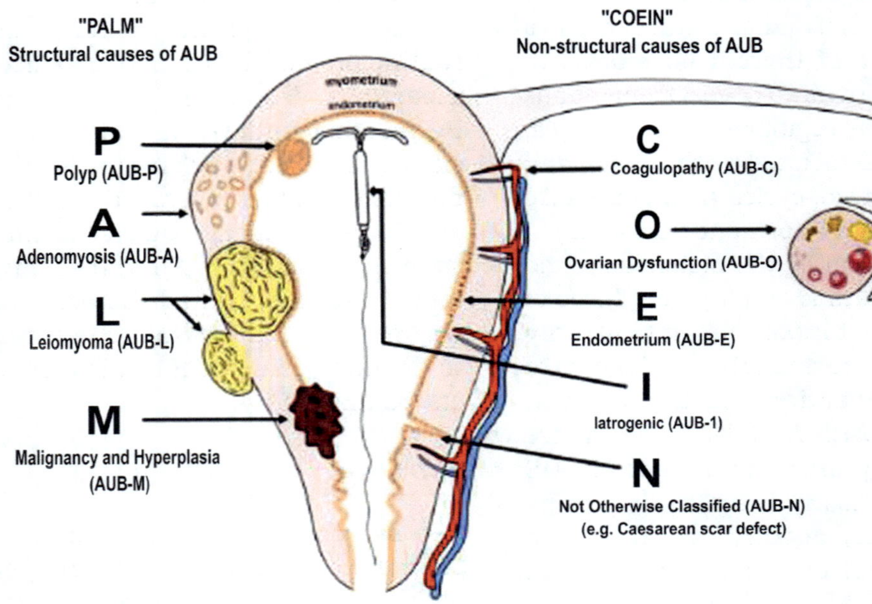

Figure 7.5. FIGO classification of abnormal uterine bleeding (AUB) – structural (PALM) and non-structural (COEIN) causes.

Source: https://www.thelancet.com/journals/ebiom/article/PIIS2352-3964%2822%2900420-0/fulltext

Management of structural defects leading to AUB entails an individualized approach considering the particular characteristics of identified defects. The treatments also vary widely, ranging from conservative therapy such as hormonal therapy for menstrual cycle regulation to targeted medical treatment for symptom resolution. Surgical interventions are reserved for more severe presentations, for example, myomectomy in the case of fibroids or polyp removal in the case of polyps. Treatment choice typically relies on the reproductive requirements of patients, severity of symptoms, and risk of malignant change in certain anomalies. Successful treatment accordingly relies not just on accurate diagnosis but also on careful consultations with patients regarding their options to maximize their health and quality of life (Cantarelli *et al.*, 2024).

7.2.3. Medical Conditions and Medications

Management of Abnormal Uterine Bleeding (AUB) is tricky in itself, particularly when the patient also has underlying medical conditions, such as Chronic Kidney Disease (CKD). CKD is a chronic progressive disease of the kidneys characterized by reduced kidney function, and this can lead to an imbalance in hormones affecting menstruation and could predispose to AUB. CKD patients often experience menstrual irregularities that can cause severe anemia, a worsening of an already precarious health condition. Such complications can drastically impair quality of life and complicate treatment. For such patients, the appropriate interventions are a matter of closely examining both the medical and surgical interventions for AUB because declining renal function typical of CKD can complicate medical and surgical interventions. The subtleties in the management of AUB in this population are often understudied in the literature, highlighting a clear need for more research and more specific treatment regimens (Ramu *et al.*, 2024).

Iron deficiency anemia (IDA) is prevalent in women with AUB, reflecting the interconnectedness of these health conditions. The prevalence of AUB in women of reproductive age is greater than 30%, and iron deficiency will often be a severe complication of chronic blood loss. The impact of IDA not only carries clinical significance, such as fatigue and diminished quality of life, but also reflects broader public health issues since it contributes to the disease burden worldwide. Treatment of IDA in combination with management of AUB is critical because studies have established that effective therapy can result in considerable modifications of hematological parameters. For instance, a multicenter clinical observational investigation documented the effectiveness of the regimen Vojea in women with signs of latent iron deficiency. The patients, following treatment, demonstrated marked increases in the concentration of serum ferritin and red blood cell folate, substantiating the importance of a comprehensive approach to therapy (Kononova *et al.*, 2024). The approach to therapeutically managing AUB against the backdrop of coexisting pathology requires a critical analysis of both medical and pharmacotherapeutic interventions. The incorporation of the role played by some drugs that can manage heavy menstrual bleeding is one such consideration. In AUB women, especially those with concomitant chronic diseases like CKD or iron deficiency, careful selection of drugs is necessary to achieve efficacy as well as safety. Pharmacodynamics with these drugs can be intricate in the context of renal impairment, leading to unpredictable drug clearance and potentially adverse effects. This highlights the importance of individualized treatment regimens according to patient-specific characteristics and conditions. Further research is also vital to uncovering the most effective treatment protocols not just to treat the symptoms of AUB but also to mitigate associated complications such as anemia, thereby improving overall patient outcomes (Ramu *et al.*, 2024; Kononova *et al.*, 2024).

Test Your Knowledge

1. What structural abnormalities of the uterus are commonly linked to AUB?
2. Which medical conditions or medications can lead to abnormal uterine bleeding?

7.3. Symptoms Associated with AUB

Learning Outcome

1. Discuss the changes in menstrual Cycle Patterns
2. Define physical symptoms (e.g., fatigue, pain)
3. Identify the psychological impact of AUB

Abnormal uterine bleeding (AUB) symptoms are varied and can significantly affect a woman's quality of life. Heavy menstrual bleeding (HMB) is one of the most common presentations in nearly 60% of women with AUB, according to clinical surveys. HMB can manifest as overflow during menses or excessive bleeding that exceeds the typical duration of menstrual flow. Irregular menstrual bleeding, which is seasonless or out-of-season menstrual periods, is also typically observed, impacting women's daily functioning and hormonal balance. The presence of dysmenorrhea, or cramping menstrual pain, also adds to the clinical picture by provoking pain that can interfere with physical and psychological function. All these symptoms underscore the importance of understanding AUB not only as a benign state but also as a state that requires proper investigation and management strategies (Banmeru *et al.*, 2025). In addition to the physical signs, AUB can initiate psychological effects, including depression and anxiety. The unpredictability and volatility of the bleeding pattern may cause emotional distress, causing interpersonal relationships and mental health to suffer.

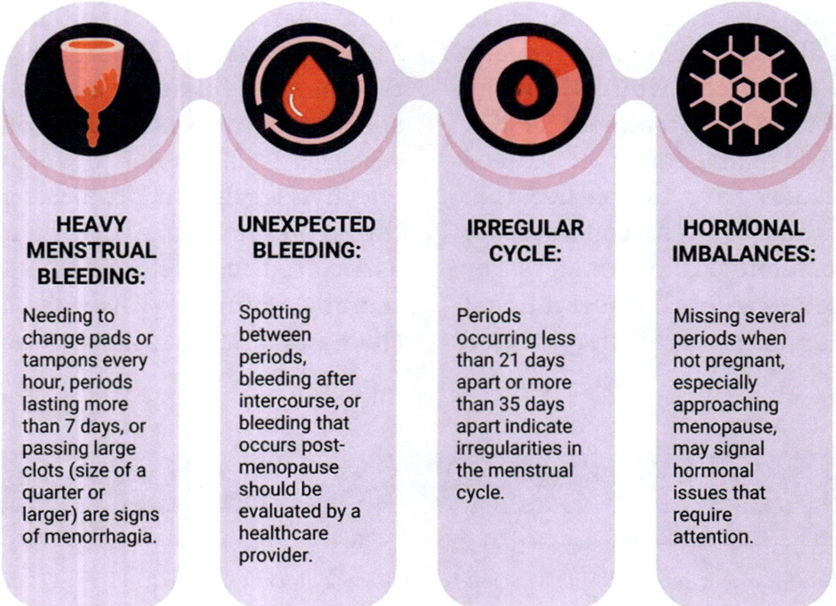

Figure 7.6. Common symptoms of abnormal uterine bleeding (AUB).

Source: https://nycgyne.com/wp-content/uploads/2025/01/common-symptoms-of-abnormal-uterine-bleeding.jpg.webp

They may feel embarrassed or stigmatized about their condition and therefore experience a decline in their quality of life. They may develop avoidance behaviors, such as limiting exercise or social activity, due to fear of menstruation bleeding. Chronic AUB may also result in complications such as iron-deficiency anemia, adding to the physical burden of the condition. The coordination between psychological stress and physical symptoms highlights the intricate nature of AUB and requires a general multidisciplinary approach to treatment and patient management (Ahmed *et al.*, 2024). The potential etiologies of AUB are many, as testified by the categories established within the PALM-COEIN system, enabling an objective diagnosis of this condition. Polycystic ovarian syndrome, uterine fibroids, and endometrial pathologies are the culprits of choice and can cause a myriad of symptoms, including HMB and irregular cycles. Clinically appreciated co-existing pathologies such as adenomyosis also play significant roles in symptomatology. Accurate diagnosis is crucial as it dictates treatment, ranging from pharmacologic therapy to surgery in the form of hysterectomy. As clinical practice shows, symptom presentation is highly correlated with histopathological findings, supporting the call for tailor-made therapeutic regimens. Understanding the symptoms and their meaning ensures better management in conjunction with the overall requirement of women presenting with AUB (Banmeru *et al.*, 2025).

7.3.1. Changes in Menstrual Cycle Patterns

The intricate cycles of menstruation are at the hub of the understanding of abnormal uterine bleeding (AUB). Menstrual cycles typically run 28 days, but may be far from that in different women. Changes in flow duration, intensity, and frequency are most often indicative of pathologic conditions. AUB may be intermenstrual bleeding, menorrhagia, or prolonged periods, for which investigation is required. The perimenopause phase, especially, sees dramatic changes in the hormone levels that can be responsible for irregular cycle patterns. In this transitional phase, women may experience various symptoms, primarily due to estrogen and progesterone imbalance, affecting endometrial stability and thus leading to alterations in bleeding patterns. Such variability leads one to suspect the necessity of a proper assessment to separate normal physiological change and possibly pathological conditions of AUB. The evaluation of endometrial tissue in females complaining of abnormal bleeding patterns is important in diagnosis. From research, the histopathology of endometrial biopsies ranges from normal endometrial tissue to abnormal findings such as hyperplasia and malignancy. Most notably, perimenopausal age is the most vulnerable to such changes; a significant proportion of cases have proliferative and secretory endometrium, as would be anticipated with the menstrual cycle alterations of this life stage. For instance, one study illustrated that the most common symptom identified among perimenopausal women with AUB was excessive menstrual bleeding, highlighting the urgent need for maximized clinical evaluation and treatment protocol (*et al.*, 2017). This critical correlation of cycle changes and histological presentation helps clinicians formulate patient-specific treatment plans. Furthermore, familiarity with the clinical management of AUB needs a holistic approach reflecting the physiological as well as psychological aspects of abnormal menstruation. Women presenting with menstrual cycle changes report increased anxiety and distress due to disordered bleeding patterns. This psychological impact further worsens the challenges these women face, and hence, it is crucial that medical professionals engage patients in supportive counseling along with medical treatment. In the management of these challenges, an interdisciplinary approach, which includes medication and surgery, as evidenced by clinicopathological examination, is necessary. As background research shows, implementing patient education on menstruation and creating customized management plans can successfully improve overall results (Gulia *et al.*, 2020). Lastly, it is important to have awareness and knowledge of menstrual cycle variation in order to avoid the adverse consequences of AUB and improve the quality of life for individuals suffering from it.

7.3.2. Physical Symptoms (e.g., Fatigue, Pain)

The physical symptomatology of Abnormal Uterine Bleeding (AUB) has a broad impact on the overall well-being and quality of life of patients with the condition. Fatigue is one of the top symptoms, yet it is further exacerbated in instances of heavy menstrual bleeding that could lead to profuse loss of blood. This blood loss results not only in decreased levels of energy but can also result in anemia, creating a vicious circle in which the fatigue becomes increasingly more difficult to manage. Those who suffer from AUB may experience debilitating fatigue, disrupting daily activities and impacting work performance, leading to a lower quality of life. Additionally, such tiredness can affect social interactions and lead to loneliness since people tend to avoid participating in activities because of their physical condition.

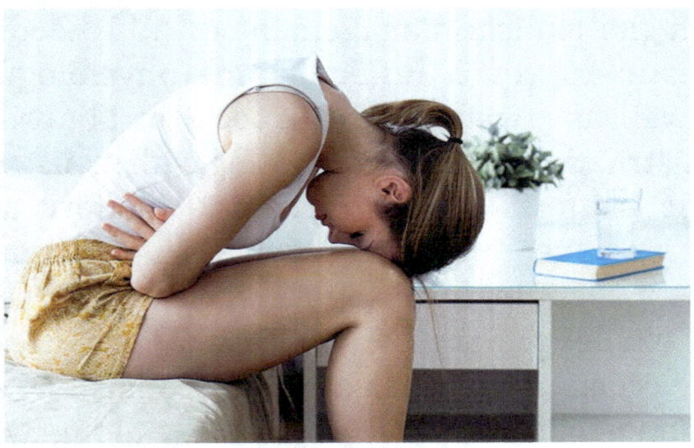

Source: https://www.draliabadi.com/wp-content/uploads/2020/12/abnormal-bleeding.jpg

In addition to fatigue, pain, particularly pelvic pain, is another key symptom that is encountered in patients with AUB. The pain may be as mild as it is severe and typically accompanies underlying conditions of the uterus, such as fibroids or polyps. The presence of pain introduces a new level of complexity because it can be transient or chronic, introducing an additional level of challenge to managing AUB. Patients can experience pain not only during the time of heavy bleeding but also at other times during their cycle. This can cause added stress and anxiety, which can make the pain seem greater, thus causing a cycle of vice between physical and emotional symptoms. The division between the management and treatment of pain and AUB is necessary since treatment of either alone may not improve the overall status of the patients very much. Management of the physical symptomatology resulting from AUB is crucial to the restoration of quality of life in affected individuals. Treatment varies with etiology, with medications such as ulipristal acetate (UPA) being effective symptom management agents. According to research, UPA not only reduces bleeding but also shrinks fibroids, which are most often a primary source of symptomatology for AUB, thereby eliminating associated pain and discomfort. Additionally, surgical interventions, including hysteroscopic interventions, offer more choices in effectively managing structural etiologies of AUB. While these strategies may provide relief and improve emotional well-being, one must involve patients in a shared decision-making process to tailor treatment regimens to fit their unique physical complaints and quality-of-life goals. Overall, diagnosis and effective management of physical symptoms constitute a vital component of AUB treatment (Fauser *et al.*, 2014; *et al.*, 2022).

7.3.3. Psychological Impact

The psychological impact of abnormal uterine bleeding (AUB) extends far beyond the physical symptoms that women endure. AUB most typically inflicts severe emotional distress on a woman's quality of life and mental well-being. Women frequently complain of anxiety, depression, and frustration because of the unpredictability and severity of their bleeding attacks. This psychological burden can lead to a decreased sense of mastery of routine and social contact because the fear of unexpected bleeding can restrict their involvement in routines or outside the home. The psychosocial impact can be profound, as women may avoid individuals or situations that may ultimately lead to embarrassment. These psychological implications require a holistic regimen of treatment that not only addresses the physical manifestations of AUB but also the concomitant emotional burden, thereby emphasizing the role of mental health care in therapeutic treatment (. *et al.*, 2016). The correlation of AUB with reproductive health problems further complicates the psychological context for women with these concerns. Conditions such as fibroids and adenomyosis, presenting in the form of AUB, could have fertility implications, thus adding to emotional effects. The knowledge that AUB could interfere with future reproductive plans creates heightened states of anxiety and feelings of inadequacy among women, particularly those who desire pregnancy. Such a relationship highlights the coexistence of hormonal disturbances and psychiatric states since the distress of dealing with a chronic illness will worsen symptoms of depression and anxiety. Medical professionals should then take into account supplementing therapy for AUB with psychological treatment, such as counseling or support groups. This sort of strategy may not only liberate the psychological burden but may also lead to improved overall health consequences among these women (Barra *et al.*, 2023).

Finally, education and awareness of the psychological impact of AUB can play an essential role in prevention and management. Increased recognition of the affective aspects of AUB can facilitate dialogue between women and clinicians, enabling patients to convey their distress and seek assistance. Support groups comprised of peers can also be an enormous source of comfort for women, providing a platform where they can share coping mechanisms and experiences, thus minimizing feelings of loneliness. Furthermore, the inclusion of mental health assessments during routine gynecological checkups can help identify women who are prone to psychological distress for AUB. Prioritizing mental health, in conjunction with medical treatment, can enable clinicians to provide a balanced approach to the care of patients. The multidisciplinary strategy can possibly facilitate improved coping mechanisms, empower women, and eventually enhance their quality of life while addressing the complex issues of AUB (. *et al.*, 2016).

Test Your Knowledge

1. How can changes in menstrual cycle patterns help identify abnormal uterine bleeding (AUB)?
2. What are common physical symptoms associated with AUB, such as fatigue or pelvic pain?

7.4. Diagnosis of Abnormal Uterine Bleeding

Learning Outcome

1. Define medical history and physical examination
2. Discuss the diagnostic tests (e.g., ultrasound, blood tests)

Diagnosis of abnormal uterine bleeding (AUB) demands a careful and systematic process to determine its causes accurately. Physicians typically start this process with a comprehensive history of the patient, which ought to cover menstrual cycles, previous medical illnesses, and factors most likely to influence bleeding, such as medication and lifestyle. Once a history has been obtained, the physical exam is performed in full, occasionally even a pelvic exam to check for any anatomical abnormalities, such as fibroids or polyps. Laboratory studies like complete blood counts and hormone level testing also play an important role in diagnosing AUB since they can diagnose thrombocytopenia or hormonal imbalance as the etiology of AUB. In others, imaging studies like transvaginal ultrasound can be applied to increase the visualization of ovaries and uterus, thus rendering diagnostic identification of the patient's condition even more effective. In certain situations, when less invasive diagnostic methods are inconclusive, more advanced methods like hysteroscopy can be required. This method facilitates direct visualization of the inner uterine cavity of the endometrium so that health care professionals are able to diagnose and perhaps treat endometrial disease like hyperplasia or polyps. The importance of appropriate diagnosis cannot be overstated, as it directly affects the treatment plan as well as patient management. To put it into context, the presence of an endocervical polyp, as researched in malignancy diagnoses such as Non-Hodgkins lymphoma, may be an indicator of the need for further intervention, for example, biopsy or surgical excision, to rule out cancerous changes (Kaler *et al.*, 2012). Effective diagnostic practices thus extend beyond symptom relief and actually prevent more serious complications of undiagnosed or undertreated AUB conditions. Besides, with the emergence of new techniques offering innovative options, interventional treatment has been touted as a fundamental intervention for managing advanced cases of AUB complicated by conditions like abnormal placental implantation. These include pelvic artery embolization (PAE), which has been shown to effectively control postpartum hemorrhage in such complications, and hence its potential in managing AUB complications. As per reviews evaluating PAE effectiveness, the treatment is capable of preventing more invasive procedures such as hysterectomy by efficiently managing acute bleeding attacks without posing any risk to the patient (Renzo *et al.*, 2015). Thus, the use of both interventional and diagnostic techniques is critical in the overall management of AUB, highlighting the need to remain abreast of developments in the specialty to maximize patient outcomes.

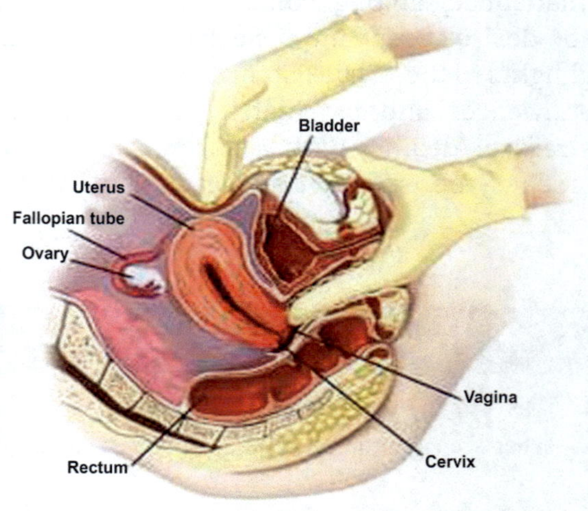

Figure 7.7. A pelvic exam.

Source: https://www.singhealth.com.sg/patient-care/conditions-treatments/menorrhagia-heavy-menstruation

7.4.1. Medical History and Physical Examination

In the assessment of abnormal uterine bleeding (AUB), it is most important to get a complete medical history. This first step provides information regarding the patient's menstrual cycle, including patterns like frequency, duration, and quantity of bleeding. Obtaining precise information regarding associated symptoms such as pelvic pain, intermenstrual bleeding, and history of previous gynecological problems helps in formulating a differential diagnosis.

Such variables as the patient's age may play a significant role in the likelihood of a given underlying condition. Young women, for instance, may present with endocrine abnormalities or polycystic ovary syndrome, while perimenopausal patients tend to present with structural lesions like leiomyomas or adenomyosis, based on research that applied the FIGO PALM-COEIN classification system to categorize AUBs etiologies based on patient history (Asudani *et al.*, 2025). Physical examination is the single most crucial antidote to the medical history and is utilized to augment the assessment of AUB. It includes a thorough abdominal examination and a pelvic examination to determine any masses or tenderness that would suggest underlying pathology. Transvaginal ultrasonography as a first imaging choice is highly valuable in the visualization of the reproductive organs and detection of structural abnormalities such as fibroids and endometrial abnormalities.

Histopathological examinations, particularly through endometrial biopsy, are helpful in situations where there is atypical presentation, most significantly in older women. They are able to elucidate secretory or proliferative period changes, such as in the cases that were explored in various age groups where endometrial hyperplasia was prevalent in the perimenopausal group (Abhilasha *et al.*, 2024).

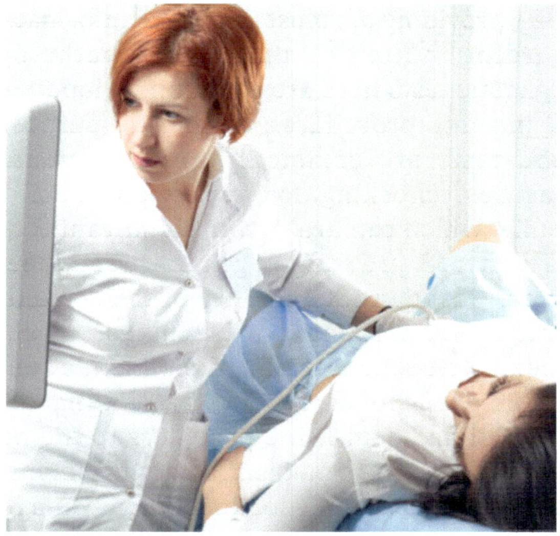

Source: https://pac-md.com/wp-content/uploads/2023/05/Dysfunctional-Uterine-Bleeding.png

With the integration of medical history and physical examination results into a clinical framework, AUB management is enhanced. With this organized presentation, an individualized treatment plan directed against the determined cause from clinical findings is enabled. The uniform application of surgery and hormonal therapy, for example, hysterectomy in severe cases, is facilitated with appropriate knowledge of the patient's individualized presentation. Also, continuous monitoring and follow-up are crucial, particularly in women diagnosed with conditions with a malignancy risk. Through the process of detecting age-related differences in endometrial patterns, as explained in current literature, clinicians can provide well-targeted interventions not only for AUB symptoms but also for its underlying causes, thereby improving patient outcomes (Abhilasha *et al.*, 2024).

7.4.2. Diagnostic Tests (e.g., Ultrasound, Blood Tests)

Diagnostic tests hold a significant position in the investigation of Abnormal Uterine Bleeding

(AUB), providing the most important information regarding potential underlying pathology. Diagnostic tests here are commonly blood tests and imaging procedures, diagnostic purposes. Blood tests are commonly initial evaluative measures, checking for conditions such as anemia, which can arise from significant blood loss with AUB. In a study of general practitioners, anemia was identified in 36% of the screening women, emphasizing the usefulness of such screening tests in assessing the patient's status (Ankum *et al.*, 2008). Further, these initial tests aid in guiding healthcare providers to the best interventions, from medication management to more complicated diagnostic methods. Imaging tests, particularly transvaginal ultrasound, are another practical aid in diagnosis for AUB. Ultrasounds allow healthcare providers to visualize structural abnormalities, e.g., uterine fibroids or polyps, which can contribute to abnormal bleeding patterns. Ultrasound results are significant; 41% of the women who were evaluated by ultrasound in one study had fibroids detected, supporting the significance of imaging when AUB is inexplicable (Ankum *et al.*, 2008).

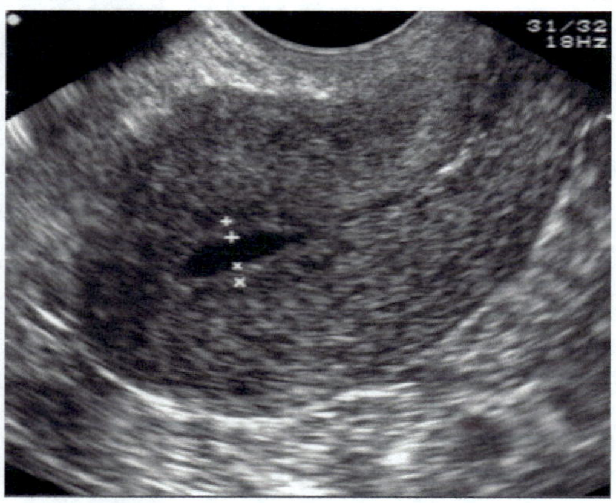

Figure 7.8. Ultrasound Imaging of Women with Abnormal Uterine Bleeding (AUB)

Source: https://media.springernature.com/lw685/springer-static/image/art%3A10.1007%2Fs10397-004-0012-5/MediaObjects/s10397-004-0012-5fhb3.jpg

Such testing not only confirms or rules out specific pathologies but also aids in future treatment planning. Each patient's case can differ greatly, thereby necessitating an individualized diagnostic plan that employs both blood testing and imaging to optimally counter the complex nature of AUB. Ultimately, the application of blood testing and ultrasound in the diagnosis of AUB illustrates the complex interaction of test modalities in the clinical setting.

The variation in diagnostic approaches among general practitioners is an indication of the requirement for differential evaluation and management guidelines. While the majority of practitioners will be inclined to a conservative approach towards AUB initially, employing systematic diagnostics will reveal salient underlying factors that need to be addressed. It is thus important to interpret findings with caution in the line of treatment, so that patients can get timely and effective interventions. Their application together not only enhances clinician understanding but also empowers females to grasp their health problems in the context of abnormal uterine bleeding.

7.4.3. Differential Diagnosis

In the differential diagnostic approach to abnormal uterine bleeding (AUB), one needs to keep in mind the broad approach brought about by the PALM-COEIN classification system. It distinguishes causes into two broad categories: structural and non-structural causes. Structural causes of the disease entities such as polyps, adenomyosis, leiomyomas, and malignancies, can be visually diagnosed through imaging and clinical presentations. Non-structural causes comprise coagulopathies, disturbances of ovulation, primary endometrial disease, and iatrogenic factors. Identification of the underlying cause is important as it guides management modalities and treatment. In the end, this enhances patient outcomes in

AUB, thereby upholding the importance of a systematic diagnosis (Viganò *et al.*, 2024).

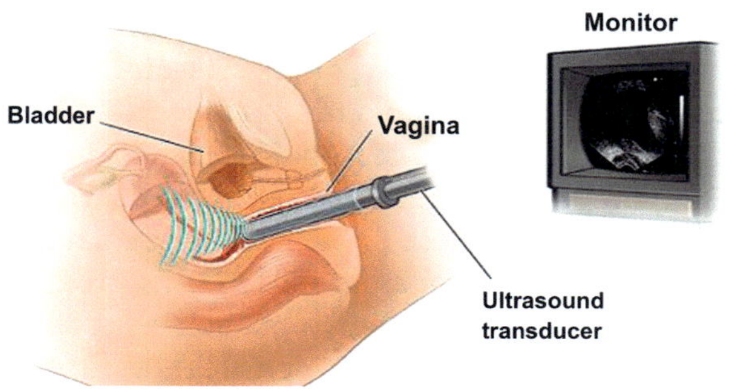

Figure 7.9. Transvaginal Ultrasound.

Source: https://content.healthwise.net/resources/14.3/en-us/media/medical/hw/h9991613_001.jpg

As imaging technology improves, transvaginal ultrasonography (TVUSG) is now a central diagnostic tool in AUB differential diagnosis. It is not invasive and is available at low cost, thus becoming a first-line assessment of endometrial pathologies. The imaging study can detect structural anomalies with moderate sensitivity but diminished specificity compared to more invasive studies. It has been proven with research that while TVUSG yields informative data on potential AUB causes, a combined method—combining dilation and curettage (D&C) and hysteroscopy—is more diagnostic. Hysteroscopy, particularly when added with biopsy, has been shown to have higher sensitivity in corroborating histopathological findings, thereby highlighting the importance of using supportive diagnostic modalities (Omurca, 2023). In order to embark on a correct differential diagnosis of AUB, the healthcare professionals have to embark on an extensive clinical history and physical exam in addition to proper imaging and procedural interventions. The clinical spectrum is broad, ranging from benign polyps to more serious malignancies, such that a complete and systematic approach is needed. The application of a stepwise evaluation strategy not only aids in the detection of the cause of bleeding but also aids in the stratification of the risk of severe underlying pathology. Furthermore, the inclusion of patient history and laboratory information in the decision-making process can assist in revolutionizing clinical thought. This interdisciplinary methodology ultimately forms the foundation for individualized treatment regimens, wherein AUB management is coordinated with the patient's unique needs and clinical evidence (Viganò *et al.*, 2024).

Test Your Knowledge

1. What are the key components of a clinical evaluation for diagnosing abnormal uterine bleeding?
2. Which diagnostic tests are commonly used to assess the cause of AUB?

7.5. Treatment Options for AUB

Learning Outcome

1. Discuss the medical management (e.g., hormonal therapy)
2. Define surgical interventions (e.g., D&C, hysterectomy)
3. Explain the lifestyle modifications and home remedies

The treatment modalities for abnormal uterine bleeding (AUB) are diverse and tailored to the patient's underlying etiology and overall condition. Medical therapy is often first-line management, especially in women presenting with dysfunctional uterine bleeding or those of reproductive age. Hormonal therapies, such as the combined oral contraceptives, progestins, and the levonorgestrel-releasing intrauterine system (IUS), have been proven to stabilize endometrial lining and decrease menstrual blood loss. Aside from the relief of bleeding, these treatments can also have effects on contraception, being generally regarded as necessary for women who want to manage their menstrual cycle. Other than this, the non-hormonal medications like tranexamic acid and NSAIDs can offer symptomatic relief from heavy menstrual bleeding without systemic endocrine effects, thus enabling treatment of patients with varying affinities and medical histories. In women in whom AUB persists despite medical treatment, surgery is the next step to be considered. Hysteroscopy plays a pivotal role in intrauterine pathology diagnosis and treatment of conditions such as polyps and fibroids, common culprits of abnormal uterine bleeding. The technique allows for chosen treatments like dilation and curettage (D&C) and polypectomy, thus providing symptomatic relief without undergoing more invasive surgical procedures. When the structural abnormalities are quite large, like fibroids or adenomyosis, uterine artery embolization can be chosen as a less invasive option compared to hysterectomy. However, in the event of severe AUB among women without response to conservative measures, hysterectomy is the definitive procedure, largely indicated in those situations with a clear pathological etiology of AUB determined, as noted in studies where leiomyoma and adenomyosis are prevalent diagnoses in surgical specimens (Banmeru *et al.*, 2025) (Asudani *et al.*, 2025). In treating AUB, a patient-centered approach is critical, not only addressing the clinical symptom of bleeding but also synchronizing with the patient's reproductive desires, particularly for younger women.

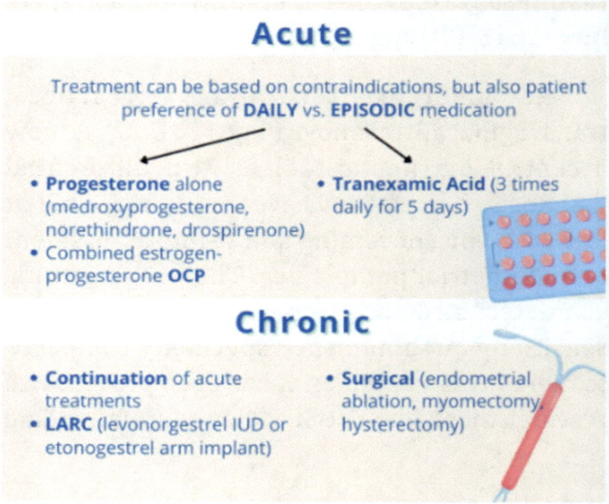

Figure 7.10. Abnormal uterine bleeding treatment.

Source: https://thecurbsiders.com/wp-content/uploads/2023/02/2-2-1.png

Awareness of the implications of various treatment modalities, their potential side effects, and risks empowers women in making their own healthcare decisions. Continuous monitoring and regular follow-up allow for modification of treatment plans according to the response of the patient and the advent of newly developed complications. As elaborated in the thorough classification systems such as PALM-COEIN, proper diagnostic workup is essential for managing AUB effectively with a quality of life in participating individuals. By an integrating combination of surgery and medicine, medical practitioners are able to offer customized, effective treatment modes that enhance the treatment of AUB (Banmeru *et al.*, 2025;Asudani *et al.*, 2025).

7.5.1. Medical Management (e.g., Hormonal Therapy)

Management of Abnormal Uterine Bleeding (AUB) has increasingly fallen into the hands of medical treatment, with hormonal treatment being at the forefront in bringing relief and menstrual regularity to the majority of women. Hormonal therapy, including the progestins, estrogens, and combinations thereof, has emerged as the first-line treatment for the majority of women with AUB. Norethisterone, a synthetic progestin, is frequently utilized because it can mimic natural progesterone and thus reverse the progesterone-deficiency effects of estrogen dominance that more frequently leads to heavy menstrual bleeding. The effectiveness of norethisterone in treating AUB is also enhanced by its ability to create a more stable endometrial lining, thereby restricting the incidence of heavy menstrual bleeding. Also, its controlled release presentations ensure prolonged drug concentration in the blood that minimizes side effects and maximizes patient compliance with treatment, as indicated by the need for innovative and patient-compliant hormone treatments in ensuring effective control of AUB (Boruah *et al.*, 2024). The challenge is further complicated by management of AUB in comorbid populations such as CKD, where disturbances in hormones and other systemic pathologies produce irregular menstrual cycles. CKD females may also present additional challenges to the management of AUB through hormonal dysregulation of their renal illness. As renal function declines, hormone clearance and metabolism are altered, resulting in anticipation of uncertain responses to standard medical therapy. This calls for a judicious assessment of the risks and advantages of hormonal therapy for AUB in this group. While medical treatment is possible, clinicians must remain vigilant and adjust treatment protocols as necessary to prevent sequelae like anemia due to excessive blood loss, thus highlighting the necessity of clearly established guidelines and individualized management protocols in this case (Ramu *et al.*, 2024). Finally, medical management of AUB, particularly with hormonal therapy, is a critical part of management planning to optimize women's well-being. Determination of the pathophysiological mechanisms of AUB and individualized hormonal therapies may lead to improved menstrual regulation and quality of life. Nevertheless, efforts like patient compliance, anticipated side effects, and comorbid health conditions need to be evaluated cautiously to maximize treatment protocols. With continuous research, the development of more effective, safer hormonal therapies takes precedence, particularly among populations with complicating circumstances like CKD. Prioritizing the expansion of treatment guidelines and streamlining the process of management demonstrates a deeper commitment from the medical field to resolving the diversified needs of women with AUB (Boruah *et al.*, 2024; Ramu *et al.*, 2024).

7.5.2. Surgical Interventions (e.g., D&C, Hysterectomy)

Surgical treatment is usually reserved when conservative treatment of Abnormal Uterine Bleeding (AUB) fails or is unacceptable to the patient. The most common among these surgical procedures is dilation and curettage (D&C). D&C is a scraping of the uterine lining performed carefully to eliminate unusual tissue or stop bleeding spells. D&C can either be diagnostic, providing lots of information about the source of bleeding, or therapeutic, establishing comfort.

Although generally safe, patients do run risks including infection or anesthetic complications. The effectiveness of D&C for AUB symptom treatment is well documented, but it is still necessary that clinicians individualize treatment to address the differential needs and concerns of AUB patients. Surgical options thus have to be evaluated not just on their potential clinical benefits but also on their compatibility with patients' preferences and values, as evidenced by treatment satisfaction studies (Daniels *et al.*, 2010).

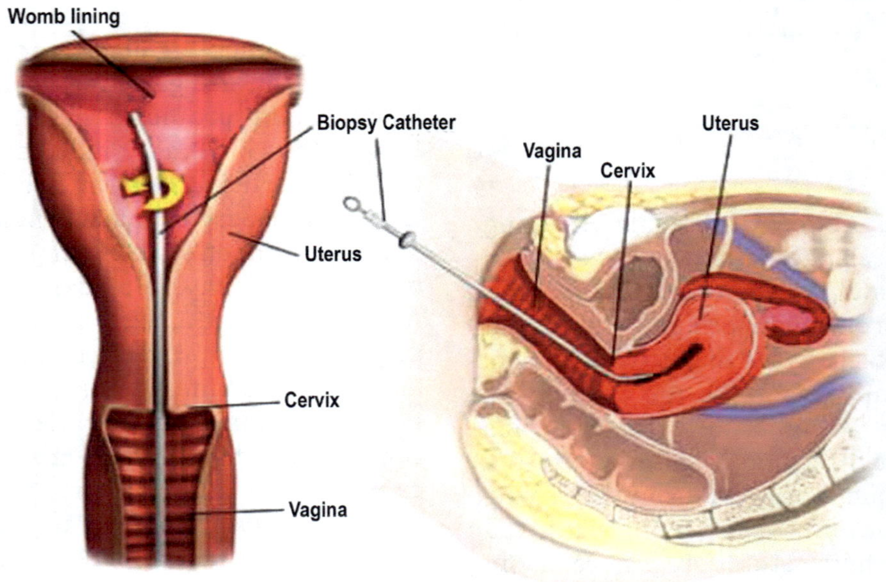

Figure 7.11. Endometrial sampling to test cells in the lining of the womb.

Source: https://www.singhealth.com.sg/patient-care/conditions-treatments/menorrhagia-heavy-menstruation

Hysterectomy appears to be a more definitive surgical procedure for AUB, particularly in patients with chronic and intractable bleeding. It involves complete removal of the uterus and may be offered to women with excessive symptoms of fibroids, endometriosis, or other etiologies. Even though hysterectomy is effective in eliminating AUB, it is crucial to consider the implications of such a surgical procedure, particularly in terms of fertility and overall quality of life. Studies have indicated that the majority of women exhibit a preference for less invasive procedures, and therefore, patient-oriented counseling is needed to explore options before considering a hysterectomy. The choice to undertake this major procedure should involve an in-depth discussion of possible complications, recovery times, and long-term outcomes so as to enable patients to make informed decisions (Byron *et al.*, 2014). Moreover, the dynamics of surgical interventions for AUB also continue to be dynamic with regard to advancements in technology and methods. Minimally invasive procedures like laparoscopic hysterectomy or endometrial ablation have gained popularity because they have shorter recovery times and, overall, fewer complications than open procedures. These procedures enable women to return to daily life sooner, which is a concern for most women. It is essential that healthcare professionals remain current on emerging strategies and their effectiveness in treating AUB, since this continues to keep them capable of delivering the most current and suitable combinations of treatments for individual cases. Shared decision-making, as emphasized by current studies, promotes patient engagement and satisfaction, ultimately leading to better outcomes for health. Hence, it is essential to have an understanding of the entire gamut of surgical procedures and to include patient preference while deciding to effectively manage AUB (Daniels *et al.*, 2010).

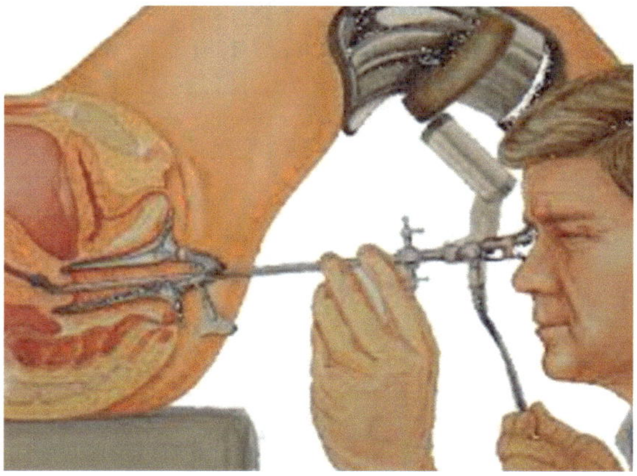

Figure 7.12. Hysteroscopic Surgeries.

Source: https://encrypted-tbn0.gstatic.com/images?q=tbn:ANd9GcQaATrXBwDxLoRwBJY8CYA5dDOmaBN-VxdZxA&s

7.5.3. Lifestyle Modifications and Home Remedies

Lifestyle changes are a crucial complement to the management of Abnormal Uterine Bleeding (AUB) since they have the potential to affect hormonal balance and overall health directly. For instance, a balanced diet that is rich in essential nutrients such as iron, vitamin C, and omega-3 fatty acids has the ability to curtail excessive blood loss and improve hemoglobin levels in individuals with AUB. A regular exercise regimen is also needed, as it has been found to reduce stress and regulate menstrual cycles. Women with AUB are typically advised to adopt a lifestyle with a focus on proper sleeping habits and stress-reduction techniques like yoga or meditation. These modifications not only enhance menstrual function but also general well-being, highlighting the harmony between lifestyle and reproductive health. In addition to dietary change, folk remedies have also gained popularity among women for the treatment of AUB.

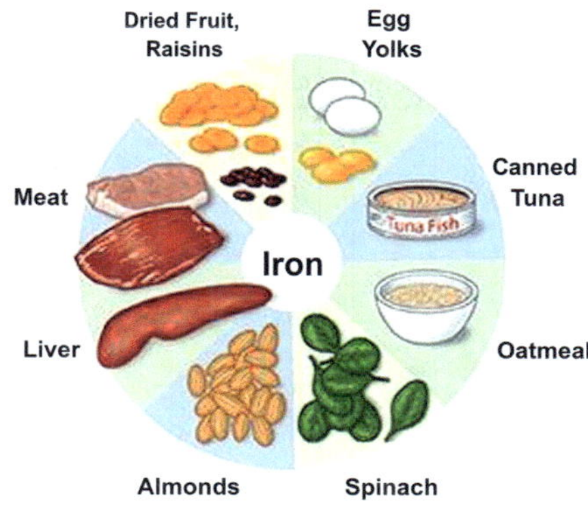

Figure 7.13. Source of iron.

Source: nutrients diet in managing Abnormal Uterine Bleeding (AUB)

Herbal supplements such as turmeric, ginger, and chamomile are also studied for their anti-inflammatory properties and role in regulating menstrual flow. Ginger, for instance, has been utilized to soothe menstrual cramps as well as regulate bleeding patterns, particularly beneficial for those with irregular cycles or heavy bleeding. It is necessary, however, that women consult medical practitioners before adding herbal treatments to their treatment program. The complex etiology of AUB means that there must be a careful and knowledgeable approach to adding natural therapy so as not to conflict with given treatments but to complement them. It is a reflection of the necessity of individualization in that it takes into account the particular needs and wishes of each patient. Education on lifestyle modification and natural cures is necessary for patients and healthcare providers with AUB. As medicine is constantly evolving, OB-GYN practitioners must know the advantages and disadvantages of adding natural cures to the treatment of patients. The literature shows that an integrated treatment approach with conventional therapy and natural remedies is crucial for effective management of women's healthcare conditions (Rahm, 2025). Such awareness not only informs women about informed treatment decisions for AUB but also promotes the inter-patient-provider collaborative partnership. Through increased awareness by healthcare providers of lifestyle modifications, they are in a better position to support women in their successful management of AUB, leading to improved quality of life and health.

Test Your Knowledge

1. What are the common hormonal treatments used to manage abnormal uterine bleeding?
2. When is surgical intervention considered necessary in the treatment of AUB?

SUMMARY

AUB pathogenesis is characterized by a multitude of pathological and physiological processes' interactions, which need to be carefully evaluated and managed. AUB prevalence, particularly in perimenopausal women, merits diagnosis of AUB signs and symptoms at the early stages for management of conditions such as endometrial carcinoma. Detection of specific risk factors like age and history of diabetes, observed in 462 perimenopausal women in this study, emphasizes the necessity for targeted screening protocols. Such prevention can significantly impact patient outcomes and enhance quality of life through the application of timely interventions that avert the progression of benign lesions to malignancies and direct attention towards the primary determinants of endometrial characteristics and arterial flow in such procedures (Wang *et al.*, 2024).

Moreover, following standard testing protocols, such as the International Endometrial Tumor Analysis (IETA) scoring system, in the clinic setting can optimize diagnostic accuracy of ultrasound scanning for AUB diagnosis. Through analysis of distinctive endometrial characteristics, the IETA system helps clinicians to distinguish between malignant and non-malignant lesions. The correlation between high IETA scores and malignancy highlights the value of a systematic approach in managing patients with AUB. Evidence for the contribution of endometrial thickness and vascular patterns towards diagnosing abnormal growth strengthens the argument for a shift towards integration of newer diagnostic modalities in everyday evaluation (Patil *et al.*, 2024). Overall, abnormal uterine bleeding requires an evidence-based, patient-centered, multi-faceted practice that is driven by diagnostic technology. Increased awareness of risk factors and application of more advanced imaging modalities may result in early detection and successful management, and reduce the number of complications such as endometrial cancer. More studies and cross-sectional collaboration are needed in formulating universal protocols tailored to the requirements of a heterogeneous population of patients, in order to manage the nuances of AUB in a successful way. By promoting these programs, the healthcare community can further enhance the quality of care received by women who experience AUB, which ultimately creates better overall health and healthier outcomes.

Abnormal Uterine Bleeding (AUB) is a significant clinical condition in a high percentage of women, and one-third of them are estimated to have such bleeding at some point in their lives. AUB is rarely caused by life-threatening causative conditions like cancer or pregnancy complications, thus it is challenging to treat. Women are mostly presented with different therapeutic options, which sometimes create confusion because the decision in most cases depends more on personal preference than on certain clinical outcomes. Shared decision-making in such a situation becomes questionable, as it places a strong focus on the right communication and preference elicitation instruments to enable patients and enhance their treatment experience (Byron *et al.*, 2014). In recent years, the use of adaptive conjoint analysis (ACA) has also been found to be an efficient way of eliciting patient preferences in AUB treatment.

Women who take part in such studies in a properly structured forum rate elements like efficacy of treatment, healing time, and expense, which are of the highest priority to them in decision-making. However, trial evidence finds that treatment satisfaction is high overall, with low decision regret even where there was use of preference elicitation tools, very similar to outcomes where conventional counseling strategies were employed. This aims to acknowledge the necessity for ongoing discussion on practice tools and raises the potential area of future research in promoting collaborative decision-making, specifically among young women who can be perceived as having a dissimilar decision outcome compared to their older peers (Byron *et al.*, 2014). Furthermore, research on the impacts of endometrial ablations yields findings on the quality of life that is associated with AUB interventions. Experiments have shown that the women who went through the treatments reported differing experiences based on the bleeding patterns, i.e., heavy/regular and heavy/irregular bleeding. Findings showed that the women who had heavy/irregular bleeding suffered more, which created a more impressive adverse effect on their quality of life. Screening instruments such as the Menstrual Bleeding Questionnaire (MBQ) are helpful in providing insight into the importance of varying bleeding patterns, and it is suggested that individualized evaluation may outrank the general concern of responding to the unique needs and distressful symptoms of these patients. Increased sensitivity of these dynamics is of utmost relevance for designing effective interventions and achieving optimal overall patient outcomes in the treatment of AUB.

KEY TERMS FROM THIS CHAPTER

- Menorrhagia
- Oligomenorrhea
- Postcoital bleeding
- Anovulatory cycles
- Endometrial carcinoma
- Uterine fibroids (leiomyomas)
- Coagulopathy
- Hormonal imbalance
- Metrorrhagia
- Intermenstrual bleeding
- Dysfunctional uterine bleeding (DUB)
- Endometrial hyperplasia
- Endometritis
- Adenomyosis
- Platelet dysfunction
- Iatrogenic causes

CRITICAL THINKING QUESTIONS

1. **Abnormal uterine bleeding (AUB) is best defined as:**
   a. Bleeding only during menstruation
   b. Any bleeding from the uterus that is irregular in volume, duration, or timing
   c. Bleeding exclusively after menopause
   d. Bleeding caused only by pregnancy complications
2. **Which of the following is NOT a common cause of AUB?**
   a. Hormonal imbalance
   b. Uterine fibroids
   c. Endometrial cancer
   d. Appendicitis
3. **The acronym PALM-COEIN used to classify causes of AUB stands for:**
   a. Polyp, Adenomyosis, Leiomyoma, Malignancy, Coagulopathy, Ovulatory dysfunction, Endometrial, Iatrogenic, Not yet classified
   b. Pregnancy, Anemia, Leukemia, Malignancy, Coagulopathy, Ovary, Endometrium, Infection, Neoplasm
   c. Polycystic ovary, Anemia, Leukemia, Malignancy, Coagulopathy, Ovulation, Endometritis, Injury, Necrosis
   d. Pelvic pain, Adenomyosis, Leukorrhea, Malignancy, Coagulopathy, Ovarian cyst, Endometriosis, Infection, Neoplasm
4. **Heavy menstrual bleeding lasting more than 7 days is called:**
   a. Oligomenorrhea
   b. Menorrhagia
   c. Metrorrhagia
   d. Polymenorrhea
5. **Which diagnostic tool is most commonly used initially to evaluate the uterine lining in AUB?**
   a. Hysteroscopy
   b. Pelvic MRI
   c. Transvaginal ultrasound
   d. CT scan

Short Answer Questions

1. What are the main types of abnormal uterine bleeding (AUB)?
2. Name two common causes of abnormal uterine bleeding.
3. What symptoms are typically associated with abnormal uterine bleeding?
4. Which diagnostic methods are used to evaluate abnormal uterine bleeding?
5. What are two treatment options for managing abnormal uterine bleeding?
6. How can hormonal imbalance lead to abnormal uterine bleeding?

Answer to Critical Thinking Questions

1. (b) 2. (d) 3. (a) 4. (b) 5. (c)

REFERENCES

1. Abhilasha, Dwivedi, G., Ashish, & Khan, N. (2024). Endometrial histopathological patterns in patients with abnormal uterine bleeding: A six months observation of 285 cases in a tertiary care hospital. *Asian Journal of Pharmaceutical and Clinical Research.* https://www.semanticscholar.org/paper/6323621a58a0c7c2fd697c45515aecf2b742f088 (accessed on 14th June 2025).
2. Ahmed, S., Ahmed, S., Gullabzada, M., Gullabzada, U., & Jobanputra, K. (2024). Abnormal uterine bleeding with leiomyomas: A case report of its natural course and therapeutic management. *Cureus, 16.* https://www.semanticscholar.org/paper/7b0b0bbad1d5e2a316709f3b86ce96e0131181e7 (accessed on 14th June 2025).
3. Ankum, W. M., Bindels, P. J. E., de Vries, C. J. H., *et al.* (2008). Abnormal vaginal bleeding in women of reproductive age: A descriptive study of initial management in general practice. https://core.ac.uk/download/pdf/8034010.pdf (accessed on 14th June 2025).
4. Arikarevula, S., Seedipally, S. R., & Ragoor, S. (2024). Causes of abnormal uterine bleeding in women of 20–60 years of age based on polyp, adenomyosis, leiomyoma, malignancy, coagulopathy, ovulatory dysfunction, endometrial, iatrogenic, and not-yet-classified at a tertiary care hospital: A cross-sectional study. *MRIMS Journal of Health Sciences.* https://www.semanticscholar.org/paper/0c278bd7984e652f77551bda8a44c71cc129ea97 (accessed on 14th June 2025).
5. Asalkar, M., Rumani, I., Supe, M., Thakkarwad, S., Ramesh, S., Shete, S. S., & Gautam, A. (2024). Endometrial pathology in abnormal uterine bleeding (AUB) & role of different techniques of endometrial sampling in evaluation of AUB: A cross-sectional study. *Indian Journal of Obstetrics and Gynecology Research.* https://www.semanticscholar.org/paper/728c4c695149ec34d39ad292573f4ece3c11f912 (accessed on 14th June 2025).
6. Asudani, N. P., Yadava, P. A., Vyas, R. C., Jani, S., Rawal, N. G., Dangar, K. V., & Patel, H. J. (2025). Evaluation of PALM–COEIN classification and management of abnormal uterine bleeding in peri-menopausal age group. *International Journal of Reproduction, Contraception, Obstetrics and Gynecology.* https://www.semanticscholar.org/paper/40dc8a7ec959de00690b37a8c761a1e556e38e12 (accessed on 14th June 2025).
7. Banmeru, A. P., & Narayanaswamy, M. (2025). From symptoms to surgery: Clinicopathological correlation in women undergoing hysterectomy for abnormal uterine bleeding. *International Journal of Reproduction, Contraception, Obstetrics and Gynecology.* https://www.semanticscholar.org/paper/a9776ff6cbd6c8bb621c4e9fc64e8e93e89f7d0d (accessed on 14th June 2025).
8. Barra, F., Bogliolo, S., Ceccaroni, M., *et al.* (2023). Current medical therapy for adenomyosis: From bench to bedside. https://core.ac.uk/download/590920564.pdf (accessed on 14th June 2025).
9. Bektaş, O., Bektas, K., Aydın, Ş., Doğan Durdağ, G., & Celik, H. (2024). The effects of the COVID-19 pandemic on abnormal uterine bleeding according to the PALM-COEIN classification. *Gynecology Obstetrics & Reproductive Medicine.* https://www.semanticscholar.org/paper/fb5a38daec183480c67b6c5e1dadd17c234e6a14 (accessed on 14th June 2025).
10. Bhadani, P. P., Gurung, P., Sinha, H. H., *et al.* (2018). Study on abnormal uterine bleeding among adult women in a tertiary care hospital in Bihar, India. https://core.ac.uk/download/544390370.pdf (accessed on 14th June 2025).

11. Boruah, A. M., Banerjee, D., Bhardwaj, F., Mallya, S., Singal, R., Sharma, S., & Gautam, A. (2024). Effect of norethisterone dose and duration in the management of abnormal uterine bleeding: A narrative review and case report. *Drugs in Context, 13*. https://www.semanticscholar.org/paper/803ba07966bb8c8c2b93adb4154fb0ef3338c619 (accessed on 14th June 2025).

12. Byron, J., Hess, L. M., Kasper, K., *et al.* (2014). Preference elicitation tool for abnormal uterine bleeding treatment: A randomized controlled trial. https://core.ac.uk/download/46962891.pdf (accessed on 14th June 2025).

13. Cantarelli, A. de L. J., Suzart Júnior, M. F., De Sá Pereira, M. C., De Queiroz, T. L., Nicácio, T. da S. L., Cardoso, L. T., Mendonça, G. C. S., *et al.* (2024). Diagnosis and treatment of abnormal uterine bleeding: A review of the literature. *Revita ft*. https://www.semanticscholar.org/paper/534f4a47c6879b939ad85f943b7fb2a4ca06f9c0 (accessed on 14th June 2025).

14. Chau, M. T., Cheung, A. N. Y., Lee, S., *et al.* (1997). A woman with persistent vaginal bleeding after suction evacuation of the uterus. https://core.ac.uk/download/37890108.pdf (accessed on 14th June 2025).

15. Chodankar, R., Critchley, H. O. D., & Munro, M. G. (2022). Historical perspectives and evolution of menstrual terminology. https://core.ac.uk/download/533464934.pdf (accessed on 14th June 2025).

16. Cocksedge, K. A., Li, T. C., & Saravelos, S. H. (2008). Prevalence and diagnosis of congenital uterine anomalies in women with reproductive failure: A critical appraisal. https://core.ac.uk/download/50624.pdf (accessed on 14th June 2025).

17. Daniels, J. P., Cooper, K. G., Khan, K. S., Middleton, L. J., Gannon, M., Hilken, N. H., null null, *et al.* (2010). Hysterectomy, endometrial destruction, and levonorgestrel releasing intrauterine system (Mirena) for heavy menstrual bleeding: Systematic review and meta-analysis of data from individual patients. https://core.ac.uk/download/9633761.pdf (accessed on 14th June 2025).

18. Renzo Di , G. C., Epicoco, G., Fischer, M., *et al.* (2015). Endovascular management of massive post-partum hemorrhage in abnormal placental implantation deliveries. https://core.ac.uk/download/141695765.pdf (accessed on 14th June 2025).

19. Effendi, K. Y., Amran, R., Zulqarnain, I., Manan, H., Abadi, A., Usman, F., Nurtjahyo, A., *et al.* (2021). Abnormal uterine bleeding in adolescent. *Bio Scientia Medicina: Journal of Biomedicine and Translational Research*. https://www.semanticscholar.org/paper/b2ed5030de647dff852f902b4c2d90e8c064496b (accessed on 14th June 2025).

20. Fauser, B. C. J. M., Brown, J., Busfield, D. H., Barlow, D., Dolan, S., Donnez, J., Donnez, O., *et al.* (2014). Long-term treatment of uterine fibroids with ulipristal acetate. *Human Reproduction, 29*(9), 2011–2021. https://core.ac.uk/download/9367119.pdf (accessed on 14th June 2025).

21. Gonzalez, S. (2017). Assessing patient satisfaction levels following endometrial ablations in the treatment of abnormal uterine bleeding to determine effectiveness. https://open.bu.edu/bitstream/2144/23801/5/Gonzalez_bu_0017N_12872.pdf (accessed on 14th June 2025).

22. Gulamali, D., & Padval, R. K. M. (2023). Hysteroscopic evaluation of menorrhagia and correlation with saline infusion sonography and histopathology of the endometrium. https://core.ac.uk/download/570905880.pdf (accessed on 14th June 2025).

23. Gulia, S. P., Kaur, S. P., Lata, G., Sharma, *et al.* (2020). Histon-pathological pattern of endometrial biopsy in females with abnormal uterine bleeding: A retrospective study in tertiary care

hospital of Haryana. https://core.ac.uk/download/539900101.pdf (accessed on 14th June 2025).

24. Iacovides, S., Avidon, I., & Baker, F. C. (2015). What we know about primary dysmenorrhea today: A critical review. *Human Reproduction Update, 21*, 762–778. https://doi.org/10.1093/humupd/dmv039 (accessed on 14th June 2025).

25. Islam, L., & Maqsood, M. (2025). The impact of thyroid dysfunction on abnormal uterine bleeding menstrual irregularities. *Insights-Journal of Health and Rehabilitation*. https://www.semanticscholar.org/paper/c52c89ad0b5ac194997e15440b4f176b30a86a3c (accessed on 14th June 2025).

26. Jain, V., Chodankar, R., Maybin, J., & Critchley, H. (2022). Uterine bleeding: How understanding endometrial physiology underpins menstrual health. *Nature Reviews. Endocrinology, 18*, 290–308. https://www.semanticscholar.org/paper/101f9d21f78ea8e7052aab065041a14bcf3f3332 (accessed on 14th June 2025).

27. Kaler, A. K., & Vasudev, D. S. (2012). Non-Hodgkin's lymphoma of the uterine cervix. https://core.ac.uk/download/pdf/13598730.pdf (accessed on 14th June 2025).

28. Kononova, I. N., Dobrokhotova, J., Kareva, E. N., Stebenyaeva, E. V., Shmakova, N., Graban, I., Krasnoshchok, E. V., *et al.* (2024). New options for replenishing the iron stores in patients with abnormal uterine bleeding. *Meditsinskiy Sovet = Medical Council*. https://www.semanticscholar.org/paper/9dfeec4ddf3485c79f98894972b12f8673687844 (accessed on 14th June 2025).

29. Omurca, F. (2023). Comparison of diagnostic techniques used in the differential diagnosis of endometrial pathologies presenting with an abnormal uterine bleeding. *Journal of Contemporary Medicine*. https://www.semanticscholar.org/paper/bfd3ba836228e3003e14c4bdc0369188fe22e302 (accessed on 14th June 2025).

30. Patil, Y., Dhande, A., Khaladkar, S., & Patil, P. P. K. (2024). Application of the International Endometrial Tumor Analysis (IETA) in ultrasound evaluation of abnormal uterine bleeding. *Cureus, 16*. https://www.semanticscholar.org/paper/ed16d9ac5e14f8c641f211cca79e65413e8a5901 (accessed on 14th June 2025).

31. Philip, F. K., Pillai, S. S., Pushpangadan, P., *et al.* (2022). Histopathological evaluation of endometrial patterns in workup of abnormal uterine bleeding. https://core.ac.uk/download/539901679.pdf (accessed on 14th June 2025).

32. Piatyhor, A. (2025). Pre-eclampsia as a risk factor for diabetes. https://repo.knmu.edu.ua/bitstream/123456789/24411/1/ISIC_2019_Piatyhor_Anastasiia%20.pdf (accessed on 14th June 2025).

33. Pooja, N., & Choudary, G. (2024). Assessing thyroid abnormalities in abnormal uterine bleeding: A comprehensive prospective study. *International Journal of Reproduction, Contraception, Obstetrics and Gynecology*. https://www.semanticscholar.org/paper/6a6bc224c96e0ba05a33d7b01cd25bbdbc30f93b (accessed on 14th June 2025).

34. Rahm, C. (2025). General obstetrics and gynecology (OB-GYN) and global traditional and natural treatment options. *Clin Med Eng Live, 3*(1), 1–38. https://www.wecmelive.com/open-access/general-obstetrics-and-gynecology-obgyn-and-global-traditional-and-natural-treatment-options.pdf (accessed on 14th June 2025).

35. Ramu, S., & Zangmo, R. (2024). Management options of abnormal uterine bleeding in chronic kidney disease: A brief review. *ASEAN Journal of Psychiatry*. https://www.semanticscholar.org/paper/905e7b79946985df41088913d9b4d8a515b7a796 (accessed on 14th June 2025).

36. Salvi, P., Aramandla, S., & Gaikwad, V. A. (2024). The correlation of hysteroscopy and histopathology in evaluating abnormal uterine bleeding: Observations from a tertiary care center. *Cureus, 16*. https://www.semanticscholar.org/paper/de0f05f824f7e6a727760ca51cadfdda9f82625f (accessed on 14th June 2025).

37. Shree, R. J., & Sailatha. (2025). The role of levonorgestrel intrauterine device in managing abnormal uterine bleeding. *International Journal of Reproduction, Contraception, Obstetrics and Gynecology*. https://www.semanticscholar.org/paper/eb0a580f7601ad60651cbb7ae5a99b07c8aa7823 (accessed on 14th June 2025).

38. Singh, M. (2024). Ormeloxifene can be used as first line drug in abnormal uterine bleeding: A cross sectional prospective interventional study. *International Journal of Reproduction, Contraception, Obstetrics and Gynecology*. https://www.semanticscholar.org/paper/4fd390614a60694d85e472e60d5f1cc8dd1d79e5 (accessed on 14th June 2025).

39. Soni, A., Patel, A., Patel, S., & Gandhi, M. (2024). To estimate the prevalence of anemia in patients of abnormal uterine bleeding (AUB) admitted in tertiary care center. *International Journal of Health Sciences*. https://www.semanticscholar.org/paper/7a78c9269131924af9bc398174cc7873e8458796 (accessed on 14th June 2025).

40. Subhashini, T., Sreelakshmi, U., & Bindu, T. (2017). Abnormal uterine bleeding in perimenopausal age group women: A study on clinicopathological evaluation and management. https://core.ac.uk/download/539901209.pdf (accessed on 14th June 2025).

41. Trivedi, F. J., Deliwala, K., Deliwala, D. J., & Patel, S. V. (2024). FIGO classification system (PALM-COEIN) for causes of abnormal uterine bleeding in non-gravid women. *International Journal of Reproduction, Contraception, Obstetrics and Gynecology*. https://www.semanticscholar.org/paper/c90f65a8723313fcd893ba125c16d7ba22e8fd87 (accessed on 14th June 2025).

42. Viganò, S., Smedile, A., Cazzella, C., Marra, P., Bonaffini, P., & Sironi, S. (2024). Abnormal uterine bleeding: A pictorial review on differential diagnosis and not-so-common cases of interventional radiology management. *Diagnostics, 14*. https://www.semanticscholar.org/paper/7c407360797ff1f78c22959846304c8df4085b6b (accessed on 14th June 2025).

43. Wang, L., Quan, S., Bai, E., Yang, X., Scollo, P., & Mereu, L. (2024). Analysis of clinical data of different endometrial pathological types in perimenopausal women with abnormal uterine bleeding. *Frontiers in Oncology, 14*. https://www.semanticscholar.org/paper/fc6410cbf667c3efc7c33fdd0c7a1a21f827dd45 (accessed on 14th June 2025).

44. Whitaker, L., & Critchley, H. (2015). Abnormal uterine bleeding. *Best Practice & Research Clinical Obstetrics & Gynecology, 34*, 54–65. https://doi.org/10.1016/j.bpobgyn.2015.11.012 (accessed on 14th June 2025).

POLYCYSTIC OVARIAN SYNDROME

8

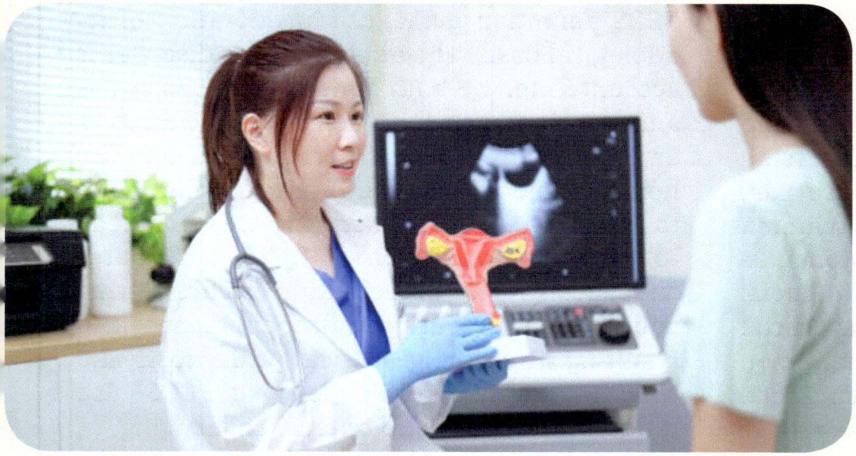

LEARNING OBJECTIVES

After studying this chapter, you will be able to:

1. Explain the causes of polycystic ovary syndrome (PCOS).
2. Identify the common symptoms of PCOS.
3. Describe the diagnostic criteria and methods for PCOS.
4. Discuss the health risks associated with PCOS.
5. Evaluate the treatment options available for managing PCOS.

Introduction

Polycystic Ovarian Syndrome (PCOS) is a prevalent endocrine disorder in women of childbearing age, occurring in approximately 5–10% of this demographic according to recent research. PCOS is characterized by a diverse set of symptoms, including light or infrequent menstruation, high androgen levels, and polycystic ovaries. Despite its prevalence, PCOS has largely been misunderstood and underdiagnosed, establishing a vast knowledge and treatment gap. The diagnostic criteria are now different, and having a more profound insight into the syndrome's etiology is significant to both the patients and healthcare professionals. This chapter tries to bring to light the nuances of PCOS diagnosis, symptoms, and long-term implications on health for creating an improved awareness path for afflicted individuals and their advocates. Understanding the causal mechanisms of PCOS is important to achieve practical interventions. Insulin resistance, genetic predisposition, and obesity are some of the causative factors that play a significant role in disease manifestation and advancement. It has been shown by studies that insulin resistance not only plays a role in poor metabolic health but also in symptoms of PCOS, including hirsutism and infertility. Current research shows that the traditional treatments, including metformin and oral contraceptives, are not necessarily for all, and treatment procedures need to be reconsidered. Current evidence supports exploring both pharmacologic and nonpharmacologic therapy, e.g., diet modification and lifestyle change, as possibilities to manage the syndrome. The worth of an interdisciplinary treatment model cannot be overstated, as tailored care can optimize both physical and mental well-being in PCOS patients. In light of these factors, it is necessary to expand the dialogue regarding PCOS by addressing the stigma and misconceptions that are part of the syndrome. The majority of women with PCOS experience physical symptoms, as well as emotional responses related to social expectations and infertility stigma. It is crucial that healthcare professionals caring for women with PCOS have knowledge of the psychosocial facets of the condition in order to give proper care. Education and advocacy are paramount in empowering women to seek appropriate treatment and support. Lastly, the chapter attempts to provide an overall analysis of PCOS, venturing into its multifactorial etiology and advocating for a holistic management approach using medical and lifestyle interventions outlined in more current studies (Bernier *et al.*, 2012; Fagg *et al.*, 2024).

Definition of Polycystic Ovarian Syndrome

The diagnosis of Polycystic Ovarian Syndrome (PCOS) is a complex endocrine disorder involving hormonal derangement affecting the female reproductive system. PCOS is a highly prevalent metabolic and hormonal disorder, affecting close to 116 million women worldwide, or 3.4% of all females, according to World Health Organization (WHO) statistics (Lahari *et al.*, 2025). The disorder is complex, typically with irregular periods, hirsutism, acne, weight gain, and infertility. The pathophysiologic mechanisms of PCOS include dysregulation of insulin and gonadotropin hormones, which results in excess production of androgens and cystic ovary formation. Therefore, the condition not only impairs reproductive function but also has significant implications in terms of metabolic health, uncovering its heterogeneity and variability of symptom expression in affected subjects. Further clarification of the PCOS definition demands consideration of its etiological basis. The etiology of the disorder is accounted for by both genetic predispositions and environmental influences, i.e., nutrition and lifestyle (Cochran *et al.*, 2024). The female subjects with PCOS are usually noted to have insulin resistance, and this may lead to complications such as type 2 diabetes and obesity. The presentation occurs during adolescence or early adulthood, hence also resulting in challenges in early diagnosis and treatment. The heterogeneity of PCOS also renders the diagnostic criteria challenging, as not all individuals who have the condition will have the classic picture of the syndrome. This in-built variability reinforces the importance of individualized treatment and assessment plans, tailored to the specific presentation and health profiles of the patients. The definition of Polycystic Ovarian Syndrome, as a whole, appears as an important factor in comprehending its broader implications for women's health. Because it is so prevalent and has such an extensive range of symptoms, PCOS has a significant impact on women's physical and psychological well-being. Contemporary literature indicates that alongside progression in treatment modalities for symptom diminution, delays in diagnosis and heterogeneous treatment plans continue to pose challenges to quality of life in women with PCOS (Cochran *et al.*, 2024). A better comprehension of PCOS thus not only aids in therapeutic choice evaluation but also empowers women to become healthcare partners. Ongoing research into novel therapeutic approaches and overall management regimens remains vital in the treatment of the underlying pathophysiologic processes of PCOS, with the end result being to improve the overall health outcome for women with PCOS.

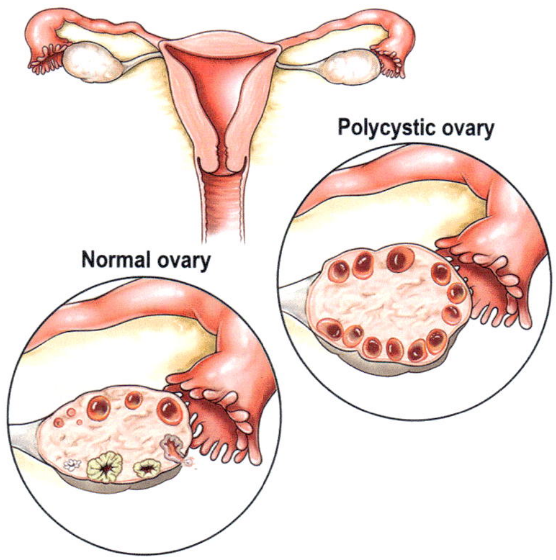

Figure 8.1. PCOS (Polycystic Ovary Syndrome).

Source: https://my.clevelandclinic.org/-/scassets/images/org/health/articles/8316-polycystic-ovary-syndrome-pcos

Prevalence and Demographics

Polycystic Ovarian Syndrome (PCOS) is recognized as the most prevalent endocrine disorder among women of reproductive age, affecting approximately 5% to 10% of women of this age group globally. The disparity in prevalence rates could be attributed to differing diagnostic criteria applied in the different studies, including the Rotterdam criteria frequently employed in clinical assessments. The syndrome's complex nature, comprising metabolic, reproductive, and psychological components, is what makes its real prevalence so complicated to determine. Additionally, diverse demographic components like ethnicity and geographical location also appear to influence the presentation of symptoms of PCOS, hence implying that this disorder does not affect everyone within all populations equally. For instance, it has been established through research that certain ethnic groups, such as South Asian women, have been shown to exhibit even higher incidence rates for PCOS, reflecting a mix of genetic, environmental, and lifestyle factors that would be worth delving into further in epidemiological research. Clinical presentation of PCOS varies widely among women, impacting diagnosis at a younger age and clinical outcomes. Women diagnosed at earlier phases of life tend to exhibit greater symptoms, such as irregular menstruation and signs of hyperandrogenia, but the same can vary across different conditions of overall well-being and lifestyle. That most have hyperandrogenism, one of the key diagnostic features, is telling when comparing these variable levels of androgen across populations. Studies have indicated that certain biomarkers, such as salivary testosterone (salT) and androstenedione (salA), are elevated in women with PCOS compared to controls, also suggesting the hypothesis that hyperandrogenism closely correlates with the disorder. The increased prevalence of metabolic disorders associated with PCOS, including insulin resistance, also complicates the demographic trend of this syndrome since the women with the worst symptoms are more likely to develop additional medical conditions in the long run, thus necessitating long-term integrated care planning. PCOS has far-reaching implications demographically beyond the realm of reproductive medicine and extends to mental health as well as quality of life in these women. PCOS women are also more likely to suffer from psychological issues such as depression and anxiety, which can be caused by the physical and hormonal manifestations of the disease, such as acne and weight. These compounded mental disorders may further be driven by social pressure regarding body image and fertility, which is another psychological burden for these patients. Further, the economic cost of treating PCOS, including medication cost, fertility treatment, and psychiatric treatment, may be substantial and may be distributed unevenly across various socio-economic groups. With ongoing studies aiming to solidify diagnostic criteria and broaden the scope of the wider health outcomes of PCOS, an understanding of the multifaceted demographics and symptom prevalence of the syndrome remains an integral part in the transition to improve treatment and care initiatives to reach women across the globe, particularly among disparate and disadvantaged populations.

Importance of Understanding PCOS

It is crucial to comprehend PCOS thoroughly as it is now a chronic endocrine disorder that impacts approximately 10% of women and female-to-female individuals globally. Comprehending PCOS is critical, not just to identify its multilingual signs such as irregular menstruation, metabolic dysregulation, and psychological signs, but also in avoiding its long-term health consequences of diabetes, cardiovascular disease, and infertility. Evidence indicates that the complexity of PCOS requires individually tailored management strategies that account for both physical and psychological health (Orr *et al.*, 2024). By an informed public and healthcare team, we can ensure early diagnosis and intervention, and then improve the quality of life for affected individuals. No less important is the role of self-management in coping with the difficulties that accompany PCOS. Most individuals with this condition are confronted with barriers to effective self-management, including a lack of information and emotional distress (Orr *et al.*, 2024). Web-based and digital interventions have emerged as strong tools for empowering patients, with the offering of lifestyle changes, dietary data, and coping skills. The establishment of integrated web-based systems, e.g., the HOPE program tailored for PCOS, is an advancement towards enhancing patients' self-efficacy and motivation. These interventions are potentially significant in prioritizing the integration of psychological care and educational resources, ultimately resulting in improved health outcomes, reduced anxiety, and overall improved quality of life (Orr *et al.*, 2024).

Further, identification of the psychological components of PCOS illuminates the importance of understanding this syndrome beyond its physical presentation. Mental disorders such as depression and anxiety are prevalent among PCOS patients, and therefore, a holistic treatment strategy should incorporate both medical and psychological intervention (Orr *et al.*, 2024). Acknowledgment of these interactive factors also highlights the necessity for healthcare providers to be well-trained and well-versed enough to treat emotional states alongside physical symptoms. While evidence grows to validate the significance of individualized self-management treatments, creating strategic healthcare models that embrace this integrated understanding of PCOS will be vital in increasing patient empowerment and maximizing equitable access to care.

8.1. Causes of PCOS

Learning Outcome

1. Define genetic factors and hormonal imbalances
2. Explain the environmental influences

The etiology of Polycystic Ovarian Syndrome (PCOS) is complex with an etiological interplay involving genetic, hormonal, and environmental factors. A genetic predisposition has been suggested by research as the underlying mechanism of PCOS development, as evidenced by familial clustering and the presence of specific genetic markers associated with PCOS. For example, family studies reveal that women with a familial background of PCOS have a higher prevalence of the disorder, supporting a potential genetic component. Moreover, hormonal imbalance, with high levels of androgens such as testosterone, forms the basis of PCOS symptoms like anovulation and irregular menstruation. These endocrine disturbances may result in hirsutism to acne-like symptoms, emphasizing the need for a deep understanding of these biochemical pathways as a foundation for addressing the condition's impact on women's health (Bernier *et al.*, 2012). The second primary contributing element of PCOS development is insulin resistance, present in a large proportion of affected women. Insulin resistance induces hyperinsulinemia, which in turn results in increased ovarian production of androgens and aggravates PCOS symptoms. Studies have identified that insulin resistance occurs in various phenotypes of PCOS, though their prevalence varies between classical and normoandrogenic forms of the disorder. For instance, it has been reported that among PCOS women, approximately 71.4% exhibit some form of insulin resistance. These findings indicate the significance of considering metabolic health in PCOS treatment, where lifestyle modifications to improve insulin sensitivity could have a revolutionary effect on people with the condition (Bonin *et al.*, 2013).

Obesity appears to be one of the main perpetrators of PCOS aetiology and its worsening, and thereby complicates the treatment and management of the disorders further. PCOS women usually present with overweight or obesity, whose extent may also increase insulin resistance and disrupt hormonal homeostasis. The increased fat mass, particularly visceral fat, results in increased androgen production, thereby creating a cycle of hormonal imbalance. This observation suggests that weight regulation needs to be an integral component of treatment protocols for PCOS women. On top of this, lifestyle and diet are also environmental influences that must be honored since they can control the severity of symptoms and overall health outcomes. For this reason, the application of a holistic lifestyle with the management of weight, dietary changes, and physical exercise is necessary in order to mitigate the impact of PCOS and improve the quality of life among individuals with PCOS (Bernier *et al.*, 2012).

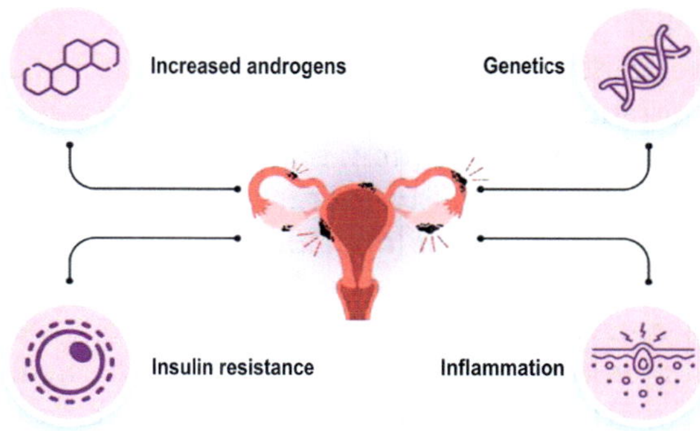

Figure 8.2. Causes of PCOS.

Source: https://images.ctfassets.net/eexbcii1ci83/6l6oDtnFmmnQw6IPpPWgOg/75aefe089b54f20395cf736fc99f1a54/Causes_of_PCOS.jpg

8.1.1. Genetic Factors

The subtle interaction between genetic elements is at the heart of Polycystic Ovarian Syndrome (PCOS) pathogenesis, and this highlights the complexity of the endocrine condition. Research shows genetic predisposition plays a significant role in the etiology of PCOS, as evidenced by its hereditary pattern. Women with a first-degree relative suffering from PCOS have a much greater likelihood of suffering from the same condition. The concept of genetic predisposition is key here. Apart from this, several candidate genes have also been involved in PCOS pathogenesis, particularly insulin signaling and androgen synthesis genes. Not only does the genetic underpinning help in validating the probable genetic nature of PCOS, but it also helps with the acknowledgment of the necessity for more research in these genetic markers so that diagnostic accuracy and therapeutic outcomes could be enhanced (Madhavi PMP *et al.*, 2025). The genetic component also covers the inheritance of metabolic and reproductive derangements that are traditionally linked with PCOS. For example, research has indicated the presence of genetic mutations that influence insulin resistance and hyperandrogenism among affected women, which in turn adds to the clinical presentation of the syndrome. These genetic factors may lead to an interruption of the hypothalamic-pituitary-ovarian axis, resulting in a subsequent hormonal imbalance that leads to the characteristic features of PCOS, such as irregular menses and hirsutism. Moreover, the interconnectedness of genetic mutations and metabolic conditions, for instance, type 2 diabetes, may elucidate the long-term health implications for women with PCOS, thus supporting the necessity of an integrative treatment regimen covering lifestyle as well as genetic factors (Zalwade *et al.*, 2025).

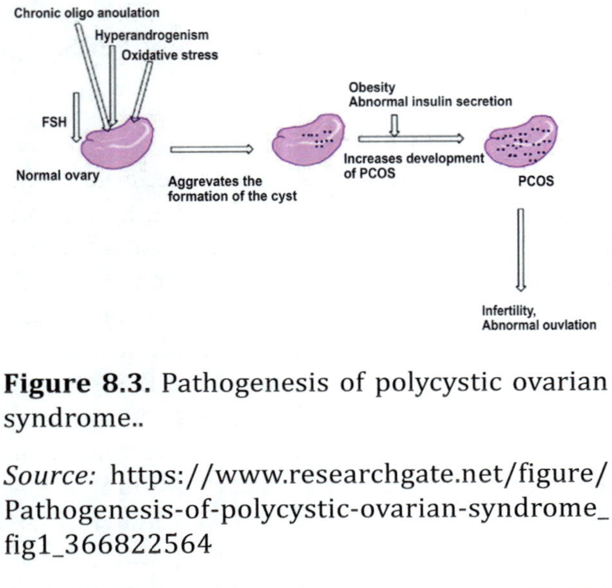

Figure 8.3. Pathogenesis of polycystic ovarian syndrome..

Source: https://www.researchgate.net/figure/Pathogenesis-of-polycystic-ovarian-syndrome_fig1_366822564

Clarification of the genetic aspects of PCOS is of utmost significance not only because it can shed light on its etiology but also for the advancement of personal medicine strategies. With further research, genetic testing can have an integrated role in the diagnosis of PCOS and tailoring treatment specifically designed for each patient. This change could prevent the limitations of conventional treatment methods, which tend not to be adjusted to the genetic makeup of the individual. Apart from that, the integration of genetic results with the newer treatment modalities, including the use of herbal medicine and dietary modification, can result in a more integrated management protocol. Finally, embracing genetics as a significant determinant in PCOS diagnosis can transform the treatment plan, resulting in improved outcomes and improved quality of life in impacted women with this multifaceted syndrome (Madhavi PMP *et al.*, 2025).

8.1.2. Hormonal Imbalances

Hormonal imbalance is the feature of Polycystic Ovarian Syndrome (PCOS), which is responsible for the syndrome's complexity. PCOS is commonly associated with elevated levels of luteinizing hormone (LH) and reduced levels of follicle-stimulating hormone (FSH), creating an unbalanced hormonal environment that disrupts the ovarian cycle. It decreases menstrual irregularity, anovulation, and opportunities for infertility. These hormonal alterations, besides acting upon ovarian function, also have a systemic impact, most commonly taking the form of acne, hirsutism, and weight gain. These symptoms underscore the importance of an understanding of hormonal dysregulation in the management of PCOS, in that the reversal of such imbalances can significantly improve the quality of life for such women, including their reproductive health outcomes (Dhamija *et al.*, 2025).

The management of PCOS also often consists of attempting to rebalance the hormones through intervention. Some research has recently explored the addition of dietary control to conventional treatments in an effort to balance out the hormonal imbalance. For instance, seed cycling has proven effective in balancing out estrogen and progesterone. Such nutritional modulation intends to harness the endogenous phytestrogens in foods like flaxseeds and pumpkin seeds during the follicular phase, while sunflower and sesame seeds are recommended for the luteal phase. All these interventions, when combined with drug therapy like Myo-inositol and folic acid supplementation, can lead to significant improvement in endocrine profiles, menstrual cyclicity, and overall metabolic function. The etiologically complex nature of PCOS demands a multi-dimensional approach to its treatment with a combination of lifestyle modification and medication therapy (Satkar *et al.*, 2024). Complementary therapies with natural products have also gained popularity as a successful alternative to conventional hormonal medications in the treatment of PCOS. Herbal products with estrogen-modulating effects, such as spearmint and fenugreek, are gaining widespread acceptance for their use in the treatment of hormonal deregulations associated with PCOS. These herbal remedies may enhance insulin sensitivity, a consideration in particular since insulin resistance tends to accompany hormonal dysregulation in PCOS. Adding these herbs to lifestyle modifications can have beneficial effects on the balance of the hormones as well as on symptoms. With growing research into the efficacy of such complementary therapies, it becomes evident that an integrated treatment approach not only addresses the hormonal dysregulations at the cause of PCOS but also allows women to become active participants in their health management (Satkar *et al.*, 2024).

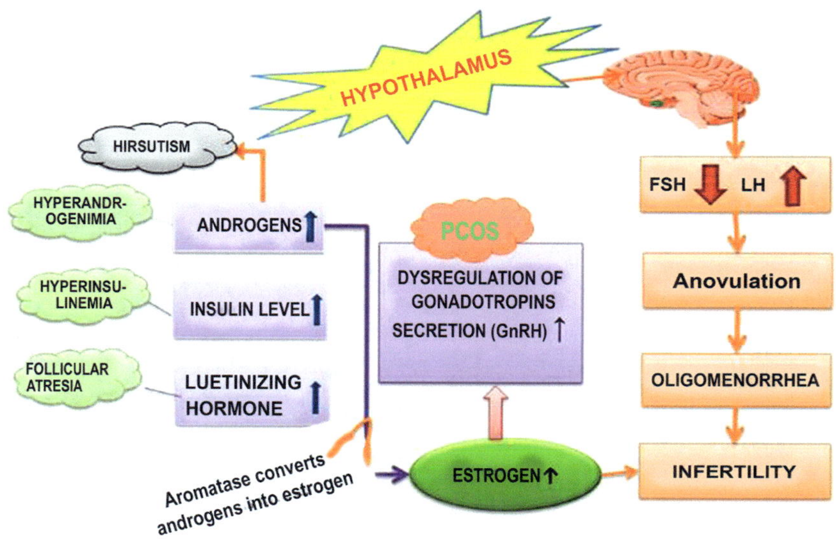

Figure 8.4. Hormonal imbalance associated with PCOS.

Source: https://www.researchgate.net/figure/Hormonal-imbalance-associated-with-PCOS_fig3_362070744

8.1.3. Environmental Influences

Environmental factors have a major impact on the development and worsening of Polycystic Ovarian Syndrome (PCOS), combining with genetic susceptibility to determine the clinical presentation of the disorder. Diet, exercise, and endocrine-disrupting chemical exposure have effects on the hormonal imbalance characteristic of PCOS. For instance, including a high-calorie diet, which is often rich in refined carbohydrates and saturated fat, can lead to increased insulin resistance, a feature of the disease. It has been established that lifestyle intervention, including diet therapy and exercise intensification, will enhance symptoms and reproductive performance in women with PCOS, further affirming that environmental determinants play a substantial role in disease control and progression. This interaction between environment and genetics suggests a multifactorial etiology that needs to be explored further in order to develop effective treatment interventions for the disorder. Environmental stressors also need to be considered when investigating the pathophysiology of PCOS. Psychological stress, which is present in many women with the syndrome, is able to worsen symptoms like androgen excess and menstrual disturbance. Higher stress hormone levels, particularly cortisol, have been known to disrupt normal hormonal control and worsen insulin resistance, resulting in weight gain. It has been shown through experiments that PCOS women are more anxious and depressed, indicating that mental health plays a significant role in the overall impact of the conditions. Psychological health, discussed in terms of stress management competencies and counseling, can therefore be an integral component of a comprehensive treatment plan, highlighting the role of environmental factors in shaping the experience of PCOS.

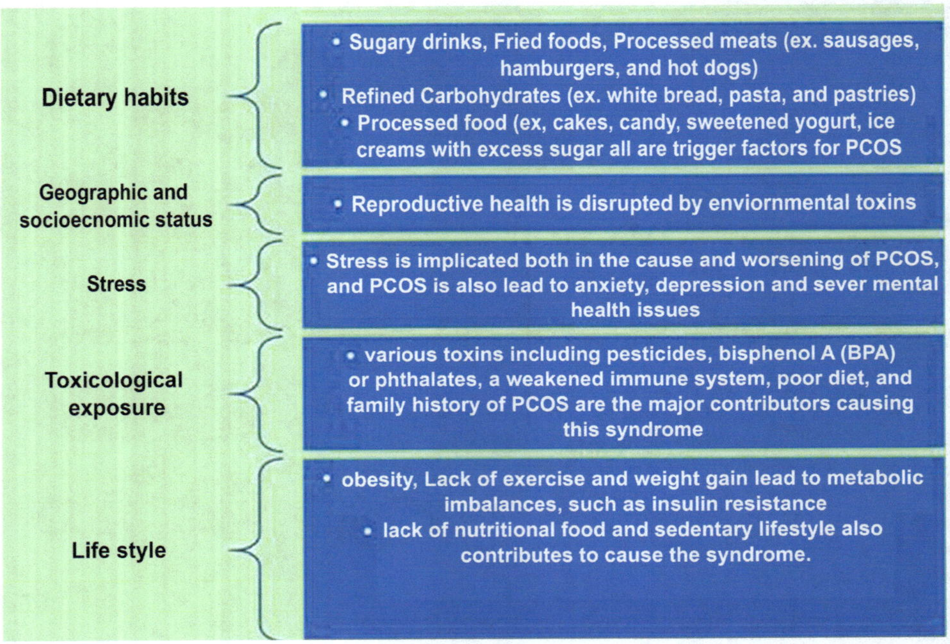

Figure 8.5. Environmental factors affecting PCOS.

Source: https://www.researchgate.net/figure/Environmental-factors-affecting-PCOS_fig1_362070744

In addition, exposure to certain environmental toxins, like endocannabinoids and phthalates, has been found to have an association with reproductive issues, including PCOS. Studies have found that such chemicals affect endocrine functions to result in irregular menstrual cycles and suboptimal ovarian function. PCOS is also associated with increased levels of such pollutants among the affected groups, with this implying that environmental pollutants may be contributing to the syndrome's occurrence in specific groups. With additional research being conducted on the connections between environmental exposures and hormonal disturbances, it further becomes clear that neutralizing these effects is a potential way to treat PCOS. Addressing these environmental factors enables clinicians to empower patients with useful information aimed at reducing risk factors associated with the syndrome while improving overall reproductive well-being (Boomsma *et al.*, 2006; Kumari *et al.*, 2024).

Test Your Knowledge

1. What hormonal imbalances are commonly associated with the development of PCOS?
2. How can genetics contribute to the risk of developing PCOS?

8.2. Symptoms of PCOS

Learning Outcome

1. Discuss the irregular menstrual cycles
2. Define physical manifestations (e.g., hirsutism, acne)
3. Understand the psychological effects (e.g., anxiety, depression)

The presentations of Polycystic Ovarian Syndrome (PCOS) are varied and potentially have a wide-ranging impact on the physical and mental well-being of women. Common presentations are menstrual irregularities, which can take the form of infrequent or prolonged periods. They are a result of endocrine derangements, commonly in the form of elevated androgen levels, which can disrupt regular ovarian function. PCOS also characteristically presents with anovulation in most women, causing fertility problems and adding to reproductive health issues. Moreover, these disturbances may cause a cascade of metabolic symptomatology, underlining the complexity of PCOS because this syndrome encompasses reproductive and metabolic components, affecting diagnosis and treatment plans for patients affected by it (Bernier *et al.*, 2012). Another characteristic symptom of PCOS is the development of hirsutism, or overgrowth of hair at locations typically associated with male-pattern hair growth, including the face, chest, and back. This symptom is attributed to the high levels of androgens present in PCOS and has grave psychological effects on the victims, including embarrassment, low self-esteem, and anxiety. Apart from hirsutism, women can also experience acne, oily complexion, and male-pattern baldness, all of which bear testimony to the elevated dermatological stakes in this syndrome. Although the visibility of these signs completely differs from individual to individual, their cumulative effect poses issues that transcend the physical structure of the body, bearing testimony to the psychosocial stakes involved in PCOS living (Khan *et al.*, 2014). Weight gain or increased body mass index (BMI) is another prominent symptom often associated with PCOS, where most women have difficulty with their weight. This aspect of PCOS is usually linked with insulin resistance, which is a widespread condition among this population, that can hinder effective metabolic functioning. Insulin resistance also predisposes patients to developing type 2 diabetes and cardiovascular disease, adding to the myriad of complexities in the health history of PCOS patients. Lifestyle modification in the form of dietary correction and exercise is thus an effective real-world management tool that can improve symptoms and quality of life. By appreciating the interconnected nature of these signs, it also becomes evident that an all-round approach encompassing both hormonal and metabolic issues is required in managing PCOS (Bernier *et al.*, 2012).

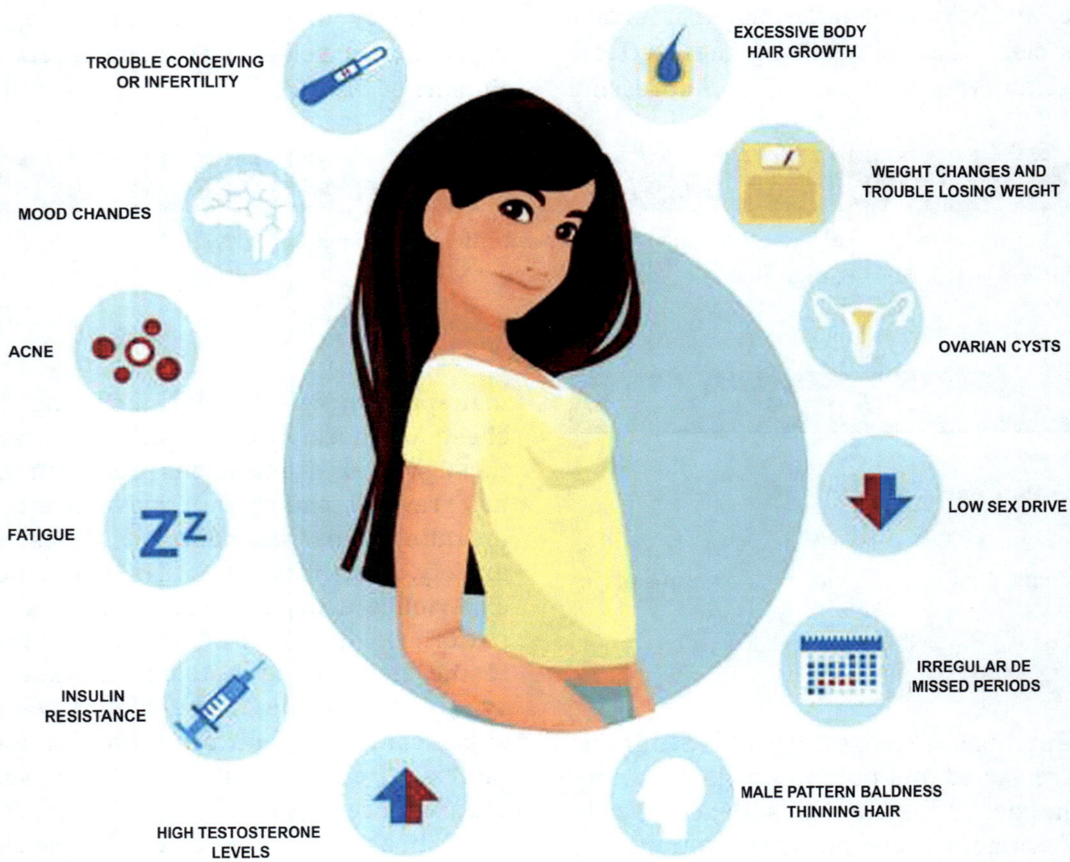
TROUBLE CONCEIVING OR INFERTILITY
EXCESSIVE BODY HAIR GROWTH
MOOD CHANDES
WEIGHT CHANGES AND TROUBLE LOSING WEIGHT
ACNE
OVARIAN CYSTS
FATIGUE
Zz
LOW SEX DRIVE
INSULIN RESISTANCE
IRREGULAR DE MISSED PERIODS
HIGH TESTOSTERONE LEVELS
MALE PATTERN BALDNESS THINNING HAIR

Figure 8.6. PCOS Symptoms.

Source: https://images.squarespace-cdn.com/content/v1/5c319e0d25bf02353683db93/1569122403100-ZAIVQ0YC8E702MOUQJG1/shutterstock_1035434050-1-e1532966569521.jpg

8.2.1. Irregular Menstrual Cycles

Irregular menstruation is among the most common signs of Polycystic Ovarian Syndrome (PCOS) that can affect women's reproductive health profoundly, with irregularities in the flow and duration of menstruation, hormonal imbalance, which is inherent in PCOS, can cause them. Women with the syndrome have elevated levels of androgens—male hormones that occur in lower levels in females—which disrupt normal ovulatory function. Consequently, the cycle from one month to another can be unstable, leading to prolonged periods of amenorrhea or irregular ovulation. For this purpose, understanding the hormonal interaction responsible for such unpredictable cycles in both the diagnosis and treatment of PCOS is crucial so that clinicians can adopt appropriate management strategies in affected women, thus addressing critical issues pertaining to reproductive health and fertility (Faqih *et al.*, 2024). The connection between abnormal menstrual cycles and other illnesses in women with PCOS is multifaceted and often reciprocal. The majority of women with PCOS will not only have irregular menstrual cycles but also concomitant symptoms such as weight gain, acne, and excess hair growth—all indicative of the syndrome's hormonal imbalance. Irregular cycles can be an initial warning sign for general metabolic disease, including insulin resistance, which is prevalent in this population and has the potential to raise cardiovascular disease and type II diabetes mellitus risk (Bernier *et al.*, 2012).

Therefore, the diagnosis and treatment of irregular menstruation are important not just to enhance menstrual regularity but also in attenuating related long-term health repercussions of PCOS, necessitating a multidisciplinary treatment approach involving lifestyle intervention and medical treatments. Along with the chief complaint of irregular menstrual cycles, psychological and emotional ramifications for women with PCOS cannot be overlooked. A majority of women are afflicted by anxiety, depression, and impaired quality of life due to the seemingly related symptoms of the syndrome, which occur regularly along with menstrual irregularities. This uncertainty of their cycle can heighten stress and concern about infertility and cause an emotional torture cycle. It is of the highest necessity for medical professionals not just to offer physiological treatments but also psychological guidance, given the impactful influence of PCOS on the psychological realm. Through education, counseling, and support care, practitioners can help women understand the complexity of the condition, thus adopting a holistic approach towards the physical as well as the psychological condition of having abnormal cycles (Faqih *et al.*, 2024; Bernier *et al.*, 2012).

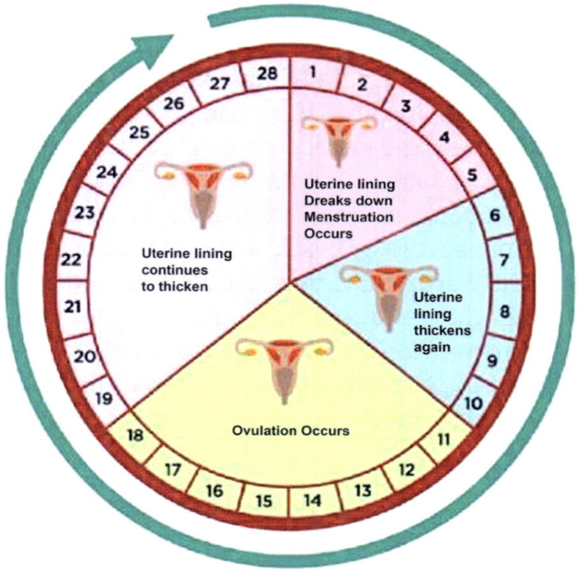

Figure 8.7. Irregular Menstrual Cycles.

Source: https://www.ovumhospitals.com/blog/dealing-with-irregular-menstrual-cycles

8.2.2. Physical Manifestations (e.g., Hirsutism, Acne)

Polycystic Ovarian Syndrome (PCOS) is usually detected by a range of physical characteristics, which can have a very significant impact on the self-worth and overall health of an individual. Among them, hirsutism—a development of hair in locations that are typically found to contain male-pattern hair distribution—is particularly prevalent. The condition arises due to high levels of androgens, which are the hallmark of PCOS. The psychological effect of hirsutism is considerable, and those who are affected may develop shame, anxiety, and depression. Visibility of the symptoms will likely lead to social stigma and emotional distress and will thus require holistic management strategies that cater to both the physiological and psychological needs of this syndrome (Bernier *et al.*, 2012). Acne is a common physical symptom of PCOS as a result of hyperandrogenism, leading to overproduction of sebum and clogging of follicular plugs. The skin ailment most often begins at puberty but persists well into adulthood in the majority of women with PCOS. The long length of time acne persists, particularly when combined with other symptoms of the syndrome, can further enhance feelings of inadequacy and social pressure to achieve conventional standards of beauty. In addition, severe or cystic acne, as seen in PCOS, can cause scarring and additional psychological effects that require the implementation of specific treatment strategies aimed not only at relieving the physical symptoms but also at promoting emotional adjustment (Bernier *et al.*, 2012).

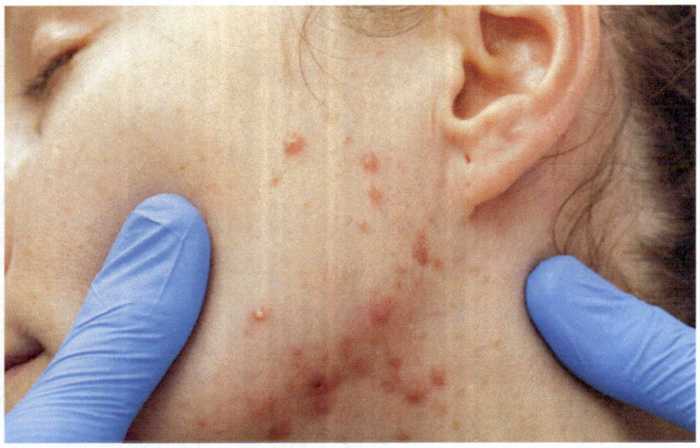

Source: https://www.nwhjournal.org/cms/10.1016/j.nwh.2020.01.011/asset/7cd02bbb-21a4-4c13-8ce2-a12700781fce/main.assets/fx1_lrg.jpg

Moreover, treating these physical symptoms goes beyond symptom relief; it includes a comprehensive knowledge of how metabolic and psychological health interact in women with PCOS. A dual treatment regimen often includes lifestyle modification, such as dietary modification and weight control, coupled with pharmacological regimes directed toward the attainment of normal hormone levels. There is evidence that early diagnosis and appropriate therapeutic management may reduce the impact of hirsutism and acne significantly, going on to prevent the emotional distress and quality of life impairment so commonly associated with these symptoms (Bagatin *et al.*, 2011). Therefore, an integrated approach to managing PCOS is essential in helping the affected individuals reclaim their identity and well-being.

8.2.3. Psychological Effects (e.g., Anxiety, Depression)

The psychological effect of Polycystic Ovarian Syndrome (PCOS) is significant and pervasive, most often manifesting as heightened levels of depression and anxiety. PCOS patients report a significantly higher prevalence of these mood disorders than unaffected women. Research asserts that 78.3% of PCOS-afflicted women have anxiety versus the 35% of the control population, and 60% have signs of depression versus 30% of the controls. The findings stand as testament to the imperative need to include mental health screening as part of the therapeutic strategy in managing women with PCOS. Without such evaluations, worldwide management of PCOS is inadequate, even exacerbating the psychological impacts of the disease and overall quality of life (Fatima *et al.*, 2019). In addition to depression and anxiety, women with PCOS are also at risk for a range of psychological disturbances that can complicate both their physical and mental health. The metabolic derangement and hormonal imbalances that accompany PCOS not only affect reproductive issues but also mood disorders. Mood disorders manifest differently along the spectrum of PCOS cases, varying based on such factors as weight gain and infertility. The endocrine and psychological profiles of such patients need to be targeted with intervention; psychologists and medical practitioners must work in concert to create personalized care plans that deal with both the endocrine and psychological profiles of these patients. With these factors in mind, it is clear that the correspondence between somatic symptoms and psychological health has a powerful impact on women's experiences with this condition (Falbo *et al.*, 2015). Additionally, the stigma that is sometimes associated with PCOS will enhance the psychological distress of the affected women. Most of these individuals will feel stigmatized or marginalized due to the nature of the symptoms they bear, such as irregular menses, obesity, and acne. It will trigger a pervasive sense of inadequacy that enhances feelings of depression and anxiety. Therefore, educational interventions towards the destigmatization of PCOS and education about its psychological effects are essential. Increased awareness will generate an enabling environment where patients will not be stigmatized and will be more willing to visit therapists and reveal their experiences. In the long term, managing the psychological effects of PCOS in a holistic way is necessary to improve patient outcomes and offer a good quality of life to those afflicted by this multifaceted condition (Fatima *et al.*, 2019).

Test Your Knowledge

1. How do irregular menstrual cycles manifest in individuals with PCOS?
2. What are common physical signs of PCOS, such as hirsutism and acne?

8.3. Diagnosis of PCOS

Learning Outcome

1. Explain the clinical criteria for diagnosing PCOS, including the Rotterdam criteria.
2. Interpret laboratory test results relevant to PCOS
3. Analyze imaging study findings, particularly ultrasound, used in the diagnosis of PCOS

Diagnosis of Polycystic Ovarian Syndrome (PCOS) is a multifaceted process that employs several clinical features, hormonal assessments, and imaging techniques to arrive at the diagnosis of this complex condition. As per the Rotterdam criteria, PCOS is diagnosed based on the presence of two of three fundamental characteristics: ovulatory dysfunction, hyperandrogenism, and polycystic ovaries on ultrasound. The prevalence of these manifestations can vary considerably in different patients, leading to different phenotypes of PCOS. To illustrate, in one study, 84.7% of women with PCOS demonstrated both hyperandrogenism and chronic oligo-anovulation, and 89% demonstrated polycystic ovarian morphology. The variability in manifestations demonstrates the need for a non-rigorous strategy for diagnosis based on careful evaluation of the patient and clinical acumen, in contrast to a protocol-based approach. In addition to the clinical presentation, metabolic profiling is a critical component of PCOS diagnosis. Insulin resistance is prevalent among the patients and has been reported to affect approximately 71.4% of them, according to existing literature. The prevalence of insulin resistance has been noted to vary by PCOS phenotypes, such that in patients with the classic phenotype, compared to those with normoandrogenic phenotypes, it is especially high. This heterogeneity provides the opportunity to utilize these phenotypic assessments to not only diagnose PCOS but also to initiate proper metabolic screens. With this, the clinician can gain insight into the associated metabolic risk of each phenotype and utilize targeted treatment strategies to address the reproductive as well as metabolic aspects of the disorder, ultimately improving patient outcomes. Recent advances in molecular diagnosis have widened further the diagnostic realm of PCOS, particularly through the study of circulating microRNAs as potential biomarkers. Notably, it has been found that circulating miRNA-93 and miRNA-223 are elevated in women with PCOS compared with matched controls. These microRNAs were not found to be insulin-resistance or testosterone-dependent, even though their roles in the syndrome's pathophysiology are clear. Their potential use in diagnosis is based on their capacity to enhance PCOS diagnostic specificity, and the area under the receiver operating characteristic curve is considerable for miR-93. With ongoing research further exposing the genetic and molecular etiology of PCOS, microRNA analysis has the potential to become an element in delivering more precise diagnostic criteria in addition to improved management of the affected subjects, with the end result being a clearer understanding of this multifaceted disease (Bonin *et al.*, 2013; Atkin *et al.*, 2015).

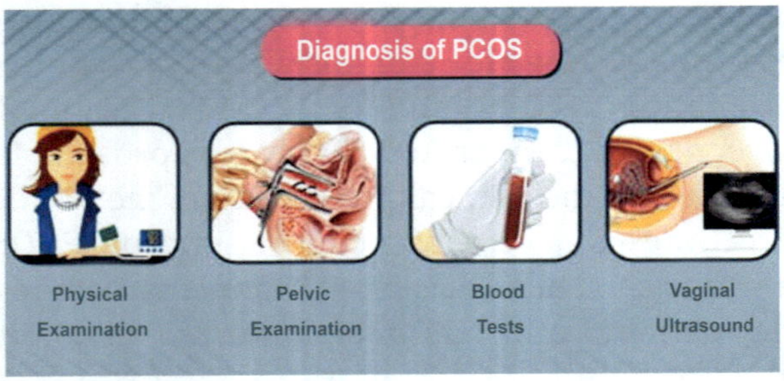

Figure 8.8. Different diagnosis of PCOS.

Source: https://images.medindia.net/infographics/article-images/450_237/diagnosis-of-polycystic-ovarian-syndrome.jpg

8.3.1. Clinical Criteria (Rotterdam Criteria)

The Rotterdam criteria, established in 2003, form the cornerstone of the diagnosis of polycystic ovary syndrome (PCOS), a complex endocrine disorder in women globally. The agreement focuses on the multifactorial model, whereby two of the three criteria need to be fulfilled for diagnosis: hyperandrogenism, ovulatory disturbance, and polycystic ovaries on imaging. This model allows broader inclusion of phenotypic heterogeneity, as PCOS can manifest differently in different individuals. Specifically, the criteria have been refined to better describe the syndromes' disparate presentations, removed from an overly reductionist focus on ovarian morphology alone. This subtle categorization aids clinicians in the identification of successful treatment modalities for individual patients, including both the reproductive and metabolic ramifications of the disorder, which is essential to effectively treat PCOS (Bonin *et al.*, 2013). More recent evidence illuminates the clinical utility of the Rotterdam criteria in establishing metabolic health in women with PCOS. Evidence indicates that PCOS phenotypes have a high association with insulin resistance, a common comorbidity of the syndrome. For instance, women diagnosed under the traditional PCOS phenotype, characterized by clear hyperandrogenism and anovulatory ovulations, presented with a higher frequency of insulin resistance compared to their normoandrogenic counterparts. This is significant because it informs healthcare providers about the necessity of screening for metabolic complications in the affected. The various metabolic risk profiles of various phenotypes underscore the necessity of employing the Rotterdam criteria not only for diagnosis but also in interpreting the broader implications of PCOS on global health, thereby enhancing patient care and outcomes (Bonin *et al.*, 2013). The implication of the Rotterdam criteria extends beyond diagnosis, defining a model for strategic intervention and effective management of PCOS. An awareness of the interrelations between hormonal derangement, metabolic derangement, and late-life health consequences, such as cardiovascular disease and type II diabetes, directs clinicians to the need for integrated treatment approaches. Evidence suggests that changes in lifestyle, as well as pharmacologic interventions, can enhance co-morbid symptoms and metabolic status in women with PCOS. As elaborated in the current reviews, taking into account insulin resistance as a shared underlying aspect can lead to more effective interventions, wherein weight and lifestyle modification are accorded prominence in treatment modalities. By applying these standards to practice, clinicians can deliver customized care that is matched to the different presentations and health risks of PCOS and ultimately enhance patient outcomes.

8.3.2. Laboratory Tests (Hormone Levels, Glucose Tolerance)

Hormone and glucose tolerance evaluation by diagnostic tests is the focal point of diagnosis for Polycystic Ovarian Syndrome (PCOS). It is a disorder of hormonal imbalance in reproductive hormones, specifically elevated levels of androgens, resulting in various reproductive and metabolic disorders. Estimation of serum testosterone and androstenedione is a routine clinical measure for these hormones as they play a significant role in determining hyperandrogenism, one of the primary diagnostic criteria for PCOS. Research indicates that salivary testosterone (salT) concentrations can complement standard blood tests, demonstrating significant elevations in PCOS-diagnosed women compared to controls. This discovery underscores the potential for non-invasive testing methods to boost PCOS accuracy, thereby facilitating earlier intervention and better management alternatives for affected individuals (Adaway *et al.*, 2017).

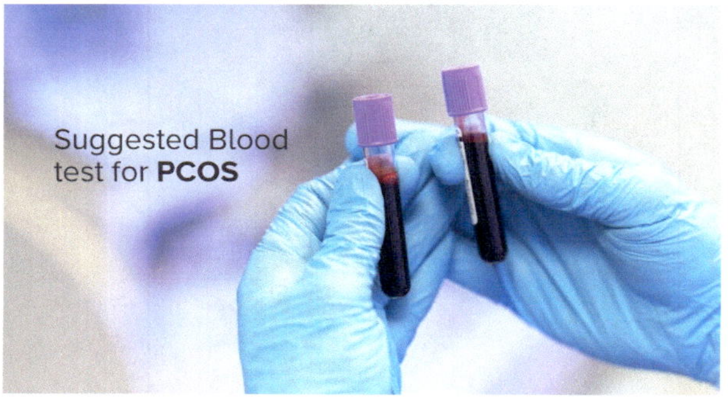

Source: https://ampath.com/category/1706683800.jpg

Besides hormonal testing, measurement of glucose tolerance is key to understanding the metabolic impact of PCOS. The majority of women with the syndrome are insulin resistant, which in turn is related to overweight and can enhance the clinical picture of PCOS. Laboratory tests such as the oral glucose tolerance test (OGTT) measure how well the body processes glucose, providing data regarding the subject's insulin sensitivity. An abnormal glucose tolerance test is not only indicative of a higher risk of the development of type 2 diabetes but also indicative of an underlying metabolic phenotype routinely found in PCOS patients. The fight against insulin resistance through dietary modification and drug therapy, such as metformin, becomes the rationale behind effective control of the disease (Matzke *et al.*, 2011). The correlation of findings from hormone level and glucose tolerance testing guides an integrated therapeutic strategy for PCOS management. These tests are not only crucial to establishing a correct diagnosis, but they also provide significant information regarding a patient's health and comorbid risk overall. The recognition that both hormonal dysregulation and insulin resistance are intertwined supports the need for multiple disciplines in planning treatment. By characterizing PCOS on a biochemical level through directed laboratory testing, clinicians can provide customized treatment plans that might include dietary changes, medication, or both. Finally, the enhancement of diagnostic procedures through the application of advanced laboratory techniques has the potential not only to improve patient outcomes but also to bring about increased public awareness about PCOS and its complex relationship with metabolic health (Matzke *et al.*, 2011).

8.3.3. Imaging Studies (Ultrasound Findings)

Imaging studies, particularly ultrasound, have a significant role in diagnosing Polycystic Ovarian

Syndrome (PCOS). Transvaginal ultrasound is the gold standard in assessing ovarian anatomy, which enables clinicians to see the numerous cystic structures within the ovaries. In a classic case of PCOS, ultrasound will reveal large ovaries containing numerous small follicles, also known as the string of pearls sign. Such typical morphology aligns with the Rotterdam consensus diagnostic criteria, wherein identification of 12 or more follicles in one or both of the ovaries is a key feature of PCOS. Ultrasound is not only a tool used for diagnosis but for assessment of associated complications, such as endometrial thickening that may arise as a consequence of chronic anovulation prevalent in PCOS individuals. In addition, ultrasound evidence can give us clues regarding PCOS's metabolic consequences, particularly concerning insulin resistance. It is found that studies have outlined that PCOS women exhibit characteristic ovarian morphology that is favorable for hormonal dysregulation, which is known to amplify metabolic derangements, as seen in studies of biochemical hyperandrogenism (Adaway *et al.*, 2017). Ultrasound scanning can thus serve a dual purpose; while it validates the diagnosis of PCOS via morphological characteristics, it also alerts doctors to the need for metabolic testing since there is an increased risk for complications like type 2 diabetes. Through this interface, the importance of a multidisciplinary approach to management policy is emphasized in determining how imaging data complements biochemical testing to treat every aspect of PCOS in patients. Moreover, ultrasound technology has improved the diagnostic accuracy of PCOS. Three-dimensional ultrasound and Doppler studies provide more accurate measurements of ovarian perfusion and follicular behavior (Kumari *et al.*, 2024). Improved technology is able to differentiate between common PCOS presentations and other conditions with similar ultrasound features, such as functional ovarian cysts or cystic teratomas. Also, it is important to realize these differences for the purpose of directing proper therapeutic interventions. The simultaneous application of sophisticated imaging modalities not only facilitates diagnostic workflow but also helps devise individualized management plans for women with PCOS, leading to enhanced patient outcomes by means of customized treatment plans derived from extensive imaging studies.

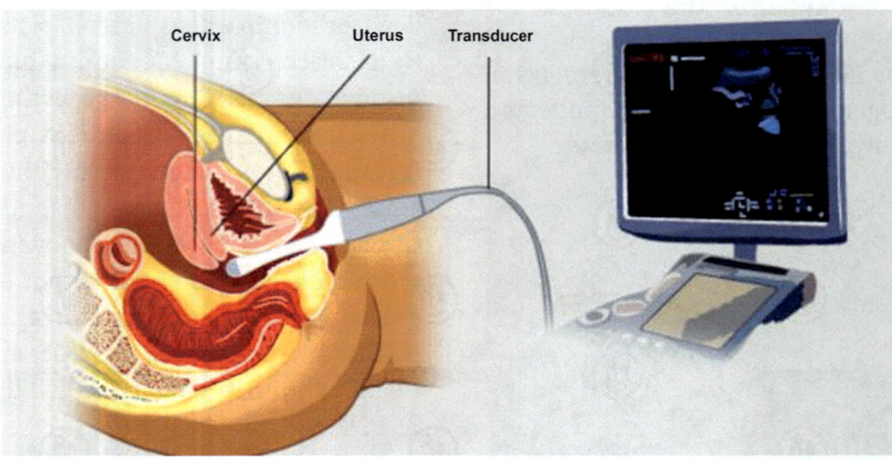

Figure 8.9. Ultrasound Aids PCOS Treatment.

Source: https://ultrasoundplus.co.uk/trole-of-ultrasound-in-monitoring-pcos-treatment/

Test Your Knowledge

1. Which laboratory tests are commonly used to assess hormone levels and glucose tolerance in PCOS diagnosis?
2. What ultrasound findings are typically observed in patients with PCOS?

8.4. Health Risks Associated with PCOS

Learning Outcome

1. Describe the infertility and reproductive challenges associated with PCOS.
2. Explain the link between PCOS, metabolic syndrome, and the increased risk of diabetes.
3. Assess cardiovascular health concerns related to PCOS.

The medical complications of Polycystic Ovarian Syndrome (PCOS) go beyond reproductive problems, reaching a gamut of metabolic and cardiovascular disorders that may have far-reaching effects on women's general health. Perhaps the most alarming feature of PCOS is insulin resistance, which afflicts around 71 percent of women with the condition, based on the latest research. This metabolic impairment not only increases the risk of type 2 diabetes development but is also included in overall metabolic syndrome development. The connection between PCOS and insulin resistance underlines the need for early screening and intervention strategies to manage these medical risks, given that the disease impacts a considerable percentage of women of reproductive age (Bernier *et al.*, 2012). In addition, cardiovascular disease also emerges as a pertinent issue of health among women with PCOS. The interaction between chronic oligo-anovulation and metabolic dysregulation results in deterioration in cardiovascular health, with women who present with features of metabolic syndrome being at increased risk of cardiovascular-related complications. Indeed, studies have established that there exist variations in the prevalence of metabolic syndrome between PCOS phenotypes, implying that women are not equally at risk for cardiovascular disease. The classic phenotype of PCOS, with the associated development of hyperandrogenism and chronic oligomenorrhea, is more prone to metabolic syndrome and therefore deserves to be monitored and intervened strictly (Bonin *et al.*, 2013).

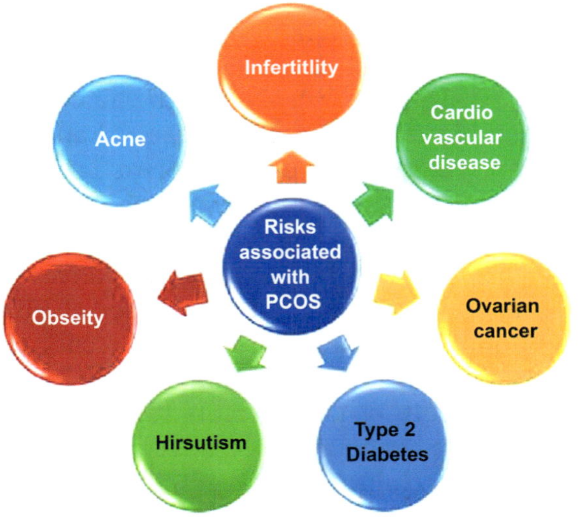

Figure 8.10. Risks associated with PCOS.

Source: https://www.researchgate.net/figure/Risks-associated-with-PCOS_fig1_367612177

Long-term complications of PCOS also include an increased risk of endometrial cancer because of long-standing anovulation and exposure to unopposed estrogen. The intrinsic hormonal disturbances in PCOS can predispose to an abnormal endometrial growth, with significantly elevated cancer risks if left uncontrolled. Ultrasonography and endometrial biopsies are recommended for routine follow-up in women with chronic anovulation or amenorrhea. This emphasis on routine screening and preventive treatment is key to minimizing the long-term health implications of PCOS, upholding the merit of an integrative treatment and monitoring method (Bernier *et al.*, 2012; Bonin *et al.*, 2013).

8.4.1. Infertility and Reproductive Challenges

Infertility as well as reproductive disorders are huge challenges for ladies with Polycystic Ovarian Syndrome (PCOS). The endocrine disturbances underlying PCOS tend to lead to abnormal ovulation, as well as to conception problems. Females suffering from this disorder commonly experience anovulation, a condition where no eggs are released from the ovaries, and thus significantly decrease their chances of pregnancy. Besides, the presence of cystic ovaries and elevated androgen levels exacerbates such fertility issues, creating a chaotic interaction between increased hormonal disturbance and impaired ovarian function. The onset of PCOS symptoms, such as hirsutism and acne, can also contribute to stress and psychological tension, resulting in a cumulative impact on reproductive health. As PCOS affects about 10% of women in childbearing years, the syndrome not only presents issues with conception but also general aspects of women's health and wellbeing (Ghazeeri *et al.*, 2021).

Dietary and lifestyle changes are central in addressing the fertility problems of PCOS. Management of weight through dietary means is the first-line therapy for the majority of affected women. An optimally balanced diet with a focus on unsaturated fats and the minimum amount of saturated fat will improve insulin sensitivity and, consequently, hormone regulation. High glycemic index food intake, which may exacerbate insulin resistance, must be controlled to optimize total metabolic health. Daily exercise, integrated into the daily routine, is also essential in weight management and increasing insulin sensitivity. With a shift towards a healthier lifestyle and nutrition-based diet, women with PCOS not only control symptoms such as irregular menstruation but also optimize their chances of conceiving. This multifaceted approach speaks volumes about the importance of whole-person care in controlling the reproductive challenges that accompany PCOS (Ghazeeri *et al.*, 2021).

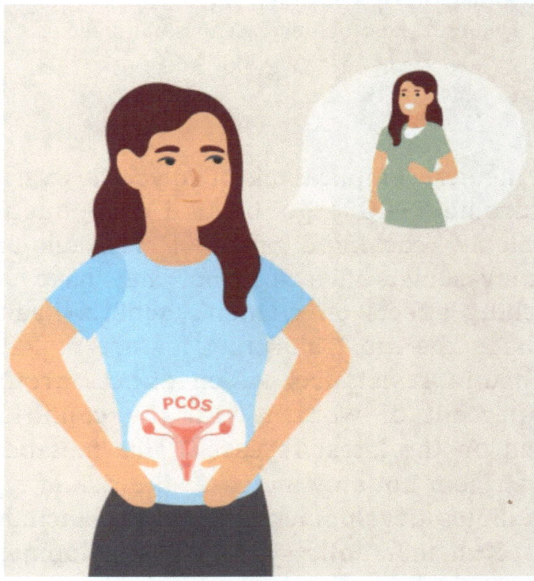

Source: https://www.fertility.com/content/dam/web/healthcare/biopharma/fertility/global/psp/fertilitypatient/resources-articles/501_PEP_Sep_Article_Single_pcos.png

Apart from this, breakthroughs in medical therapies hold hope for women suffering from infertility because of PCOS. Clomiphene citrate is a potent drug that has been employed as a fertility drug in women with problematic aberrant cycles. In cases where Clomiphene does not work, other regimens like insulin-sensitizing agents such as metformin have been employed to manage the ensuing insulin resistance, which is prevalent among PCOS patients. Interventions have been shown to often lead to improved ovulatory function and conception rates by various studies. Furthermore, reproductive technologies like IVF are increasingly being viewed as plausible substitutes for women whose fertility is severely compromised by PCOS. The diverse therapeutic options exemplify the logic of individualized approaches in reproductive health, such that women confronted with infertility caused by PCOS are given holistic and personalized care interventions (Coutinho *et al.*, 2019).

8.4.2. Metabolic Syndrome and Diabetes Risk

The intersection of diabetes risk and metabolic syndrome is particularly fervent in women with Polycystic Ovary Syndrome (PCOS) and highlights grave health concerns. Metabolic syndrome, a group of characteristics that comprises insulin resistance, elevated blood pressure, dyslipidemia, and obesity, is prevalent among patients with PCOS. Investigations reveal that a very high percentage of women with PCOS possess some degree of insulin resistance, which is among the basic features of metabolic syndrome. Uniquely, the phenotyping of PCOS steers risk stratification towards metabolic issues. The classic phenotype, which encompasses the majority of women diagnosed, is most commonly linked to insulin resistance alongside other phenotypes and therefore needs to have specific monitoring and management plans for metabolic conditions for this group (Bonin *et al.*, 2013). Furthermore, the effects of metabolic syndrome extend beyond acute insulin resistance and potentially lead to long-term health effects like type II diabetes mellitus and cardiovascular disease. Such intricate interaction between obesity and PCOS lends continuity to this risk for metabolic syndrome; the majority of PCOS women are further affected by hyperandrogenism and metabolic disturbances that do little to mitigate their convoluted health profiles. Lifestyle factors, like nutrition and physical activity, play a significant role in managing these risks. Effective. weight management may improve insulin sensitivity and reduce the risk of diabetes and cardiovascular disease development. Current studies highlight the necessity of an active response in treating metabolic syndrome in PCOS women since early interventions may profoundly alter the direction of their health status (Bernier *et al.*, 2012). With these challenges, there is no doubt that clinicians should prioritize metabolic screening for women diagnosed with PCOS, particularly those presenting with signs of insulin resistance.

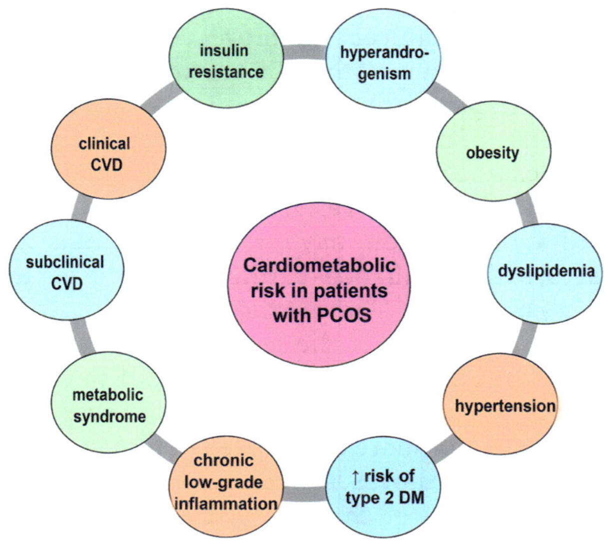

Figure 8.11. Cardiometabolic risk in patients with polycystic ovarian syndrome (PCOS).

Source: https://www.mdpi.com/medicina/medicina-60-01656/article_deploy/html/images/medicina-60-01656-g003.png

The findings from a variety of studies indicate that the diagnostic features of PCOS alone cannot be used to predict the complexity of metabolic health. Instead, a multidimensional approach to phenotypes enables more precise identification of those who are at higher risk for metabolic syndrome and diabetes. With the utilization of thorough screening devices and preventive care, health practitioners can maximize early interventions that are capable of mitigating the development of severe metabolic complications. Such personalized treatment is an indication of the recognition that PCOS is not a monolithic condition but a spectrum of complaints that must be addressed through multispectral approaches for effective management (Bonin *et al.*, 2013).

8.4.3. Cardiovascular Health Concerns

Polycystic Ovarian Syndrome (PCOS) and cardiovascular pathology have become subjects of growing interest in more contemporary research. Women with PCOS are at a higher risk for developing cardiovascular disease due to the presence of metabolic derangements that have been classically associated with the syndrome. Specifically, insulin resistance, hyperlipidemia, and hypertension have been identified as factors that enhance cardiovascular risk in this population. The overlap of these factors serves to underscore the need for an integrated understanding of the way in which PCOS not only impacts reproductive health but also serves as a precipitant for more severe metabolic disorders as well as cardiovascular disease. Through the understanding of the correlations, healthcare providers can more effectively individualize treatments targeting the reproductive and metabolic aspects of PCOS, ultimately towards stemming the risk for cardiovascular disease as part of an integrated treatment plan. It is noteworthy to mention that lifestyle modification plays a significant role in the management of cardiovascular disease conditions associated with PCOS. Evidence suggests weight loss, healthy eating, and exercise are very beneficial in increasing insulin sensitivity and reducing the risk of cardiovascular complications in affected women. For instance, a low-glycemic index diet that contains high whole grains, vegetables, and lean proteins can normalize insulin levels and combat obesity—a widespread issue among PCOS patients. Physical activity, in the form of a minimum of 150 minutes each week, has been proven to have beneficial effects on cardiovascular health through the optimization of lipid profiles and lowering blood pressure. Implementation of these lifestyle changes not only enhances several of the symptoms of PCOS but also makes a profound impact on cardiovascular health over the long term, highlighting the interconnectedness of these conditions for women with the syndrome. Additionally, treatment of PCOS by physicians should also involve attempts to mitigate cardiovascular health risk. Clinical practice guidelines recommend the management and monitoring of risk factors such as hypertension and dyslipidemia as part of routine management in PCOS women. Medication, if needed, might include the administration of insulin-sensitizing drugs and lipid-lowering agents, thereby facilitating an aggressive strategy to minimize cardiovascular events. As PCOS is a chronic disorder, continuous assessment of cardiovascular risk is necessary, as prevalence can lead to tremendous morbidity in adulthood. By concurrent consideration of cardiovascular and reproductive factors, women with PCOS may enjoy better quality of life, and in the long term decrease the risk of cardiovascular disease and metabolic syndrome (Bernier *et al.*, 2012; Ghazeeri *et al.*, 2021).

Test Your Knowledge

1. What reproductive challenges are commonly associated with infertility in women with PCOS?
2. How does PCOS increase the risk of developing metabolic syndrome and diabetes?

8.5. Treatment Options for PCOS

Learning Outcome

1. Analyze the role of lifestyle modifications, including diet and exercise, in managing PCOS
2. Evaluate the use of medications (hormonal treatments, insulin sensitizers)
3. Discuss the effectiveness and applications of alternative therapies, including supplements and acupuncture, for PCOS.)

The treatment modalities of Polycystic Ovarian Syndrome (PCOS) are heterogeneous and must be tailored on an individual basis to suit the requirements of the patients. The most successful method is through addressing insulin resistance, which is a common underlying etiology in most females with this disorder. Antidiabetic medications, particularly metformin, have increasingly been acknowledged for their benefit in managing metabolic parameters as well as enhancing reproductive outcome. Studies reveal that if metformin is prescribed along with hormonal therapies such as oral contraceptives, the dual action considerably diminishes hyperandrogenism symptoms and menstrual dysfunction. Through its treatment of the metabolic and reproductive deficiencies of PCOS, this combination treatment provides a holistic regimen for management that can yield enhanced long-term health outcomes for women with the condition (Nandikola *et al.*, 2025). Apart from pharmacological treatment, changes in lifestyle are also a major contribution to the management of PCOS symptoms, particularly in cases with excessive weight or obesity. One study recently highlighted the immense potential of lifestyle modification, such as diet and regular physical activity, in reducing body mass index (BMI) in PCOS patients. Apart from assisting the patient in controlling weight, these lifestyle modifications are also useful in improving insulin sensitivity and hormonal balance. Interestingly, the results showed that a combination of lifestyle changes and drug therapy yielded greater benefits than either solution in itself. This highlights the importance of an integrated treatment protocol with lifestyle change as key to the effective management of PCOS (Krishna *et al.*, 2024). Also, PCOS is a complicated disorder that requires tailored treatment and can incorporate a variety of solutions besides medication and lifestyle change. Psychological therapy and counseling are also part of the comprehensive care that needs to be addressed for women with PCOS, since the condition extends to profound impacts on mental health and quality of life. Addressing the psychological and emotional aspects may be key to enhancing adherence to treatment protocols and patient self-esteem and body image. As research evolves in this arena, health professionals must begin to adopt more holistic and patient-centered care that recognizes the complexities of PCOS and supports more favorable results in a variety of areas of health and well-being (Nandikola *et al.*, 2025).

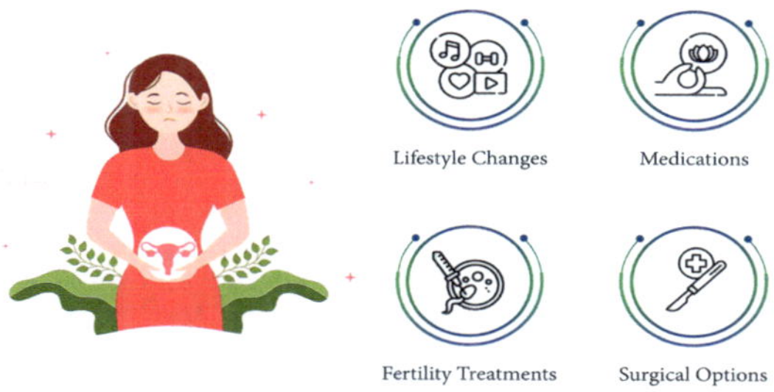

Figure 8.12. Treatment of PCOS.

Source: https://drshreyaendocrinologist.com/assets/img/treatment/pcos/treatment-of-pcos.jpg

8.5.1. Lifestyle Modifications (Diet and Exercise)

Management of PCOS requires an all-round approach, with lifestyle modification being a significant component. Nutrition and physical activity can have a great impact on the symptoms as well as on the accompanying health risks of PCOS, particularly by targeting insulin resistance, which is a universal factor among patients. It has been reported through research that even modest weight loss can equate to considerable improvement in the metabolic status, menstrual cyclicity, and ovulatory function. For instance, 5-10% weight loss improves insulin sensitivity as well as reduces cardiovascular risks associated with PCOS. Thus, integrating broader lifestyle changes, particularly diet and exercise, is essential to maintain the proper control as well as prevention of long-term complications such as type II diabetes and metabolic syndrome (Bernier *et al.*, 2012).

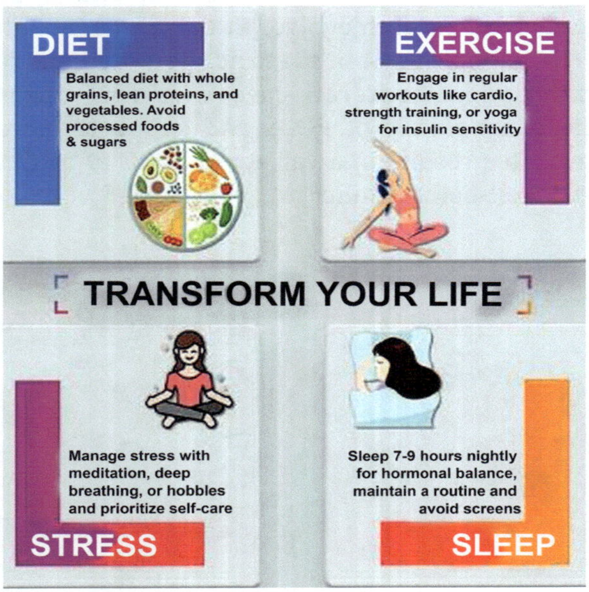
DIET
Balanced diet with whole grains, lean proteins, and vegetables. Avoid processed foods & sugars
EXERCISE
Engage in regular workouts like cardio, strength training, or yoga for insulin sensitivity
TRANSFORM YOUR LIFE
Manage stress with meditation, deep breathing, or hobbles and prioritize self-care
STRESS
Sleep 7-9 hours nightly for hormonal balance, maintain a routine and avoid screens
SLEEP

Figure 8.13. Lifestyle change PCOS management.

Source: https://www.instagram.com/drmadhugoel/p/DEMDV7jTa_6/

With regard to dietary modifications, emphasis should be laid on a balanced diet for metabolic well-being. A low GI diet is preferable in PCOS patients because it lowers insulin spikes and raises insulin sensitivity. This approach incorporates the reduction of high-GI food consumption, which is often linked to an enhanced risk of type 2 diabetes. Besides, attention to macronutrient proportion is also needed; the dietary fat composition should prioritize unsaturated fats over limiting saturated fats. Protein consumption should be within certain limits, preferably contributing to approximately 20% of the total caloric consumption. By adjusting diet in this manner, one is able to manage the hormonal dysregulation associated with PCOS and also improve such signs as hirsutism, acne, and infertility (Ghazeeri *et al.*, 2021). Additionally, the addition of regular physical activity constructs a central element of the management of PCOS. At least 30 minutes of moderate exercise, performed five days a week, can greatly improve insulin sensitivity and enable weight control. There are several forms of exercise, including aerobic exercise and resistance training, that have been shown to effectively impact metabolic function and control weight. Also, exercise is suited to mental health, something particularly beneficial given the psychiatric implications that are often associated with PCOS. With a view towards an exercise program combined with dietary adjustment, one can create an active plan that not only assists in reducing the symptoms of PCOS but contributes to overall quality of life as well (Bernier *et al.*, 2012).

8.5.2. Medications (Hormonal Treatments, Insulin Sensitizers)

The treatment of Polycystic Ovarian Syndrome (PCOS) is usually multisystemic, particularly in the management of menstrual imbalance and insulin resistance, because these are the typical presentations of the syndrome. Treatment with hormone therapy in the form of oral contraceptive pills is the most popular way of replacing menstrual cyclicity and relieving hyperandrogenic symptoms such as hirsutism and acne. These medications function by releasing man-made hormones that mimic the actions of natural estrogen and progesterone and thus restore menstrual balance. However, while hormonal therapy may alleviate symptoms, it fails to address the root issues of insulin resistance, which are prevalent among most PCOS women. This interwoven relationship of hormonal regulation makes it imperative to know the proper treatment techniques that can simultaneously address both hormonal and metabolic dysfunction in PCOS. Aside from hormonal treatment, insulin sensitizers such as metformin also take center stage in PCOS management, particularly in insulin-resistant individuals. Metformin has been found to enhance insulin sensitivity and, by extension, normalize ovulatory function. More recent information also indicates that if metformin is supplemented with myo-inositol—a naturally occurring substance thought to enhance ovarian function—much-improved ovulation and pregnancy rates are achieved over the use of metformin alone. For instance, in PCOS women with insulin resistance, PCOS women who were given a combination of metformin and myo-inositol both showed a notable increase in the number of mature follicles as well as progesterone levels, thus again confirming the therapeutic potential of this combination for enhancing fertility in PCOS patients. These findings point towards the central role played by insulin sensitizers in the overall treatment scheme of PCOS, not just with regard to reproductive wellness but also metabolic wellness (Akter *et al.*, 2022). The research on alternative treatments, such as herbal medication, also presents a hopeful direction for the management of PCOS, particularly in patients who are interested in complementary therapy to the primary treatments. Recent research on *Hunteria umbellata*, a traditional antidiabetic herbal medicine, shows that it can reduce the physiological manifestations of PCOS, such as development of ovarian cysts and insulin resistance. In animal models, administration of *Hunteria umbellata* showed a reduction in the frequency of ovarian cysts and also in metabolic parameters concerning insulin sensitivity, reiterating its role as an adjuvant treatment. Although more in-depth investigation is required in larger clinical trials, these findings suggest that herbal treatments may prove to be a useful adjunct to conventional hormonal treatments, and insulin sensitizers, and create an overall blueprint for exploring the sensitivity of PCOS (Ineza *et al.*, 2024).

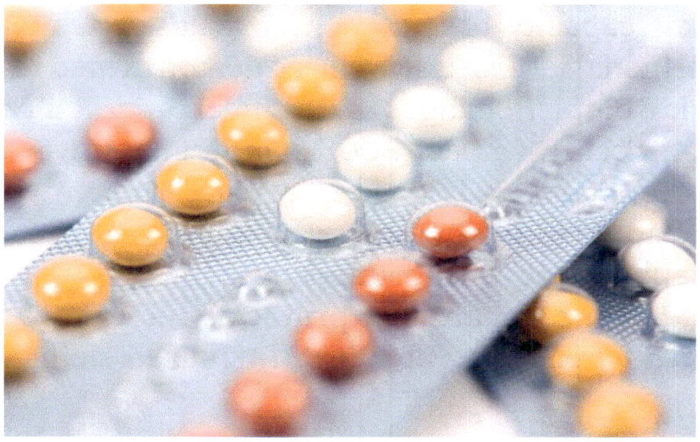

Source: https://images.squarespace-cdn.com/content/v1/54b53631e4b04ebefeb14d13/1616950903576-VP355PNZLN8SLN6U2PRD/treatments-for-PCOS-birth-control-pills.jpg

8.5.3. Alternative Therapies (Supplements, Acupuncture)

Alternative medicine has gained popularity as an adjuvant modality in the treatment of Polycystic Ovarian Syndrome (PCOS), a multifactorial endocrine disorder that can lead to infertility and other complications. Of all the alternative treatments, acupuncture has been very promising. This traditional Chinese medicine therapy attempts to rebalance the body by stimulating some points along channels of energy. Much research has shown that acupuncture may have a positive impact on PCOS women's reproductive function. For example, it is believed to induce the development of the ovarian follicle and also increase insulin sensitivity, both of which are the most important factors in treating the syndrome.

Integrating acupuncture into standard therapy may yield an overall remedy for those who wish to improve their symptoms and quality of life. In addition to acupuncture, nutritional supplements have been extensively researched to manage PCOS. Nutritional supplements such as inositol, a B-vitamin-like compound, have proven to be of beneficial value in reducing insulin resistance and normalizing ovarian function. Other vitamins such as omega-3 fatty acids and vitamin D are also being studied for their capacity to control menstrual cycles and hormonal levels. Research has demonstrated that some dietary changes and supplementation can significantly impact PCOS symptoms. However, these alternatives need to be undertaken with caution; while evidence nowadays suggests their efficacy, rigorous clinical trials must establish standardized protocols for their use in the treatment of PCOS. Increased demand for complementary and alternative medicine (CAM) for treating PCOS-associated infertility reflects a larger movement toward integrative health care. As illustrated in the latest studies, many CAM modalities, including acupuncture and nutritional supplementation, have been shown to be effective, but much more research remains to be done. On comparison of the available randomized controlled trials (RCTs) on these therapies, acupuncture and some of the supplements such as selenium have consistently shown to positively influence fertility parameters (Al-Bader *et al.*, 2013). Nevertheless, evidence currently available needs more stringent trials to determine the optimal use of these treatments. Lastly, while complementary treatments may offer women with PCOS support management options, they should supplement rather than substitute conventional medical treatments (Hu *et al.*, 2017).

Test Your Knowledge

1. What are the common hormonal treatments used to manage PCOS symptoms?
2. How can lifestyle changes help in the treatment of PCOS?

SUMMARY

In summary, polycystic ovarian syndrome (PCOS) is a multi-factorial endocrine disorder that significantly impacts a large percentage of the female population, particularly in the reproductive years. PCOS, being multi-factorial with diverse presentations and long-term health consequences, requires a deeper understanding of its pathogenesis. The first chapter of this study described the intricate interaction between obesity, genetics, and insulin resistance, which are important etiologic contributors to PCOS. Furthermore, the likelihood of unfavorable health outcomes like metabolic syndrome, cardiovascular disease, and type II diabetes mellitus increases the importance of early detection and treatment plans tailored in accordance with individual requirements (Bernier *et al.*, 2012). Together, these results reveal the necessity for ongoing research and education regarding PCOS. Treatment of PCOS remains a point of interest, as current research demonstrates lifestyle modification and pharmacologic management to be efficacious. The second chapter of this research assessed numerous treatment modalities, revealing that an integrated approach could lead to a significant improvement in quality of life in patients with PCOS. Notably, incorporating lifestyle changes alongside medical therapies can alleviate many symptoms associated with insulin resistance, which is central to the condition (Bernier *et al.*, 2012). This suggests that an interdisciplinary approach, integrating diet, exercise, and medication, can empower women to manage their symptoms more effectively. Ultimately, the ongoing exploration of PCOS treatment demonstrates promise in enhancing health outcomes and fostering an improved understanding of this prevalent condition. Continued research, funded by grants from entities such as the Australian National Health and Medical Research Council, also stresses the necessity of revising our knowledge regarding PCOS and treatment techniques. As fresh facts come to light through research, it is imperative that doctors keep themselves abreast of current developments and alter their methods according to new information. The pathophysiology of PCOS is evolving, but there is still much that is not known. Constant dialogue among healthcare practitioners, scientists, and patients is instrumental to developing more effective models of care that address not only clinical manifestations but the emotional and psychological aspects of living with PCOS. In that partnership, it is possible to develop a more comprehensive strategy for managing the condition, effectively leading to improved health among the women suffering from polycystic ovarian syndrome.

Polycystic Ovarian Syndrome (PCOS) is a heterogeneous endocrine disorder with a significant effect on women's reproductive and metabolic health, affecting approximately 5-10% of women in the reproductive age group. Awareness of the key facts regarding PCOS is essential for diagnosis and management. The pathogenesis of PCOS is multifactorial, traditionally associated with insulin resistance, obesity, and genetics. The most recent research focuses on the prevalence of metabolic syndrome among women with PCOS, referring to the importance of the disorders' broader health effects, i.e., increased risks for type II diabetes mellitus and cardiovascular diseases. Their interaction emphasizes the necessity for early and accurate diagnosis in an attempt to avoid the syndrome's long-term consequences (Bernier *et al.*, 2012). In investigating vascular complications of PCOS, recent studies have produced alarming findings with regard to arterial function. Testing the elastic reserve of carotid arteries reveals a significant decrease in compliance and enhanced stiffness in symptomatic and asymptomatic PCOS women relative to normal controls. Specifically, both groups of women with PCOS exhibited radically altered vascular parameters that suggested an underlying risk for stroke and coronary artery disease. The findings indicate that PCOS may not only affect reproductive functions but also have high cardiovascular risks. Understanding such vascular dysfunctions is important in the promotion of clinical approaches to the management of PCOS, as they are necessary for making interventions more particular to women with this syndrome (Hardiman *et al.*, 2002). Moreover, management and treatment of PCOS must be founded on a thorough comprehension that includes lifestyle changes along with pharmacological interventions. Effective control of PCOS tends to include weight loss, food regimen, and physical training, all aimed at increasing insulin sensitivity and reducing androgen secretion. Evidence is on our side that addressing lifestyle modification will benefit most symptoms of PCOS without the sole use of medicines. Nonetheless, an integrated treatment approach involving drug therapies, such as hormonal contraceptives and insulin-sensitizing medications, is also required in most women to achieve relief of symptoms as well as restore fertility. Thus, a good understanding of both treatment modalities and the pathophysiology of PCOS is needed to develop effective, individualized treatment of the affected people (Bernier *et al.*, 2012).

KEY TERMS FROM THIS CHAPTER

- Hyperandrogenism
- Acne
- Polycystic ovaries
- Hyperinsulinemia
- Infertility
- Rotterdam criteria
- Oral contraceptives
- Hirsutism
- Anovulation
- Insulin resistance
- Dyslipidemia
- Menstrual irregularity
- Lifestyle modification

CRITICAL THINKING QUESTIONS

1. **Which of the following is a common hormonal feature of PCOS?**
   a. Decreased luteinizing hormone (LH)
   b. Increased follicle-stimulating hormone (FSH)
   c. Elevated androgens (testosterone)
   d. Low insulin levels
2. **The typical ultrasound finding in PCOS is:**
   a. Enlarged ovaries with multiple small follicles arranged peripherally ("string of pearls")
   b. Enlarged uterus with thickened endometrium
   c. Ovarian cyst larger than 10 cm
   d. Absence of follicles
3. **Which of the following is NOT a common symptom of PCOS?**
   a. Irregular menstrual cycles
   b. Hirsutism
   c. Weight gain
   d. Excessive bleeding during menstruation
4. **Insulin resistance in PCOS primarily contributes to:**
   a. Hyperandrogenism
   b. Increased estrogen production
   c. Increased progesterone levels
   d. Decreased LH secretion
5. **Which of the following is a first-line treatment for managing menstrual irregularities in PCOS?**
   a. Antibiotics
   b. Oral contraceptive pills
   c. Insulin injections
   d. Surgery

Short Answer Questions

1. What are some common causes of Polycystic Ovary Syndrome (PCOS)?
2. List three typical symptoms experienced by individuals with PCOS.
3. Which tests are commonly used to diagnose PCOS?
4. Name two health risks associated with untreated PCOS.
5. What lifestyle changes can help manage PCOS symptoms?
6. What are common medical treatment options for PCOS?

Answer to Critical Thinking Questions

1. (c) 2. (a) 3. (d) 4. (a) 5. (b)

REFERENCES

1. Adaway, J., Al-Qaissi, A., Atkin, S., *et al.* (2017). Salivary testosterone measurement in women with and without polycystic ovary syndrome. https://core.ac.uk/download/151156463.pdf (accessed on 14th June 2025).
2. Akter, S., Banu, J., Chowdhury, P., *et al.* (2022). Effects of metformin plus myo-inositol compared to metformin alone as pre-treatment of ovulation induction in polycystic ovary syndrome with insulin resistance. https://core.ac.uk/download/544390427.pdf (accessed on 14th June 2025).
3. Al-Bader, T., Cakmak, H., Chan, L., de Klerk, C., Dieterle, S., Domar, A., *et al.* (2013). A systematic review of the evidence for complementary and alternative medicine in infertility. *International Journal of Gynecology & Obstetrics.* http://deepblue.lib.umich.edu/bitstream/2027.42/135426/1/ijgo202.pdf (accessed on 14th June 2025).
4. Atkin, S. L., David, R., Gooderham, N. J., *et al.* (2015). Increased expression of circulating miRNA-93 in women with polycystic ovary syndrome may represent a novel, non-invasive biomarker for diagnosis. https://core.ac.uk/download/151157243.pdf (accessed on 14th June 2025).
5. Bagatin, E., Costa, D. L. M., Manela-Azulay, M., *et al.* (2011). Polycystic ovary syndrome: A dermatologic approach. https://core.ac.uk/download/37709652.pdf (accessed on 14th June 2025).
6. Bernier, D. (2012). Polycystic ovary syndrome: Pathogenesis, health consequences, and treatment of PCOS in relation to insulin resistance. https://core.ac.uk/download/72048051.pdf (accessed on 14th June 2025).
7. Bhattacharya, S., Costello, M. F., Johnson, N. P., *et al.* (2017). Treatment strategies for women with WHO group II anovulation: Systematic review and network meta-analysis. https://core.ac.uk/download/77052590.pdf (accessed on 14th June 2025).
8. Bonin, C., Bonora, E., Dall'Alda, M., *et al.* (2013). Divergences in insulin resistance between the different phenotypes of the polycystic ovary syndrome. https://core.ac.uk/download/55800175.pdf (accessed on 14th June 2025).
9. Boomsma, D. I., Lambalk, C. B., Sadrzadeh, S., *et al.* (2006). Heritability of polycystic ovary syndrome in a Dutch twin-family study. https://core.ac.uk/download/pdf/15457246.pdf (accessed on 14th June 2025).
10. Broom, J., Johnston, K. L., Love, J. G., *et al.* (2016). The experiences of women with polycystic ovary syndrome on a very low-calorie diet. https://core.ac.uk/download/131024400.pdf (accessed on 14th June 2025).
11. Cochran, L., Nadolny, R., Garcia, K., Kluglein, K. A., Yagoda, A., Gandhi, P., Dressel, J., *et al.* (2024). Available treatments and adjunctive therapies for polycystic ovarian syndrome (PCOS) patients of reproductive age: A scoping review. *Cureus, 16.* https://www.semanticscholar.org/paper/9244e585d8c9a2541b4a8a874f480787827d81bb (accessed on 14th June 2025).
12. Coutinho, E. A., & Kauffman, A. S. (2019). The role of the brain in the pathogenesis and physiology of polycystic ovary syndrome (PCOS). https://core.ac.uk/download/323065551.pdf (accessed on 14th June 2025).

13. Dhamija, P., More, A., Choudhary, N., Wadhe, T., Barai, J., & Shah, D. (2025). Seed cycling and hormonal balance: A case study of successful fertility intervention in polycystic ovarian syndrome. *Journal of Pharmacy and Bioallied Sciences*. https://www.semanticscholar.org/paper/37073f5bcfabca5762ee25bd200c8d79f2529b92 (accessed on 14th June 2025).

14. Dominguez, J. N., & Pallasigui, A. I. M. A. (2024). Mixed methods study of physical and affective self-concept among Filipino adolescents with polycystic ovarian syndrome (PCOS). https://core.ac.uk/download/620076782.pdf (accessed on 14th June 2025).

15. Dybciak, P., Humeniuk, E., Raczkiewicz, D., Krakowiak, J., Wdowiak, A., & Bojar, I. (2022). Anxiety and depression in women with polycystic ovary syndrome. *Medicina, 58*, 942. https://doi.org/10.3390/medicina58070942 (accessed on 14th June 2025).

16. Fagg, E. (2024). Effects of nonpharmacological and pharmacological interventions on the management of polycystic ovarian syndrome. https://core.ac.uk/download/613192591.pdf (accessed on 14th June 2025).

17. Falbo, A., La Sala, G. B., Palomba, S., *et al.* (2015). Complications and challenges associated with polycystic ovary syndrome: Current perspectives. https://core.ac.uk/download/80172069.pdf (accessed on 14th June 2025).

18. Faqih, A., Nurdiawan, O., & Susana, H. (2024). Deep learning for polycystic ovarian syndrome classification using convolutional neural network. https://core.ac.uk/download/599386529.pdf (accessed on 14th June 2025).

19. Fatima, A., Fatima, U., Naz, M., *et al.* (2019). Psychological complications of polycystic ovarian syndrome and women's health. https://core.ac.uk/download/539911943.pdf (accessed on 14th June 2025).

20. Fehring, R. (2009). Current medical research winter 2008–spring 2009. https://core.ac.uk/download/213086359.pdf (accessed on 14th June 2025).

21. Ghazeeri, G., Hmedeh, C., *et al.* (2021). Nutritional management in polycystic ovary syndrome: Challenges and opportunities. https://core.ac.uk/download/161103740.pdf (accessed on 14th June 2025).

22. Gregory, J. W., Cameron, F., Joshi, K., Eiswirth, M. E., Garrett, C., Garvey, K. C., Agarwal, S., *et al.* (2022). ISPAD clinical practice consensus guidelines 2022: Diabetes in adolescence. *Pediatric Diabetes, 23*, 857–871. https://doi.org/10.1111/pedi.13408 (accessed on 14th June 2025).

23. Hardiman, P., Lakhani, K., & Seifalian, A. M. (2002). Impaired carotid viscoelastic properties in women with polycystic ovaries. https://core.ac.uk/download/1676676.pdf (accessed on 14th June 2025).

24. Hu, W. L., Hung, Y. C., & Liao, Y. N. (2017). Complementary and alternative therapy with traditional Chinese medicine for infertility. https://core.ac.uk/download/322429385.pdf (accessed on 14th June 2025).

25. Ineza, N. (2024). Effects of aqueous extract of *Hunteria umbellata* on hormonal, metabolic, and hematological parameters of polycystic ovarian syndrome in Sprague-Dawley rat model. https://core.ac.uk/download/615522945.pdf (accessed on 14th June 2025).

26. Khan, N. A., Mirza, S. M., Qureshi, M. A., *et al.* (2014). Association between circulating adiponectin levels and polycystic ovarian syndrome. https://core.ac.uk/download/42352677.pdf (accessed on 14th June 2025).

27. Krishna, U. R. N., Nazrin, T. M. S., Biju, A., & Joseph, M. (2024). A comparative study on the effect of different management options on body mass index in overweight polycystic ovarian syndrome patients at a tertiary care hospital. *Acta Medica International*. https://www.semanticscholar.org/paper/27f0443512a9949fd782620440d34d624a2758a5 (accessed on 14th June 2025).

28. Kumari, A., & Jha, S. N. (2024). Unraveling the complexities of polycystic ovarian syndrome: A comprehensive review. https://core.ac.uk/download/617167612.pdf (accessed on 14th June 2025).

29. Maheshwari, A., Ayyad, A., Balen, A. H., Bellver, J., *et al.* (2010). The impact of female obesity on the outcome of fertility treatment. *Human Reproduction Update*. https://core.ac.uk/download/4193248.pdf (accessed on 14th June 2025).

30. Matzke, A. (2011). The underdiagnosis of polycystic ovarian syndrome in normal weight adolescent females. https://core.ac.uk/download/200291160.pdf (accessed on 14th June 2025).

31. Nandikola, J. R., Wayal, S. R., Vijayabanu, S., Ravindra, B. N., Keshava, K. S., Chatterjee, A., Jaganmohan, C., *et al.* (2025). Antidiabetic management strategies for treatment of polycystic ovarian syndrome. *Journal of Neonatal Surgery*. https://www.semanticscholar.org/paper/5cb9dc3cd9a009a0d7bec8eba338237f20e7bce5 (accessed on 14th June 2025).

32. Orr, C., Percy, C., & Turner, A. (2024). Developing a novel web-based self-management support intervention for polycystic ovary syndrome: Mixed methods study with patients and health care professionals. https://core.ac.uk/download/603360980.pdf (accessed on 14th June 2025).

33. Pillalamarri, M., Patnala, V. G., Singam, A., Bhavani, B. S. J., & Gugulothu, B. (2025). A comparative review of herbal medicinal plants and synthetic drugs in the treatment of polycystic ovarian syndrome (PCOS). *International Journal of Pharmaceutical Research and Applications*. https://www.semanticscholar.org/paper/f50e3c183c71e98a6a5fde319ad274ef027ffa3c (accessed on 14th June 2025).

34. Sanchez, N. (2015). Polycystic ovary syndrome, absent from national surveillance and present online: Implications for mental and behavioral health. http://deepblue.lib.umich.edu/bitstream/2027.42/113329/1/ninive_1.pdf (accessed on 14th June 2025).

35. Satkar, S. S., Sonawane, M. D., Kumbhar, P. M., & Gurav, M. V. (2024). Herbal arena for treatment of polycystic ovarian syndrome (PCOS). *Asian Journal of Pharmaceutical Research*. https://www.semanticscholar.org/paper/1bb6aed75a0ef4bdad7c71ef5b6d9dde63133405 (accessed on 14th June 2025).

36. Surisetty, L., & Kumar, K. S. (2025). Polycystic ovarian syndrome (PCOS)–An overview. *International Journal of Pharmaceuticals and Health Care Research*. https://www.semanticscholar.org/paper/0c4f633b16b328d0d82db508b8212a3be8355104 (accessed on 14th June 2025).

37. Zalwade, P., Darunde, D., & Turke, A. (2025). Polycystic ovary syndrome (PCOS): A complex endocrine disorder. *International Journal of Pharmaceutical Research and Applications*. https://www.semanticscholar.org/paper/f7d80cab6438ccdecf40a87588016d93e87b6adc (accessed on 14th June 2025).

DYSMENORRHEA AND PREMENSTRUAL SYNDROME

9

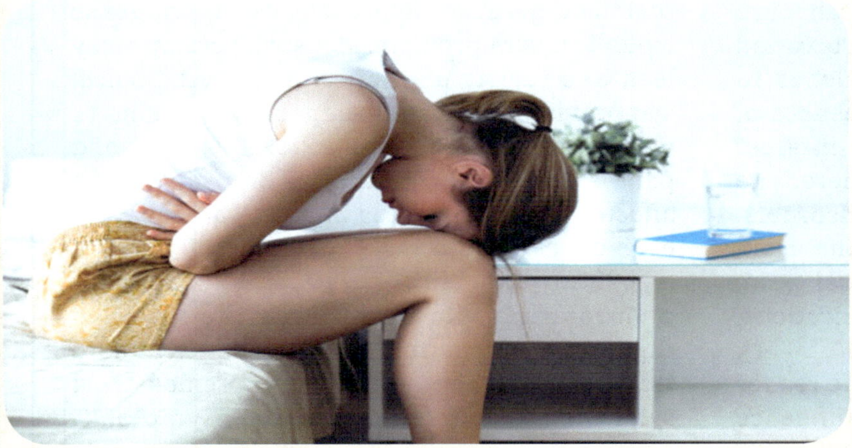

LEARNING OBJECTIVES

After studying this chapter, you will be able to:

1. Explain the overview and characteristics of dysmenorrhea.
2. Describe the overview and symptoms of premenstrual syndrome (PMS).

Introduction

Chapter introduction of premenstrual syndrome (PMS) and dysmenorrhea is essential in the actualization of the overall implication of these widespread women's health disorders. Dysmenorrhea, characterized by painful menstrual cramps, affects a significant percentage of women, particularly adolescents and early adults. According to Katib *et al.* (2024), the prevalence of primary dysmenorrhea has an alarmingly high rate of 83.7%, which reflects its universality. Such discomfort is usually beyond physical and tends to impact emotional status and function in daily living, both of which are important for working women and students. The introduction also lays the groundwork for the examination of the interaction between primary dysmenorrhea and PMS because, if each condition is comprehended, therapeutic strategies can be established and clinical outcomes improved. The introduction also opens up the possibility of examining the basis of menstrual health, which has received little research attention previously. Even though menstruation, with its cyclical pattern, occurs in millions of people worldwide, menstrual health is a relatively underdeveloped field of reproductive medicine, highlighted in Critchley *et al.*, (2020). The paucity of knowledge on the physiology and pathology of menstruation has hindered progress in the care. By highlighting the need for ongoing research into ailments like dysmenorrhea, PMS, and other menstruation syndromes, the introduction establishes the platform for an understanding of the need to apply patient voice and experience to research. This call for further research into menstrual well-being can pave the way for more effective fertility preservation strategies and individualized approaches to care. Finally, considering the consequences of dysmenorrhea and PMS transcends interest in personal health into the public sphere. The physical and emotional effect of such disorders, as seen in 76.3% of women suffering from emotional problems due to menstrual pain, has school and work productivity implications, especially for young women (Katib *et al.*, 2024). The introduction serves to enlighten the reader as to how menstrual disorder issues influence not only personal health but also society's views of women's health. Additionally, with societal movements for menstrual equity and visibility gaining momentum, it is increasingly imperative that one positions these conditions in the broader picture of health literacy and access. Doing so allows the introduction itself to provide a complete approach to understanding dysmenorrhea and PMS as problems worthy of study and discussion.

Definition of Dysmenorrhea

Dysmenorrhea, or menstrual cramping, is typically described as painful and crampy during menses. Dysmenorrhea is divided into primary and secondary dysmenorrhea. Primary dysmenorrhea is typically associated with the release of prostaglandins, which cause uterine contractions that result in pain in otherwise healthy women. This form of dysmenorrhea typically occurs soon after menses has begun and may continue for several days. Conversely, secondary dysmenorrhea is linked with inherent medical disorders such as endometriosis, pelvic inflammatory disease, or fibroids that complicate the menstrual cycle and aggravate pain experiences. These differences are noteworthy to recognize because they have implications for treatment strategies and symptom management overall for dysmenorrhea. The prevalence of dysmenorrhea is high, occurring in as many as 95% of women of childbearing age throughout their lifetime, thus emphasizing its importance as a public health problem. Menstrual cramps may lead to a variety of physical and psychological symptoms, significantly impacting a woman's quality of life. Symptoms generally go beyond pain in the body, with the majority of women affected by disturbances in mood, anxiety, and even depression in cases where dysmenorrhea is painful and chronic. The intersection of dysmenorrhea with mental health is essential to explore, as evident from studies trying to explore treatment validity in relation to premenstrual syndrome (PMS) and associated symptoms. These issues raise the importance of not only treating the physical symptoms of dysmenorrhea but also the emotional and psychological issues women face during menstruation (Leonard *et al.*, 1985).

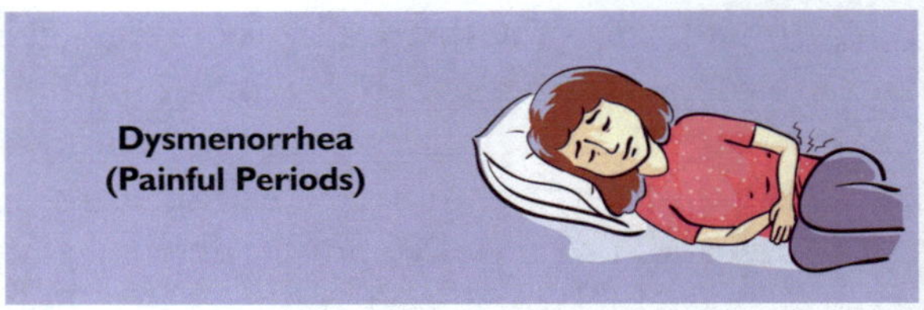

Source: https://www.medicoverhospitals.in/woman-and-child/images/diseases/wc-dysmenorrhea-bnr.webp

To manage dysmenorrhea symptoms, various treatments have been established, from pharmacologic treatments, lifestyle modification, to complementary treatment. Conventional treatment has involved prescribing nonsteroidal anti-inflammatory drugs (NSAIDs)

or hormonal contraceptives that aim to reduce pain and regularize menstrual cycles. However, increasing interest in complementary and alternative medicine (CAM) says it's all about new approaches that appeal to the majority of women seeking integrative treatment alternatives. Of special interest is the Arvigo Techniques of Maya Abdominal Therapy™, a non-invasive massage of the belly to correct uterine alignment and address menstrual cramping. Measurement has begun to capture the effectiveness of such therapies, using pain assessment tools to track decreases in menstrual distress before and after treatment (Burchett *et al.*, 2013). This interdisciplinary perspective on the management of dysmenorrhea opens up an integrated understanding of women's health-related concerns.

Definition of Premenstrual Syndrome (PMS)

The Premenstrual Syndrome (PMS) is a luteal phase syndrome of physical, emotional, and behavioral symptoms that appear during the premenstrual phase of the menstrual cycle, typically one or two weeks prior to menstruation. PMS affects approximately 41.2% of women belonging to certain age groups and is the etiology of a wide range of impairments capable of significantly interfering with quality of life. Symptoms can significantly vary from patient to patient, with changes in mood, irritability, fatigue, bloating, and physical discomfort, all as reminders of the hormonal shifts that occur within the body. The cyclical nature of PMS renders it more of a syndrome than a single disorder whose complexity of presentation and impact is mirrored according to recent research on menstrual health (Greydanus *et al.*, 2012). Understanding about PMS is significant not just for diagnosis but also for therapeutic intervention and management. The condition is thought to be influenced by hormonal changes, particularly variations in the estrogen and progesterone levels. The hormone changes can lead to alterations in neurotransmitter systems, which could be the etiology for reported emotional symptoms in PMS. The prevalence of PMS places emphasis on awareness and education on menstrual disorders, as the symptoms affect the majority of women and hinder their work and personal activities. Also, it has been found through research that women suffering from PMS will turn to alternative therapies to manage their symptoms and hence demonstrate greater interest in complementary and alternative medicine (CAM) therapy (Chapple *et al.*, 2016). Management of PMS can be through lifestyle modifications, diet, and application of various pharmacological interventions. As the popularity of an integrated model of healthcare increases, increasingly women approach alternate modes of treatment as a means to combat PMS symptoms. Severity of symptoms and personal preference are extremely influential aspects in the choice of appropriate interventions. Through investigation of both the physical and mental components of PMS, medical professionals are better positioned to develop holistic treatment plans that address both the somatic and affective components of the syndrome. Thus, the definition and understanding of PMS remain essential for physicians and women seeking to improve their condition and receive appropriate treatment, so they can better deal with the complexities of their menstrual cycle.

Importance of Understanding These Conditions

An understanding of the complexities of dysmenorrhea and premenstrual syndrome (PMS) is important for a variety of reasons, most significantly women's health and well-being. Both are not merely physical afflictions; they can be emotionally, socially, and economically debilitating. As described in recent research, a spectrum of women who experience PMS also experience irritability and anxiety, reducing their standard of living and daily engagement in both home and work life. Repeated consumption of over-the-counter pain medications, which are often taken for symptom relief, can only worsen these conditions while ignoring the underlying causative factors that cause the pain. An integrated knowledge of dysmenorrhea and PMS can facilitate more effective treatment strategies, such as magnesium supplements, which can improve overall functioning and quality of life in sufferers (Baumer *et al.*, 2024). Further, rates of dysmenorrhea and PMS in teenage girls indicate the importance of understanding the conditions. Dysmenorrhea was the most common condition in 57.5% of the sample in one study of 215 teenage girls presenting for medical attention. This high incidence means that there is a requirement to intervene and provide care to the population, given that many menstrual abnormalities are likely to influence future reproductive health. Education and familiarity with these conditions are critical to facilitating early diagnosis and effective management. Furthermore, appreciating the potential co-association of dysmenorrhea, PMS, and other health conditions, such as hypothyroidism or anemia, highlights the importance of an integrative approach strategy (*et al.*, 2020). By appreciating the multifaceted nature of PMS and dysmenorrhea, medical professionals, educators, and policymakers can also work together to offer supportive environments for victims. Focusing on research and education can ensure greater access to resources, educational interventions, and medical evaluation that respond to young women's unique needs. By promoting open conversation about menstrual health, the stigma associated with these conditions can be eliminated, allowing women to seek help and become more attuned to their bodies. Ultimately, a better understanding of dysmenorrhea and PMS not only heals the physical but fosters a culture of education and compassion towards women suffering from these common yet complex health issues. This cultural transformation can have long-term effects on both public and individual health outcomes.

9.1. Overview of Dysmenorrhea

Learning Outcome

1. Differentiate between the types of Dysmenorrhea: Primary and Secondary.
2. Identify the symptoms and diagnostic methods for Dysmenorrhea.
3. Explain the prevalence of Dysmenorrhea and its impact on daily life.
4. Analyze the causes of Dysmenorrhea.
5. Evaluate the treatment options available for Dysmenorrhea.

Dysmenorrhea, or painful menstruation, is a condition that has a high incidence among a wide percentage of the female population, particularly young women and teens. Entailing cramps and pelvic pain during menstrual periods, dysmenorrhea has physiological as well as psychological impacts. The condition typically presents in two forms: primary dysmenorrhea, as a result of menstrual cycles themselves, and secondary dysmenorrhea, as a result of underlying reproductive complications such as endometriosis or fibroids. Consistent with the study carried out in Central Jakarta, 87.5% of the participants reported having had dysmenorrhea, with manifestations between mild and severe, confirming its incidence among adolescents and highlighting the necessity for targeted interventions for the relief of such a common condition (Juniar *et al.*, 2015). The impact of dysmenorrhea is not restricted to physical discomfort only, but affects daily functioning and general well-being as well. In the above study, participants reported that approximately 43.75% of them reported that dysmenorrhea obstructed their involvement in daily activities, thus emphasizing the need for appropriate management. Self-medication was common among the respondents because most of them used over-the-counter drugs against pain without seeking professional' help.

Such behavior reflects a dire educational gap in healthcare provision on menstrual health since most women do not have access to full information resources educating them about the options available, including medical visits. The intricate relationship between dysmenorrhea, mental health, and social support necessitates more awareness and education among medical professionals to address patients' needs more effectively (Juniar *et al.*, 2015). Moreover, studies on the application of alternative therapies for dysmenorrhea have become quite trendy in recent years, and numerous women have also turned to complementary and alternative medicine (CAM) treatments. Clinical findings show that therapies such as herbal medicine, nutrient supplements, and massage therapy are usually applied by women who need to be relieved of the perimenstrual pain symptoms. A critical review noted that the majority of women self-medicate with these CAMs, often without professional advice, illustrating a universal trend of seeking independence in controlling their health. While individual reports typically characterize positive assessments of the efficacy of CAM, the lack of evidence regarding patterns and reasons for CAM use poses the imperative to continue pursuing research to ensure safety and optimal outcomes for women using such alternative practices. Their integration with conventional treatment might have the potential to enhance treatment strategies for dysmenorrhea and facilitate more integrated care.

9.1.1. Types of Dysmenorrhea: Primary and Secondary

Dysmenorrhea, being a very frequent gynecological disorder, occurs in two primary forms: primary dysmenorrhea and secondary dysmenorrhea. Primary dysmenorrhea is menstrual pain that does not occur with any other reproductive health issue. This type typically occurs as a result of the release of prostaglandins, hormones that are responsible for bringing about uterine contractions, thus leading to pain and discomfort. A majority of teenagers and young adults experience this form of dysmenorrhea during their menstrual cycles, which means that it is common among reproductive-aged women.

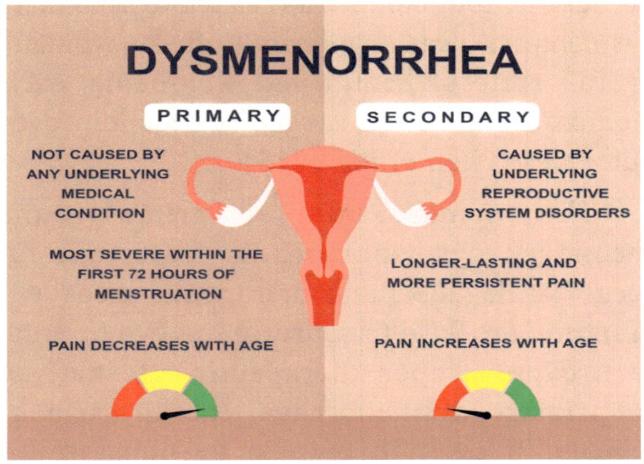

Figure 9.1. Types of Dysmenorrhea

Source: https://s.guavahealth.com/article-img/understanding-menstrual-cramps/period-types.png

Results indicate that about 87.5% of the interviewed teens stated that they had been suffering from some form of dysmenorrhea, as well as the high prevalence of the condition among young individuals (Juniar *et al.*, 2015). It is worth recognizing the nature and relevance of primary dysmenorrhea, as it immediately influences women's ability to function daily and enjoy quality of life. Secondary dysmenorrhea, on the other hand, refers to pain resulting from anunderlying reproductive disease, such as endometriosis, uterine fibroids, or pelvic inflammatory disease. Unlike primary dysmenorrhea, which typically begins shortly after the onset of menses, secondary dysmenorrhea can develop at any point in the menstrual cycle and can be associated with other symptoms such as heavy menstrual flow and abnormal menstrual cycles. This type can also develop with a slow development of pain, but a persistent one that worsens as the disease process continues. The importance of women's health is great; secondary dysmenorrhea may be an indicator of a more debilitating medical condition requiring full evaluation and treatment. Because various conditions related to secondary dysmenorrhea can significantly affect a woman's overall state of health and well-being, early medical intervention is required for improved outcomes (Chen *et al.*, 2015).

The demarcation of primary and secondary dysmenorrhea is important for accurate diagnosis and therapeutic measures. Practitioners have to separate the two in order to provide proper therapeutic alternatives. In primary dysmenorrhea, therapy usually involves alleviation of pain by nonsteroidal anti-inflammatory drugs (NSAIDs) and lifestyle modifications, such as exercise and diet. On the other hand, the treatment of secondary dysmenorrhea involves a rigorous examination of the underlying causes, which may include hormonal therapy, surgery, or medication to cure specific conditions of the reproductive tract. Because the psychosocial impact of dysmenorrhea may be far-reaching—impacting mental health as well as school or work performance—the categorization of types and their ensuing challenges can better equip medical practitioners to enhance the quality of life for women suffering from such painful menstrual experiences (Juniar *et al.*, 2015; Chen *et al.*, 2015).

9.1.2. Symptoms and Diagnosis

Understanding symptoms of dysmenorrhea and premenstrual syndrome (PMS) is important in the diagnosis and treatment of these two. Dysmenorrhea is cramping pain during menses and may start one to two days prior to menses and persist for a few days. Lower abdominal pain extending to the thighs and lower back, as well as gastrointestinal discomfort, nausea, and headache, are commonly felt. PMS, on the other hand, encompasses a broad range of emotional and physical symptoms that range from mood swings and irritability to fatigue, bloating, and breast tenderness. The common characteristics shared by the syndromes can cause diagnosis to be challenging, necessitating a detailed evaluation involving both physical and psychological well-being in order to confirm the specific symptoms of the patient. The diagnosis of dysmenorrhea and PMS can be challenging since the symptoms are subjective and can differ among individuals.

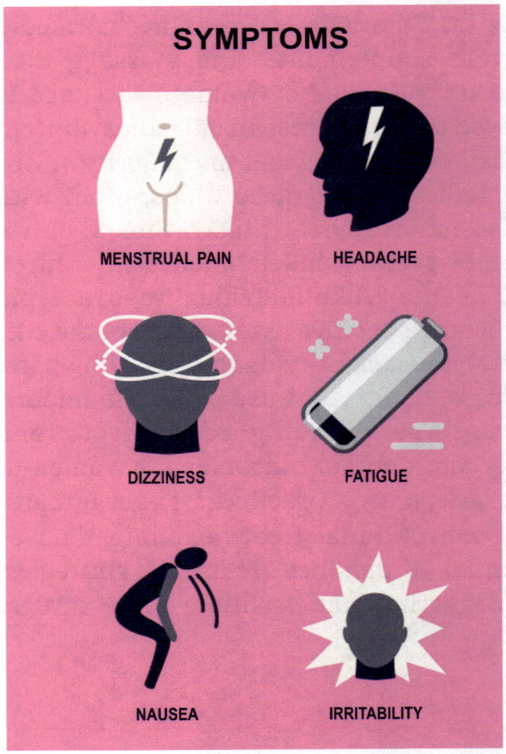

Figure 9.2. Symptoms of dysmenorrhea.

Source: https://www.alhilalhealthcare.com/wp-content/uploads/2022/05/Dysmenorrhea.jpg

Patient history and symptom diaries are utilized by clinicians to determine the patterns that assist in diagnosis. There is a need to distinguish between primary and secondary dysmenorrhea because the latter is largely attributed to elevated prostaglandins, while the former may be caused by inherent reproductive pathology like endometriosis or fibroids. Furthermore, PMS diagnosis adheres to DSM-5, which requires that there be the presence of at least five symptoms from a listed set within a specified time frame before menstruation. The intricacy of this stipulation highlights the appropriateness of multidimensional assessment in considerations for diagnosis, incorporating both the interrelatedness of symptoms as well as their impact on functioning. Recent studies have looked at whether treatments for both PMS and dysmenorrhea are possible, highlighting advances in understanding what works to cure. To illustrate, some research has demonstrated that vitamin D supplementation can lead to a statistically significant reduction in the symptomatology of PMS and dysmenorrhea, as results have shown a decrease in prevalence rates after supplementation (Bahrami *et al.*, 2018). Besides, a number of women have resorted to complementary and alternative medicine (CAM) for symptom management. CAMs like herbal medicine, nutritional supplements, and alternative therapies like massage have become familiar, usually practiced without professional advice (Abdul-Razzak *et al.*, 2016). This indicates a primary need for medical professionals to tackle patients' demand for CAM alongside conventional treatment, advocating for an integrative approach to effectively treat dysmenorrhea and PMS symptoms.

9.1.3. Prevalence and Impact on Daily Life

The prevalence of dysmenorrhea and premenstrual syndrome (PMS) has caused serious concerns about their impact on the daily life of the sufferer. A recent survey revealed that approximately 60.8% of female health sciences students self-report PMS, thus underlining the magnitude of this problem among young women. The effects of PMS extend beyond physical health; students exhibited declining academic performance, which manifested itself in lower levels of concentration, increasing absenteeism, and even failing marks. The multi-dimensionality of PMS symptoms—affective, behavioral, and somatic occurrences—speculates the impacts not just transient but also with the potential to significantly alter one's quality of life as such interferences have the ability to hinder engagement in academia and social processes, which eventually affects the trajectories of lives and mental well-being outcomes (Kustriyanti *et al.*, 2020). Similarly, dysmenorrhea is a problem in itself, with reports that 87.5% of female adolescents experience it to some degree or another. Interference with daily life is most conspicuous, with 43.75% of the sample reporting symptoms that interfere with normal functioning activities, suggesting an implication between severe menstrual pain and reduced functionality in school and social interactions. This disturbance has the potential to perpetuate a cycle of self-medication and inappropriately managed health, since the vast majority do not receive professional medical attention despite the incapacitating nature of their symptoms. It is crucial to be informed about dysmenorrhea: not only does it disrupt personal functioning, but it also impinges upon society in terms of labor force engagement as well as educational attainment (Juniar *et al.*, 2015). Dysmenorrhea and PMS both need an approach based on current prevalence and experience. Educational institutions and medical practitioners need to integrate proactive management procedures for both of these conditions to tackle the specified demand for interventions and resources. The dissemination of information about symptoms and potential treatment could stem the unwanted effects on educational performance and social life. Apart from that, speaking openly about menstrual health will reduce stigmas, encouraging the sufferers to seek help and incorporate coping strategies as part of their daily lives. By giving these programs high priority, society can enhance the safeguarding of the quality of life of suffering young women with dysmenorrhea and PMS and thus promote healthier lives (Kustriyanti *et al.*, 2020; Juniar *et al.*, 2015).

9.1.4. Causes of Dysmenorrhea

The multifactorial etiology of dysmenorrhea encompasses varied physiological as well as pathological processes with a strong impact on the lives of patients. Primary dysmenorrhea, which is the most prevalent type, is most often brought about by an exaggerated production of prostaglandins, which are hormone-like chemicals that trigger uterine contractions. Elevated levels of prostaglandins tend to cause more intense menstrual cramping, resulting in severe pain during menstruation. In addition, secondary dysmenorrhea results from the existence of an underlying condition such as endometriosis, pelvic inflammatory disease, or fibroids that causes aggravated menstrual discomfort. It is of utmost significance to assess the prevalence of such underlying conditions, as can be seen in a study that revealed 57.5% of adolescent girls experience dysmenorrhea, further requiring medical evaluation in this age group (Bahrami *et al.*, 2018). Apart from hormonal etiology, lifestyle and dysmenorrhea play a role as well. Stress, lack of physical activity, and poor diet have been blamed for increasing menstrual cramping. As an interesting fact, deficiency of vitamin D has also been proposed as a causative agent for dysmenorrhea, and hence, supplementation can decrease symptoms. A clinical trial with vitamin D supplementation showed a statistically significant reduction in premenstrual syndrome and dysmenorrhea in adolescents along with improved physical and psychological health (Bahrami *et al.*, 2018). The correlation points to the importance of adopting an integrative model that incorporates nutrition and lifestyle modifications along with medication to promote menstrual wellness in adolescent females. Hormonal imbalance and anemia also play critical roles in the causation of dysmenorrhea. It was discovered that a significant percentage of adolescent girls experiencing menstrual disorders also have anemia, which exacerbates the experience of menstrual pain. Hypothyroidism was statistically linked to menstrual irregularities, adding to the experience of dysmenorrhea among adolescents (*et al.*, 2020). It is crucial to recognize and treat these underlying medical conditions with the appropriate medical attention, as untreated menstrual disorders can have a negative impact on future reproductive well-being. Lastly, a complete understanding of the pathogenesis of dysmenorrhea can give way to more efficient ways of managing it, improving the quality of life for those affected by this common but frequently debilitating disorder.

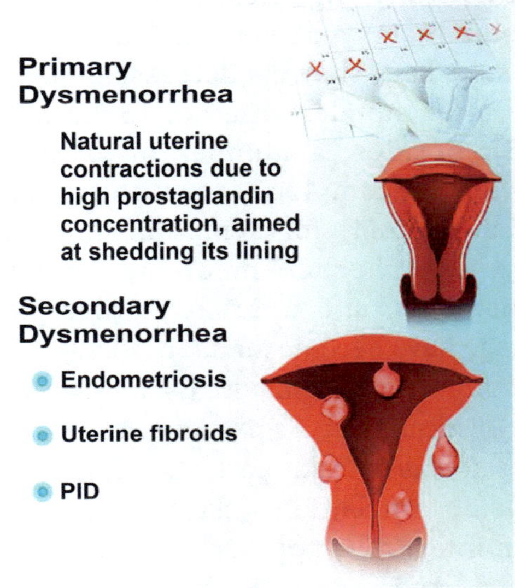

Figure 9.3. Dysmenorrhea causes.

Source: https://www.shecares.com/imgs/5/1/f/118088/dysmenorrhea-causes.png

9.1.4.1. Hormonal Factors

Endocrine influences play an important role in the causation and severity of dysmenorrhea and premenstrual syndrome (PMS), with several hormones influencing physiological and psychological functioning. The menstrual cycle is primarily regulated by estrogen and progesterone, the fluctuations of which may give rise to a spectrum of PMS-related symptoms. During the luteal phase, increased levels of progesterone will lead to increased sensitivity to such changes in the form of mood swings, anxiety, and bodily discomfort. Dysmenorrhea is most frequently linked with increased levels of prostaglandins, hormone-like substances that stimulate uterine contractions. The higher the concentrations of prostaglandins, the more forceful the contractions and, hence, the pain experienced. Hormonal regulation is important in the treatment of the effects of dysmenorrhea and PMS since the treatment options can be uniquely designed depending on the hormonal content. PMS is noted by a large percentage of women of reproductive age, especially impacting academics and psychological life. One study determined that the prevalence of PMS among female students of health science was at 60.8%, having significant interference with physical, health, and psychological domains, such as concentration and social relationships (Kustriyanti *et al.*, 2020).

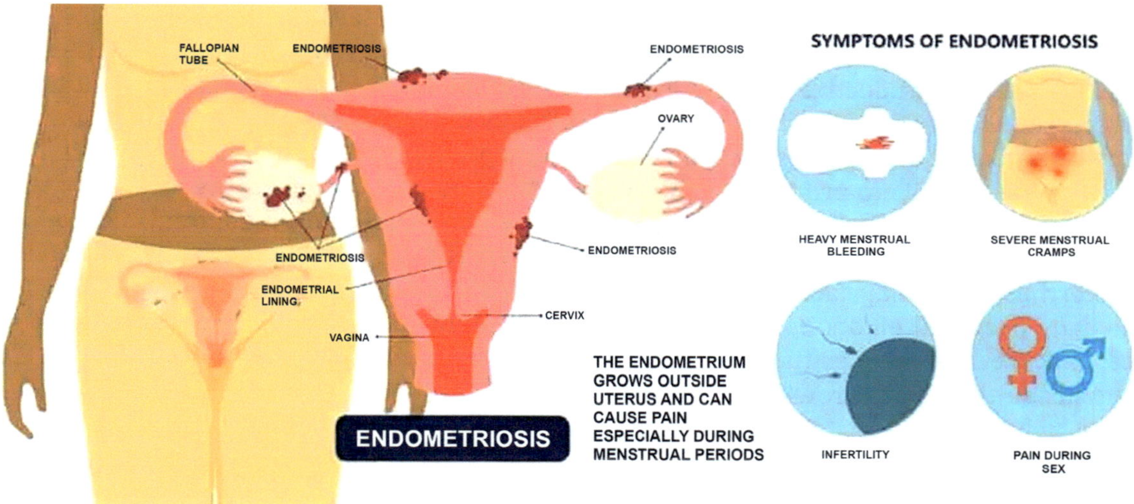

Figure 9.4. The tissue that functions somewhat like the lining of the uterus grows outside it – on the fallopian tubes, pelvis, and ovaries.

Source: https://birlafertility.com/blogs/what-is-dysmenorrhea/

These are clear signs of the severity of these hormone effects and the importance of awareness and education. Furthermore, adolescent girls are particularly at risk of the effects of hormonal change, as exemplified by the impact on their education and social life. The incorporation of such issues not only promotes personal quality of life but also public health policy more generally applied to women's health in terms of a sense of hormonal issues in building effective interventions. Evidence shows that menstrual history in mothers can affect daughters' experiences of PMS, pointing to the genetic component of hormonal influences. A study found a 39.6% prevalence of PMS among college women, which was negatively correlated with any maternal history of menstrual disorders (Badkur *et al.*, 2018). This similarity underscores the applicability of family patterns in PMS expression and possibly dysmenorrhea expression as well. By knowing these genetic links, healthcare professionals can provide individualized education and guidance to young women proactively to help them manage their symptoms more efficiently. Additionally, encouraging communication among mothers and daughters regarding menstruation can lead to increased awareness and coping strategies, ultimately diminishing the plight of hormonal changes associated with this significant phase of life.

9.1.4.2. Underlying Medical Conditions

The pathophysiology of dysmenorrhea, premenstrual syndrome (PMS), and accompanying medical diseases is interactive and multifactorial. Pelvic pain and pelvic reproductive organ disorders can increase the severity of dysmenorrhea and PMS. Endometriosis, adenomyosis, and uterine fibroids have been shown to produce significant menstrual pain and discomfort. These women are most likely to have a higher frequency and severity of dysmenorrhea, and it may have severe impacts on their daily lives and emotional stability. For instance, endometriosis makes tissue similar to the lining inside the uterus grow in other areas within the pelvis, and it leads to excruciating pain, especially when menstruation occurs. This underscores the importance of accurate diagnosis and management of underlying conditions to ensure relief from dysmenorrhea and symptoms of PMS. Further complicating the clinical picture, pre-existing medical conditions have the potential to influence women's perceptions of PMS. Research has revealed that physiological changes and psychological factors associated with PMS are potentially exacerbated by underlying health conditions. Depression and anxiety have been seen to be common in cases of PMS, leading to increased mood swings and irritability. Along with this, endocrine imbalances that cause the physical and emotional symptoms of the luteal phase may be influenced by such mental ailments. Among a sample of college students, findings portrayed approximately 99.3% of the participants with some of the symptoms of PMS, further affirming the extent of this condition among young women. Such findings further support the need to learn about psychological as well as physiological factors involved in managing PMS and improving overall health status (Raule *et al.*, 2025). Also, lifestyle issues and environmental stressors may combine with underlying medical issues and increase the intensity of dysmenorrhea and PMS. For instance, those who have menstrual cycle irregularities may feel higher stress levels and anxiety due to their conditions and thus end up creating a vicious cycle that further intensifies symptoms. Experiments with female students indicated a correlation between levels of stress and severity of PMS symptoms, which suggests that environmental factors play an important role in controlling the conditions. The study demonstrated variations in dysmenorrhea symptoms caused by ethnicity and lifestyle attitudes, and therefore, the validity of the one-size-fits-all solution is doubtful. Hence, specific interventions to address both medical and lifestyle issues are required to guarantee effective symptom control and quality of life in patients with dysmenorrhea and PMS (Suri *et al.*, 2024).

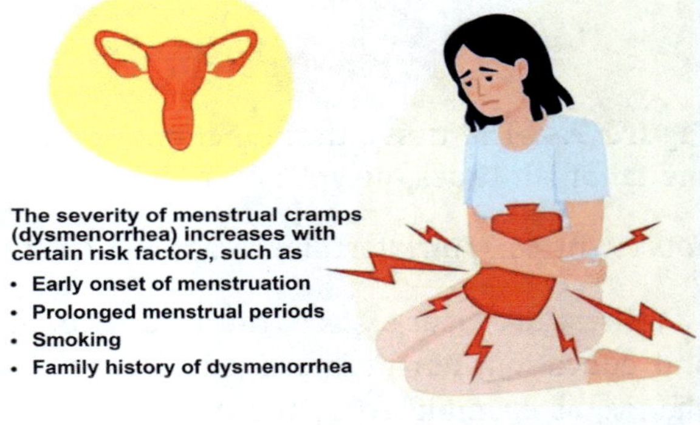

Figure 9.5. Risk factors of Dysmenorrhea.

Source: https://lirp.cdn-website.com/69c0b277/dms3rep/multi/opt/Risk+factors+of+Dysmenorrhea+-+PACE+Hospitals-640w.jpg

9.1.4.3. Lifestyle and Environmental Influences

The sophisticated framework of lifestyle variables and perception of premenstrual syndrome (PMS) and dysmenorrhea is of great academic concern. Physical activity, in particular, has been an important factor in influencing menstrual health. Research has established that adolescent girls, women, and menstruating individuals engage in less physical activity compared to their male counterparts. As previously integrated in Cooper *et al.*, (2024), poor physical activity can increase the severity of menstrual-related symptoms, including mood changes and cramps. Therefore, promoting more exercise not only improves overall health but may also serve as a therapeutic tool in reducing the severity of these menstrual disorders. This emphasizes the need for special interventions to enable women to engage in physical exercise during their menstrual cycle, which could counteract the disabling effects of dysmenorrhea and PMS as well as enhance a healthier lifestyle. Environmental factors add complexity to the dynamic of lifestyle factors on menstrual health. Socioeconomic status, culture, and access to healthcare resources can have a significant impact on women's experience of dysmenorrhea and PMS. For instance, social stigma related to menstruation often discourages women's reporting of their menstrual health, thereby causing ignorance and self-medication, as reaffirmed in Johnson *et al.*, (2023). Stigmatization has the potential to force someone to eschew medical consultation or talking about symptom alleviation. Enhanced education and sensitization efforts may overcome these barriers by empowering women to resist societal pressures. Moreover, communities that openly promote discussion of menstrual health can establish a health-promotive environment under which women can manage the psychological and physical stress of dysmenorrhea and PMS more adequately. Lifestyle characteristics and diet also have a significant influence on deciding menstrual health and symptom control. Lack of some nutrients or a poor diet can contribute to higher intensity of PMS symptoms such as fatigue, mood swings, and physical discomfort. Several studies point to the use of micronutrients like calcium, magnesium, and vitamin B6, which have been found to alleviate some of the problematic symptoms associated with premenstrual syndrome. In addition, the inflammatory or anti-inflammatory quality of food consumption may affect the body's response to changing hormones in the menstrual cycle. Educational interventions educating women about the role of nutrition in menstrual health could potentially offer better management methods for dysmenorrhea and PMS, validating the role of lifestyle options in minimizing these conditions. In this context, a strategy integrating lifestyle modifications like diet and exercise can benefit women's quality of life during the menstrual cycle.

9.1.5. Treatment Options For Dysmenorrhea

Dysmenorrhea treatment is typically separated into pharmacological and non-pharmacological therapy, each with various modalities to provide relief from menstrual cramps. Non-steroidal anti-inflammatory drugs (NSAIDs) remain one of the most common first-line treatments due to their ability to effectively reduce menstrual pain and inflammation. Medications such as ibuprofen and naproxen have been shown to work by inhibiting prostaglandin synthesis, chemical messengers responsible for contracting the uterine muscle and producing pain. Timing of administration is critical; administration with the onset of menses is recommended for optimal effectiveness. Additionally, the use of lifestyle modification and alternative therapies, such as exercise and acupuncture, has gained widespread popularity as adjuncts to the treatment of dysmenorrhea symptoms. More recently, novel treatments have taken center stage due to their potential to treat the root causes of dysmenorrhea. Biologic and new pharmacologic agent studies are promising, particularly in cases where conventional interventions have failed. One of these bioactive molecules, DLBS1442, from *Phaleria macrocarpa*, has also demonstrated potential in alleviating endometriosis- and adenomyosis-related pain. Clinical trials show that DLBS1442 significantly inhibits pain by modulating estrogen receptor function and enhancing progesterone gene expression, which may be pivotal in treating dysmenorrhea associated with these illnesses (Harzif *et al.*, 2015). Thus, research into such new agents could significantly contribute to the therapeutic armamentarium of practitioners. While pharmacotherapy is prevalent, other patients also employ complementary therapies in an attempt to manage dysmenorrhea symptoms. Techniques of yoga, herbal preparations, and dietary changes have been spontaneously reported as easing menstrual pain. An emphasis on total management is especially pertinent for adolescent girls who may resort to alternatives to conventional medication due to concerns about side effects or prescriptions. Additionally, understanding the biological underpinning of menstrual dysfunctions is essential for effective treatment; for instance, understanding the role of dysfunctional uterine bleeding and other menstrual dysfunctions enables the tailoring of treatment protocols to individual patients (Greydanus *et al.*, 2012). With the improvement in research, the integration of both mainstream and alternative disciplines provides a comprehensive strategy for effective management of dysmenorrhea.

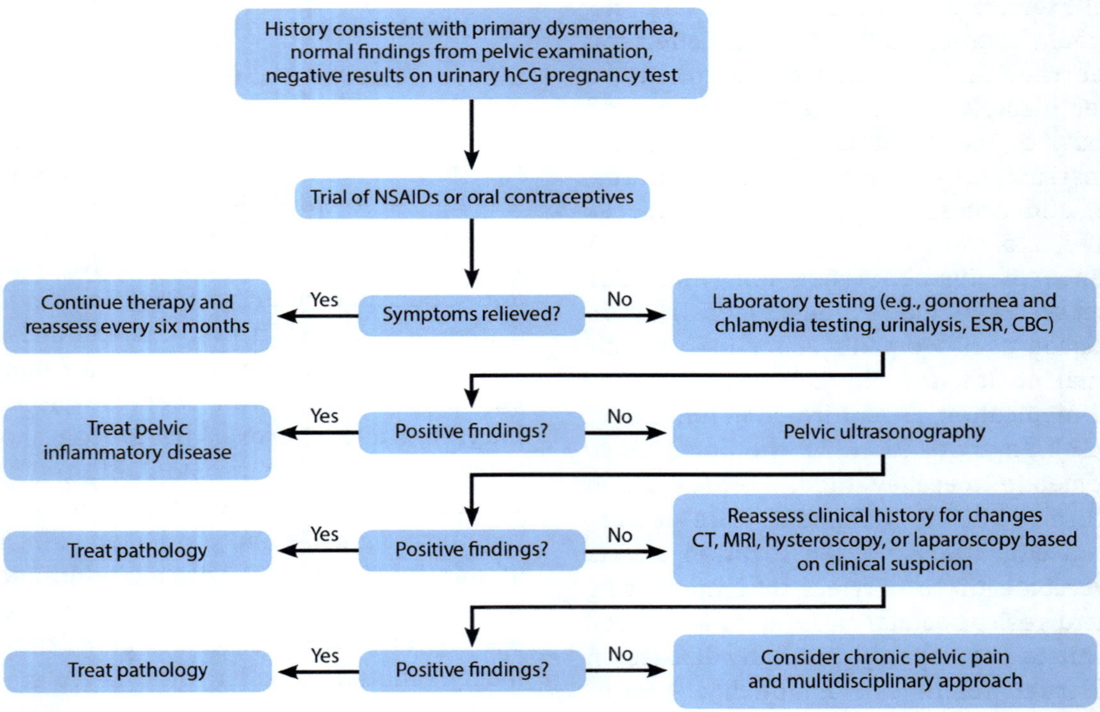

Figure 9.6. Evaluation and treatment of dysmenorrhea.

Source: https://wbhf.walterbushnell.com/images/Bush-Beats-2016/image2.jpg

9.1.5.1. Over-The-Counter Medications

Over-the-counter (OTC) medications play a significant role in the alleviation of pain due to dysmenorrhea and premenstrual syndrome (PMS). The majority of women take OTC pain relievers, including nonsteroidal anti-inflammatory drugs (NSAIDs), to alleviate menstrual cramps and other symptoms such as headache and muscle pain. Commonly prescribed medications, including ibuprofen and naproxen, work by inhibiting prostaglandin synthesis, body chemicals that are responsible for inflammation and pain. Even though such drugs can grant immediate relief, excessive use can result in side effects, such as gastrointestinal upset and long-term problems. Moreover, because PMS is a range of symptoms that are both emotional and physical in nature, sensations such as irritability and mood swings are typically not adequately addressed by these medications, and more integrated treatment plan with behavioral and nutritional approaches is necessary, thus emphasizing the complexity in addressing women's health issues comprehensively (Baumer *et al.*, 2024). While OTC medications can be beneficial to some women, they do not address the underlying causes of PMS and dysmenorrhea and have a tendency to produce a cycle of reliance on the medication. Studies have shown that frequent ingestion of pain medicine can lead to diminishing returns in efficacy, where the same doses produce progressively weaker effects. This raises uncertainty about the syndromes' long-term management and suggests that women may resort to alternative or complementary therapy. Herbal foodstuffs and supplements are increasingly used as potential adjuvants to OTC drugs. For instance, drugs like ginger and turmeric, characterized by their anti-inflammatory properties, are promising alternatives. As such, a treatment regimen that covers various aspects that include both OTC and alternative therapies could provide a more comprehensive response in symptom management associated with PMS as well as dysmenorrhea and thus improve women's quality of life (Areefin *et al.*, 2024).

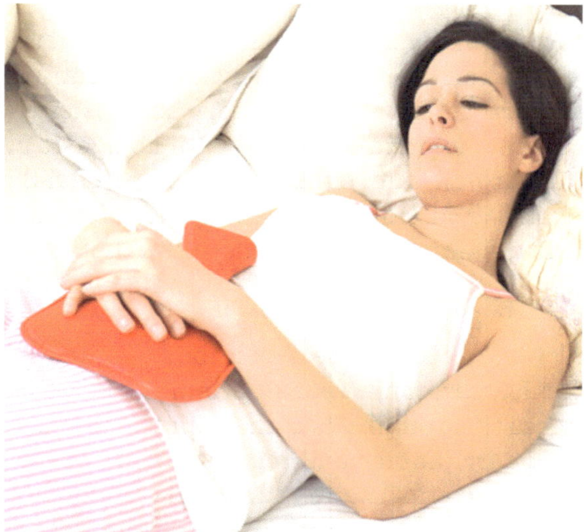

Source: https://www.clinicaladvisor.com/wp-content/uploads/sites/11/2018/12/feat_dysmen_1110_127943.jpg

The need for additional studies on the effectiveness of OTC drugs, in combination with other therapies, is imperative to maximize management strategies for dysmenorrhea and PMS. While OTC medications are ubiquitous and safe, miscalculation of their boundaries can lead to poor symptom management and more side effects. Furthermore, the search for safer, more effective alternatives such as herbal remedies helps to accentuate a movement toward individualized treatment modalities in women's health care. Directed clinical trials and meta-analyses will provide the information required to substantiate the use of these remedies in conventional practice. This developing situation calls for an integrative, patient-centered approach that takes into consideration individual choice and differential symptomatology. Thus, optimization of dysmenorrhea and management of PMS relies on continuous communication between researchers, doctors, and affected individuals to adopt well-balanced treatment protocols with both pharmacological as well as holistic components (Baumer *et al.*, 2024).

9.1.5.2. Prescription Medications

Therapy of dysmenorrhea and premenstrual syndrome (PMS) often necessitates the use of prescription medication, which can greatly alleviate the debilitating symptoms of these disorders. Nonsteroidal anti-inflammatory analgesics (NSAIDs) are typically prescribed as first-line treatment for dysmenorrhea since they are analgesic and anti-inflammatory drugs. These medications, such as ibuprofen and naproxen, are beneficial pain reducers and quality-of-life enhancers during menstruation. However, the majority of women may not visit medical facilities for dysmenorrhea due to the assumption of normalcy with their symptoms or preference to take care of themselves, which is highlighted in the study as women would rather suffer than consult medical advice (Carpenter *et al.*, 2017). Thus, there is a necessity to encourage discussion regarding menstrual well-being and relief that can be prescribed. For many women with PMS, prescription medications such as selective serotonin reuptake inhibitors (SSRIs) can be highly beneficial in reducing emotional and physical symptoms. The antidepressants have been found to reduce mood-related PMS symptoms, such as irritability and anxiety. While SSRIs are effective, their use must be balanced against the risk of side effects and individual choice. The cause of resistance to receiving medical care for PMS is perhaps a strategy to prevent using conventional therapies with putative unwanted effects, a trend that has been observed in patients.

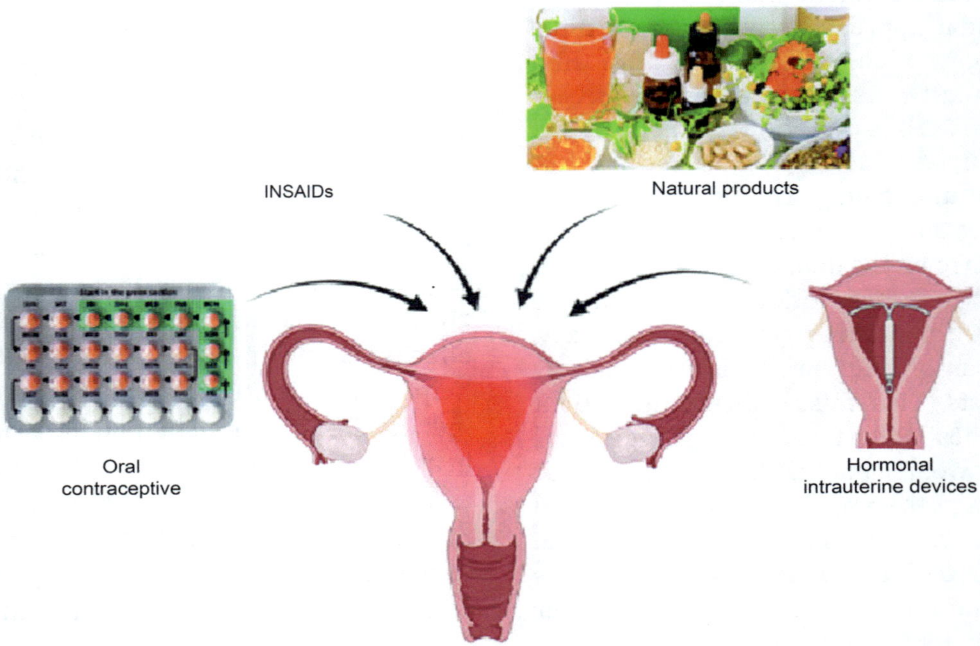

Figure 9.7. Pharmacological treatments for dysmenorrhea.

Source: https://www.researchgate.net/figure/Pharmacological-treatments-for-dysmenorrhea_fig4_371471994

Thus, complementary medicines like herbal medicines in the form of ginger and saffron are gaining prominence as supplementary or adjunctive therapy that may improve the symptoms of PMS without doing much harm (Areefin *et al.*, 2024). Through the creation of a balanced approach that utilizes both conventional prescriptions and alternatives, healthcare providers can best address patient needs. Furthermore, the integration of holistic care methods remains vital in efficient management of dysmenorrhea and PMS. Patients feel neglected as they present to healthcare providers with symptoms, making it necessary to have regular screening and open discussion of menstrual well-being (Carpenter *et al.*, 2017)..

By teaching women about treatment options, clinicians can empower women to explore the usefulness of prescription medication alongside lifestyle modification and complementary modalities. Such an integrative approach not only facilitates better symptom management but also promotes a better understanding of each woman's unique experience of dysmenorrhea and PMS. As the medical profession continues to develop, characterizing and addressing women's issues for drug risk and effectiveness can offer more educated decisions and, subsequently, improve their overall well-being. Combining evidence-guided prescribing decisions and patient-centered care can offer a route to improved control of these prevalent conditions.

9.1.5.3. Alternative Therapies

High prevalence of dysmenorrhea and premenstrual syndrome (PMS) in women has led to extensive research into alternative forms of treatment as viable treatment modalities. Conventional medical therapies incline towards pharmacologic management, yet most women seek relief through complementary and alternative medicine (CAM) treatment modalities. Growing interest in CAM also arises from the need for more holistic approaches involving physical, psychological, and lifestyle factors. Research has indicated that many other methods, including herbalism, dietary therapy, and massage, are used by women with cyclic perimenstrual pain and discomfort. This practice of self-prescription is an indication of the necessity for increased understanding and control of the use of CAM to ensure safe and effective treatment of those suffering from such conditions, since users are too often receiving no expert guidance in the selection of therapies (Abdul-Razzak *et al.*, 2016). In a study of the use of CAM, studies have found significant patterns of use among women who suffer from dysmenorrhea and PMS. Worthy of mention, women suffering from endometriosis and menstrual heaviness are apt to use the services of complementary health practitioners such as acupuncturists and masseurs. Based on data from the Australian Longitudinal Study of Women's Health, patients of PMS are more inclined to use the services of a variety of CAM providers than symptomatic women (Chapple *et al.*, 2016).

This suggests a correlation between symptom severity and desire for alternative therapies, underlining the absolute significance of healthcare providers considering such alternatives when writing prescriptions. Understanding what drives women to choose therapy can help treatment plans be tailored to meet specific needs and facilitate an integrative model of menstrual health. The effectiveness of CAM therapies in the management of dysmenorrhea and PMS symptoms is an active area of research. Although anecdotal benefits and positive self-reported results have been noted, there are as yet sparse empirical data available to support the efficacy of specific therapies. Women's CAM use is likely to yield perceived symptom relief, but rigorous clinical trials are needed to confirm these results and determine which modalities produce the greatest benefit. By placing value on both professional management and informed use, decision-makers in women's health can work toward creating complete, integrated models of care for safe integration of alternative therapies as a legitimate adjunct to mainstream medical treatment. Such a strategy not only respects women's choice but also fosters evidence-based use of CAM in the treatment of incapacitating menstrual disorders (Abdul-Razzak *et al.*, 2016).

Test Your Knowledge

1. What is the difference between primary and secondary dysmenorrhea?
2. How does dysmenorrhea affect the daily life of those who experience it?

9.2. Overview of Premenstrual Syndrome (PMS)

Learning Outcome

1. Identify the symptoms and diagnostic criteria of Premenstrual Syndrome (PMS)
2. Describe the prevalence and demographic patterns of PMS
3. Analyze the psychological and physical effects of PMS
4. Explain the causes of Premenstrual Syndrome (PMS)
5. Evaluate the treatment options available for managing PMS

The Premenstrual Syndrome consists of a variety of physical and mood disturbances occurring during the luteal phase of the menstrual cycle, typically resolving with menstruation. Characterized by a range of symptoms, including mood shifts, irritability, depression, physical discomfort, and changes in appetite, PMS afflicts a high percentage of menstruating women, with prevalence estimates ranging from 50% to 80% of women experiencing some aspect of these symptoms. The etiology of PMS is also multifactorial, involving changes in hormones, genetic predispositions, and psychosocial stressors as contributing factors to the severity of symptoms and diverse individual experiences. Understanding the complexities associated with PMS is important for medical practitioners in order to manage and treat patients with PMS. The management of PMS, in most instances, entails holistic practice through lifestyle modification, stress management, and dietary interventions, which are effective in eliminating the severity of symptoms in patients with PMS. Recent research puts a large proportion of attention on the importance of dietary interventions as effective measures for the treatment of PMS symptoms. Systematic review of important nutrients mentioned some supplements, such as vitamin D, zinc, calcium, and omega-3 fatty acids, that had measurable effects on alleviating symptoms of PMS and dysmenorrhea. The close relationship between diet and menstrual health makes it essential for healthcare providers to include nutritional assessment in a wider management plan. By integrating these nutritional recommendations, practitioners can empower patients with concrete steps on how to manage PMS, raising the quality of life for those afflicted with it. Moreover, educating patients on the likely role of nutrition can help improve patient knowledge and adoption of healthier lifestyle choices that can boost menstrual well-being and diminish the severity of PMS (Motzko *et al.*, 2024). In addition, knowledge about the effect of PMS on mental health is also crucial, as symptoms have been shown to have a significant impact on psychological well-being in addition to physical symptoms. Mood swings, anxiety, and depression are commonly used to describe individuals with

PMS, resulting in heavy disruption of daily life and interpersonal relationships. Thus, treating the psychological features of PMS is included in the overall treatment. Intervention may take the form of counseling, cognitive-behavioral therapy, and support groups, all of which provide people with coping strategies for emotional problems. PMS exacerbations of pre-existing mental illness are also possible, emphasizing the value of an active management plan. By integrating physical and psychological treatments in the same care field for PMS, practitioners are able to offer a more educated and integrated patient care that is necessary to effectively treat symptoms and enhance well-being overall (Greydanus *et al.*, 2012).

9.2.1. Symptoms and Diagnosis

Symptoms of dysmenorrhea and premenstrual syndrome (PMS) are physically and emotionally disabling, and they significantly diminish a woman's quality of life. Dysmenorrhea is best characterized by severe cramps during menstruation, which can radiate to the lower back, thighs, or abdomen. In addition to pain, others report gastrointestinal symptoms, headache, and fatigue with menstruation.

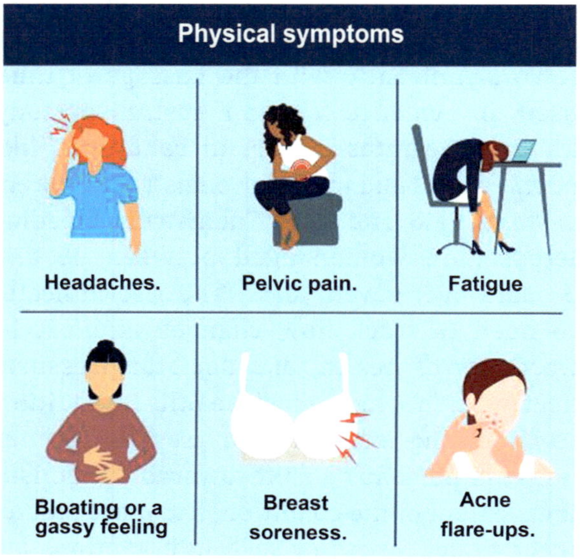

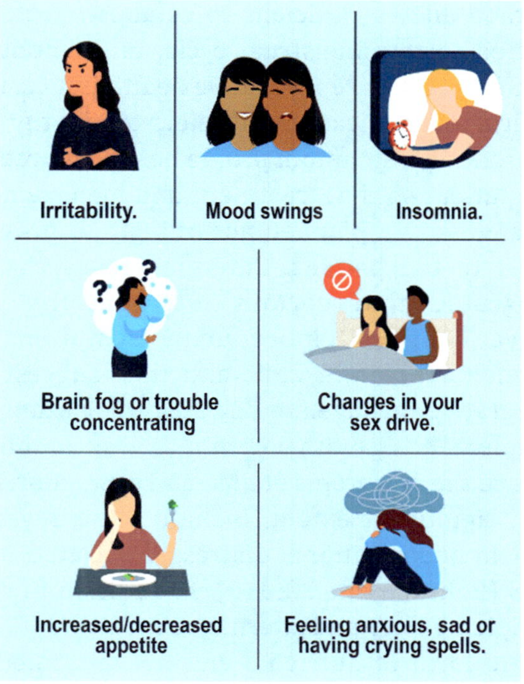
Irritability.
Mood swings
Insomnia.
Brain fog or trouble concentrating
Changes in your sex drive.
Increased/decreased appetite
Feeling anxious, sad or having crying spells.

Figure 9.8. Common physical and emotional symptoms of PMS.

Source: https://my.clevelandclinic.org/-/scassets/images/org/health/articles/24288-pms-premenstrual-syndrome

PMS has more symptoms, with mood swings, irritability, depression, and physical symptoms like bloating, breast tenderness, and headaches.

The coincidence of the two conditions necessitates careful differential diagnosis, as women may experience both PMS and dysmenorrhea concurrently, complicating the clinical presentation and management.

Clinical history and symptom appraisal commonly provide the groundwork for PMS and dysmenorrhea diagnosis because there are no definite laboratory tests for these conditions. Physicians usually employ a symptom diary in which women document their menstrual cycle, the onset time, duration of symptoms, and severity of symptoms to help aid diagnosis. This method allows clinicians to establish patterns related to the menstrual cycle, differentiating PMS from other reproductive health issues. It is critical for medical practitioners to identify the international symptom profile being endured by the patient so that treatment and management modalities are planned accordingly to provide relief to the patient. Emerging research has suggested that certain interventions can prove beneficial in reducing symptoms of dysmenorrhea and PMS, and thus suggest an integrative management strategy. For example, supplementing with vitamin D was found to reduce the symptoms of PMS and dysmenorrhea to a significant extent, including the severity of pain and emotional distress associated with PMS (Bahrami *et al.*, 2018). In addition to this, complementary and alternative medicine (CAM) in the form of nutrients and herbal remedies is widely employed in the management of the symptoms, with a number of women reporting beneficial efficacy from independently initiated CAM interventions (Abdul-Razzak *et al.*, 2016). A full understanding of such symptoms and the mechanisms underlying them can translate into more effective and focused care practices, ultimately facilitating improved patient outcomes and satisfaction.

9.2.2. Prevalence and Demographics

The prevalence of premenstrual syndrome (PMS) and dysmenorrhea is established in a range of groups and has significant relevance to the health and quality of life of women. Research indicates that most women experience both of these conditions during their reproductive lifetime, with research indicating 50% to 80% of menstruating women experiencing symptoms of PMS and dysmenorrhea. Interestingly, the occurrence of these conditions appears to differ with age and way of life. That is, younger females, particularly those aged in their late teens and early twenties, tend to complain of more severe symptoms, which has encouraged a few researchers to propose that differences in hormones and life stresses are major factors contributing to their symptomatology.

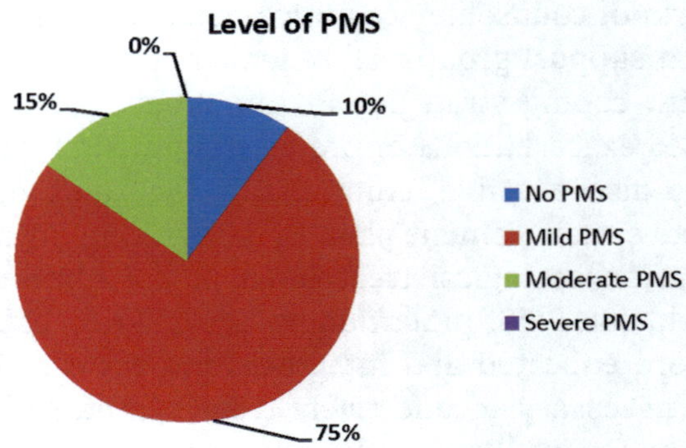

Figure 9.9. Prevalence of PMS among adolescent girls.

Source: https://www.semanticscholar.org/paper/Prevalence-of-Premenstrual-Syndrome-(-PMS-)-Among-Joseph-Nandini/9ff731809952babed80c42bd1682f8e48f9f0581/figure/1

Thus, it is important to know the demographic profile of the afflicted individuals in order to plan efficient intervention programs and create awareness about these prevalent health conditions. The longitudinal trend in women's health indicates that the prevalence rates for PMS and severe menstrual pain have grown significantly with the passage of time. Based on evidence from an Australian study, although the rates of certain conditions like endometriosis and irregular menstruation were constant, PMS and heavy menstrual bleeding increased in women aged between 28 and 33 years over seven years. The rise indicates the need to track how changes in lifestyle, awareness of health, and societal pressures affect women's menstrual health. In addition, the increasing trend of CAM usage by women with PMS portends a shift towards the holistic management of the condition, and more studies on the effectiveness of such interventions are required. The evolving profile of menstrual well-being necessitates ongoing exploration of demographic trends and symptom prevalence, as these factors can guide health practices and education.

Furthermore, the impact of PMS and dysmenorrhea has a broader reach than individual health, affecting women's activity levels in everyday life, such as participation in sports and education. Most athletes have reported feeling constrained by symptoms of menstruation, according to evidence that shows the overwhelming majority stating they cannot fully participate in sport activities during their periods. This reality has necessitated research into potential interventions, such as magnesium supplementation, that can address these conditions and improve performance. With the multifaceted adolescent athlete population, symptom prevalence and effective dietary interventions may be utilized to yield critical information to maximize physical well-being and sports participation. With the persistent struggle with PMS and dysmenorrhea in a variety of populations, this research must be a top priority to not only enhance women's quality of life but also to allow them to become empowered throughout every area of life.

9.2.3. Psychological and Physical Effects

Psychological effects of premenstrual syndrome (PMS) and dysmenorrhea are significant and have a far-reaching effect on a woman's overall health. Most women also develop emotional sensitivity in the luteal phase, leading to states of irritability, anxiety, and depressed moods. Hormonal disturbances present in these states further perpetuate mood instability, leading to interpersonal and professional relationship issues. Furthermore, chronic pain that arises from dysmenorrhea also leads to coping mechanisms to manage discomfort, such as avoidance behaviors, further depleting quality of life. As such, the concomitant effect of physical pain and emotional distress is thus cyclical in nature, which can have significant impairment on daily functioning and mental health outcomes and requires effective therapeutic interventions to treat both dimensions of these illnesses. Physically, PMS and dysmenorrhea are brought about by a range of manifestations, including severe abdominal cramping, headache, weakness, and gastrointestinal distress.

These presentations often wax and wane in intensity and have the potential to interfere with daily functioning tasks like work or social performance. In other cases, the pain is so debilitating that it leads to absenteeism, ultimately affecting academic or work performance. Additionally, new studies also mentioned the pharmacological benefit of curcumin, an extract of the spice Curcuma longa, in diminishing the severity of symptoms in PMS and dysmenorrhea. Curcumin, according to research, has been noted to possess anti-inflammatory and antioxidant properties, and these are potentially capable of alleviating pain and restoring hormonal balance, thereby improving physical symptoms as well as mood stability (Boroujeni *et al.*, 2024; Sharifipour *et al.*, 2024). Given the multidimensional effects of PMS and dysmenorrhea, it is necessary to treat them in an interdisciplinary style. Psychiatric treatment supplemented by physical therapies might be the optimum line of treatment for people affected by these disorders. It has been seen that lifestyle modifications, such as regular exercise, dietary optimization, and stress management, can be beneficial in reducing the symptomology of these illnesses. Further, consumption of dietary supplements, including curcumin, has also been shown to have beneficial impacts on relieving the physical and psychological dimensions of dysmenorrhea and PMS, and therefore, more extensive research in this regard is warranted. In the future, highlighting a multidisciplinary treatment strategy will be inevitable in the management of the complex relationship between psychological and physical impacts and ultimately enhancing the quality of life in women suffering from such common reproductive health conditions.

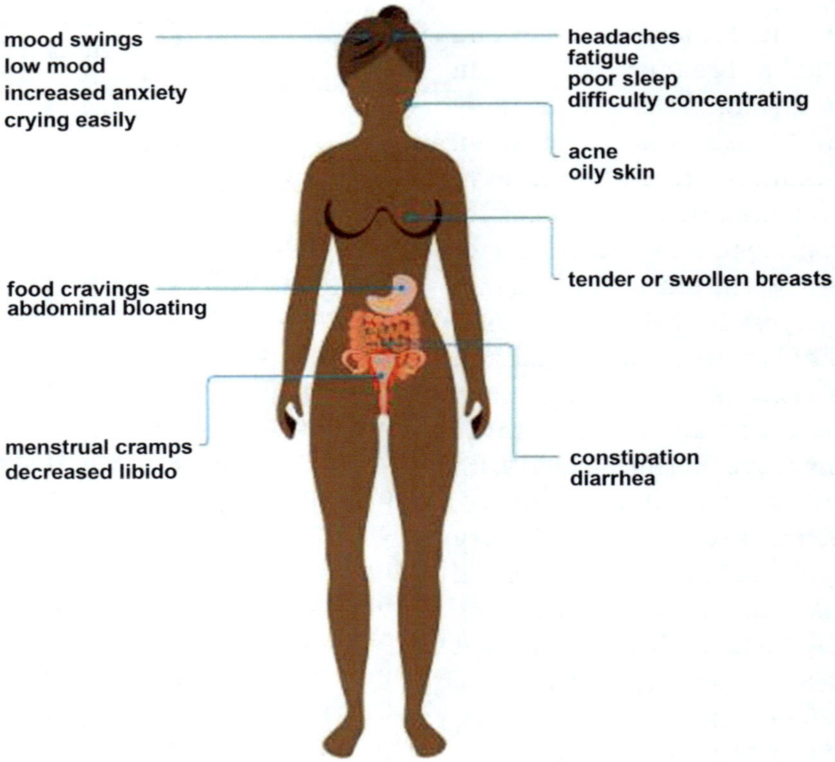

Figure 9.10. Effects of body of Premenstrual Syndrome (PMS).

Source: https://cdn-prod.medicalnewstoday.com/content/images/articles/325/325314/premenstrual-syndrome-pms-symptoms-illustration-in-different-areas-of-the-body.jpg

9.2.4. Causes of Premenstrual Syndrome (PMS)

The etiology of Premenstrual Syndrome (PMS) remains multifactorial and complex, including hormonal fluctuations, psychopathology, and lifestyle. The key feature is the cyclical variation of estrogen and progesterone during the menstrual cycle, which may influence the neurotransmitter systems concerned with mood regulation. Research has shown that such hormonal changes may alter the level of serotonin and other neurochemicals within the brain, leading to the physical and emotional symptoms of PMS. Women with pre-existing anxiety disorders or mood disorders are also more likely to have severe symptoms of PMS, implying some interaction between the hormonal changes and susceptibility at the psychological level. It is important to comprehend these interactions to design focused intervention strategies that deal with both the physiological and emotional sides of this syndrome.

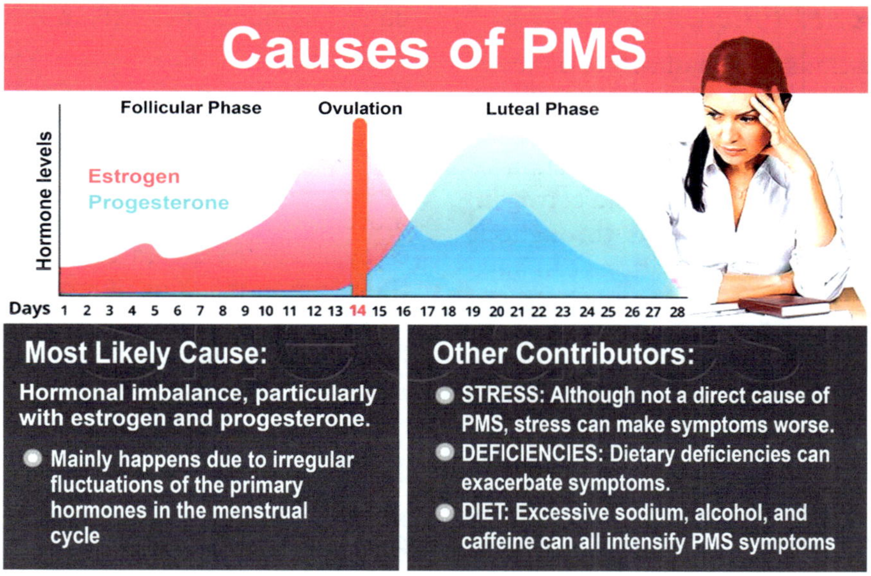

Figure 9.11. Causes of PMS.

Source: https://external-content.duckduckgo.com/iu/?u=https%3A%2F%2Fwww.shecares.com%2Fimgs%2F9%2F7%2Fd%2F38836%2Fpms-causes.jpg&f=1&nofb=1&ipt=b1622f638c03cc33c2909bc5459469a24ae79388c06fab88d74a5ae10bdea13b

Moreover, lifestyle and environmental aspects contribute importantly to the severity and timing of PMS. Stress, lack of sleep, bad eating habits, and physical inactivity can aggravate symptoms of PMS, as they show the interdependent nature of psychosocial health and physical well-being. It has been indicated by research that alcohol consumption in excess and caffeine consumption in excess possess the potential to augment symptoms of PMS, further highlighting the status of eating habits as reversible risk factors. Also, lack of exercise and obesity have been associated with increased severity of PMS, and this points toward the importance of life management in symptom control. Therefore, addressing these extrinsic factors by life modification, such as dietary changes and measures for control of stress, can offer beneficial effects in managing PMS in affected women. Polycystic ovary syndrome (PCOS) is an illness that may complicate the experience of PMS, commonly influencing its presentations. While the pathophysiology of PCOS is unknown, factors such as insulin resistance and hyperandrogenism have been observed to contribute to menstrual disturbance and psychoneurosis. The complexity illustrates the necessity for a multi-faceted approach to PMS, considering other coexistent reproductive disorders since they may worsen symptoms or complicate treatment regimens. Recent conference presentations highlight up-to-date research in this area, showing new methods of diagnosing menstrual-associated pain and the psychological implications involved with long-standing disorders like endometriosis. As a result, interdisciplinary models and personalized treatment regimens for both the physiological and psychosocial features of PMS and its syndromic equivalents like dysmenorrhea are coming under increasing prominence (Sadeghi *et al.*, 2022; Lamvu, 2021).

9.2.4.1. Hormonal Fluctuations

Hormonal fluctuations are an absolute concern when describing both premenstrual syndrome (PMS) and dysmenorrhea. The menstrual cycle is characterized by an intricate equilibrium of hormones, including progesterone and estrogen, that rise and fall at specific points throughout the cycle. These hormonal fluctuations can have a very significant influence on mood, sensitivity to pain, and physiological reaction. For example, under the influence of luteal progesterone elevation, most people experience an increase in emotional sensitivity and bodily aching. This dysregulation of hormones can worsen symptoms of PMS as well as dysmenorrhea, cause bothersome physical and psychological ramifications. Therefore, studying hormonal fluctuations is key to planning effective treatment modalities for these prevalent disorders. Hormonal change has end-organ manifestations that extend beyond simple distress and are significant for women's health. Dysmenorrhea, painful menstrual cramps, may be intensified by the release of prostaglandin, which is responsive to fluctuations in estrogen and progesterone. Increased prostaglandin levels lead to increased uterine contractions and enhanced sensitivity to pain. Also, research shows that vitamin D may play a role in controlling such hormonal fluctuations and in lowering symptoms associated with menstrual issues. When the role of vitamin D on menstrual symptoms was studied, participants were revealed to exhibit a considerable decline in the frequency of PMS and dysmenorrhea, possibly suggesting the role of hormonal balance in lowering symptoms (Bahrami *et al.*, 2018). Understanding the hormonal etiology of dysmenorrhea and PMS also lays out where interventions can be applied. As argued in the literature, vitamin D is a secosteroid hormone that can potentially suppress symptoms of PMS through its function in hormonal balance (Dabbagh *et al.*, 2017). Improvement following vitamin D supplementation indicates that balancing hormones will improve both physical and mental symptoms associated with the menstrual cycle. By placing emphasis on the significance of hormonal shifts, clinicians and researchers can more precisely design therapies, going beyond symptom management to a more holistic strategy that treats the causes of dysmenorrhea and PMS rather than merely their symptoms. This perspective highlights the need for ongoing research and clinical studies into effective therapies that can enhance well-being for sufferers.

9.2.4.2. Neurotransmitter Changes

Neurotransmitter fluctuations are key to the pathophysiology of dysmenorrhea and premenstrual syndrome (PMS), which directly affect the physical and emotional symptoms women experience. Throughout the menstrual cycle, changing levels of neurotransmitters such as serotonin, dopamine, and gamma-aminobutyric acid (GABA) can make the mood and pain response change. For example, serotonin, also known as the feel-good neurotransmitter, is involved in mood control and pain modulation. Decreased levels of serotonin tend to worsen depressive symptoms and enhance sensitivity to pain, aggravating dysmenorrhea. A sense of these changes in neurotransmitters is paramount in researching effective treatment measures to alleviate symptoms of PMS and dysmenorrhea, as highlighted in evidence validating the significant emotional weight these conditions create over quality of life (Franco-Antonio *et al.*, 2025).

Moreover, the way lifestyle affects neurotransmitter fluctuation further displays the complexity of PMS and dysmenorrhea. Evidence indicates that certain health habits, such as diet and exercise, influence the synthesis and function of neurotransmitters. For example, adherence to a healthy diet such as the Mediterranean diet has been associated with optimal balance in neurotransmitters, which can avert symptoms of dysmenorrhea and PMS. However, greater consumption of salty foods and sweets during the menstrual period is linked with heightened severity of dysmenorrhea, because such diets can lead to dysregulation of neurotransmitters. The interrelationship of exercises and mood also comes into focus, where exercise on a regular basis has been shown to enhance mood through enhanced serotonin levels, thereby reducing the severity of premenstrual emotional changes (Alatorre-Cruz *et al.*, 2024). In conclusion, the intricate connection between neurotransmitter changes and symptoms of dysmenorrhea and PMS renders a multi-dimensional treatment strategy not just preferable, but essential. By altering neurotransmitter imbalance through the process of adjusting lifestyle, women can be relieved of dysmenorrhea's symptoms and improve their emotional well-being. For instance, incorporating regular exercise and a healthy diet can enable better neurotransmitter function, ultimately improving the quality of life for the affected individuals. Furthermore, such comprehension can pave the way to novel therapeutic interventions of neurotransmitter pathways, with the promise of better control of PMS and dysmenorrhea. Further research on the matter will be significant in order to tailor effective treatment interventions for addressing such very prevalent conditions among women globally (Franco-Antonio *et al.*, 2025).

9.2.4.3. Genetic Predisposition

Genetic predisposition is also a significant factor in explaining the complexities of premenstrual syndrome (PMS) and dysmenorrhea. Family histories have determined that individuals with a family history of PMS are at higher risk of developing symptoms themselves. Familial clustering of such cases suggests that there are some genetic factors involved in influencing the severity and frequency of these conditions. For instance, studies have established that the incidence of PMS disorders is far greater in the event that the women have relatives experiencing such conditions, demonstrating the importance of genetic testing in the management of such menstrual disorders. In addition, the prevalence of mood swings and other symptoms that are typically suffered by PMS patients can also be partly explained through genetic predispositions, which would suggest that inherited traits might trigger emotional dysregulation during the menstrual cycle (Adedapo *et al.*, 2022).

We should also seek to broaden our viewpoint of PMS by examining neurotransmitter concentrations and hormonal fluctuations that are most likely influenced by genetics. Hormonal disturbances, particularly between estrogen and progesterone, have been implicated in the dysregulation of mood and somatic symptoms of PMS. Genetic influences can be on the synthesis and metabolism of hormones that, in turn, influence PMS symptomatology. Additionally, certain gene polymorphisms that influence neurotransmitter function, such as serotonin and dopamine, have been mentioned as potential causes of PMS experiences, testifying to genetic susceptibility being the foundation of biological reactions to hormonal changes (Atim *et al.*, 2022). In-depth exploration of these genetic factors can guide specific interventions and individualized treatment. The implication of genetic susceptibility not only impinges on individual clinical presentation but also on public health policy in managing dysmenorrhea and PMS. As an awareness of the genetic determinants of these menstrual conditions grows, clinicians will begin considering genetic screening as a routine component of evaluation in affected patients with refractory symptoms. Knowledge of individuals who are at high genetic risk can lead to earlier intervention and targeted therapeutic interventions, ultimately improving patient outcomes. Besides, further research on the genetic etiology of PMS and dysmenorrhea can be extended to training programs that aim at destigmatizing both, thus granting relief to those afflicted by them with appropriate care and attention for their well-being (Adedapo *et al.*, 2022; Atim *et al.*, 2022). Awareness of genetic susceptibility not only enhances treatment strategies for patients but also enhances public health discourse regarding women's reproductive health.

9.2.5. Treatment Options for Premenstrual Syndrome (PMS)

Treatment of the symptoms and impact of premenstrual syndrome (PMS) is a challenging process that could significantly enhance the quality of life in affected individuals. Lifestyle modifications, dietary modification, drug therapy, and complementary therapy may all be part of treatment. For instance, regular exercise has been reported to alleviate certain PMS symptoms, particularly emotional disturbances such as irritability and mood swings. In addition, the inclusion of a proper diet with high intake of complex carbohydrates, fiber, and essential vitamins and minerals can also prevent bodily symptoms accordingly, i.e., bloating and tiredness. Thus, patients are generally advised to live lives with lower stress levels, bringing overall health to the patient, thus making a comprehensive plan for managing the syndrome that includes physical as well as emotional aspects. Medications are an important aspect of treating PMS, particularly for people with severe symptoms. Non-steroidal anti-inflammatory drugs such as ibuprofen can be effectively utilized to alleviate pelvic pain and somatic symptoms associated with PMS. Also, genetic therapies in the form of oral contraceptives are typically employed to stabilize the hormonal disturbances that cause the symptoms of PMS. New research has explored new treatments, such as DLBS1442, a bioactive *Phaleria macrocarpa* extract, which targets hormonal imbalance through estrogen receptor regulation. Preliminary findings show that DLBS1442 has the potential to relieve PMS and PMS disorder menstrual cramps, presenting a hopeful direction of treatment intervention (Harzif *et al.*, 2015). The development of more specific drugs has the potential to improve treatment outcomes as work in this direction goes on. Aside from conventional remedies, complementary therapies are increasingly being considered as a potential source of relief for PMS symptoms. Therapies such as acupuncture, yoga, and herbal supplements have proved to be effective in reducing physical as well as psychological symptoms. The success of the treatment varies with individuals in most cases, and therefore, management needs an individualized approach. Interestingly, the understanding of various menstrual disorders like PMS has reconfirmed the importance of understanding the physiological origins of these disorders (Greydanus *et al.*, 2012). This overall knowledge is beneficial for better integration of conventional and alternative care and ultimately improves the overall management of PMS and allows individuals to receive quality care according to their specific needs.

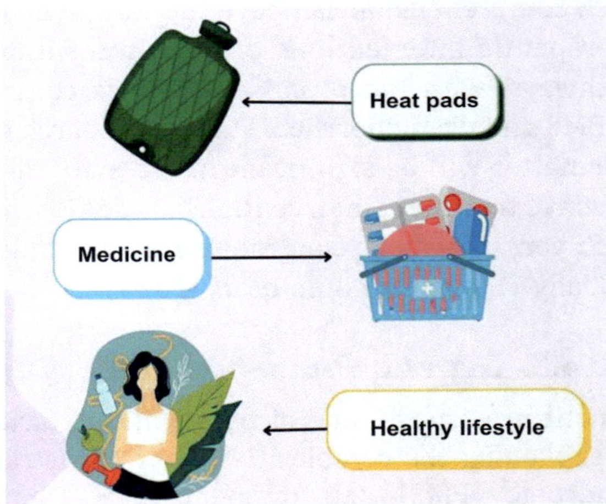

Figure 9.12. Treatment for premenstrual syndrome (PMS).

Source: https://bunny-wp-pullzone-kugxoqmv29.b-cdn.net/wp-content/uploads/2024/03/treatments-for-pms-1024x1024.jpg

9.2.5.1. Lifestyle Modifications

Lifestyle modification is necessary for managing premenstrual syndrome (PMS) and dysmenorrhea. Both are conditions with extreme pain and emotional distress that can largely affect a woman's quality of life. Research has established that stress plays a significant role in the severity of menstrual symptoms. Severe levels of stress can exacerbate menstrual disorders, including PMS and dysmenorrhea, thereby necessitating effective stress-reduction measures. Through life changes, such as regular exercise, sleep, and relaxation strategies, stress levels among women can be reduced, thus potentially remitting menstrual symptoms. Healthcare providers should instruct patients in stress self-behaviors directed at stress, which can be positively related to the menstrual cycle and health (Gilbrech *et al.*, 2020). Besides stress management, nutrition modification is required to alleviate dysmenorrhea and symptoms of PMS. A healthy diet with nutrients can positively affect hormonal balance and alleviate pain. Specific dietary elements like omega-3 fatty acids, calcium, and magnesium are said to have anti-inflammatory and analgesic effects against menstrual pain. The avoidance of caffeine, sugar, and excessive sodium intake may also alleviate bloating and mood swings during PMS. Studies show that women undergoing these dietary modifications see their frequency of menstrual pain and mood disturbance diminish. Thus, enhancing nutrition education can allow women to adopt healthy eating habits that promote reproductive health and reduce menstrual disorders (Rajipet *et al.*, 2021). In addition, physical exercise also serves as another lifestyle modification that may reverse the effects of dysmenorrhea and PMS. Exercise not only helps relieve stress but also has direct effects on menstrual symptoms. Physical activity increases blood flow and releases endorphins, which are the body's analgesics. Thus, women who incorporate even small amounts of physical activity into their routine have reported that there is an enhancement in their pain perception and mood during the time of menstruation. In addition, team sports such as aerobics or yoga can also give social support, contributing to mental health. Combining these physical activity interventions is a significant step towards developing an integrative treatment plan for dysmenorrhea and PMS, demonstrating that lifestyle change is a robust intervention (Gilbrech *et al.*, 2020).

9.2.5.2. Medications and Supplements

The management of dysmenorrhea and premenstrual syndrome (PMS) may include a combination of medication and supplements with the intention of symptomatic improvement and general health. Nonsteroidal anti-inflammatory agents (NSAIDs) like ibuprofen and naproxen are often used since they can alleviate pain by reducing inflammation. They are effective in managing the menstrual cramps that come with dysmenorrhea and also provide some relief for symptoms of PMS. Furthermore, hormonal contraceptives are frequently used because they regulate menstrual cycles and have the potential to reduce the severity of dysmenorrhea by suppressing ovulation. However, medication choice needs to be personalized and take into account the history and preferences of each patient, as some patients can develop side effects or contraindications to using standard pharmaceutical preparations. Besides the usual drugs, more and more studies corroborate that some dietary supplements have the capacity to alleviate PMS and dysmenorrhea as well. Studies indicate that simple nutrients such as omega-3 fatty acids, zinc, calcium, and vitamin D can help provide symptom relief for both menstrual diseases. These supplements have been shown to help with hormonal balance and the reduction of inflammation, both factors that are significant components in both PMS and dysmenorrhea outcomes. Omega-3 fatty acids, for instance, often found in fish oil, were discovered to be linked with diminished menstrual pain and improved mood stability. Application of these supplements as a part of the treatment protocol can provide an adjunctive approach, allowing patients to address their symptoms from a holistic stance while potentially reducing pharmacological therapy dependency (Motzko *et al.*, 2024). The search for herbal remedies for PMS also provides a means to enhance traditional treatments. Ginger, turmeric, and Ashwagandha, these ancient herbs, have proven to have analgesic, anti-inflammatory, and mood-enhancing properties.

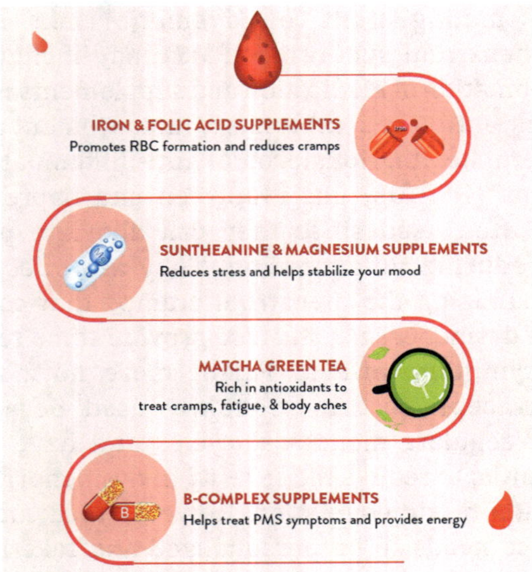

Figure 9.13. Four Supplements to Make PMS Bearable.

Source: https://cdn.shopify.com/s/files/1/0240/2942/9840/files/4_Supplements_to_Make_PMS_1_2048x2048.jpg?v=1672995178

These therapies are potential options for women seeking natural means of alleviating PMS symptoms while minimizing the side effects associated with pharmacological interventions. Research indicates that these herbal therapies can improve both the physical and emotional components of PMS, with enhanced quality of life in patients. However, additional scientific studies are required to establish standard doses, evaluate long-term safety, and elucidate the mechanisms of action of these natural interventions in order to validate their effectiveness in the clinical setting (Areefin *et al.*, 2024).

9.2.5.3. Psychological Interventions

The psychological dimensions of dysmenorrhea and premenstrual syndrome (PMS) deserve to be taken into serious account because the interaction between emotional state and pain symptomatology can exacerbate the composite experience of those suffering from them. Psychological interventions such as cognitive-behavioral therapy (CBT), mindfulness training, and relaxation therapies have emerged as stronger contenders as effective alternatives to traditional pharmacological management. By focusing on the reversal of negative thinking patterns and enhancing coping mechanisms, these therapies cover the emotional aspects that are involved in menstrual-associated disturbances. Evidence suggests that women undergoing psychological therapy demonstrate a reduction in both the intensity and frequency of PMS symptoms, attesting to the efficiency of such procedures in their removal. These psychological treatments not only guarantee the reduction of the physiological manifestations of dysmenorrhea but also aim to empower women by learning to manage their symptoms more effectively in the long term.

When researching the effectiveness of various psychological treatments, it is clear that learning from individual experiences is essential for effective treatment. The hypothesis for treatment validity underlies the premise that individually designed interventions, directed at PMS-specific target behaviors, will yield improved outcomes. The case of distinguishing between symptoms of depression and behavioral change illustrates a targeted approach, raising the probability of reducing turmoil related to PMS. By assessing those symptoms, clinicians can implement more targeted methods, which lead to dramatic quality-of-life improvements. The requirement for specific therapies highlights the limitations of non-specific treatments and necessitates rigorous assessment to manage the multivariate manifestations of PMS (Leonard *et al.*, 1985). This will not only promote better symptom management but also assist in the development of resilience in the psychological condition of women with these illnesses.

A combination of herbal medicines along with psychological therapies is a novel way of managing dysmenorrhea and PMS. There are a number of traditional herbal treatments, such as ginger, yellow turmeric, and Ashwagandha, with extensive documented therapeutic effects that can be employed to complement psychological measures. These encompass analgesic, anti-inflammatory, and mood-stabilizing effects, which play a central role in alleviating physiological pain and emotional distress caused by menstrual disorders. Recent literature calls for the investigation of action mechanisms of the above herbal treatments to delineate safety and efficacy (Areefin *et al.*, 2024). Moreover, the integration of psychological therapies and herbal remedies might also enable women to take power through enhanced self-control strategies. With ongoing progress in research, the effectiveness of this integrated method may pave the way for more tailored treatment options for addressing the multifaceted nature of dysmenorrhea and PMS.

Test Your Knowledge

1. Which demographic groups are most commonly affected by Premenstrual Syndrome (PMS)?
2. What are the common psychological and physical effects experienced during PMS?

SUMMARY

The subtle interaction between dysmenorrhea and premenstrual syndrome (PMS) underscores the necessity for tailored management regimens that meet the unique needs of afflicted patients. Dysmenorrhea, or cramping pain with menses, often co-occurs with PMS, a constellation of psychological and somatic complaints that can potentially significantly influence functioning. Understanding this interaction is crucial in order to institute appropriate treatment regimens. Recent research identifies the potential of new treatments, such as phytotherapeutic diet supplements, that have been seen to efficiently reduce symptoms of PMS without adverse effects. Hence, exploring integrative systems can enhance women's quality of life, with it being a major component in curing these common reproductive system issues (Herrera *et al.*, 2024). Drug therapy is also a crucial component in treating PMS and dysmenorrhea. Recent evidence regarding the efficacy of 0.5 mg dienogest has shown declining, and in some cases dramatic, decreases in PMS-like symptoms compared to conventional treatments such as combined oral contraceptives. The compelling evidence that appears to indicate that the majority of women experienced a marked reduction of symptoms over a six-month period also serves to emphasize the place of individualized treatment regimens. Such comparative effectiveness studies are essential to guiding clinical practice and informing treatment decisions that are specific to individual women (Yokosuka, 2024). As the research evolves, these results can pave the way for therapies focusing on both symptom improvement and quality of life. Finally, the need for ongoing research into the psychosocial symptoms of both dysmenorrhea and PMS cannot be overstated. Variables such as stress, lifestyle habits, and affect all contribute significantly to symptom severity and quality of life in the patient. A multidisciplinary approach that incorporates both clinical management and global well-being modalities, stress reduction, and dietary changes is essential. In understanding the complexity of these conditions, health providers are better positioned to help women manage their experiences more effectively, ultimately developing a supportive climate that promotes physical and mental well-being. Through higher levels of awareness and understanding, the potential for marked improvement in care and outcomes for women suffering from dysmenorrhea and PMS is even more probable.

Premenstrual syndrome (PMS) and dysmenorrhea are significant health conditions in the majority of menstruating individuals, affecting their quality of life. Dysmenorrhea can be divided into primary or secondary and is characterized by the presence of painful menstruation that regularly affects regular daily activities. The condition is quite common among women in the reproductive age group, according to available evidence, with age and lifestyle influencing its prevalence rate. The effects of dysmenorrhea extend beyond short-term pain, possibly leading to the development of long-term reproductive health issues if ineffective. The multifaceted nature of dysmenorrhea is critical to grasp in order to develop effective interventions for reducing symptoms as well as quality of life overall, particularly through evidence-based measures of symptoms that capture the multifaceted illness experience of women with menstrual pain and interference in daily functioning (Chen *et al.*, 2015). In addition to dysmenorrhea, premenstrual syndrome entails a spectrum of physical and affective symptoms that occur during the luteal phase and remit with menstruation. PMS affects women's psychological status, causing significant distress and disrupting social and occupational functioning. Diagnostic assessment of PMS has led to the identification of numerous symptom dimensions in addition to severity, including frequency and duration. Interventions against these symptoms, e.g., cognitive-behavioral therapy (CBT), have shown promising effects on enhancing management strategies. A pilot study in which a CBT program was investigated in young women with intellectual disabilities recently demonstrated the potential of individualized interventions in significantly enhancing coping abilities and pain management (Kennedy *et al.*, 2014). These programs place a strong focus on appreciating the importance of establishing a comprehensive understanding of the psychological aspects of premenstrual syndrome that may impact symptom expression and quality of life. In addition, accurate measurement of dysmenorrhea and PMS symptoms is key to effective management and intervention. Several self-report symptom measures have been used to examine these conditions, but the available literature indicates that none of them is optimal for assessing the full range of symptoms of dysmenorrhea. Dysmenorrhea-specific measures may be more helpful, but they often require revision and further psychometric testing to ascertain their value. Refining the accuracy and relevance of these measures can guide studies and guide clinical practice, ultimately allowing healthcare practitioners to better treat the unique experience and needs of women with dysmenorrhea and PMS. Improved understanding of symptomatology will be crucial to the development of effective treatments that take into account both the psychological and physiological factors of these common yet disabling disorders (Chen *et al.*, 2015).

KEY TERMS FROM THIS CHAPTER

- Primary Dysmenorrhea
- Prostaglandins
- Menstrual Cramps
- Adenomyosis
- Premenstrual Syndrome (PMS)
- Irritability
- Headache
- Nausea
- Secondary Dysmenorrhea
- Pelvic Pain
- Endometriosis
- Uterine Contractions
- Mood Swings
- Fatigue
- Breast Tenderness
- Anxiety

CRITICAL THINKING QUESTIONS

1. **Primary dysmenorrhea is caused mainly by:**
   a. Pelvic infection
   b. Endometriosis
   c. Increased production of prostaglandins
   d. Uterine fibroids
2. **Which of the following is a common symptom of Premenstrual Syndrome (PMS)?**
   a. Heavy menstrual bleeding
   b. Mood swings and irritability
   c. Amenorrhea
   d. Infertility
3. **Secondary dysmenorrhea is most commonly associated with:**
   a. Structural abnormalities such as endometriosis or fibroids
   b. Hormonal imbalance only
   c. Stress alone
   d. Vitamin deficiency
4. **Which hormone fluctuation is most commonly implicated in the development of PMS symptoms?**
   a. Increased progesterone before menstruation
   b. Decreased estrogen before menstruation
   c. Fluctuations in estrogen and progesterone levels
   d. Increased testosterone levels
5. **A common treatment option for managing primary dysmenorrhea includes:**
   a. Antibiotics
   b. Nonsteroidal anti-inflammatory drugs (NSAIDs)
   c. Hormone replacement therapy
   d. Antidepressants

Short Answer Questions

1. What is dysmenorrhea and how is it classified?
2. Name two common symptoms of dysmenorrhea.
3. What causes primary dysmenorrhea?
4. What is premenstrual syndrome (PMS)?
5. List three common symptoms of PMS.
6. How do dysmenorrhea and PMS differ in their timing and symptoms?

Answer to Critical Thinking Questions

1. (c) 2. (b) 3. (a) 4. (c) 5. (b)

REFERENCES

1. Abdul-Razzak, A., Adams, J., Adegbesan-Omilabu, M., AlBraik, F., Awad, A., Baines, A., *et al.* (2016). A critical review of complementary and alternative medicine uses by women with cyclic perimenstrual pain and discomfort: A focus upon prevalence, patterns and applications of use and users' motivations, information seeking and self-perceived efficacy. https://opus.lib.uts.edu.au/bitstream/10453/47546/6/9DA1B635-C094-4659-A8E5-4E04E0420352%20am.pdf (accessed on 14th June 2025).
2. Adams, J., Fisher, C., Hickman, L., Sibbritt, D., *et al.* (2018). Cyclic perimenstrual pain and discomfort and Australian women's associated use of complementary and alternative medicine: A longitudinal study. https://opus.lib.uts.edu.au/bitstream/10453/123571/4/Cyclic%20perimenstrual%20pain%20and%20discomfort%20and%20the%20associated%20use%20by%20Australian%20women%20of%20complementary%20and%20alternative%20medicine.%20.pdf (accessed on 14th June 2025).
3. Adedapo, E. A., Eduviere, A. T., Ojezele, M. O., Wool, A., *et al.* (2022). Mood swing during menstruation: Confounding factors and drug use. https://core.ac.uk/download/544240243.pdf (accessed on 14th June 2025).
4. Alatorre-Cruz, J. M., Alatorre-Cruz, G. C., Marín-Cevada, V., & Carreño-López, R. (2024). Dysmenorrhea and premenstrual syndrome in association with health habits in the Mexican population: A cross-sectional study. *Healthcare, 12*. https://www.semanticscholar.org/paper/ede523048f26433bd7bc6949c92fb39a84f4e8db (accessed on 14th June 2025).
5. Andrews, M. A., Nishi Roshini, K., & Hibina, P. (2020). Common menstrual disorders in adolescent girls attending a tertiary care center. https://core.ac.uk/download/539902176.pdf (accessed on 14th June 2025).
6. Areefin, P., Hossen, S., Mohd Yusri, M. Y., Mohd Yunus, R., Roni, R., *et al.* (2024). Traditional herbal interventions for premenstrual syndrome management: A comprehensive literature review. https://core.ac.uk/download/613051618.pdf (accessed on 14th June 2025).
7. Atim, E., Lwanira Nassozi, C., Nabushawo Okecho, F., Ndagire, F., *et al.* (2022). Social-demographic factors associated with premenstrual syndrome among female university students in Central Uganda: A cross-sectional study. https://core.ac.uk/download/539828038.pdf (accessed on 14th June 2025).
8. Badkur, D., Chauhan, D. S., Singh, S., Sinha, R., *et al.* (2018). Premenstrual syndrome and its association with menstrual profile among female students of colleges in Ujjain City, Madhya Pradesh, India. https://core.ac.uk/download/539910259.pdf (accessed on 14th June 2025).
9. Bahrami, A., Avan, A., Rastgar-Moghadam, A., El Gilany, A., Ghasemi, F., Nejati Salehkhani, F., Ferns, G. A., *et al.* (2018). High dose vitamin D supplementation can improve menstrual problems, dysmenorrhea and premenstrual syndrome in adolescents. https://core.ac.uk/download/144580202.pdf (accessed on 14th June 2025).
10. Baumer, H., Powell, A., & Richardson, R. (2024). The effects of magnesium supplementation for adolescent female athletes with PMS or dysmenorrhea: An intervention. https://core.ac.uk/download/621633692.pdf (accessed on 14th June 2025).
11. Boroujeni, Z. S., Heidari-Soureshjani, S., & Sherwin, C. (2024). Effects of *Curcuma longa* (turmeric) and curcumin on the premenstrual syndrome and dysmenorrhea: A systematic

review. *Journal of Endometriosis and Pelvic Pain Disorders, 16*, 33–44. https://www.semanticscholar.org/paper/bf2a3884ea0ef72330e51a33b9a07e68ce5aaae6 (accessed on 14th June 2025).

12. Burchett, T. S. (2013). Efficacy of the Arrigo Techniques of Maya Abdominal Therapy on dysmenorrhea symptoms in women. https://core.ac.uk/download/214063711.pdf (accessed on 14th June 2025).
13. Carpenter, J. S., Chen, C. X., Draucker, C. B., Shieh, C., *et al.* (2017). Reasons women do not seek health care for dysmenorrhea. https://core.ac.uk/download/129148678.pdf (accessed on 14th June 2025).
14. Chapple, A., Direkvand-Moghadam, A., Fugh-Berman, A., Girman, A., Milewicz, A., Sharma, A., Steinsbekk, A., *et al.* (2016). The use of complementary and alternative medicine by 7427 Australian women with cyclic perimenstrual pain and discomfort: A cross-sectional study. https://core.ac.uk/download/pdf/81218304.pdf (accessed on 14th June 2025).
15. Chen, C. X., Kwekkeboom, K. L., & Ward, S. E. (2015). Self-report pain and symptom measures for primary dysmenorrhea: A critical review. https://core.ac.uk/download/286682354.pdf (accessed on 14th June 2025).
16. Cooper, A., Csontos, J., Edwards, A., Edwards, L., *et al.* (2024). Supporting women, girls and people who menstruate to participate in physical activity–Rapid evidence summary. https://core.ac.uk/download/621692400.pdf (accessed on 14th June 2025).
17. Critchley, H., Babayev, E., Bulun, S. E., Clark, S., Garcia-Grau, I., Gregersen, P. K., Kilcoyne, A., *et al.* (2020). Menstruation: Science and society. *American Journal of Obstetrics and Gynecology, 223*, 624–664. https://doi.org/10.1016/j.ajog.2020.06.004 (accessed on 14th June 2025).
18. Dabbagh, A., & Rajaei, S. (2017). The molecular mechanisms of vitamin D effects on alleviating premenstrual syndrome pain. https://core.ac.uk/download/483640620.pdf (accessed on 14th June 2025).
19. Franco-Antonio, C., Santano-Mogena, E., & Cordovilla-Guardia, S. (2025). Dysmenorrhea, premenstrual syndrome, and lifestyle habits in young university students in Spain: A cross-sectional study. *Journal of Nursing Research, 33*, e374. https://www.semanticscholar.org/paper/255dba09a1121deda46efff4c369452cf5720b2a (accessed on 14th June 2025).
20. Gilbrech, K. I. (2020). The impact of stress on the menstrual cycle. https://core.ac.uk/download/304636274.pdf (accessed on 14th June 2025).
21. Greydanus, D. E., Omar, H. A., & Sorrel, S. (2012). Menstrual disorders in the adolescent female. https://core.ac.uk/download/232583670.pdf (accessed on 14th June 2025).
22. Harzif, A. K., Hestiantoro, A., Natadisastra, M., Pratama, G., *et al.* (2015). The effectiveness of *Phalleria macrocarpa* bioactive fraction in alleviating endometriosis and/or adenomyosis related pain. https://media.neliti.com/media/publications/60762-EN-the-effectiveness-of-phalleria-macrocarp.pdf (accessed on 14th June 2025).
23. Herrera, A., Al Adib, M., Rodríguez, A. B., & Carrasco, C. (2024). Effects of the PREMEN-CALM® in the management of the premenstrual syndrome: A randomized, double-blind, placebo-controlled pilot study. *Journal of Dietary Supplements, 21*, 495–511. https://www.semanticscholar.org/paper/5463597c6d3380fec569e785eb5e7a2f25f9e1f4 (accessed on 14th June 2025).

24. Johnson, A. M., Menon, C. P. J., Narmadha, M., Sabu, B., *et al.* (2023). Exploring the salient factors influencing menstrual health and hygiene: A review. https://core.ac.uk/download/591404969.pdf (accessed on 14th June 2025).

25. Juniar, D. (2015). Epidemiology of dysmenorrhea among female adolescents in Central Jakarta. https://media.neliti.com/media/publications/150772-EN-epidemiology-of-dysmenorrhea-among-femal.pdf (accessed on 14th June 2025).

26. Katib, Y., Almehmadi, M., Alhajaji, F., Alqorashi, S., Almajnooni, F., Alshinawi, M. A., & Marghalani, R. (2024). Prevalence of primary dysmenorrhea and its effect on the quality of life among female students at Umm Al-Qura University. *Cureus.* https://doi.org/10.7759/cureus.72136 (accessed on 14th June 2025).

27. Kennedy, S., McGuire, B. E., O'Higgins, S., Sarma, K., *et al.* (2014). Evaluation of a group-based cognitive behavioral therapy programmed for menstrual pain management in young women with intellectual disabilities: Protocol for a mixed methods controlled clinical trial. https://core.ac.uk/download/76981093.pdf (accessed on 14th June 2025).

28. Kustriyanti, D., & Rahayu, H. (2020). Prevalence of premenstrual syndrome and quality of life among health science college students. https://core.ac.uk/download/480550077.pdf (accessed on 14th June 2025).

29. Lamvu, G. (2021). Abstracts from the International Pelvic Pain Society (IPPS) Annual Scientific Meeting on Pelvic Pain 2020. *PAIN Reports, 6*, e940–e940. https://doi.org/10.1097/pr9.0000000000000940 (accessed on 14th June 2025).

30. Leonard, S. R. (1985). The treatment validity of identifying and treating depression and behavior change symptom clusters in women complaining of the premenstrual syndrome. https://core.ac.uk/download/345088550.pdf (accessed on 14th June 2025).

31. Motzko, E. R. (2024). Accessible dietary interventions for the prevention and management of common menstrual disorders: A systematic review. https://core.ac.uk/download/624274635.pdf (accessed on 14th June 2025).

32. Rajipet, P., Rakuditti, S. R., Rathod, P., Valmeekam, S., *et al.* (2021). The prospective study on prevalence of menstrual disorders in school-going adolescents at Sangareddy district, Telangana. https://core.ac.uk/download/543137113.pdf (accessed on 14th June 2025).

33. Raule, E. B., Sapulete, I., & Engka, J. N. A. (2025). Relationship between premenstrual syndrome (PMS) and appetite in female medical students at Sam Ratulangi University. *Journal Impresi Indonesia.* https://www.semanticscholar.org/paper/bed20272d0604cf14e0278639b0dd86e61f3d1e2 (accessed on 14th June 2025).

34. Sadeghi, H. M., Adeli, I., Călina, D., Docea, A. O., Mousavi, T., Daniali, M., Nikfar, S., *et al.* (2022). Polycystic ovary syndrome: A comprehensive review of pathogenesis, management, and drug repurposing. *International Journal of Molecular Sciences, 23*, 583. https://doi.org/10.3390/ijms23020583 (accessed on 14th June 2025).

35. Sharifipour, F., Siahkal, S. F., Qaderi, K., Mohaghegh, Z., Zahedian, M., & Azizi, F. (2024). Effect of curcumin on dysmenorrhea and symptoms of premenstrual syndrome: A systematic review and meta-analysis. *Korean Journal of Family Medicine, 45*, 96–104. https://www.semanticscholar.org/paper/f63228034b783429b683ada9cfe006fa39a0f912 (accessed on 14th June 2025).

36. Suri, S., & Khuraseva, A. (2024). Statistical analysis of primary dysmenorrhea and mittelschmerz syndrome among female students of Kursk. *Special Journal of the Medical Academy and Other Life Sciences.* https://www.semanticscholar.org/paper/1de139e0ac16a82f7f5af1b3b20572bcaf2b55a2 (accessed on 14th June 2025).

37. Yokosuka, H. (2024). Efficacy of 0.5 mg dingoes' tablets in treating premenstrual syndrome-like symptoms: A comparative study with a low-dose estrogen–progestin combination. *Endocrines.* https://www.semanticscholar.org/paper/ee575c2f0fb00a07549cba171bc54d932e51c92c (accessed on 14th June 2025).

BENIGN LESIONS OF THE VULVA, VAGINA, AND CERVIX

10

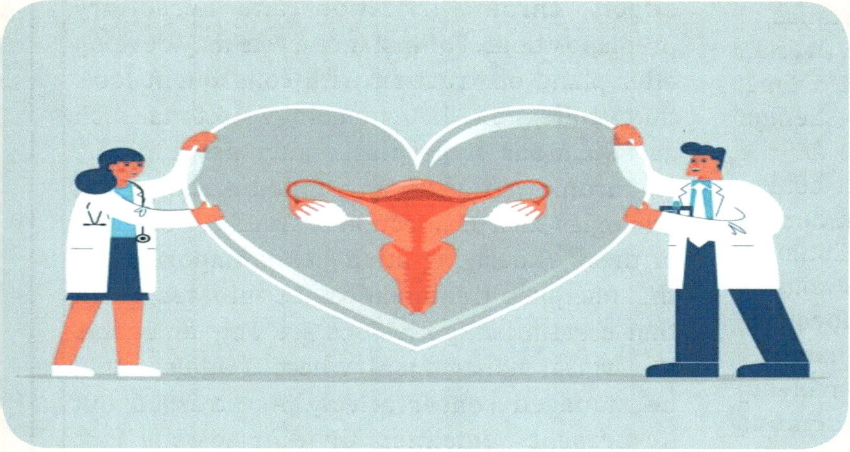

LEARNING OBJECTIVES

After studying this chapter, you will be able to:

1. Discuss the types of benign lesions
2. Explain the vulvar lesions, vaginal lesions, and cervical lesions
3. Understand the symptoms and diagnosis of benign lesions of the vulva, vagina, and cervix
4. Define treatment options for benign lesions of the vulva, vagina, and cervix

Introduction

The vulvar, vaginal, and cervical benign lesion pathology consists of a great spectrum of tumors and polypoid lesions that are not cancerous but demand clinical attention due to their impact on women's health. They may differ significantly in nature, presentation, and treatment. It is essential to recognize such conditions so that an accurate diagnosis and effective treatment can be made, as benign lesions may simulate malignant processes or have symptoms resulting in surgery. Increased awareness among clinicians of the subtle but important differences between benign and malignant conditions allows for more informed decision-making regarding patient care and management streams. This concise review will address prominent forms of benign lesions, their clinicopathologic characteristics, histology, and relevance to women's health. In the numerous benign lesions, fibroepithelial polyps of the vagina (FEPV) are sterling examples of the complexity encountered in this category. With a core of connective tissue covered by benign squamous epithelium, the polyps are rare, and there have been only a few reported cases in the literature. Their presence highlights the heterogeneity of benign lesions, composed of connective and epithelial structures that may complicate diagnosis. Fibroepithelial stromal polyps, as observed, can present in a non-vaginal environment, affecting the vulva and cervix alike, and necessitate comprehensive familiarity with their potential sites and presentations (Nongo *et al.*, 2024). Each case is a lesson in and of itself, contributing to the larger tale of benign lesions and stressing the importance of differential diagnoses in clinical practice. Ovarian neoplasms, or the serous cystadenofibroma, are yet another important category of benign lesions in demonstrating the potential for the simultaneous development of different benign tumors. Though labeled as benign, such tumors carry serious clinical consequences. Collision tumors, wherein two distinct benign neoplasms occur within the same anatomical location, are a very rare phenomenon. For instance, there have been documented cases involving serous cystadenofibromas and mucinous cysts in conjunction, which underscores the significance of thorough examination and surgical management (Kumar *et al.*, 2025). Such a case not only poses a diagnostic challenge but also makes a point regarding the overall significance of benign gynecologic disease, highlighting the clinician's need to be aware in order to effectively navigate the complexities of women's health.

Definition of Benign Lesions

In medical terminology, benign lesions refer to non-cancerous growths or abnormalities that can occur in certain tissues of the body, including the vulva, vagina, and cervix. Benign lesions are special in the sense that they cannot invade the surrounding tissues nor migrate to other sites in the body as cancerous tumors do. Certain common benign lesions of these tissues are cysts, papillomas, and hyperplastic lesions. While the majority are asymptomatic, benign lesions can, especially, disturb patients with discomfort or aesthetic distress. Recognition of the definition and classification of benign lesions is essential to ensure proper diagnosis and treatment, as their presence may, at times, mimic more threatening processes and require additional workup to offer the patient proper treatment.

The pathogenesis of benign lesions tends to encompass many causes, including hormonal effects, chronic irritation, and hereditary predispositions. For instance, cysts may develop after gland obstruction with consequent local fluid collection. In gynecology, lesions such as squamous hyperplasia may develop due to chronic irritation and inflammation from etiologies such as infection or trauma. Detection of these underlying etiologies is important so that adequate treatment can be initiated, given that certain benign lesions are only amenable to surgical management, whereas others could be managed conservatively. As stressed out by present guidelines, dividing lesions into categories based on their characteristics not only aids in the diagnosis but also directs follow-up management plans best suited for addressing individual cases of the patients (Perkins *et al.*, 2020). Since benign lesions are mostly not a risk of any extent as in the case of malignant conditions, patient education remains a major portion of their treatment. Doctors are responsible for educating people about the value of routine screenings and monitoring, particularly among groups at higher risk of cervical complications. It is core to adhering to stipulated screening guidelines, with the aim of ensuring patients engage in active practice of health. It also helps in the elimination of fear associated with potential abnormalities, thus granting women the liberty of approaching physicians without fear. Evidence-based practice development, as reflected through enhanced risk factor knowledge of related lesions, enables the capacity to answer patient questions effectively while favoring a compassionate clinical atmosphere (Oronsky *et al.*, 2017).

Importance of Studying Benign Lesions in Gynecological Health

The investigation of benign gynecologic lesions is paramount to patient outcome improvement and clinical practice. They consist of a range of non-malignant lesions, which can potentially affect women's quality of life significantly. By evaluating their prevalence, causation, and risk of complications, health practitioners are in a position to develop effective screening and treatment processes. Such practices are particularly important because some of the conditions, which are benign, if left untreated, have the potential to develop into malignancies. Studies on such lesions continue to guide the formulation of prevention programs as well as the implementation of gynecological health education, ultimately generating an environment of anticipatory care among women. Awareness of benign lesions' histological and clinical features provides vital information regarding their management. For instance, cervical intraepithelial neoplasia (CIN) is a lesion that causes cervical cancer and originates from a benign source, emphasizing the role of screening in high-risk groups. Early identification of these lesions during normal examination allows clinicians to implement adequate monitoring and, where necessary, treatment control based on patient individualization. Also, population patterns of benign lesions identify risk factors, which can be used to enhance preventive care schemes. Knowledge obtained by such research is invaluable in developing effective public health policy favoring women's health and wellbeing. The consequences of innocent lesions extend beyond the medical field, reaching into socioeconomic determinants related to women's health. Emotional suffering associated with diagnoses, even those benign, can lead to significant emotional distress and influence women's social and economic activities. As an instance, the diagnosis of benign lesions intrudes into normal life and necessitates follow-up and potential treatments that consume valuable time and resources. An in-depth investigation into these lesions underscores the importance of comprehensive care, allowing healthcare systems to attend not only to physical health but also to mental health and social impacts that accompany benign conditions of the gynecology. With the pathology of these lesions clearer, it stresses the importance of adopting an integrated approach considering the general health of women, as also pointed out in Donovan *et al.*, (2024) and Khashcha *et al.*, (2024).

Overview of the Vulva, Vagina, And Cervix

The vulva is the external female reproductive system, consisting of a number of structures like the labia majora, labia minora, clitoris, and vaginal opening. Each of these structures serves not just a role in the anatomy of the place but also functional purposes in protection, sexual arousal, and childbirth. The vulva is highly vascular and sensitive and hence liable to many benign lesions such as cysts, fibromas, and dermatoses. They usually present as swelling, itchiness, or pain, and result in clinical evaluation. Understanding of the vulva's complexity is fundamental in identifying benign lesions compared to more serious pathologies, particularly because the lesions do not necessarily exhibit alarm symptoms but require appropriate medical attention. Proceeding inward, the vagina provides an entranceway from the external vulva to the cervix and plays a key role in sexual intercourse and childbirth. The vaginal mucosa contains mucosal tissue that supports a balanced flora, which is important in the prevention of infection. Because of the specific environment, the vagina can also form benign lesions such as vaginal cysts and hyperplastic lesions. These lesions may range from asymptomatic growth to those that cause discomfort or abnormal vaginal discharge, so knowing their etiology is important. Radiologic evaluations through ultrasound and magnetic resonance imaging are used in the assessment of symptoms to help doctors decide whether lesions are benign or require further intervention. Differentiation is necessary because benign diseases, though normal, can be signs of underlying pathologies when they present with atypical features. The cervix, which is the lower part of the uterus, is an essential point of transition between the vagina and the uterine space. It plays a vital role in both reproductive health and the menstrual cycle. Benign cervical lesions, such as cervical polyps and nabothian cysts, are not uncommon in everyday practice. Whilst usually asymptomatic, the lesions may be related to abnormal bleeding or discomfort, and investigation is required. Up-to-date imaging has provided more accurate investigations with the minimum need for invasive diagnostic maneuvers. Second, an understanding of the range of cervical lesions is valuable, especially within the context of related pathology such as gastric-type lesions, which may be synchronous at many locations in the female genital tract (Wong *et al.*, 2024). Such comprehensive knowledge equips practitioners to manage benign lesions more effectively and remain vigilant for potential malignancies (Ning *et al.*, 2023).

10.1. Types of Benign Lesions

Learning Outcome

1. Identify and differentiate the common types of benign lesions, including cysts, polyps, and warts

For vulva, vagina, and cervix benign lesions, including clinicians being able to detect heterogeneity in the condition, from cystic to solid masses. Vestibular cysts and endometriomas are two examples of cystic lesions containing fluid-filled cavities and may or may not be symptomatic. They are benign structures due to gland obstruction or ectopic endometrium and manifest as localized swelling and pain. Challenging diagnosis necessitates accuracy, and thus the application of imaging modalities like ultrasound is needed, particularly when lesions are perineal in nature. Such benign lesions are typically confused with malignancy, which is more solid and larger. By recognizing these forms, physicians can better manage patients and avoid unnecessary invasive diagnostics, ultimately producing better patient care and outcomes (Ning *et al.*, 2023). Conversely, solid tumors such as leiomyomas and angiofibromas are yet another category of benign tumors of the lower genital tract. Leiomyomas, or smooth muscle tumors, may develop as a reaction to hormonal stimulation, suggesting their origin as estrogen-dependent. Although generally asymptomatic, large leiomyomas may be extremely painful or disturbing functionally. Angiofibromas, consisting of fibrous tissue and a rich supply of blood vessels, may present as soft, pedunculated masses. Despite their benign nature, they require proper assessment, as their clinical appearance can be suspicious for malignancy. Through this, the use of modalities such as MRI can be very helpful in distinguishing benign from malignant lesions, considering that some benign tumors can have uncharacteristic imaging features. This diagnostic differentiation is important in guiding proper management approaches for those presenting with such lesions (Ning *et al.*, 2023). The virus contribution of human papillomaviruses (HPVs) adds an additional layer of complexity to understanding benign lesions, particularly in relation to their evolutionary history and infection route. Most types of HPV are associated with benign proliferative disorders in the majority of instances, yet certain alpha-papillomaviruses can induce lesions on the cervix, vulva, and vagina that will develop into malignant disease. Such virus infections remain asymptomatic and, therefore, difficult to diagnose and treat early. The interaction of HPV with host cellular machinery can result in a spectrum of lesions, primarily through localized viral replication and transcription of viral oncogenes. Identification of the benign spectrum of lesions is important because it will enable the use of targeted surveillance and intervention approaches, particularly in those who are at higher risk of developing malignancy. Thus, the recognition of the forms and relevance of benign lesions associated with HPV is necessary in order to achieve optimal clinical outcomes in gynecology.

10.1.1. Cysts

Cysts represent one of the most common benign vulvar, vaginal, and cervical lesions and are characterized by sacs filled with fluid occurring in various tissues. Lesions may result from duct blockage or anatomical defects and form an accumulation of secretions. Some common types include Bartholins gland cysts, which are formed when the ducts for the Bartholins glands become blocked. Although usually asymptomatic, the cysts can be painful, distressing, or cause complications like infection. Cysts are usually evaluated by pelvic examinations, imaging tests, and biopsy, at times when differential diagnoses are an issue, as lesions of similar appearance can be representative of more sinister conditions. Cysts must be identified by practitioners to undertake the appropriate management and avoid unnecessary surgical interventions. Reproductive tract cysts can be highly varied in etiology and presentation. Endometriotic cysts, for example, which typically occur after endometriosis, illustrate the intricate interplay of physiological and hormonal factors that result in cyst development. These cysts can induce significant complications such as chronic pelvic pain and infertility, and thus, diagnosis and treatment become significant to the victims. In light of the fact that endometriosis affects so many women globally, and retrograde menstruation plays such an important role in pathogenesis, the implications extend beyond physical health and reach into general quality of life. The identification of cysts as predictive of future conditions such as endometriosis is one of the top reasons why overall clinical assessment and management on a per-case basis are essential (Smolarz *et al.*, 2021).

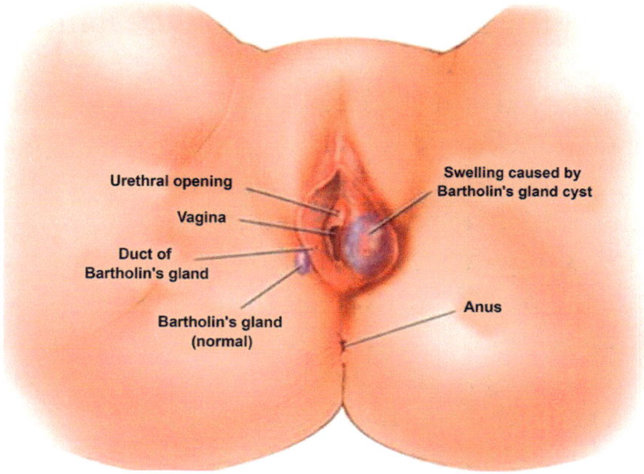

Figure 10.1. Bartholin's Gland cysts.

Source: https://azaleahealthtt.com/wp-content/uploads/2021/02/Bartholins-Gland.jpg

Additionally, while cysts are normally benign, some lesions, such as angiofibromas, may have cystic presentations but must be distinguished carefully at diagnosis. Angiofibromas, which predominantly present in middle-aged women, are vascular lesions and may be mistaken for other cystic lesions. Angiofibromas presenting in younger women emphasize the role of pathological examination and imaging, particularly if presented with abnormal presenting signs such as vaginal bleeding. Although rare in the vagina, their occurrence underscores the extensive spectrum of benign lesions to which clinicians must remain alert during differential diagnoses. Lastly, a clear and comprehensive understanding of cysts and related lesions is crucial to effective diagnosis, treatment planning, and patient education (Arega *et al.*, 2019).

10.1.2. Polyps

Among the study of benign vulvar, vaginal, and cervical lesions, polyps are outstanding structures that should receive special emphasis. These neoplastic masses, which occur from various sites of anatomy, are generally asymptomatic but can be symptomatic depending on their size and the site of occurrence. Fibroepithelial stromal polyps, for example, tend to occur in the connective tissue and can occur in the vaginal and cervical regions. Their diagnosis is often established with imaging investigations such as magnetic resonance imaging (MRI), which is necessary to comprehend their nature and separate them from malignant lesions and other pathological findings. Early diagnosis of the polyps is important, as it permits appropriate management and dispels the associated fears regarding their potential oncogenic activity.

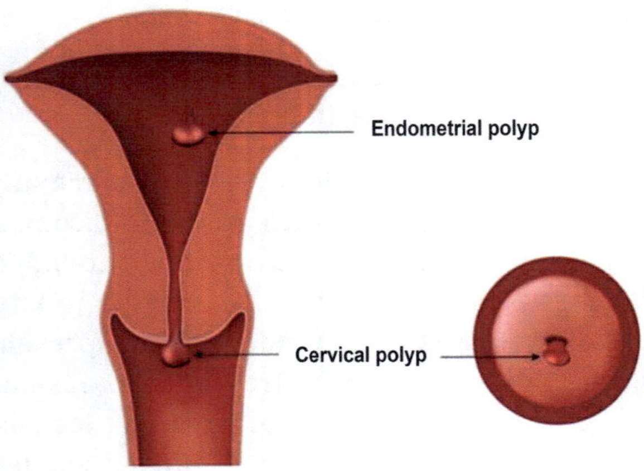

Figure 10.2. Cervical Polyp.

Source: https://healthify.nz/media/1001/cervical-polyp.jpg?width=650&height=571.6124661246613

Adding to the clinical picture are the variations in the various types of polyps. While the majority are benign and will require little or no therapy, there is a minority that can undergo dysplastic alterations, particularly when considering their relationship to the status of human papillomavirus (HPV). Cervical lesions and cancers have been identified by the World Health Organization based on their relationship with HPV, which emphasizes how clinicians must be sensitive to these nuances in the clinic. Parameters such as immunohistochemical markers, in which p16 expression serves as a surrogate for HPV association, facilitate improved prognostication and treatment planning.

Treatment of such polyps within the overall context of HPV-associated pathology also underscores the complexity inherent in cervical health and the necessity for intensive screening regimens. Treatment of polyps generally involves surgical intervention, particularly in cases where they are symptomatic or exhibit atypical features suspicious of malignancy. Surgical excision is often pursued, yielding not only therapeutic value but also diagnostic clarity through histologic study. For fibroepithelial stromal polyps, MRI findings have demonstrated that the lesions are able to exhibit varying signal intensities, allowing clinicians to distinguish between benign and potentially more sinister growths. Case reports indicate that resection can lead to favorable outcomes and resolution of symptoms, firmly establishing the role of surgery in the treatment of these benign lesions. Finally, knowledge about the implications of polyps in the context of the vulvar, vaginal, and cervical is essential for clinicians to take the lead towards individualized approaches which consider both the benign nature of these growths as well as the necessity for continued monitoring in the context of broader HPV-related discussion.

10.1.3. Warts

Warts, as condyloma acuminata, constitute a large category of benign lesions in the cervix, vulva, and vagina. They are caused by specific strains of the Human Papilloma Virus (HPV), types 6 and 11. Clinically, they appear as fleshy growths that are variable in size and shape but are usually multiple in anogenital sites. Their ease of transmission and contagiousness corroborate their status as one of the most common sexually transmitted illnesses. The prevalence of condyloma acuminata is markedly increased in subjects with compromised immune status, such as those who are infected with Human Immunodeficiency Virus (HIV), and treatment becomes difficult due to multiplicity of lesions increased and likelihood of forming larger, more aggressive tumors, exemplified by giant condyloma acuminata in some instances, emphasizing the need for judicious clinical management (Misra *et al.*, 2024).

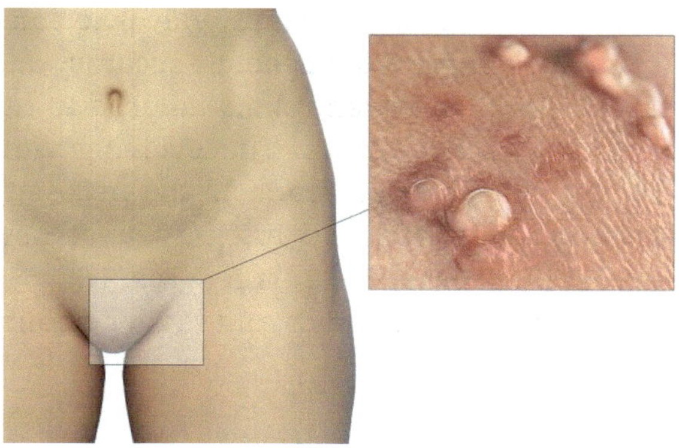

Figure 10.3. Vaginal Warts.

Source: https://dermadvance.gr/wp-content/uploads/2016/08/kondylomata-kolpou-1.jpg

The management of genital warts is a multidimensional process in which both the size of the lesions and the overall health status of the patients are taken into account. Standard treatment modalities include a range of topical agents, including podophyllin and imiquimod, as well as procedural treatments like cryotherapy and electrosurgical ablation. Another major issue is the recurrence rate of genital warts; patients may have recurrent episodes after treatment. This is particularly so for high-risk HPV-infected patients who have a higher tendency for malignant transformation (Mohamed *et al.*, 2023). Therefore, managing the high incidence of recurrences requires innovation in treatment procedures and patient education, particularly on the chronicity of the HPV infection and the importance of frequent return visits. There have been recent studies on novel ways of treating recurrent genital warts using immunotherapy as an alternative option. The needling-induced autoinoculation and intralesional injection techniques indicate the advancement of non-conventional treatment protocols. There have been encouraging outcomes observed from these treatments, and they enhance the body's immunity to HPV. These immunotherapeutic treatments try to decrease the long-term burden of lesions due to HPV by eliciting local immunity and thereby decreasing recurrence. Overall, the integration of traditional and innovative treatment methods is most important to effectively controlling the clinical and psychological burden caused by warts, ultimately improving patient quality of life and therapeutic outcomes in HPV-associated benign lesions (Misra *et al.*, 2024; Mohamed *et al.*, 2023).

Test Your Knowledge

1. What are the distinguishing features of cysts compared to other benign lesions?
2. What causes genital warts, and how are they classified as benign lesions?

10.2. Vulvar Lesions

Learning Outcome

1. Define Bartholin's cyst
2. Discuss the vulvar vestibulitis
3. Explain the lichen sclerosus

Vulvar lesion investigation is significant in the scenario of benign vulvar, vaginal, and cervical conditions. Vulvar lesions could present in the form of multiple structural imperfections like cysts, neoplasias, and inflammation, which could be a duplicate of more severe ones. Among benign vulvar lesions that are typically frequent are bartholin gland cysts, which arise from obstruction of the ducts of the bartholin gland, leading to fluid accumulation and localized swelling. They are typically symptomless but can be associated with pain and tenderness. Additionally, epidermoid cysts, derived from keratinized epithelial cells, can occur on the vulva and require differential diagnosis in order to rule out more serious entities. Recognition of these benign lesions is vital in order to provide proper treatment and management, placing a focus on the need for healthcare providers to be aware of their specific characteristics. Within the context of the overall picture of female reproductive health, the care of vulvar lesions must preserve the underlying principles of screening and intervention. As emphasized in updated guidelines, clinical decisions regarding the assessment of lesions rest on an integration of patient history, risk factors, and imaging results (Perkins *et al.*, 2020).

For example, clinicians must differentiate between benign and at-risk lesions, especially when dealing with unusual presentations. Further, the definition of benign lesions must take into account variation in demographic factors, including age and previous medical history, which influence lesion behavior and patient outcomes. The importance of distinguishing benign from malignant pathology cannot be overstated, since error may result in inappropriate anxiety or inappropriate treatment intervention. Complicating clinical management even more is the association of vulvar lesions with inflammation and STIs, both of which can alter benign lesion presentation. STIs such as herpes simplex virus and human papillomavirus can result in lesions that are difficult to differentiate from benign lesions, thus emphasizing the need for careful clinical assessment (Höhn *et al.*, 2021). Thus, a multidisciplinary approach involving gynecologists, dermatologists, and pathologists is crucial in the management of vulvar lesions. This provides improved diagnostic accuracy and ensures overall treatment plans tailored to the individual patient's needs. The evolving view of benign vulvar lesions reflects the necessity of ongoing education and integration of new research into practice, further resulting in improved patient outcomes and higher quality of care.

10.2.1. Bartholin's Cyst

Bartholin's cyst is one of the more common benign vulvar lesions, which occurs due to the blockage of the Bartholin's glands that are bilaterally located at the posterior aspect of the vaginal opening. Both these glands play an important role in secreting mucus for lubrication during coitus. When the duct system becomes obstructed—often secondary to trauma, infection, or inflammation—a cystic dilatation can ensue, which is painful or can be symptomatic if the cyst becomes infected or the abscess develops. Of note is that Bartholin's cysts cannot only be asymptomatic, with presentation either not noticed or on routine gynecological examination, but that symptoms develop if cysts become large, causing pain or pressure. Bartholin's cyst treatment typically begins with conservative observation, as long as the patient is asymptomatic.

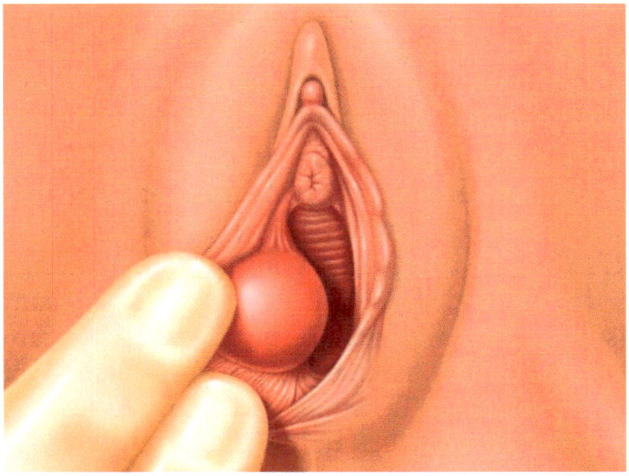

Figure 10.4. Bartholin's cyst.

Source: https://www.mayoclinic.org/diseases-conditions/bartholin-cyst/symptoms-causes/syc-20369976

After symptoms have arisen, however, several treatment options are indicated, including incision and drainage of the abscess or cyst. In selected cases, placement of a Word catheter will allow a patent fistula to exist within the cyst so that adequate drainage may occur with lower rates of recurrence. Surgical intervention would also be considered in recurrent cases, where removal of the gland itself may be a more effective solution. The treatment choice should take into account the age of the patient, the overall health of the patient, as well as the presence of any complication related to the cyst. Curiously enough, although Bartholin's cysts are more frequent in adults, there have also been occasional reports in children. Bartholin's gland abscesses were estimated to occur far less frequently in younger patients, and few have been described in the pediatric group. The therapy in such cases is typically under the same regimen as adult cases, although the rarity of occurrence necessitates conservative evaluation and planning from healthcare providers. Given the possibility of presentation overlap with more serious conditions such as tumors or infections, clinicians must diagnose and differentiate Bartholin's cysts correctly from other pathological findings to guarantee the appropriate and effective treatment procedures (Alsayed *et al.*, 2024). Besides, the recurrence of Bartholin's cysts may require examination to rule out malignancy and hence highlight the importance of proper monitoring of these benign cysts in all patient categories.

10.2.2. Vulvar Vestibulitis

Vulvar vestibulitis, an inflammatory and tender condition of the vulvar vestibule, is a notable but generally underemphasized feature of benign lesions of female genitalia. Dyspareunia, burning sensation, and local pain are generally the symptoms that patients complain of, and these often significantly compromise quality of life and psychosocial function. Although the absolute etiology is unknown, trauma, infection, or allergic response has been implicated. The syndrome is more prevalent in premenopausal women, making it significant in gynecologic practice. Because of its complexity and multiplicity of presentation, vulvar vestibulitis diagnosis is crucial to differentiate it from other conditions that share similar presentations, such as vulvar lichen sclerosus or vestibular adenitis. Vulvar vestibulitis diagnosis is primarily clinical, with a thorough patient history and physical examination. Physical examination typically reveals erythema and localized inflammation at the vestibule; thus, clinicians must conduct a thorough examination to rule out other vulvar pain etiologies. Radiologic evaluation, while not standard for vulvar vestibulitis, can be beneficial in identifying associated conditions. Tests such as MRI may be employed to determine the extent of the disease or to evaluate related benign lesions that are comprised of elementary cysts or solid tumors and may coexist with vestibulitis (Ning *et al.*, 2023). This diagnostic approach helps in the selection of appropriate management principles and ensures the delivery of targeted treatment that caters to symptoms and underlying causes. Vulvar vestibulitis treatment can be a complicated one, consisting of medical treatment along with surgery, depending on the severity and needs of the patient. Initial interventions may involve the application of topical anesthetics, corticosteroids, or dietary changes specifically made to reduce inflammation and pain. Conservative management will be ineffective in a few instances, resulting in the need for surgical methods such as vestibulectomy to excise the inflamed tissue, freeing patients from perpetual pain and dyspareunia. Moreover, patient education is a central component of care, addressing misinformation regarding the disorder and encouraging communication regarding sexual health. Overall, successful treatment of vulvar vestibulitis relies on collaboration between healthcare providers and patients, paving the way for improved results and a better quality of life for those with this disorder.

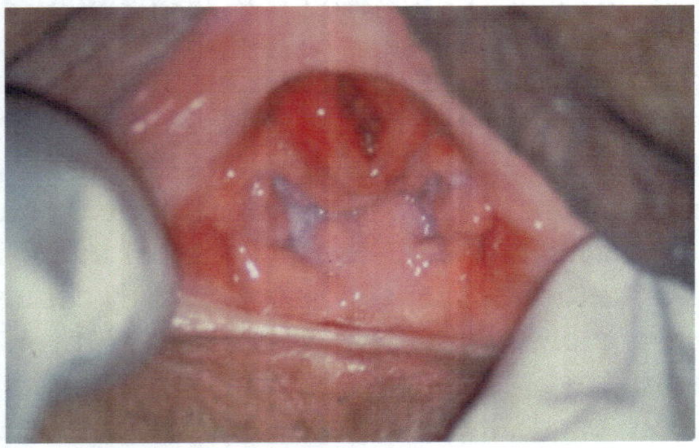

Figure 10.5. Severe vulvar vestibulitis.

Source: https://www.researchgate.net/figure/Severe-vulvar-vestibulitis-provoked-vulvodynia_fig1_26870111

10.2.3. Lichen Sclerosus

Lichen sclerosus is a chronic inflammatory condition that predominantly affects the vulvar region with whitish patches of skin, which, if left untreated, can be highly troublesome and cause complications. The condition typically affects postmenopausal women and can encompass symptoms of pruritus, pain, and pain during intercourse, significantly impairing women's quality of life. While the exact etiology is not entirely sure, there is supportive evidence for an autoimmune component, since patients can have associated autoimmune disease. Lichen sclerosus, having an insidious onset, tends to result in delayed diagnosis, so significant tissue change may have resulted and complicate therapy. Clinicians must be highly suspicious of lichen sclerosus in women with vulvar lesions in order to enable timely treatment, which is not only critical in relieving symptoms but also in the prevention of potential progression and associated morbidity. The management of lichen sclerosus is aimed at symptomatic relief and modification of the disease process. Topical corticosteroids constitute the bulk of treatment, antagonizing the inflammation and shortening the course of the symptoms efficiently.

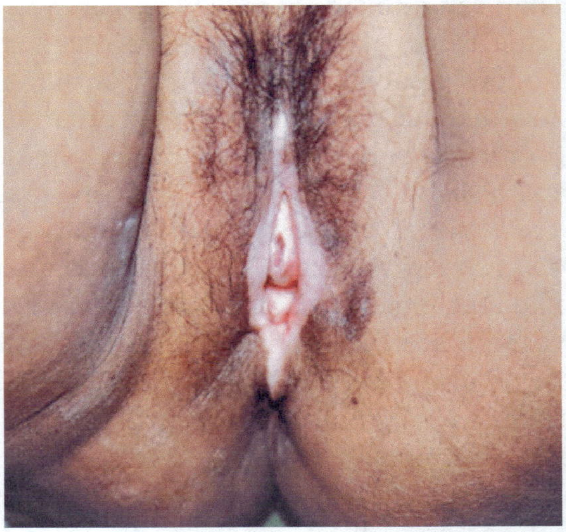

Figure 10.6. Lichen sclerosis.

Source: https://oshimu.com/wp-content/uploads/2021/07/Gynaecology-DC-Dutta.pdf

For refractory cases when corticosteroids are not enough, other immunomodulatory medications may be utilized, though they are utilized less often. Response to treatment may be unpredictable; patients can get considerably better, or they may require maintenance therapy in order to maintain skin integrity and manage symptoms. Follow-up is required to monitor for side effects, such as the risk of squamous cell carcinoma associated with chronic lichen sclerosus. With presentation sharing of the clinical presentations with other vulvar diseases, histopathology reports, and thorough clinical examination are important in making a correct diagnosis, in order to offer the most suitable management care to patients. The implications of not treating lichen sclerosus can also extend beyond the physical realm and involve the psychological and emotional states as well. Many women with lichen sclerosus report embarrassment and distress, and this can deter them from attending for evaluation. Also, the chronic pain and potential sexual dysfunction highlight the importance of a multidisciplinary treatment plan that includes psychological intervention. Both patients and physicians can become much more aware of lichen sclerosus through educational programs, thus facilitating earlier diagnosis and treatment. Besides, as suggested in recent vulvar lesion consensus reports, there is also an imperative need to keep researching the risk factors and long-term consequences of diseases like lichen sclerosus so that women receive full care dealing with both the physical and psychological impact of the disease (Preti *et al.*, 2022; Höhn *et al.*, 2021).

Test Your Knowledge

1. What is a Bartholin's cyst, and how does it commonly present in patients?
2. How does vulvar vestibulitis affect the vestibular area, and what are its typical symptoms?

10.3. Vaginal Lesions

Learning Outcome

1. Discuss the vaginal cysts and vaginal polyps
2. Define fibromas

Vaginal lesions are a collection of abnormalities of the vaginal epithelium, commonly benign conditions. Lesions can exist in many forms and include polyps, cysts, and warts, among others. Lesions in certain circumstances might need clinical management because of related symptoms or possible discomfort. Vaginal cysts, for instance, are benign lesions like Gartner's cysts, which are vestigial remnants of the Wolffian duct and typically asymptomatic. However, identification and management of such lesions are necessary, as lesions can be confused with malignancies or other potentially fatal conditions if the presentation thereof is not properly evaluated. Identification of the clinical features and potential significance of vaginal lesions is necessary for accurate diagnosis and management, thus improving patient outcomes in gynecological practice. In the context of understanding the meaning of vaginal lesions, attention needs to be drawn to their relationship with human papillomavirus (HPV) infection. Certain lesions, particularly squamous cell lesions, have been found to be associated with types of HPV and thus the need for screening and follow-up for HPV-related changes. The 2020 WHO classification provides guidance for differentiating HPV-related and HPV-independent lesions and thereby allows for more efficient clinical management strategies. For instance, management of HPV-related lesions should conform to updated guidelines placing emphasis on risk assessment and careful follow-up. A risk-based model of cervical screening and management of lesions can be applied by clinicians in order to optimize preventive interventions and optimize patient education regarding the detection of lesions and potential therapy, as in current consensus guidelines (Höhn *et al.*, 2021; Perkins *et al.*, 2020). It is also necessary to address the psychosocial impact of vaginal lesions on patients. The majority of women are disturbed and worried upon learning the risk of acquiring abnormal test results when going for routine gynecological examinations. The worry is increased by a lack of knowledge regarding vaginal lesions, what they mean, and their mode of treatment. Good communication among clinicians and patients can minimize worry and enlighten women to seek medical advice in a timely manner. Additionally, the integration of education on benign lesions and treatment in routine gynecology care can significantly enhance patient satisfaction. Continuously improving medical knowledge, additional research, and education regarding vaginal lesions still remain paramount in ensuring all facets of gynecological health and overall quality of life for those affected.

10.3.1. Vaginal Cysts

Among the benign lesions, vaginal cysts represent a significant category that needs to be carefully explored. The cysts can be formed because of various subtypes, the most significant being Gartner's duct cysts and Bartholin's gland cysts. Gartner's duct cysts represent a continuation of embryologic development and occur normally along the vagina walls on the lateral sides. Bartholin's gland cysts, on the other hand, arise due to clogging of the ducts of Bartholin glands, which provide lubrication to the vaginal opening. The clogging typically results in cyst formation due to fluid retention. The cysts, though normally benign, can be a source of clinical issues, including painful intercourse and repeated infection if infected. The clinical presentation of vaginal cysts is highly variable, and the majority of individuals are asymptomatic. However, when they occur, the effect is very high on a woman's quality of life. The manifestations can be localized swelling, pain, or pain with sexual intercourse, which is a reflection of the complexity of their occurrence. These cysts can also sometimes be encountered incidentally on routine gynecologic examination or imaging studies, raising questions regarding their management.

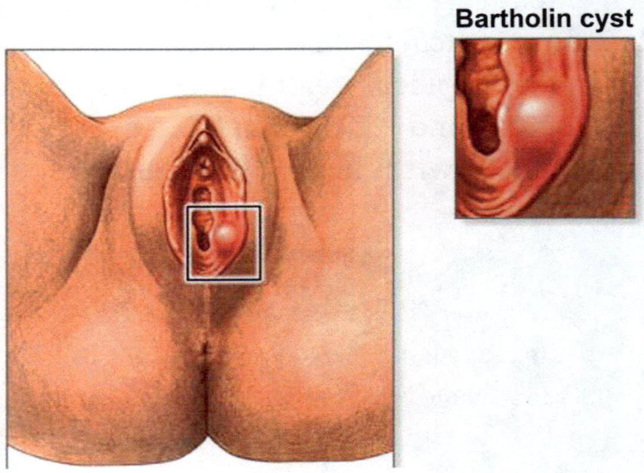

Figure 10.7. Vaginal cysts.

Source: https://ufhealth.org/assets/adam/24347.jpg

Particularly, the management is typically conservative in nature; with asymptomatic cases having watchful waiting marshaled and surgical treatment possibly being reserved for symptomatic or complicated cysts. This conflict between intervention and observation merely serves to underscore the need to be aware of the nature and implications of vaginal cysts within the framework of benign gynecological lesions. In exceptional cases, vaginal cysts are liable to be mistaken for other pathological conditions, and thus diagnostic accuracy is compromised. For example, cystic masses may appear as more serious diagnoses such as tumors or even endometriosis, which is characterized by the presence of endometrial tissue outside its normal location (Smolarz *et al.*, 2021). The issue is determining the proper differentiation because incorrect diagnosis can lead to unnecessary surgeries and undue stress to patients. Besides, angiofibromas, which are a rare type of benign tumor that has vascular connective tissue, can also present as cyst-like masses, predominantly in the vagina (Arega *et al.*, 2019). It is these various presentations that demonstrate the importance of detailed assessments by medical professionals in order to enable accurate diagnoses and the formulation of proper treatment plans.

10.3.2. Vaginal Polyps

Vaginal polyps are benign growths that may occur within the vaginal canal, typically from the epithelial lining. They are generally smooth, spherical lesions and are generally asymptomatic, hence not easy to see on normal examination. Though etiology is unclear, hormonal influence, particularly estrogen, has been reported to be significant in their development. As with other benign lesions of the female genital tract, these polyps can be found in conjunction with underlying disease, for example, hormonal disturbances or inflammation. Clinically, vaginal polyps not only vary in size but may also be single or multiple and need to be properly evaluated to exclude more serious lesions, particularly because they may be related to atypical cervical cytology or even pre-cancerous lesions due to HPV (Höhn *et al.*, 2021). Diagnosis of vaginal polyp is most often a pelvic exam during which the practitioner is able to visualize these lesions either visually or on palpation. Often, a follow-up with imaging tests, such as ultrasound, is performed to evaluate the nature of the polyps and to rule out malignancy. Sometimes, colposcopy is also employed for more detailed evaluation, especially if the polyp is cervical-adjacent or is discovered with suspicious cytological findings. It must be appreciated that while most vaginal polyps are benign, certain histological types, e.g., atypical ones, will need biopsy. This precaution finds support in even broader cervical screening guidelines that emphasize the importance of looking out for potential precursors to cervical cancer and, as such, perfection in patient care as well as adherence to screening protocols (Perkins *et al.*, 2020). Management of vaginal polyps is typically a policy of expectant management if asymptomatic, but is indicated by excision if symptomatic or exhibiting unusual features. Exeneration of vaginal polyps is a relatively simple procedure, frequently performed on an outpatient basis.

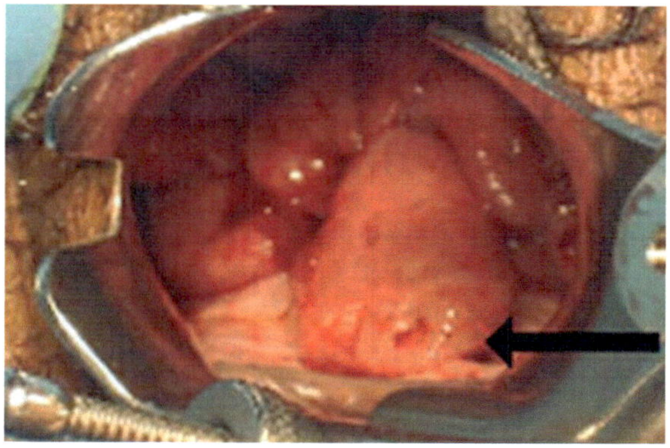

Figure 10.8. Vaginal polyps at the time of surgery. The majority of these large polyps protruded from the vaginal mucosa of the posterior fornix as a 'beard-like' linear array. Notice the ulceration at the tip of the largest polyp (arrow).

Source: https://www.researchgate.net/figure/aginal-polyps-at-the-time-of-surgery-The-majority-of-these-large-polyps-protruded-from_fig1_49675971

Close follow-up after treatment needs to be provided since recurrence of vaginal polyps can occur, although in the majority of patients, the malignant potential of vaginal polyps is low. Also, the suggestion of vaginal polyps in other benign vulvar and cervical lesions renders the acquisition of the necessary knowledge about female reproductive health by the masses a priority. Monitoring for potential concurrent illnesses such as cervical intraepithelial neoplasia enhances the effectiveness of management interventions and reminds us to be aware of the significance of community health education of regular gynecological check-ups and early detection protocols in aiding the overall outcome for women (Höhn *et al.*, 2021).

10.3.3. Fibromas

Fibromas or fibroepithelial stromal polyps are one of the benign lesions that can arise in the vulvar, vaginal, and cervical regions. By virtue of their spindle cell composition, the lesions are typically of mesenchymal origin. Clinically, they can appear as palpable nodular masses that are often asymptomatic, but in other cases can lead to pain or cosmetic disturbance for the affected patients. Their benign nature makes fibromas distinguishable from cancerous tumors, but their occurrence necessitates careful clinical screening in order to arrive at the correct diagnosis. Because of their histologic variability, pathologists are sometimes faced with challenges in distinguishing fibromas from other lesions. The potential overlap of features with benign and malignant lesions necessitates having a correct histopathological examination in order to establish the diagnosis and formulate appropriate management strategies (Shaaban *et al.*, 2013). The gynecologic practice role of fibromas is not just their diagnostic and therapeutic significance, but also the physical and emotional suffering that they induce. Although most of the fibromas are benign, one cannot underestimate their effect on the patient. These lesions may, on rare occasions, cause presentations that are imitative of more severe conditions, and therefore, a careful strategy in clinical evaluation is required. For example, although fibromas are usually not symptomatic, large lesions can cause pressure on surrounding structures and result in symptoms of dyspareunia or frequency. Surgical management, which in most cases involves excision, can offer relief. Additionally, follow-up by close-up inspection is important after treatment to monitor for any recurrence of symptoms or occurrence of lesions. The importance of differentiating between fibromas and other vulvar region lesions is maintaining overall reproductive health and quality of life in females (Chalya *et al.*, 2013). Lastly, management of the occurrence of fibromas among vulvar, vaginal, and cervical benign conditions needs to be a holistic approach that caters to both clinical and pathological manifestations. Clinicians should be continuously informed about the most current information about fibromas, continuously striving to use evidence-based practice that ensures the best possible outcomes for patients. As fibromas are benign, informing patients about fibromas can facilitate empowerment, which reduces anxiety about malignancy. Besides, routine gynecological check-ups should be emphasized by health practitioners as a means of detecting such lesions early. This foresight increases improved patient awareness of individual patient needs, hence improving overall management and patient outcomes in the area of gynecological health (Shaaban *et al.*, 2013).

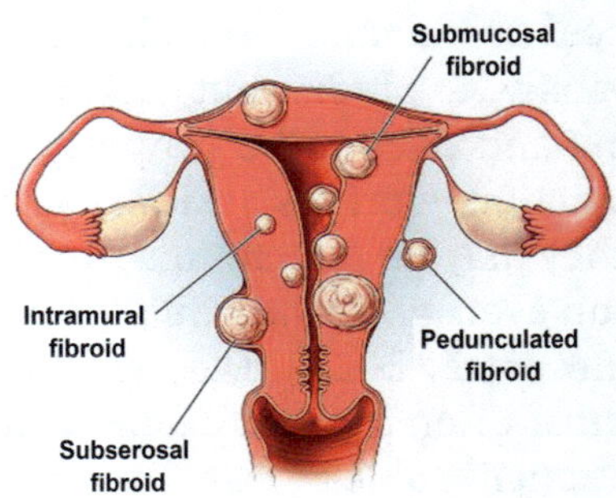

Figure 10.9. Uterine fibroids are growths made up of muscle and connective tissue. Symptoms can include heavy menstrual bleeding, back pain, frequent urination, and pain during sex.

Source: https://my.clevelandclinic.org/-/scassets/images/org/health/articles/9130-uterine-fibroids

Test Your Knowledge

1. How do vaginal polyps typically present, and are they usually symptomatic?
2. What distinguishes fibromas from other benign vaginal lesions in terms of composition and clinical features?

10.4. Cervical Lesions

Learning Outcome

1. Discuss the cervical polyps
2. Define nabothian cysts
3. Explain the squamous metaplasia

Cervical lesions, particularly benign, form a key concern of gynecologic wellness that is frequently detected by routine screening such as Pap smears or colposcopy. These methods allow physicians to visually examine the cervix and identify irregularities that may indicate pre-cancerous or benign pathology. Colposcopy, although a more intricate process, achieves maximum diagnostic capability by providing an enlarged view of the cervix, vagina, and vulva such that it is possible to ascertain the character, size, and extent of any lesion. As documented in colposcopic literature, the comparison between these visual findings and histopathological results is critical in assisting with the reliable differentiation between malignant and benign lesions, thereby guiding subsequent management (Asati *et al.*, 2022). Early detection and accurate evaluation of cervical lesions can significantly improve patient outcomes as well as decrease the risk of cervical cancer development. Histologic examination of cervical lesions shows a large variety of benign lesions, some being diverse cervical polyps and stromal lesions. Atypical stromal cells (ASCs), whose morphology might lead to misdiagnosis as malignant, are a good example of this diversity. Although ASCs are in themselves not harmful, their presence can lead to misinterpretation and hence should be examined extensively histopathologically. In the presence of atypical cervical stromal cells, the pathologist must pay attention to their typical features, including their large size and hyperchromatic nuclei, which may prove deceitful to clinical interpretation if poorly appreciated (Kurekar *et al.*, 2021). Detection of ASCs in cervical specimens is an indicator of the significance of reliable pathology techniques and the importance of the education of gynecologists about benign entities, which can mimic malignancy. Treatment of benign cervical lesions, moreover, is also complicated, typically calling for a watchful waiting approach with serial follow-up in anticipation of possible changes. In certain cases, therapy such as excisional therapy can be required in cases of lesions with suspicious features despite being initially considered benign. Understanding various cervical lesions, their clinical features, and potential implications helps provide an informed decision-making process for both patients and healthcare professionals. By drawing attention to the distinction between malignant and benign lesions and employing extensive diagnostic methods, medical practitioners can enhance educational methods with regard to women's health issues unique to the cervix and promote proactive care. Increased awareness and education can ultimately lead to lesions not being mismanaged and ensuring women are provided with necessary care specific to their own conditions.

10.4.1. Cervical Polyps

Cervical polyps are a significant characteristic of benign cervical lesions, in that they are defined by their appearance and their clinical behavior. Cervical polyps generally appear as soft, finger-like masses of tissue from the canal of the cervix. While typically asymptomatic, some patients may have abnormal vaginal bleeding or discharge during coitus, which requires further medical investigation. The prevalence of cervical polyps is variable, and evidence indicates that they occur most commonly in women of childbearing age but are present in any age category. It is important to differentiate them from other cervical lesions, particularly since benign polyps can be associated with more perilous disorders, such as cervical cancer. Hence, a good knowledge of their clinical presentation and histopathological features is necessary in order to treat and reassure patients adequately (Wang *et al.*, 2025). The histology of cervical polyps is generally a mixture of fibrous tissue, blood vessels, and glandular epithelium. In most cases, the above-mentioned polyps are benign and have little potential for malignant transformation; however, atypical presentation may require extensive observation and histopathological analysis. Recently acquired evidence shows that tumors discovered in the cervix may exhibit unusual behavior under specific situations. For example, development of atypical stromal cells in a rapidly developing polyp raises questions about their classification as malignant or otherwise (Wang *et al.*, 2025). This elevates the importance of regular gynecologic assessment and follow-up, particularly in populations that possibly are more at risk for multifactorial cervical disease. Having a clear diagnosis and treatment protocol can offer improved patient outcomes as well as put an end to ongoing controversy regarding these lesions.

Treatment of cervical polyps is straightforward and founded primarily on excisional procedures that can be performed on an outpatient basis. Polypectomy, performed under colposcopy as a rule, allows for the removal of the polyp with minimal discomfort and proper examination of the excised tissue. Post-procedure complications are rare; the patient nonetheless requires education about potential symptoms and follow-up visits. From retrospective reviews, it can be noted that the recurrence rate of cervical polyps is low following complete removal, proof of the efficacy of this procedure (Tirkaso *et al.*, 2024). Despite their innocuous nature, healthcare practitioners must maintain a watchful attitude towards cervical polyps, especially in those patients with abnormal bleeding or other sinister signs that might indicate underlying malignancy. Ultimately, ongoing study and education will serve to guide the evolving knowledge on these lesions in the context of gynecologic health.

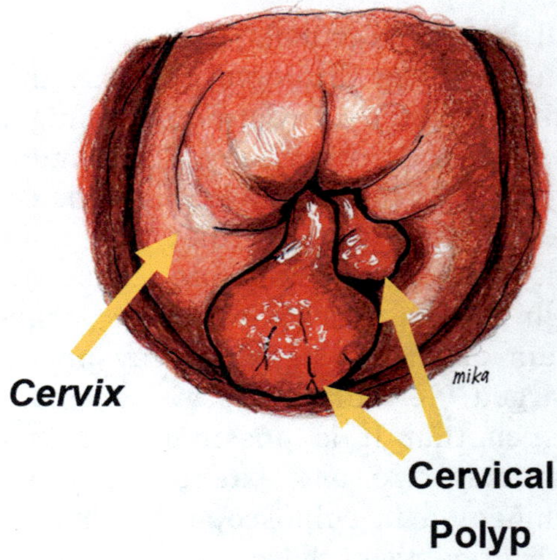

Figure 10.10. Cervical Polyps

Source: https://obgyn.com.my/wp-content/uploads/2022/12/cervical-polyp-drawing-by-Mika-edited-FINAL.png

10.4.2. Nabothian Cysts

Nabothian cysts, which are the most common to occur in the cervix, are benign lesions that result from the obstructed mucous glands of the endocervical canal. The cyst develops when the gland openings are occluded and the mucus accumulates and distends the gland. Nabothian cysts are typically asymptomatic on clinical presentation and are incidentally detected by routine gynecologic exam or imaging studies. Their low malignant potential and benign nature underscore their classification as benign lesions, contributing to their overall prevalence in women of childbearing age. While the cysts themselves are not dangerous, they may be symptomatic and thus cause concern at the time of pelvic exam, most often necessitating further evaluation to exclude other more serious pathologies. Diagnosis of nabothian cysts is mainly done by physical examination and imaging procedures like ultrasonography or colposcopy. These methods enable doctors to differentiate between nabothian cysts and other cervical lesions like cervical polyps or neoplasias. Nabothian cysts are usually not associated with any morbidity, but their detection may sometimes lead to further examination in terms of pathologies of the cervix. In some cases, healthcare providers may use visual examination with acetic acid (VIA) as part of a complete workup for cervical lesions, but nabothian cysts usually won't demonstrate the abnormal characteristics that such a procedure would call for, as evidenced by evidence from cervical cancer screening modalities research data (Nouhet *al.*, 2022). It is worth considering the clinical relevance of nabothian cysts, more so regarding their treatment and potential complications. Treatment in most instances is not required for asymptomatic cysts, but, in some rare instances where they become symptomatic, operative removal can be called for. This is a call for ongoing education on gynecologic health, given that both patients and clinicians need to know that such cysts are harmless. Also, though cervical lesions have been mapped by research as benign to malignancy, nabothian cysts are a specific indication of the varied nature of cervical conditions, and they promise continued research into their pathophysiology and their classification in the broader context of benign vulvar, vaginal, and cervical lesions (Wang *et al.*, 2022).

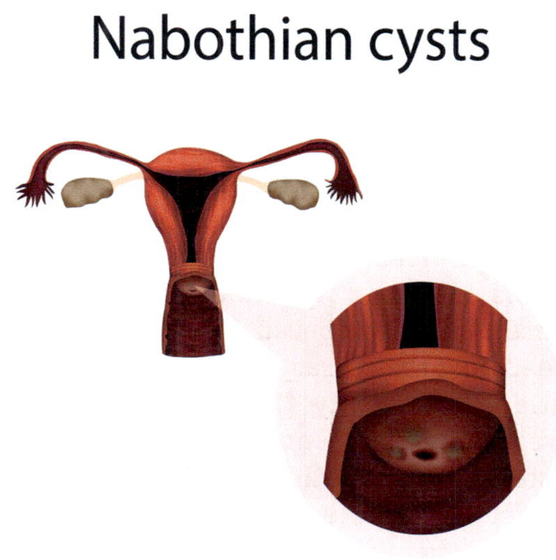

Figure 10.11. Nabothian cysts.

Source: https://www.statpearls.com/CmeImg/RetrieveImage/25504

10.4.3. Squamous Metaplasia

Squamous metaplasia is a significant pathological process located within the female genital canal, particularly in the vulva, vagina, and cervix. It is a process whereby one cell type is replaced by squamous cells, typically as a response to prolonged irritation or inflammation. It is most often seen where there exists normally columnar epithelium lining, such as in the endocervical canal. The occurrence of squamous metaplasia plays a protective function in creating a barrier against incoming pathogens and environmental abuse. It is significant because it needs to be identified, particularly between distinguishing benign from harmful conditions, as it can at times mimic neoplastic lesions' histological appearance and thus present difficulty in diagnosis and management. Clinical relevance of squamous metaplasia is also highlighted by its correlation with various benign disorders including infection with human papillomavirus (HPV) and other inflammatory disorders. In cervical tissues, squamous metaplasia is a preneoplastic alteration preceding cervical intraepithelial neoplasia (CIN), emphasizing the need for regular screening and follow-up. Histologically, metaplastic areas may possess cellular atypia that can be mistaken for malignancy, especially in the context of the presence of underlying infection or inflammation. Pathologists are therefore particularly vital in making accurate diagnoses of benign squamous metaplasia and precancerous lesions because a wrong diagnosis will lead to unnecessary intervention, adding to patient complexity (Mondal *et al.*, 2024). Also, research has widened the understanding of the different presentations of benign glandular lesions of the female genital tract that could be associated with squamous metaplasia. Recent literature shows the recently developed category of such lesions, including gastric-type adenosis and other premalignant lesions (Wong *et al.*, 2024). These findings underscore the value of a complete diagnostic workup, since morphologically squamous metaplasia resembles other lesions. The distinction between these entities warrants an elevated understanding of both clinical presentation and histological characteristics. Consequently, enhancement of immunohistochemical staining techniques as well as molecular pathology is paramount in maximizing diagnostic accuracy, thereby ensuring appropriate treatment measures for patients with such benign lesions.

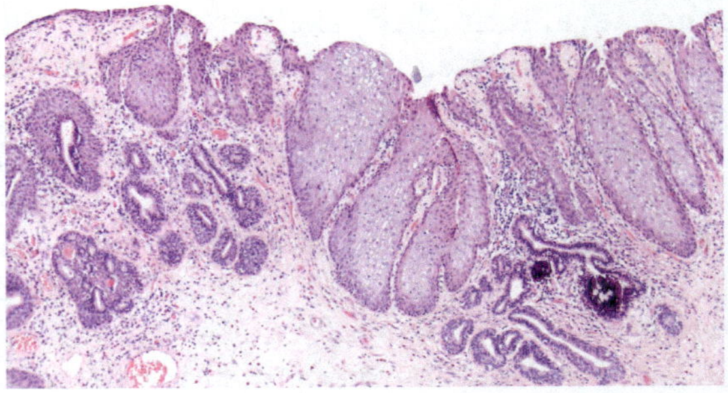

Figure 10.12. Squamous metaplasia.

Source: https://www.pathologyoutlines.com/imgau/bladdersquamousmetaplasiaTretiakova04.jpg

Test Your Knowledge

1. What are cervical polyps, and how are they typically diagnosed and treated?
2. What causes nabothian cysts to form on the cervix, and are they clinically significant?

10.5. Symptoms and Diagnosis

Learning Outcome

1. Identify common symptoms associated with benign lesions of the female reproductive tract.
2. Explain diagnostic approaches used for detecting benign lesions, including physical examinations and imaging techniques.
3. Discuss the importance of differential diagnosis in distinguishing benign lesions from malignant conditions.

It is critical to note the signs of benign vulval, vaginal, and cervical lesions for early identification and effective treatment. The symptoms may be nonspecific and can present with localized pain or discomfort, pruritus, leading to a visit to medical experts. Excessive or unusual discharge or noticeable changes in the consistency of the vaginal discharge are also signs of benign lesions. In asymptomatic presentations, routine gynecologic examination and routine screening are worth their weight in gold to detect lesions such as cysts, warts, or fibromas. Patient history and presenting complaints are employed to guide health care professionals in constructing appropriate workups. The importance of early detection of non-specific symptoms cannot be overemphasized since it allows practitioners to differentiate benign from sinister disorders and institute timely intervention while alleviating patient anxiety regarding malignancy. Benign lesions are typically diagnosed by a combination of clinical assessment and diagnostic testing. Providers will typically begin with a thorough physical examination, often augmented by colposcopy, visual inspection, and cervical cytology. Where indicated, the latter is supplemented by colposcopy. These methods yield direct visualization of the lesions and can enable directed biopsy, which is required for histological examination. Using these protocols is important, especially when prior cervical abnormality is present, since patients with such a history have an increased risk for future complications. New diagnostic technologies, such as high-resolution imaging and HPV testing, have enhanced the ability to accurately assess lesion characteristics and select the optimal treatment. The use of multidimensional diagnostic testing allows individuals to receive accurate diagnoses that have a significant impact on the effectiveness of treatment and management of long-term health. For cervical lesions, recent updates in screening guidelines emphasize a risk-based approach to diagnosis and management, acknowledging the place of HPV testing in guiding clinical decision-making. According to revised recommendations, HPV-associated lesion detection involves close assessment of risk factors, including a patient's test history and most recent results. For instance, individuals with previously abnormal results may be subject to more comprehensive surveillance than those who are at low risk. Such guidelines, as highlighted by the latest consensus findings, are designed to optimize management choices according to advancing cervical cancer pathophysiology knowledge and thus improve patients' care. By incorporating such individualized approaches, medical professionals are able to eschew unwarranted interventions and better direct resources toward those at higher risk, actually mapping the difficult ground of benign and precancerous cervical lesions in clinical practice (Perkins *et al.*, 2020; Bhatla *et al.*, 2018).

10.5.1. Common Symptoms Associated With Benign Lesions

The presence of benign lesions in the vulva, vagina, and cervix commonly manifests by way of a variety of common presenting symptoms, sensitive to the pathophysiology of the diseases. A majority of individuals will not experience any symptoms at all, particularly with small lesions, and may not notice them until a follow-up check-up. But, as lesions grow in size or become inflamed, symptoms such as localized discomfort or pruritus ensue. These symptoms can be induced by irritation due to friction or inflammation, which may affect the quality of life of patients and necessitate further inquiry or intervention. Identification of these symptoms is crucial to ensure medical professionals intervene on time and alleviate patients' worries while ensuring proper diagnosis of benign conditions, thus improving overall care outcomes. Abnormal vaginal discharge is another frequently reported symptom with benign lesions. This discharge is normally variable in nature and color based on the nature and location of the lesion. Sebaceous cysts or Bartholin's gland cysts, for instance, may result in an increase in vaginal discharge, which at times may be mistaken for infection. In addition, some lesions are associated with HPV infection, which carries cervical health consequences and needs strict monitoring following updated guidelines (Perkins *et al.*, 2020). Identification of such discharge's nature is critical in order to separate benign from serious conditions because abnormal discharge could need further diagnostic workup. The covert description of these symptoms is crucial in the successful management of benign lesions as well as in the relief of patients' concerns. Dyspareunia, or painful sex, is another common symptom seen in benign lesions in the vulvar and vaginal regions. Pain may be caused by a number of conditions of benign nature, such as vulvar vestibulitis or bulky lesions that may exert pressure within the channel of the vagina. Dyspareunia etiology should be addressed, as not only is sexual health affected, but also psychological distress may be induced. For the most part, there are treatments available that can correct symptoms effectively, enhancing the quality of life for the patient. Moreover, patient education of these symptoms by the clinician can prompt individuals to seek earlier reporting of these issues, thus allowing appropriate management practices to be applied (Bhatla *et al.*, 2018). Considering the effect on physical as well as emotional well-being, a thorough knowledge of these symptoms is necessary for gynecological healthcare professionals.

10.5.2. Diagnostic Methods (e.g., Physical Examination, Imaging)

The diagnostic methods employed for assessing benign lesions of the vulva, vagina, and cervix play a crucial role in establishing appropriate treatment protocols. Physical examination remains fundamental, allowing health professionals to visualize abnormalities, palpate lesions, and assess associated symptoms. A thorough inspection of the external and internal pelvic regions can provide immediate insights into the nature of these lesions, aiding in the differentiation between benign and potentially malignant conditions. Additionally, the patient's history, including any previous health issues or symptoms, is invaluable during initial assessments. This comprehensive approach facilitates timely intervention and helps mitigate any associated complications, emphasizing the importance of a well-rounded diagnostic process in gynecological care. Imaging techniques also significantly enhance the diagnostic landscape for benign lesions. Ultrasound, for instance, is a non-invasive method that provides real-time visualization of soft tissues, enabling healthcare providers to delineate lesions with clarity. This tool is particularly beneficial for identifying cysts, fibromas, or other anomalies within the pelvic region.

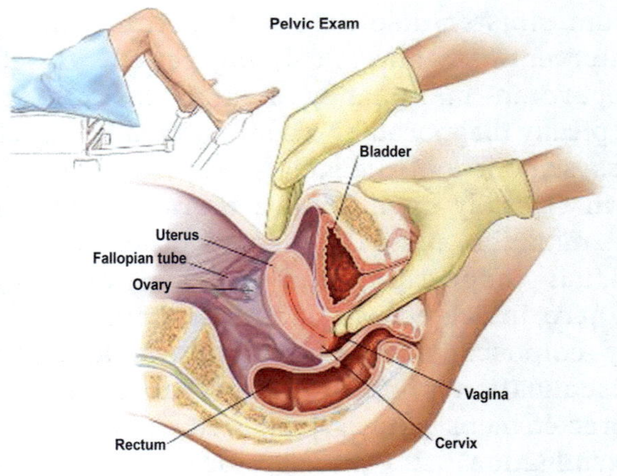

Figure 10.13. Pelvic exam. A doctor or nurse inserts one or two lubricated, gloved fingers of one hand into the vagina and presses on the lower abdomen with the other hand. This is done to feel the size, shape, and position of the uterus and ovaries. The vagina, cervix, fallopian tubes, and rectum are also checked.

Source: https://www.cancerhelpessentiahealth.org/Cancer_Types/cervical_200103E1_01.html

Besides, advanced imaging modalities such as magnetic resonance imaging (MRI) afford accurate cross-sectional images to define complex lesions or conditions such as endometriosis, which can readily be missed during primary physical examinations. Implementation of imaging in the diagnostic work-up allows for better stratification of the lesions in case they carry any risk of malignancy, and thus also helps in clinical management in a better way. Histologic inspection, often in conjunction with imaging and clinical features, is essential to the diagnosis of many lesions. In tissue specimens taken by techniques such as biopsy, there are absolute clues to the cellular makeup of a lesion, making it possible to differentiate benign from early malignancies. Of specific note is the use of standard Papanicolaou tests that have been vital to early diagnosis of cervical intraepithelial neoplasia (CIN), an initial phase of cervical cancer. Given the wide preinvasive spectrum of CIN-like diseases, early diagnosis efficiently reduces cervical cancer-related mortality, thereby indicating the value of employing multi-directional diagnostic strategies. The additional value of such comprehensive evaluations as improving outcomes for patients, besides that they ease treatment modalities, makes proactive gynecological care therefore encouraging (Smolarz *et al.*, 2021; Šarenac *et al.*, 2019).

10.5.3. Importance of Differential Diagnosis

The importance of differential diagnosis of benign vulvar, vaginal, and cervical lesions cannot be overstated. Accurate diagnosis of lesions is paramount for initiating appropriate management plans and optimizing patient outcomes. The process involves separating the benign conditions of cysts and benign tumors from more complex pathologies like endometriosis or malignancies. The implications of a hostile differential diagnosis extend beyond the momentary delivery of care; misinterpretation can lead to unnecessary intervention or omission in the diagnosis of a serious condition. Endometriosis, for instance, while often misinterpreted, is one of the most common causes of infertility and chronic pain and dictates keen investigation of any pelvic lesion that mimics its presentation (Smolarz *et al.*, 2021). By taking time to do differential diagnosis, health practitioners enhance the quality of care. Additionally, greater awareness of various adenocarcinomas of the lower female genital tract also underscores the importance of scrupulous differential diagnosis. Even though high-risk human papillomavirus (HPV) infection is universally accepted as a primary reason for cervical adenocarcinomas, non-HPV-associated forms are also being seen, and therefore, this suggests a spectrum, which is confounding.

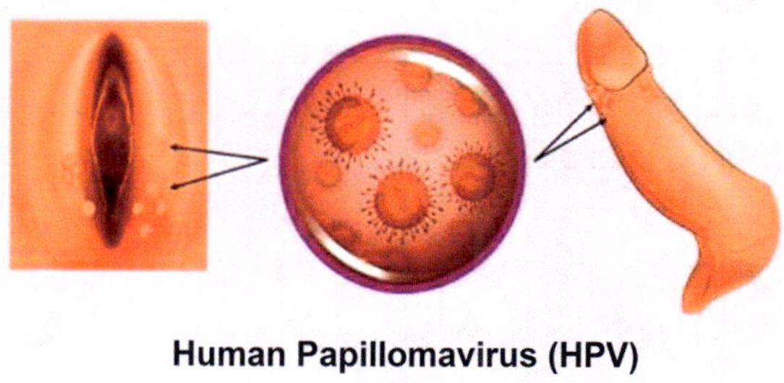

Figure 10.14. Human papillomavirus (HPV) infection.

Source: https://vitrosens.com/wp-content/uploads/2023/12/Warts-the-most-common-symptom-of-the-HPV-in-the-male-and-female-genitalia.-640x350.jpg

Gastric-type cervical adenocarcinomas and other glandular neoplasms can simulate benign processes, and therefore, they should be very closely investigated histologically (McCluggage, 2015). If these lesions cannot be distinguished, they can have catastrophic consequences, such as delayed treatment of malignancy, which in the majority of cases, presents more drastically once well-established. Therefore, there is a need for a broad differential diagnosis to understand the delicate subtleties that can guide clinicians to make effective management decisions. Here, the role of education through differential diagnosis among health professionals is also significant. Continued education in recognizing and distinguishing between benign and malignant lesions can enhance diagnostic accuracy significantly. Practical experience is complemented with research-evidenced knowledge to gain a skill in detecting the anomalies otherwise missed in standardized exams. Furthermore, access to new clinical guidelines for benign lesions and their mimics may aid in differential diagnosis. Through the integration of data from recent literature and case histories, professionals can better understand complex conditions like endometriosis and atypical adenocarcinomas, leading to earlier and more accurate diagnosis (Smolarz *et al.*, 2021; McCluggage, 2015). Ultimately, through establishing an environment in which differential diagnosis is paramount, care for patients can be improved with reduced complication rates from misdiagnosis and increased general effectiveness in treatment.

Test Your Knowledge

1. What are some common symptoms that may indicate the presence of benign lesions in the female reproductive tract?
2. Which diagnostic methods are commonly used to identify and evaluate benign lesions?

10.6. Treatment Options

Learning Outcome

1. Describe methods for observation and monitoring of benign lesions of the vulva, vagina, and cervix
2. Explain surgical intervention techniques used in the treatment of benign lesions in these areas
3. Discuss medical management strategies for benign lesions of the vulva, vagina, and cervix.

The management of benign vulval, vaginal, and cervical lesions embraces the use of various treatments based on the nature and type of lesion. For instance, small, symptom-free lesions such as condylomata acuminata can be conservatively managed with observation, especially if the patient is young and healthy. But for symptomatic larger lesions, application of topical treatments like podofilox and imiquimod or procedural therapies like cryotherapy or excisional surgery is necessary. Such a decision is guided by factors like patient preference, comfort, and medical history, emphasizing the importance of a model of shared decision-making towards treatment. This personalized paradigm with regular monitoring and timely intervention enhances patient experiences while treating their clinical settings effectively. For cervical lesions specifically, the new American Society of Colposcopy and Cervical Pathology guidelines bring in a risk-based policy of treatment. The guidelines propose substituting traditional test result-based algorithms with risk estimates for the development of significant lesions such as cervical intraepithelial neoplasia (CIN) and cervical cancer. In the management of known cervical lesions, clinical action thresholds set the treatments as per the patient's history and recent screening test. Accelerated treatments, for instance, excisional procedures, can be given without waiting for colposcopic confirmation where there is a high-risk lesion, particularly in situations where there is a very high risk for advanced disease. All such risk stratification facilitates intervention towards relevant lesions, leading to appropriate and early care with a focus on early detection and treatment of precancerous changes (Perkins *et al.*, 2020).

Besides this, the introduction of human papillomavirus (HPV) vaccine programs has transformed the landscape of cervical cancer prevention, impacting the treatment of benign cervical lesions. With the inclusion of HPV vaccination in the national health policies of most countries, including low- and middle-income countries, there is a concerted effort to prevent cervical lesions due to high-risk types of HPV. Screening advances, particularly nucleic acid testing for HPV, complement vaccination by enhancing the detection of precancerous lesions at earlier stages. Thus, this confluence of vaccination and preventive intervention upstream provides a more integrated model for the management of benign lesions and leaves health systems intact to deal with future threats to cervical health. As the effectiveness of these interventions is further established, it is hoped that treatment paradigms will further evolve and come into line with global efforts towards the elimination of cervical cancer as a significant public health issue (Bhatla *et al.*, 2018).

10.6.1. Observation and Monitoring

Good observation and monitoring are key aspects in the management of benign vulvar, vaginal, and cervical lesions. The adoption of risk-based guidelines after the 2019 consensus changes the trajectory of patient care by calling for individualized evaluation against the one-size-fits-all tradition. Individuals who enter with cervical abnormalities, such as atypical squamous cells, benefit from closely individualized follow-up practices that consider both their current pathology and their histories of past screening. For instance, individuals who have low-grade lesions can be followed without immediate treatment, which aligns with the principle of equal management for equal risk as outlined in Perkins *et al.*, (2020).

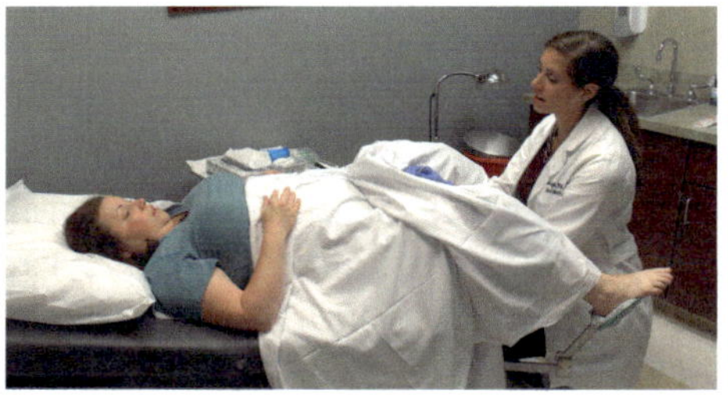

Source: https://external-content.duckduckgo.com/iu/?u=https%3A%2F%2Fcdn.ymaws.com%2Fnpwh.site-ym.com%2Fresource%2Fresmgr%2Fher%2Fpelvic-exam.jpg&f=1&nofb=1&ipt=f11e32daf24816fd9741a1c9e7c8ab62d0ef66984342c568eb5b6b2349df2e9d

The emphasis on individualized surveillance not only decreases unwarranted psychological burden on patients but also decreases overtreatment, which guarantees that it is aimed at people who require more aggressive treatment. Regular follow-up and normal cervical cancer screening are important in patients with benign lesions to prevent deterioration to severe diseases. The transition from the previous result-based algorithms to risk-based management has allowed more sensitive decision-making for follow-up durations. As an example, guidelines propose closer follow-up for patients with a previous history of high-grade lesions or immunosuppression because their risk for cervical intraepithelial neoplasia grade 3 or greater (CIN 3+) remains much higher. However, low-risk patients may be safely followed up at longer intervals between visits for provision of fair patient care and effective allocation of health resources, as in Tadir *et al.*, (2017). Such stratification offers a healthcare environment with a focus on preventive interventions in addition to responsiveness to every patient's requirements. The inclusion of new technologies and techniques in the practice of monitoring further enhances the effectiveness of cervical cancer prevention measures. Improvement in energy-based devices offers further ways through which patients can be treated, particularly through the management of lesions, but still emphasizing observation in its control. For instance, fractional lasers and radiofrequency devices are explored for their efficiency in reversing changes in vaginal tissues with aging, and additional investigation and validation with clinical trials are indicated. The modalities can potentially not only enhance the quality of life of the patient but also be used as an adjunct to conservative management if indicated. As the field advances, the continued fusion of evidence-based innovations will be essential to further optimize observation and surveillance protocols in gynecologically relevant benign lesions to provide effective care as well as enable the patient to be empowered in health decision-making.

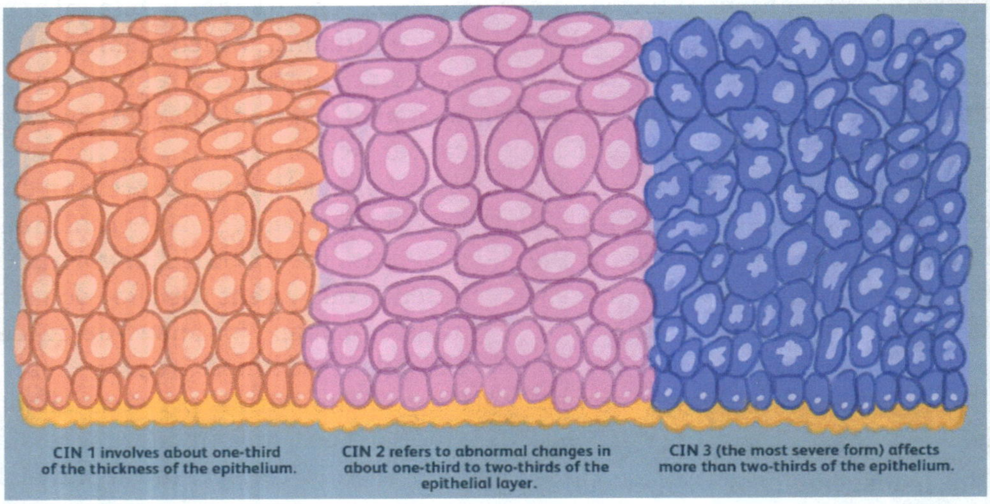

Figure 10.15. Cervical Intraepithelial Neoplasia (CIN).

Source: https://www.verywellhealth.com/thmb/clRX37siJT-kaZZ93TkPX4ZA7Lg=/1500x0/filters:no_upscale:max_bytes(150000):strip_icc()/cervical-intraepithelial-neoplasia-signs-symptoms-5199010-FINAL-433c047146ec402da496f5a5e2bf45bf.jpg

10.6.2. Surgical Interventions

Surgical management is of prime significance in the treatment of vulval, vaginal, and cervical benign lesions, with judicious evaluation underlying the best results. Of all the lesions, the Buschke-Löwenstein tumor (BLT) is of particular concern due to its local aggressiveness despite being benign. Surgical excision is usually the primary treatment of BLT, necessitating total extirpation with evident margins to prevent recurrence and reduce complications. The multifaceted nature of such interventions often requires involvement of multidisciplinary teams including plastic surgeons, gynecologists, and pathologists to facilitate successful removal and reconstruction, which can be the deciding factor in maintaining the integrity of the adjacent tissues as well as overall quality of life for the patient, as highlighted in reports of successful procedure outcomes (Grosu-Bularda *et al.*, 2024). Other than BLT, several benign lesions need surgery, particularly among immunocompromised individuals who can have worse disease progression. Vulvar condylomatosis, for instance, poses a significant challenge, particularly among those patients who have received suboptimal treatment regimens previously. Surgical excision remains the norm in such patients, especially in the case of large or refractory lesions that cannot be managed by other forms of treatment, such as topical agents that might be beyond reach for others. Intentional preoperative formulation of surgical interventions, for example, whether to leave lesions open to secondary intention healing or perform reconstructive techniques, can maximize patient rehabilitation and reduce the scope for complications. Outcomes of such operations can particularly be encouraging, as in cases where patients enjoyed a long-term disease-free status following successful excisional treatment (Monteiro *et al.*, 2022).

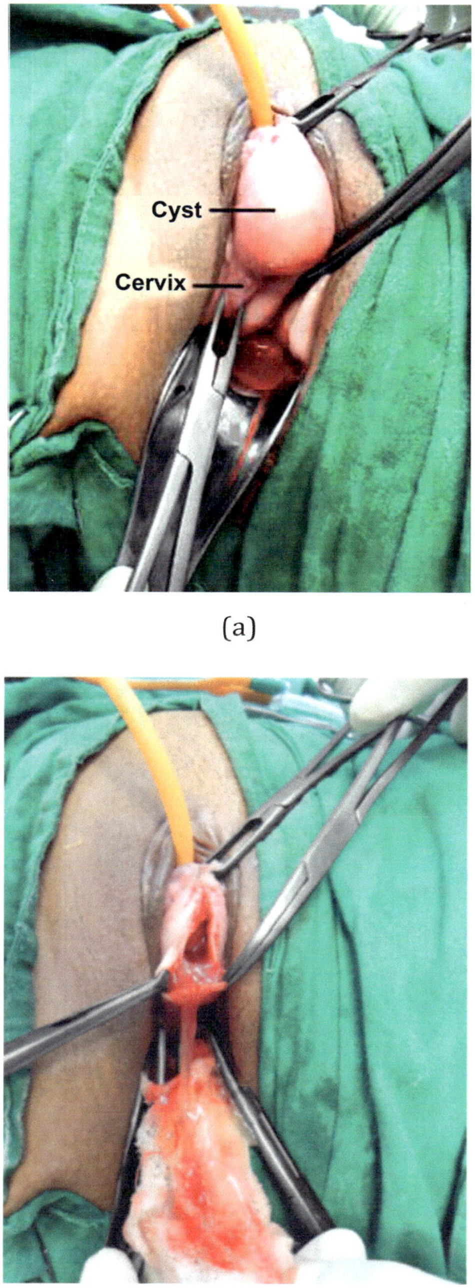

(a)

(b)

Figure 10.16. A: Vaginal wall inclusion cyst B: Same cyst is being excised

Source: https://oshimu.com/wp-content/uploads/2021/07/Gynaecology-DC-Dutta.pdf

Lastly, the decision on surgery is made from complete knowledge of not only the lesion itself but also the systemic factors that can affect patient outcomes in one way or another. Surgical interventions can significantly reduce the recurrence rate of benign lesions, particularly in conditions such as BLT and condylomatosis, which experience high rates of recurrence. The use of new surgical techniques combined with excellent post-operative care practices has the potential to facilitate improved healing and improved long-term health status. Therefore, in an evolving clinical experience and medical technology, there is a necessity to modify treatment protocols so that interventions remain in line with optimal practices, allowing for preferred outcomes in patients with benign vulvar, vaginal, and cervical lesions.

10.6.3. Medical Management

Treatment of benign vulval, vaginal, and cervical lesions mandates a careful approach that is equally mindful of patient health and safety. Prompt detection and proper classification of these lesions significantly influence subsequent medical management. The current guidelines emphasize the importance of individual risk stratification, with consideration for both screening history and patient factors such as age and immunosuppression. For instance, the 2019 ASCCP guidelines emphasize a shift from result-only algorithms to risk-based guidelines that utilize a mix of screening test findings and medical histories to inform the management strategy. This shift provides for more personalized interventions, subjecting the patient only to the necessary procedure while avoiding overtreatment, thereby sparing patient autonomy and maximizing healthcare resources (Perkins *et al.*, 2020). With cervical lesions, medical management practices have been revolutionized through the introduction of HPV testing, and it is now possible to detect precancerous changes at an earlier point than was previously possible. Beyond new screening innovations, these advancements have also facilitated the development of risk stratification protocols that are employed by clinicians to guide decisions for patient care. For example, the recommendations imply that those with low-risk findings can wait on colposcopy and have less frequent follow-up, and those with high-risk may require accelerated treatment modalities. This risk factor awareness is a useful determinant of a move towards more preventative measures, where lesions are treated before they become more advanced problems. Through continuous updating of management standards to incorporate new evidence, physicians can enhance the quality of care given to women at risk of cervical lesions (Bhatla *et al.*, 2018). Additionally, management of benign lesions extends beyond screening to encompass minimally invasive but effective therapeutic interventions. This applies particularly because there is growing concern for the psychological and physical impact of treatment on the patient. Advances in imaging modalities and minimally invasive methods in recent times have provided choices for successful treatment of such lesions with added emphasis on quality-of-life concerns. By adopting an all-around care approach for the patient by incorporating palliative measures and emotional care, improved overall treatment outcomes can be attained. With changing paradigms, ongoing engagement with updated guidelines, for instance, WHO's proposed changes for cervical cancer elimination, will be pivotal in framing future trends of medical management of benign vulvar, vaginal, and cervical lesions (Rebecca B Perkins *et al.*, 2020; Bhatla *et al.*, 2018).

Test Your Knowledge

1. What are the common treatment options for managing benign lesions in the vulva, vagina, and cervix?
2. When is surgical removal indicated in the management of benign reproductive tract lesions?

SUMMARY

The study of vulval, vaginal, and cervical benign lesions provides valuable insights into their presentation, pathophysiology, and clinical management. Accurate knowledge of these lesions is necessary to avoid misunderstanding them and taking the wrong treatment measures, which would only increase patient anxiety and compromise outcomes. Most benign conditions, including vulvar cysts, vaginal adenosis, and cervical polyps, share similar symptoms with malignancies, so healthcare professionals need to evaluate them carefully. Overall, the majority of these lesions never develop into cancer; however, diagnosis and differentiation from malignant processes form the very cornerstone of gynecologic practice. Broad education and awareness in both clinicians and patients cannot be overstressed, as it ensures that benign conditions are managed optimally without excessive interventions or distress. With ongoing new evidence emerging, it is increasingly important to examine the effect of viral pathogenesis on benign lesions. The burgeoning understanding of the human papillomavirus (HPV) and its many strains is that it serves to illustrate the complex interconnections between viral pathology and epithelial pathology. Those strains that produce benign lesions, such as genital warts, possess specific immune evasion characteristics by which they are able to reside within the host. A better comprehension of such mechanisms could be revolutionary to clinical practice, including the rechanneling of prevention strategies such as vaccination and screening protocols. Further, insight derived from the observation of HPVs' dissimilar patterns of expression could shape the way benign lesions are viewed in cervical health and disease prevention and thus dictate future therapeutic practices and patient management. In conclusion, the studies on vulvar, vaginal, and cervical benign lesions emphasize the complexity and importance of these conditions in female health. The future will necessitate a multidisciplinary approach combining molecular biology, virology, and clinical practice developments. As emphasized in the existing literature, expanding our knowledge of benign disease can facilitate more precise and effective treatment, thus improving overall patient outcomes. Ongoing involvement in ongoing research and clinical education will be paramount to continued knowledge regarding benign lesions, potentially impacting treatment of related conditions such as neuroendocrine neoplasms, which are not as frequently encountered but no less significant to gynecologic health (Oronsky *et al.*, 2017). Through syncretic learning from other disciplines, the gynecological fraternity can enhance their performance in patients who present with these diverse conditions while overcoming the intrinsic psychological as well as physical challenges they pose (Egawa *et al.*, 2015).

The observation of benign vulvar, vaginal, and cervical lesions shows the complex interplay between microbiological and pathological factors that play an overwhelming role in women's health. The progress in next-generation sequencing (NGS) technology in recent years has flung open the door to comprehending the pivotal role played by the cervical and cervico-vaginal microbiota (CM and CVM) in the case of diseases such as human papillomavirus (HPV) infection. Interferences of CMV and CVM are more and more known as having the capability to act as precursors to HPV persistence and secondary cervical dysplasia, justifying the need for ongoing research into microbial diversity in association with benign lesions. Thus, characterization of the cervical microbiome through methods like bacterial 16S rRNA gene sequencing offers a promising pathway for the development of customized diagnostic devices and interventions that will optimize cervical health and decrease the risk for malignant transformation of benign lesions (Maria Głowienka *et al.*, 2024). Moreover, benign lesions could have ramifications broader than local pathology, impacting reproductive health in general. Fresh evidence indicates that HPV not only induces cervical lesions but also has an effect on male reproductive function, hence depicting the interdependence of women's and men's health when it comes to HPV. Particularly, studies have indicated that HPV infection can adversely affect the sperm parameters such as DNA integrity, motility, number, and morphology, thereby contributing to fertility complications among couples (Sucato *et al.*, 2023). This thus points to the necessity of great knowledge in benign lesions within the reproductive health debate. Preventive interventions, including gender-neutral vaccination programs, can actually combat the spread of HPV and eventually eliminate fertility issues brought about by benign lesions, further reinforcing the connection between cervical health and reproductive outcome. In brief, a comprehensive view of vulvar, vaginal, and cervical benign lesions calls for an interdisciplinary approach in considering microbiological, pathological, and reproductive health. The examination of the cervical microbiome is critical in deconstructing the intricate dynamics that have the potential to predispose an individual to benign and more severe conditions. Evolution of research in this area, based on the use of NGS technology, holds promises for new preventive and therapeutic strategies against HPV-related diseases. Moreover, inclusion of information on the male reproductive health indicates the broader consequences of benign cervical lesions, enhancing the importance of addressing HPV as a significant determinant of male and female fertility. Collective learnings made from these analyses pave the way for more targeted interventions and enhanced public health measures related to cervical well-being and reproductive health (Maria Głowienka *et al.*, 2024; Sucato *et al.*, 2023).

KEY TERMS FROM THIS CHAPTER

- Bartholin's Cyst
- Nabothian Cyst
- Condyloma Acuminata
- Cystadenofibroma
- Papillomas
- Cervical intraepithelial neoplasia (CIN)
- Comprehensive care
- Clitoris
- Gartner's Duct Cyst
- Cervical Polyp
- Fibroepithelial polyps of the vagina (FEPV)
- Gynecologic disease
- Hyperplastic lesions
- Socioeconomic determinants
- Labia majora
- Dermatoses

CRITICAL THINKING QUESTIONS

1. **Which of the following is a common benign lesion of the vulva characterized by small, benign cysts near the vaginal opening?**
   a. Bartholin cyst
   b. Cervical polyp
   c. Condyloma acuminatum
   d. Endometriosis
2. **Nabothian cysts are benign lesions found in the:**
   a. Vulva
   b. Vagina
   c. Cervix
   d. Endometrium
3. **Which benign lesion of the cervix appears as a smooth, red, pedunculated growth often causing vaginal bleeding?**
   a. Cervical polyp
   b. Cervical carcinoma
   c. Endometrial polyp
   d. Fibroid
4. **Condyloma acuminatum is caused by infection with which virus?**
   a. Herpes simplex virus
   b. Human papillomavirus (HPV)
   c. Epstein-Barr virus
   d. Cytomegalovirus
5. **Gartner's duct cysts are benign cysts located in the:**
   a. Vulva
   b. Vagina
   c. Cervix
   d. Uterus

Short Answer Questions

1. What are the common types of benign lesions found in the female reproductive tract?
2. Name two types of benign vulvar lesions.
3. What symptoms are commonly associated with benign vaginal and cervical lesions?
4. Which diagnostic methods are used to identify benign lesions of the vulva, vagina, and cervix?
5. What are typical treatment options for benign vulvar lesions?
6. How are benign cervical lesions usually managed?

Answer to Critical Thinking Questions

1. (a) 2. (c) 3. (a) 4. (b) 5. (b)

REFERENCES

1. Alsayed, A. S., Elkadi, T. T. H., Alshamari, M. S., & Attallah, A. T. (2024). Prepubertal female Bartholin's gland abscess: A comprehensive case report study. *Case Reports in Pediatrics, 2024*. https://doi.org/10.1155/2024/8812350 (accessed on 14th June 2025).
2. Arega, C., Girma, W., & Sanchez Diaz, J. M. (2019). Angiofibroma of the vagina presenting with abnormal vaginal bleeding: A case report from Ethiopia and review of the literature. *Case Reports in Obstetrics and Gynecology, 2019*, 1–4. https://doi.org/10.1155/2019/1486387 (accessed on 14th June 2025).
3. Asati, P., Sultan, S., Nigam, R., & Asati, S. (2022). Study of colposcopy and histopathological correlation for cervical lesion at tertiary care: Original research. *International Journal of Health Sciences*. https://www.semanticscholar.org/paper/0fb2e61d09e1f37bed5bcd2ca1d56a630c99c7e6 (accessed on 14th June 2025).
4. Bhatla, N., Aoki, D., Sharma, D. N., & Sankaranarayanan, R. (2018). Cancer of the cervix uteri. *International Journal of Gynecology & Obstetrics, 143*, 22–36. https://doi.org/10.1002/ijgo.12611 (accessed on 14th June 2025).
5. Chalya, P. L., Mabula, J. B., Rambau, P., & Mchembe, M. D. (2013). Sister Mary Joseph's nodule at a university teaching hospital in northwestern Tanzania: A retrospective review of 34 cases. *World Journal of Surgical Oncology, 11*. https://doi.org/10.1186/1477-7819-11-151 (accessed on 14th June 2025).
6. de Oliveira, C. M. (2018). Adaptation of alpha-papillomavirus over millennia. *Acta Cytologica, 63*, 97–99. https://www.semanticscholar.org/paper/b2cda2cf8682a49919da423353c5f3f7ed84be67 (accessed on 14th June 2025).
7. Dellino, M., Magazzino, F., Domenici, L., Cicogna, S., Miano, S. T., Pignata, S., Mangili, G., *et al.* (2024). Aggressive angiomyxoma of the lower female genital tract: A review of the MITO Rare Tumors Group. *Cancers, 16*, 1375. https://doi.org/10.3390/cancers16071375 (accessed on 14th June 2025).
8. Donovan, E. K., Lo, S. S., Beriwal, S., Chen, H., Cheung, P., Keller, A., Nwachukwu, C., *et al.* (2024). Stereotactic ablative radiotherapy for gynecological oligometastatic and oligoprogressive tumors. *JAMA Oncology*. https://www.semanticscholar.org/paper/8452a3354d6622e2ba074c5d875bb748d52ccd60 (accessed on 14th June 2025).
9. Egawa, N., Egawa, K., Griffin, H., & Doorbar, J. (2015). Human papillomaviruses; epithelial tropisms, and the development of neoplasia. *Viruses, 7*, 3863–3890. https://doi.org/10.3390/v7072802 (accessed on 14th June 2025).
10. Głowienka, M., Bagińska, K., Szubert, S., Hennig, E. E., Horała, A., Dąbrowska, M., Micek, M., *et al.* (2024). Human papillomavirus infections and the role played by cervical and cervical-vaginal microbiota—Evidence from next-generation sequencing studies. *Cancers, 16*, 399. https://doi.org/10.3390/cancers16020399 (accessed on 14th June 2025).
11. Grosu-Bularda, A., Hariga, C., Dumitru, C. Ș., Calcaianu, N., Creangă, C., Enache, V., Tache, S. E., *et al.* (2024). Clinicopathological findings and comprehensive review of Buschke–Lowenstein tumors based on a case study. *Journal of Personalized Medicine, 14*. https://www.semanticscholar.org/paper/c2be26a9f0514114bc1764f50da36f26e3b15946 (accessed on 14th June 2025).

12. Höhn, A. K., Brambs, C. E., Hiller, G. G. R., May, D., Schmoeckel, E., & Horn, L. C. (2021). 2020 WHO classification of female genital tumors. *Geburtshilfe und Frauenheilkunde, 81*, 1145–1153. https://doi.org/10.1055/a-1545-4279 (accessed on 14th June 2025).
13. Khashcha, I., Sozanska, M. A., Mitsoda, R. M., & Korchynska, O. (2024). Cervical dysplasia, cervicitis and inflammatory bowel disease–Is there a relationship? (Literature review). *Reproductive Health of Woman*. https://www.semanticscholar.org/paper/996dc662293802f30158efee3dea38ffb8990032 (accessed on 14th June 2025).
14. Kumar, N., Rath, A., Setty, A., Rathod, P. T., & Aparna, J. (2025). Cystadenofibroma and contralateral collision lesions: A unique ovarian case report. *Oncoscience, 12*, 26–33. https://www.semanticscholar.org/paper/5139431bf1dbe27328cbc43df466a12e4928eac0 (accessed on 14th June 2025).
15. Kurekar, S. A., Chaudhari, J., Shenoy, A., & Chaturvedi, R. (2021). Atypical cervical stromal cells masquerading as malignancy. *Annals of Pathology and Laboratory Medicine, 8*. https://www.semanticscholar.org/paper/901f99c7b019809aab9ac80406610522b81a5dcd (accessed on 14th June 2025).
16. McCluggage, W. G. (2015). Recent developments in non–HPV-related adenocarcinomas of the lower female genital tract and their precursors. *Advances in Anatomic Pathology, 23*, 58–69. https://doi.org/10.1097/pap.0000000000000095 (accessed on 14th June 2025).
17. Misra, A., Madzhia, P., Malebana, T., Muavha, D., Boshomane, J., & Baloyi, K. (2024). Surgical management of giant condyloma acuminata involving vulva, perineum and perianal area. *Journal of Gynecology and Obstetrics*. https://www.semanticscholar.org/paper/495ef4fc5586fb10e0908b3f49cbb5f7113cb34b (accessed on 14th June 2025).
18. Mohamed, N. G., Zu El-Fakkar, N. M., & El-Khateeb, E. A. (2023). Comparative study of intralesional measles–mumps–rubella vaccine versus needling-induced autoinoculation in the management of genital warts. *QJM: An International Journal of Medicine*. https://www.semanticscholar.org/paper/159dbd4e61600f955fffee88b39e104fb856e6f0 (accessed on 14th June 2025).
19. Mondal, S., Pradhan, R., Chakraborty, A., & Chatterjee, S. (2024). Osseous metaplasia of cervix mimicking cervical cancer–A rare case report. *Journal of Mid-Life Health, 15*, 122–124. https://www.semanticscholar.org/paper/4d879467a9ca39a9d8d6f8ca9aa154ca01848d23 (accessed on 14th June 2025).
20. Monteiro, D., Varejão, A. M., Sampaio, J., & Rodrigues, M. (2022). Vulvar condyloma of Buschke and Löwenstein: An unusual tumor in developed countries. *BMJ Case Reports, 15*. https://www.semanticscholar.org/paper/10c1c91cc0e34cdcff73b1715a4e182cf2f7accc (accessed on 14th June 2025).
21. Ning, Y., Ling, R., Zhang, F., Zhang, G., & Zhang, H. (2023). Common and uncommon lesions of the vulva and vagina on magnetic resonance imaging: Correlations with pathological findings. *BJR Open, 5*. https://www.semanticscholar.org/paper/d5d3c8c6ece3ca96a08002abd7eb4180f9a65488 (accessed on 14th June 2025).
22. Nongo, B., Isah, D. A., & Abdul, O. A. (2024). Fibroepithelial polyp of the vagina in pregnancy: A case report. *Journal of the West African College of Surgeons, 14*, 238–240. https://www.semanticscholar.org/paper/680092ee9e6d2b10bb0b94816c048b62a25a70c4 (accessed on 14th June 2025).

23. Nouh, A. A. A. E. S., El Din, E. T. N., Abd El-Razik, E. A. E. R., & Ahmed, K. E. A. (2022). Accuracy of naked eye visual inspection in early detection of cervical intraepithelial neoplasia at Zagazig University Hospitals. *The Egyptian Journal of Hospital Medicine, 88*, 3481–3487. https://doi.org/10.21608/ejhm.2022.248820 (accessed on 14th June 2025).

24. Ogura, N., Inagaki, M., Yasuda, R., Yoshida, S., & Maeda, T. (2022). A vaginal fibroepithelial stromal polyp: A case report with magnetic resonance images. *BJR|Case Reports, 8*. https://doi.org/10.1259/bjrcr.20210189 (accessed on 14th June 2025).

25. Oronsky, B., Patrick, C., Morgensztern, D., & Carter, C. A. (2017). Nothing but NET: A review of neuroendocrine tumors and carcinomas. *Neoplasia, 19*, 991–1002. https://doi.org/10.1016/j.neo.2017.09.002 (accessed on 14th June 2025).

26. Perino, A., & Capra, G. (2023). Human papillomavirus and male infertility: What do we know? *International Journal of Molecular Sciences, 24*, 17562. https://doi.org/10.3390/ijms242417562 (accessed on 14th June 2025).

27. Perkins, R. B., Guido, R. S., Castle, P. E., Chelmow, D., Einstein, M. H., García, F., Huh, W. K., *et al.* (2020). 2019 ASCCP risk-based management consensus guidelines for abnormal cervical cancer screening tests and cancer precursors. *Journal of Lower Genital Tract Disease, 24*, 102–131. https://doi.org/10.1097/lgt.0000000000000525 (accessed on 14th June 2025).

28. Preti, M., Joura, E. A., Vieira-Baptista, P., van Beurden, M., Bevilacqua, F., Bleeker, M., Bornstein, J., *et al.* (2022). The European Society of Gynecological Oncology (ESGO), the International Society for the Study of Vulvovaginal Disease (ISSVD), the European College for the Study of Vulval Disease (ECSVD) and the European Federation for Colposcopy (EFC) consensus statements on pre-invasive vulvar lesions. *Journal of Lower Genital Tract Disease*. https://doi.org/10.1097/lgt.0000000000000683 (accessed on 14th June 2025).

29. Šarenac, T., & Mikov, M. (2019). Cervical cancer, different treatments and importance of bile acids as therapeutic agents in this disease. *Frontiers in Pharmacology, 10*. https://doi.org/10.3389/fphar.2019.00484 (accessed on 14th June 2025).

30. Shaaban, A. M., Turton, E. P., & Merchant, W. (2013). An unusual case of a large fibroepithelial stromal polyp presenting as a nipple mass. *BMC Research Notes, 6*. https://doi.org/10.1186/1756-0500-6-345 (accessed on 14th June 2025).

31. Smolarz, B., Szyłło, K., & Romanowicz, H. (2021). Endometriosis: Epidemiology, classification, pathogenesis, treatment and genetics (Review of literature). *International Journal of Molecular Sciences, 22*, 10554. https://doi.org/10.3390/ijms221910554 (accessed on 14th June 2025).

32. Tadir, Y., Gaspar, A., Lev-Sagie, A., Alexiades, M., Alinsod, R., Bader, A., Calligaro, A., *et al.* (2017). Light and energy-based therapeutics for genitourinary syndrome of menopause: Consensus and controversies. *Lasers in Surgery and Medicine, 49*, 137–159. https://doi.org/10.1002/lsm.22637 (accessed on 14th June 2025).

33. Tirkaso, B. H., Bayisa, T. H., & Desta, T. W. (2024). Histopathologic patterns and factors associated with cervical lesions at Jimma Medical Center, Jimma, Southwest Ethiopia: A two-year cross-sectional study. *PLOS ONE, 19*. https://www.semanticscholar.org/paper/41796d6493fccc28a288478f0df45520d2614cc8 (accessed on 14th June 2025).

34. Wang, J., Yang, Q., Wang, D., Li, M., & Zhang, N. (2022). Case report: Gastric-type endocervical adenocarcinoma mimicking submucosal myoma under hysteroscopy. *Frontiers in Medicine, 9*. https://doi.org/10.3389/fmed.2022.845445 (accessed on 14th June 2025).

REPRODUCTIVE TRACT INFECTIONS

11

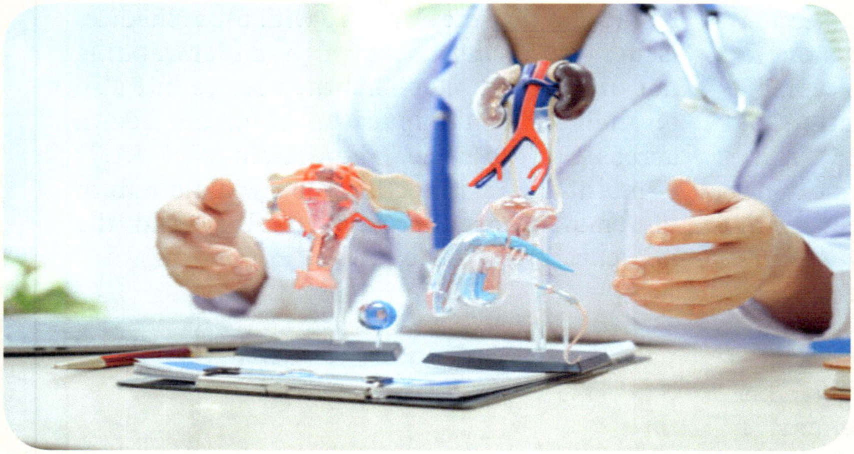

LEARNING OBJECTIVES

After studying this chapter, you will be able to:

1. Identify the common types of reproductive tract infections
2. Explain the causes and risk factors associated with reproductive tract infections
3. Recognize the symptoms and diagnostic methods for reproductive tract infections
4. Evaluate treatment options available for reproductive tract infections
5. Describe effective prevention strategies for reproductive tract infections

Introduction

Female reproductive tract infections (RTIs) are a significant public health issue, particularly among women of childbearing age in urban poor communities. RTIs lead to significant morbidity, affecting not only the physical health of women but also their socioeconomic status. The timely treatment and diagnosis are essential, but late intervention is a result of a combination of inadequate health-seeking behavior and socioeconomic constraints. For instance, in slums of urban cities like Agra, barriers in terms of financial constraints, embarrassment, and lack of support can hamper access to essential health care services among women. All these barriers combined contribute to an elevated burden of RTIs, and therefore, there is a requirement for specialized interventions in terms of increased awareness and healthcare access for vulnerable populations (Yadav *et al.*, 2025). In examining the health-seeking behavior of married women in urban slums, research has determined that the majority of those presenting with symptoms of RTIs fail to get treated. Specifically, one study discovered that a paltry 57.92% of women went for medical attention, leaving a significant proportion untreated. The barriers include not only financial, but also the subjective unreality of symptoms, stigma around reproductive health, and inadequate family support, which all exacerbate the health hazards that these women expose themselves to. These dynamics need to be appreciated in order to formulate effective public health interventions to improve treatment-seeking behavior. Interventions should be directed towards enhancing education on RTIs and facilitating open discussion to overcome stigma, thus empowering women to make decisions about prioritization of reproductive health (Yadav *et al.*, 2025). Also, the consequences of untreated RTIs can extend far beyond individual health outcomes, with implications for overall community health. Complications of RTIs can lead to severe consequences like infertility and susceptibility to sexually transmitted infections (STIs), which continue to burden public health systems. This underlines the necessity of comprehensive healthcare interventions that address not only the medical sequelae of RTIs but also the socio-cultural determinants that influence health-seeking behavior. A multi-faceted approach involving enhanced access to care, reproductive health education, and social support systems is necessary to stem the incidence of RTIs among women in such high-risk settings. By treating the symptoms as well as the root barriers, public health programs can significantly improve the health condition for women with reproductive tract infections (Yadav *et al.*, 2025).

Definition of Female Reproductive Tract Infections

Female reproductive tract infections (FRTIs) define a spectrum of infections that affect the anatomical structure in the female reproductive system, encompassing the vagina, cervix, uterus, fallopian tubes, and the ovaries. The infections are caused by exposure to a spectrum of pathogens, including bacteria, viruses, fungi, and parasites, leading to conditions from bacterial vaginosis and vulvovaginal candidiasis to sexually transmitted infections (STIs) like chlamydia and gonorrhea. The pathogenic mechanisms typically encompass destruction of normal flora, inflammatory responses, and alterations in the microenvironment, which may lead to discomfort, disorders of reproductive health, and even fulminant morbidity. The complexity of these infections is brought out by the fact that they overlap with other medical issues, requiring a thorough understanding not only of the infections themselves but also of their overall impact on women's health across the life cycle. The aetiology of FRTIs is multifaceted, reflecting the dynamic nature of female reproductive physiology and the influence of extrinsic factors.

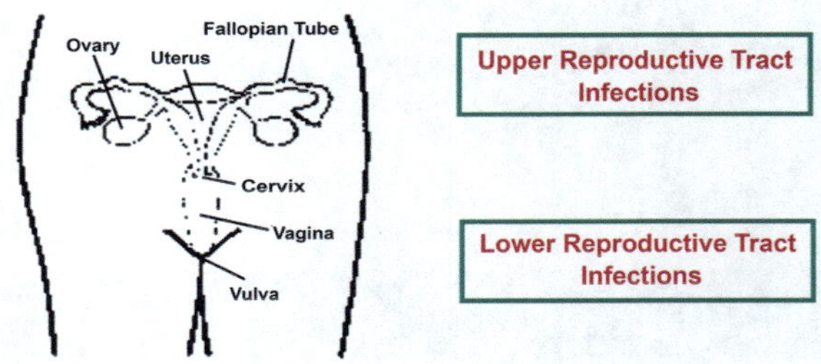

Figure 11.1. The diagram illustrates the reproductive tract of women. Infections in the area of the vulva, vagina, or cervix are referred to as lower reproductive tract infections. Infections in the uterus, fallopian tubes, and ovaries are considered upper reproductive tract infections.

Source: https://knowledgecommons.popcouncil.org/cgi/viewcontent.cgi?article=2870&context=departments_sbsr-rh

Hormonal fluctuations, such as those occurring during menstruation, pregnancy, and menopause, have a fundamental influence upon the vaginal environment and, therefore, the predisposition to infection. Research indicates that a healthy vaginal microbiota, which is largely composed of *Lactobacillus* species, plays an essential role in maintaining reproductive health by preventing the proliferation of pathogens. For instance, dysbiosis is at a greater risk of developing bacterial vaginosis as well as other infections, and thus, it is crucial to maintain an optimized microbial population (Adams *et al.*, 2025).

Besides, lifestyle, socioeconomic factors, and underlying conditions like diabetes and obesity also compromise the female reproductive tract's resistance against infection, which emphasizes the significance of targeted public health interventions for eliminating risk factors for these infections. In order to comprehend the clinical significance of FRTIs, a general evaluation of their impact on reproductive health and quality of life has to be conducted. Chronic or repeated infection can lead to severe health consequences, including pelvic inflammatory disease, ectopic pregnancy, and infertility (Adams *et al.*, 2025). Furthermore, untreated infections can expose women to severe effects, including complications during pregnancy or the progression of some cancers associated with chronic inflammation, like human papillomavirus (HPV)-associated cervical cancer (Vinitha *et al.*, 2025). Thus, early diagnosis and proper treatment of FRTIs play a key role in preventing long-term health complications. The inclusion of reproductive health education, the necessity of regular screenings, and the accessibility of treatments is paramount in enabling women to take charge of their reproductive health and prevent them from catching infections.

Importance of Understanding Infections

Understanding infection within the framework of the female reproductive tract is necessary in order to address both individual health and public health. The female reproductive system is especially susceptible to infection due to the biological and anatomical characteristics inherent in the reproductive organs. Infection may cause serious outcomes like pelvic inflammatory disease (PID), infertility, and pregnancy complications. By understanding the mechanisms by which pathogens act, medical and healthcare practitioners are better able to apply preventative interventions and treatments. Such knowledge is important for educating patients about risk factors and prodromal symptoms that could be indicative of an underlying infection. Furthermore, since infections frequently overlap with social determinants of health, reproductive tract infection education needs to be inclusive and framed for diverse populations to allow for successful outreach and intervention planning. The effects of untreated infections in the female reproductive tract go beyond the problems to individual well-being; they influence larger communities and society. They include such things as infertility caused by untreated STIs, which have long-term social and psychological impacts, especially in cultures where fertility is highly valued. Here, understanding the causal relationship between infections and infertility comes into play because it promotes the advancement of the advocacy for reproductive health services. Medical practitioners' role comes into play in de-stigmatizing such relations in order to promote healthy management. Additionally, by opening up discussions around reproductive health that include information on infections, medical practitioners can promote the advancement of the knowledge of reproductive rights and health equity in society. It is shown through studies that information regarding infections also goes a long way in the enactment of useful public health policies. With local and global health agencies working towards curtailing the transmission of reproductive tract infections, policy-making informed by evidence is crucial. Information regarding the epidemiology of infections is useful for resource allocation and the development of targeted intervention programs. Organization guidelines, such as those of the World Health Organization, recommend mainstreaming infection prevention and treatment strategies into broader reproductive health care models. These actions emphasize the importance of understanding infections as not just medical issues but also as public health problems that require a collaborative effort. To treat these infections, therefore, is a responsibility that involves individual health behaviors and policy change at the system level, critical to the achievement of universal reproductive health outcomes (N/A, 2021) (Baumgartner *et al.*, 2020).

11.1. Common Types of Reproductive Tract Infections

Learning Outcome

1. Discuss the bacterial vaginosis
2. Explain the yeast infections
3. Define sexually transmitted infections (STIs)

The prevalence of reproductive tract infections (RTIs) in females has emerged as a serious public health concern, based on their effect on overall health and reproductive capability. Among the most common types of RTIs are those produced by bacterial pathogens, mostly by Chlamydia trachomatis (Ct) and Neisseria gonorrhoeae (NG). Chlamydia, in particular, has been a well-documented causative factor in the development of pelvic inflammatory disease (PID) and infertility. Vaccination against this infection remains crucial but inconclusive, with no licensed vaccine yet available despite ongoing research into specific proteins engaged in infection adhesion, such as the polymorphic membrane protein D (PmpD) (Collar *et al.*, 2025). The implications of untreated infections can be devastating, involving increased vigilance and access to sexually active women across all demographics to screen for disease reduction and related health complications. HSV II infections also significantly impact women's reproductive health, with the virus being a frequent issue. HSV II can cause painful blisters, repeated infections, and complications during childbirth, presenting infected individuals with significant psychological and physiological burdens. More recent studies have highlighted the varying infection rates of HSV II across different age groups; adolescent women are the most vulnerable. Besides that, outpatient studies have indicated that although UU is predominantly found in infertile men, the overall trend of RTIs illustrates women displaying a greater frequency of viral infection of infections like HSV II compared to their male peers, thereby establishing the need for targeted prevention among at-risk youth populations (Zeng *et al.*, 2024). The correlation between reproductive tract infections and infertility is a critical challenge to health workers. Chlamydia and Ureaplasma infections, among others, lead to occlusion of the fallopian tubes, with attendant complications of ectopic pregnancy and chronic pelvic pain. Also, the age distribution of such infections indicates that young women, particularly in late adolescence and early adulthood, are most likely to be at highest risk for Ct infection, and this is a critical group to target within intervention programs. There is a need for health systems to place value on awareness and information in facilitating prevention and early identification efforts. This anticipatory measure may not only decrease the prevalence of STIs but also enhance reproductive health among women, hence enhancing overall health trends as they progress through their reproductive lifespan.

11.1.1. Bacterial Vaginosis

Bacterial Vaginosis (BV) is a common form of female genital tract infection, characterized by the disruption of regular lactobacilli-dominant vaginal microbiota. *Lactobacillus* spp. assume important roles in acidifying the vagina and forming a protective barrier against invasive pathogenic microbes in the uninfected condition. However, in BV, there is a shift to an overgrowth of anaerobic bacteria, including *Gardnerella vaginalis* and *Prevotella* species, at the expense of *Lactobacillus* numbers. This dysbiosis can produce symptoms of clinical disease, including thin, grayish-white discharge and fishy odor, but may not always be symptomatic. The prevalence of BV is prevalent among women in the reproductive age group, and studies have shown that it affects nearly 30% of such women, thus necessitating increased awareness and information about the condition in terms of overall reproductive health. The implications of BV extend beyond the immediate impact on the localized presentation and have overall implications for women's reproductive health, with a risk of adverse consequences. Research has demonstrated that women with BV are more susceptible to sexually transmitted infections (STIs), such as HIV, due to the imbalanced vaginal flora that diminishes mucosal defenses.

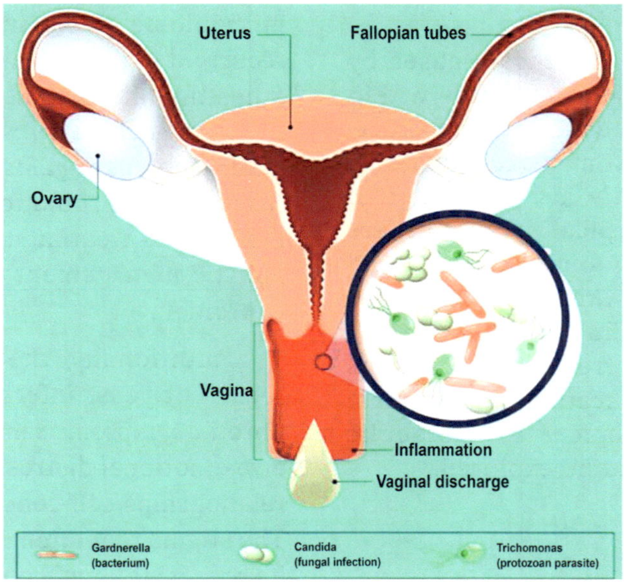

Figure 11.2. Bacterial Vaginosis.

Source: https://healthandvitalitycenter.com/medical-conditions/chronic-bacterial-vaginosis/

Also, BV has been linked to pregnancy complications, such as preterm labor and chorioamnionitis, demonstrating the systemic character of this infection. The association of BV with adverse reproductive outcomes emphasizes the need for effective screening and treatment strategies, particularly among high-risk populations. As the function of the microbiota is elucidated in the establishment of reproductive health, the investigation of therapeutic treatments that could potentially reverse the healthy bacterial flora of the vagina gains significance in minimizing risks for BV and maximizing reproductive outcome. Bacterial vaginosis is treated through the use of antibiotics like metronidazole and clindamycin. However, the recurrence of BV is the biggest challenge since studies have shown that reinfection rates could be as high as 60% following three months of treatment. Such continuity leads to the necessity to expand knowledge about vaginal microbiome dynamics and the influence of lifestyle on balance. Future studies project that the inclusion of probiotics can provide an adjunct treatment for reestablishing normal flora and reducing recurrence rates.

The interference of host immune responses and endogenous microbes is an area that is yet to be discovered, as the revelation of these variables may result in the formation of new therapies that not only cure symptoms of BV but also lead to a better long-term status of the vagina and inhibit other infections in the female reproductive tract, including those in the larger domain of female reproductive tract infections (Vinitha *et al.*, 2025; George *et al.*, 2024).

11.1.2. Yeast Infections

Fungal infections, particularly those caused by Candida albicans, are a significant issue within the context of female reproductive tract disease. They are found mostly in women of childbearing age and most commonly as vulvovaginal candidiasis. The most typical symptoms are intense itching, burning on urination, and deviant discharge, all of which have a serious effect on quality of life. While sporadic infections are mostly innocuous, frequent infections have broader health implications in the form of underlying immunological or metabolic abnormalities that need to be explored.

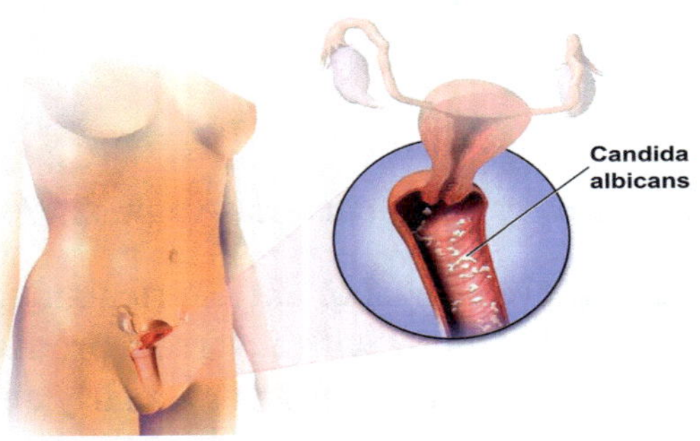

Figure 11.3. Yeast infection.

Source: https://ezraclinic.sg/wp-content/uploads/800px-Yeast_Infection.webp

Furthermore, certain high-risk groups such as pregnant women and diabetic or immunocompromised individuals are more susceptible to such infections, suggesting the need for risk-factor-specific prevention and treatment policy. Treatment of yeast infections is commonly in the form of antifungal medications, taken orally or applied topically.

Yet with the advent of antifungal resistance, treatment regimens need to be reconsidered and novel remedies sought. In the background of rising fear of side effects and return of symptoms with traditional antifungal therapy, there is increasing interest in delineating the vaginal microbiome's role in prevention, as well as recurrent vulvovaginal candidiasis. For instance, a healthy microbiome with beneficial bacteria such as *Lactobacillus* species can serve as a natural defense against Candida infection. Thus, research on probiotics and other microbiota-modulating treatments is important to develop holistic management plans for yeast infection in women.

Additionally, the psychosocial impact of recurrent yeast infection cannot be neglected. Chronic symptoms can not only produce pain but also emotional distress and affect interpersonal relationships, self-concept, and sexual well-being. The stigma that often accompanies reproductive health problems could make it difficult for patients to gain early medical advice, thereby hastening the progress of the disease. The interplay between mental health and infections of the female reproductive organs, e.g., yeast infections, also underscores the importance of integrative delivery of healthcare. Through the establishment of a culture where discussions of reproductive health are destigmatized, healthcare providers are in a better position to allow for better educational materials, triggering awareness and proactive management of yeast infection within the wider context of female reproductive tract health.

11.1.3. Sexually Transmitted Infections (STIs)

Sexually transmitted disease (STD) prevalence is a public health issue of great concern, particularly to females compared to males, because STDs have far-reaching consequences for reproductive health. STDs such as chlamydia, gonorrhea, and syphilis are largely silent, leading to late presentation and treatment. STDs, if untreated, will lead to significant complications such as pelvic inflammatory disease (PID), infertility, and even ectopic pregnancy. The complexity of the woman's reproductive system, as well as the health of the vaginal microbiome, is the crucial factor in susceptibility to STIs. Altering this balance of microbes, particularly a depletion of defensive Lactobacilli, will make a woman susceptible to pathogenic microbes associated with STIs. Understanding interactions between STIs and the female reproductive tract emphasizes the need for education and preventive healthcare interventions aimed at prevention and early intervention.

The interaction of sexually transmitted infections and the vaginal microbiome is fundamental to understanding the dynamics of female reproductive tract infection. *Lactobacillus* species regulate the healthy vaginal environment, maintaining low pH and releasing antimicrobial substances that inhibit pathogenic microorganisms. The balance is disrupted by conditions such as bacterial vaginosis (BV), allowing pathogenic microorganisms to overgrow. BV is characterized by the reduction of *Lactobacillus* and elevation of anaerobic bacteria, both of which expose individuals to STIs and exacerbate any present infection. Studies indicate that women with BV are at higher risk of acquiring and transmitting STIs, hence highlighting the importance of microbiota balance in sex. Interventions that replace and maintain a healthy vaginal microbiome can be an essential step in reducing STI infection rates and overall reproductive health outcomes.

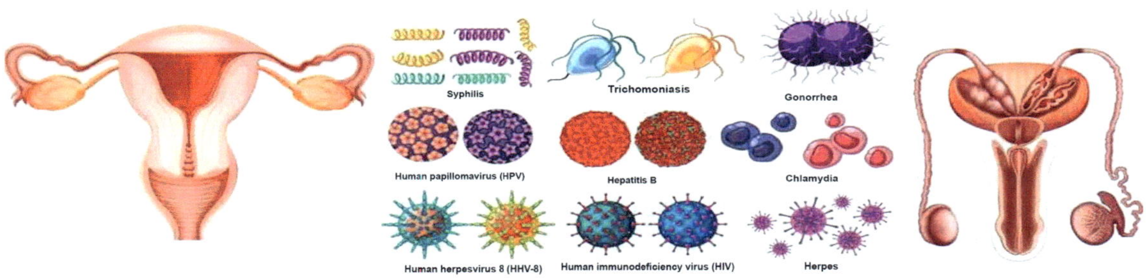

Figure 11.4. Common Sexually Transmitted Infections (STIs).

Source: https://www.drbenmedical.sg/wp-content/uploads/2024/07/image8-1024x344.jpg

Moreover, the influence of STIs extends beyond the direct danger to subsequent immediate health into long-term reproductive health and outcomes. Untreated STIs in females result in serious gynecologic consequences, including chronic pain and infertility, as well as preterm labor risk. The physiological change of hyperestrogenic states like pregnancy may also amplify the impact of STIs. For instance, the endocrine alterations of pregnancy could perpetuate a condition of pro-inflammatory states that not only aggravates existing infections but also poses an increased risk of vertical transmission to the fetal child. The latest body of evidence underscores the need for routine screening and individually directed treatments to mitigate such risks. Ensuring education access, testing, and healthcare services is crucial in reducing the occurrence of STIs and promoting healthier reproductive behaviors among women and ultimately improving reproductive health results (Chen *et al.*, 2021; Amabebe *et al.*, 2018).

Test Your Knowledge

1. What are the common causes and symptoms of bacterial vaginosis in reproductive tract infections?
2. How do yeast infections differ from bacterial vaginosis in terms of symptoms and treatment?

11.2. Causes and Risk Factors

Learning Outcome

1. Explain how bacterial imbalances contribute to reproductive tract infections
2. Analyze the impact of sexual activity and practices on reproductive health
3. Define hormonal changes and health conditions

Understanding the etiology and risk factors of female reproductive tract infections (RTIs) is essential to planning successful prevention and treatment strategies. Sociodemographic determinants such as age, socioeconomic status, and education significantly contribute to making a woman's exposure to RTIs more probable. For instance, women with less knowledge of reproductive health are more at risk, as revealed by research in which only 7.6% of the examined women had good knowledge of RTIs (Verma *et al.*, 2024).

Further, cultural menstrual and hygiene beliefs raise vulnerability; compromised sanitation and unavailability of sanitary products boost susceptibility. The merging of these social determinants creates a mixed model that necessitates targeted interventions for educating the vulnerable population. Behavioral risk factors also make a huge contribution to the occurrence of female RTIs. Poor personal hygiene, unprotected sex, and multiple partners are risk factors that increase the risk of infection. Evidence has shown that the use of barrier methods during menstruation severely reduces RTI attacks; however, very few women employ these preventive methods frequently (Verma *et al.*, 2024). Additionally, high parity, or having more than three children, is often linked to various reproductive morbidity and infections (Verma *et al.*, 2024). Women who do not use proper family planning practices are particularly at risk. This emphasizes the necessity for complete education and access to reproductive health services, empowering women to be active agents in their sexuality. Moreover, inherent physiological factors can make women prone to specific infections. For instance, urinary tract infections, prevalent among the female sex, are governed by anatomical features such as a shorter urethra, through which it becomes easier for bacteria to access. The consequence of untreated infections in older women can lead to severe complications like urosepsis, which can eventually raise the death rate. Identifying clinical features of infections, along with comorbidities present, while treating RTIs in susceptible age groups, needs to be taken into consideration. Clinicians should comprehend the multifactorial etiology and risk factors to administer effective intervention strategies and ultimately reduce the rate of female reproductive tract infections.

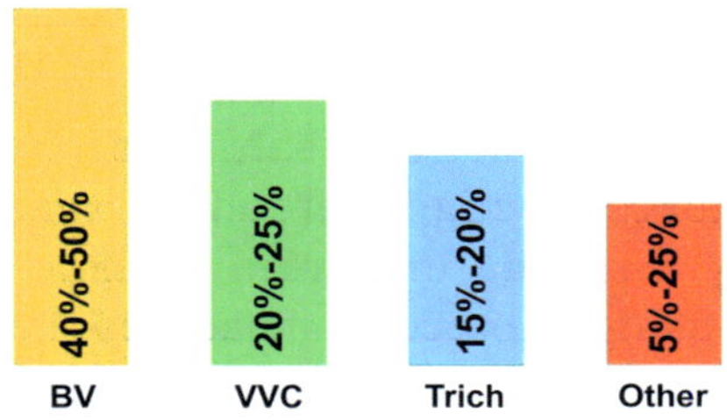

Figure 11.5. Top causes of vaginal infections.

Source: https://www.streamlinesci.com/blog/vaginal-infections-and-maternal-child-health

11.2.1. Bacterial Imbalance

The concept of dysbiosis, or bacterial imbalance, within the female genitourinary system is central to the understanding of numerous infections within this fragile environment. A normal vaginal flora contains primarily *Lactobacillus* species that help maintain a low pH and inhibit the growth of harmful pathogens. But, the equilibrium is disturbed by such influences as hormonal alterations, antibiotics, and living habits, leading to greater diversity of bacteria, potentially disease-producing varieties among them. This dysbiosis is directly attributed to infections such as bacterial vaginosis (BV) and vulvovaginal candidiasis (VVC), infections that are defined by their discomforting symptoms and potential sequelae, including increased susceptibility to sexually transmitted diseases (STIs) and adverse pregnancy outcomes, affirming the importance of microbial homeostasis upkeep in reproductive health (Vinitha *et al.*, 2025).

The implications of bacterial imbalance extend beyond symptomatic infection, having significant repercussions on overall health consequences. Changes in the vaginal microbiota can accumulate risk for upper genital tract infections that can lead to severe reproductive health impairment, such as pelvic inflammatory disease (PID) and infertility. In addition, research shows that dysbiosis contributes to the etiology of certain cancers, for instance, human papillomavirus (HPV)-associated cervical cancer, thereby showing how significant a properly balanced microbial community is.

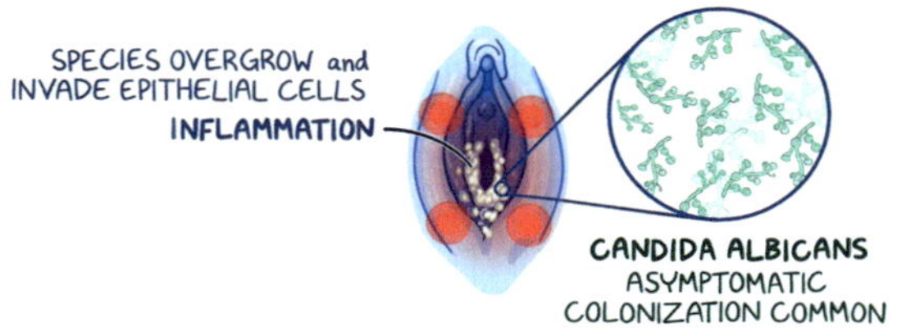

Figure 11.6. Vulvovaginal candidiasis (VVC).

Source: https://www.osmosis.org/_next/image?url=https%3A%2F%2Fd16qt3wv6xm098.cloudfront.net%2FWrq1f8fbQMmh32J0_HdVz3uPRcqLXXq2%2F_.jpg&w=3840&q=75

Combined with non-communicable disease states such as diabetes and obesity, which also affect microbial content, the implications of bacterial imbalance are wide-reaching and complex. Understanding these dynamics is important for the development of preventive strategies and therapeutic interventions in order to maximize female reproductive health (Faisal, 2025). Prevention and management of bacterial imbalance within the female reproductive tract need a multifaceted approach that includes changes in lifestyle, probiotic treatment, and customized medical treatment. Probiotics, particularly those containing *Lactobacillus* species, have been documented as promising in the restoration of normal vaginal flora and combating dysbiosis. Moreover, knowledge of antibiotic usage—both in the healthcare and daily settings—can help to avoid the risk of upsetting microbial balance. The embracing of dietary practices that favor a balanced microbiome, such as an increase in the intake of fiber and avoiding sugar, can also play a crucial role in maintaining vaginal health. By using such measures together, it is possible to develop a healthy vaginal microbiota that not only guards against infection but also supports general reproductive health (Vinitha *et al.*, 2025).

11.2.2. Sexual Activity and Practices

Sexual habits and activities greatly influence the prevalence and incidence of female reproductive tract infections (RTIs). Unprotected sexual relations are a significant risk factor for the transmission of sexually transmitted infections (STIs), which may lead to subsequent RTIs. Sex workers and women who have more than one partner are at risk because frequent exposure to different pathogens increases the risk of infection. In addition, particular sexual practices, such as anal intercourse, can increase vulnerability to infection with conditions like bacterial vaginosis or pelvic inflammatory disease. These relationships are significant in making an effort to solve the public health challenges of RTIs and designing prevention measures that emphasize safer sex behavior among sexually active young women, who in most instances happen to be more at risk for STIs and their effects. Effective sexual health communication will be instrumental in promoting safe sex and preventing RTIs. Clinicians' role is not only treating patients but also ensuring they are educated on the use of barrier methods, regular testing, and open conversation about their sexual health. Notably, frequent condom use not only inhibits STIs but also serves as a shield against infection by various pathogens in RTIs. Patients, if they are understood and cared for, would most likely be comfortable practicing safe sex, further lowering the risk for infection. Combined efforts from health professionals, educators, and community leaders can create an environment in which people are empowered to make decisions about their sexual behavior and health, an essential approach towards addressing the arising problems of female RTIs. Awareness of the psychosocial dynamics of sexual intercourse also plays a key role in achieving the complexities of female RTIs. Cultural attitudes towards sexuality, availability of sexual health care, and mental well-being can control sexual activity and thus influence women's reproductive health. For instance, the existence of stigma around sexual health talk may dissuade one from seeking proper care or using protective measures. Secondly, emotional or psychological problems for women may dissuade them from using protective practices for their sexual health. To address such interlinked factors, emphasis lies in introducing all-encompassing sexual education programs that, apart from educating individuals on safe practice, also build supportive environments that counter stigmatization and promote positive attitudes towards feminine sexuality. Such a multi-faceted approach is quintessential to assisting in mitigating the risk of female reproductive tract infections and overall reproductive health outcomes (Murray *et al.*, 2022; Sarkar *et al.*, 2020).

11.2.3. Hormonal Changes and Health Conditions

Hormonal variations throughout a woman's life exert a significant influence on her reproductive health and susceptibility to infection. Sex hormones such as estrogen and progesterone, specifically, play a role in modulating immune responses within the female reproductive tract (FRT). Sex hormones play central roles in pregnancy and the menstrual cycle, modulating vaginal and cervical tissue barrier functions and mucosal immunity. Understanding how hormonal changes influence the host-pathogen interactions will advance the prevention of FRT infections. Moreover, studies have demonstrated that alterations in the endocrine environment throughout pregnancy modulate susceptibility to ascending infection. Study of these dynamics is required as it lays the groundwork for grasping the temporal aspects of infection vulnerability under different hormonal states, as highlighted in recent studies that necessitate longitudinal assessments of these processes in pregnant and non-pregnant women (Collins *et al.*, 2022).

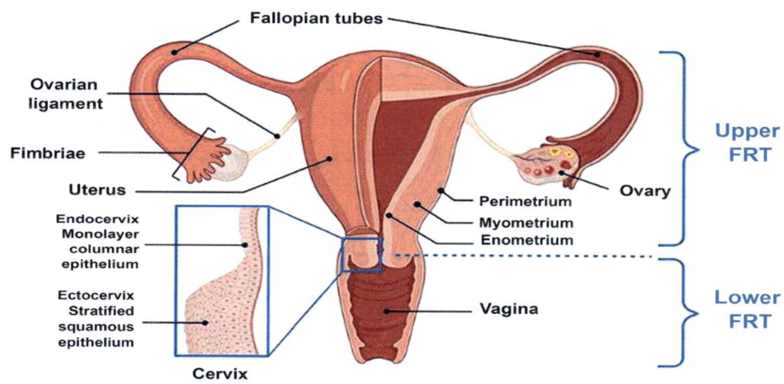

Figure 11.7. Anatomy of the female reproductive tract. A visual depiction of the female reproductive tract (FRT), further subdivided into the upper and lower reproductive tract.

Source: https://www.frontiersin.org/files/Articles/963752/frph-04-963752-HTML-r1/image_m/frph-04-963752-g001.jpg

Besides, aging is a period when hormonal change has a very significant impact on the immune landscape of the FRT. At menopause, as women undergo it, there is a noticeable decline in estrogen levels, which alters mucosal immunity and affects the body's ability to resist infection. Experiments have revealed that menopause and immunosenescence are the culprits for a compromised immune function in the FRT, making older women more susceptible to sexually transmitted infections, urogenital infections, and even gynecological cancer. Aging-induced site-specific alterations in the epithelial cells, the immune cells, and the stromal fibroblasts also further augment the vulnerability to FRT infections. Stress on interdependence between hormonal status and immune health underlines the need for interventions aimed at enhancing immune function in a bid to minimize the risk of infection among elderly populations (Rodríguez-García *et al.*, 2021). The influence of endocrine change on states of health, female reproductive tract infections in particular, extends beyond mere susceptibility. Hormonal contraceptives also play an equally important role in controlling reproductive health outcomes. Hormonal contraceptives change the hormonal landscape and, consequently, the immune reaction in the FRT. While they have an effective way of preventing unwanted pregnancies, their impact on infection risk is a double-edged sword. Some studies show that the application of hormonal contraceptives can boost or inhibit mucosal immunity to certain pathogens. Hence, it is critical to know the interactions between hormonal contraceptives and the immune system when planning comprehensive health measures. Addressing these variables is to empower women with knowledge regarding their reproductive health so that they can make knowledgeable decisions, taking into account the effectiveness of contraception and potential vulnerability to infections in light of changed hormonal conditions.

Test Your Knowledge

1. In what ways can sexual activity and practices influence reproductive tract infections?
2. How do hormonal changes and certain health conditions contribute to the risk of reproductive tract infections?

11.3. Symptoms and Diagnosis

Learning Outcome

1. Identify the common symptoms of infections
2. Understand the diagnostic methods
3. Explain the importance of early detection

Recognition of symptoms of female reproductive tract infection is crucial to ensure timely treatment and intervention. The majority of infections, particularly due to sexually transmitted organisms, are likely to be associated with some array of symptoms. Vaginal abnormal discharge, pelvic pain, irritation, and dysuria are typical pointers. The asymptomatic nature of certain infections could be a barrier to diagnosis and a source of delay in seeking appropriate treatment. By identifying and knowing these symptoms, medical practitioners are able to devise successful diagnostic strategies, including physical examinations, laboratory tests, and imaging studies, to confirm the presence of infection. Additionally, as quoted in recent studies, denial of the relationship between genital infection and reproductive health has dire long-term consequences, including infertility. Delayed diagnosis or misdiagnosis may exacerbate the illness and lead to more serious reproductive complications in adulthood (Patnaik *et al.*, 2025). Female reproductive tract infection diagnosis is a multidimensional process that involves integrating clinical findings with laboratory confirmation. Physical examination usually reveals symptoms such as pelvic tenderness or vaginal canal abnormalities. Diagnostic testing may involve nucleic acid amplification tests or culture, which help identify specific pathogens responsible for the infection. In most cases, health practitioners are also required to consider the patient's medical history, particularly in complex cases involving comorbidities. For instance, complex cases involving women with congenital anomalies may present special challenges because repeated infections may be due to structural defects. So is the situation in recurrent urinary infections overlying pregnancy in true bladder exstrophy (Batkoska *et al.*, 2025). There is a need for heightened awareness in the diagnostic practice to avert mismanagement and provide better health outcomes for women. Thus, the relationship between symptoms and diagnosis is central to treating female reproductive tract infections effectively. The presence of reliable point-of-care diagnostic instruments would greatly contribute to enhanced healthcare responses and diminish the long-term effects of these infections. Because the majority of genital infections are silent, it is critical to get women educated to identify minor symptoms and receive immediate medical attention. Furthermore, integration of multidisciplinary care can even enhance the management of complex cases, where women receive holistic treatment that not only addresses the current infection but also any reproductive health issues. This holistic approach will ultimately improve patient outcomes and promote the importance of proactive measures in women's reproductive health (Patnaik *et al.*, 2025; Batkoska *et al.*, 2025).

11.3.1. Common Symptoms of Infections

Infections of the female lower genital tract have the tendency to cause a broad variety of symptoms with considerable impact on overall health and quality of life. Abnormal vaginal discharge, which can vary in consistency and color depending on the causative infection, is one of the most frequent indicators. For instance, bacterial vaginosis (BV) traditionally causes a thin gray, fishy-smelling discharge, and vulvovaginal candidiasis presents as a white, cottage cheese-like discharge. These signs and symptoms can be vital warning signs that result in clinical presentation for assessment. Besides, the presence of marked changes in discharge alongside other symptoms can be a signal of an infection that is bound to escalate into major health complications, and thus the necessity for early treatment and diagnosis in the context of women's reproductive health. Other symptoms alongside infections also encompass genital itching, burning during urination, and pelvic discomfort. Genital pruritus occurs most frequently in vulvovaginal candidiasis, causing considerable discomfort and distress. Dysuria, which is painful urination, usually precedes infection, like cystitis or sexually transmitted disease, that may complicate treatment protocols. Lower abdominal pain can also be a feature of PID, which is more severe and needs to be managed early since it has long-term reproductive consequences. Hence, their characterization is critical in a bid to help health care providers in the diagnosis and treatment of female reproductive tract infections, with the ultimate long-term goal of safeguarding women's reproductive health. The prevalence of such symptoms testifies to the complexity of reproductive tract infections and their multiple etiologies. Statistical data indicate that high infection prevalence is found among women since research indicates up to 69% of symptomatic female patients are infected with conditions such as BV and vulvovaginal candidiasis (Sethi *et al.*, 2022).

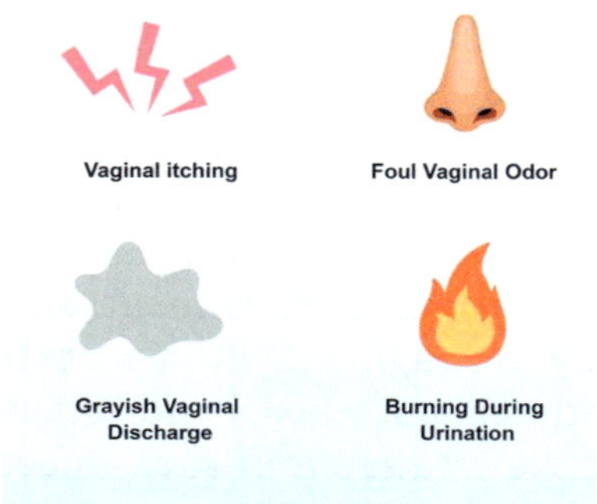

Figure 11.8. Common symptoms of bacterial vaginosis (BV).

Source: https://cdn.shopify.com/s/files/1/0063/4529/3909/files/image15-1024x1024.png?v=1724693641

These findings confirm the significance of extensive screening and education campaigns, particularly in risk populations. Furthermore, the application of preventive interventions, such as prophylactic vaccination against certain pathogens like HPV, has a key role in reducing the occurrence of potential complications (Michał Paluch *et al.*, 2023). By addressing these common symptoms and their causes, medical practitioners are better placed to prepare women for taking an active role in managing their reproductive health, with improved outcomes and reduced morbidity due to these infections.

11.3.2. Diagnostic Methods

The diagnostic methods employed in the diagnosis of female reproductive tract infections (RTIs) play a very crucial role in managing and treating the patient. Clinical evaluation can begin with the taking of a thorough medical history and physical examination of the patient, with particular attention to signs of abnormal discharge, itchiness, or pain. Laboratory tests become necessary after a preliminary evaluation. Microscopic examination of swabs obtained from the vagina verifies the existence of microbes and also helps in the identification of the specific category of infection, whether it is vulvovaginal candidiasis (VVC) or bacterial vaginosis (BV). These are necessary diagnostic tools since some of these infections can be asymptomatic or only indicate overlapping infections. Thus, accurate and timely diagnosis is critical in resolving the underlying cause of the microbiome imbalance that causes RTIs, subsequently impacting the treatment regimen and outcomes. Precise detection of the causative agents makes possible the employment of specific therapeutic modalities to successfully restore the equilibrium state of vaginal microecology. Vaginal Microecology Evaluation System (VMES) is a new diagnostic approach to female RTIs that represents an exhaustive examination of the vaginal microbiome. VMES employs both morphological and functional criteria for assessing the health of vaginal flora. A few of the key parameters are the concentration of bacteria, flora diversity, and the presence of specific markers indicating inflammation or pathogen presence.

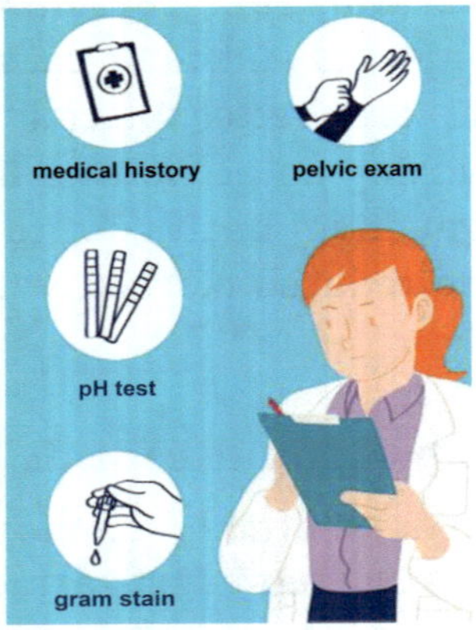

Figure 11.9. Bacterial vaginosis diagnosis.

Source: https://www.verywellhealth.com/bacterial-vaginosis-diagnosis-3132745

Evidently, the VMES may be used to perform differential diagnosis between different infections, for example, between BV and other conditions, so that patients are provided with proper therapeutic treatments. In applying VMES in the clinical practice, clinicians are able to appreciate the vaginal microbiome's complexity better and hence enhance their diagnostic ability and reduce the risk of misdiagnosis or treatment that would further exacerbate already present microbiome derangements (Baumgartner *et al.*, 2020; Li *et al.*, 2019). Also, the integration of molecular diagnostic techniques into routine clinical practice allows for rapid and reliable detection of pathogens responsible for female RTIs. Techniques such as PCR can detect specific bacterial DNA or RNA and allow for the detection of infections that resist traditional culture. These newer molecular techniques allow for quicker turnaround times, which result in timely interventions, particularly in acute disease where symptom resolution is important. Additionally, advances in point-of-care testing systems allow clinicians to obtain results within the patient visit. This instantaneity not only enhances patient satisfaction but also treatment plan adherence because patients feel more engaged in their care. The evolving diagnostic environment emphasizes the necessity of sophisticated technologies in maximizing results for women with reproductive tract infections (Baumgartner *et al.*, 2020; Li *et al.*, 2019).

11.3.3. Importance of Early Detection

Early detection of female reproductive tract infections (RTIs) is crucial in avoiding potential health risks and enhancing therapeutic outcomes. Various infections, such as Chlamydia trachomatis and Candida albicans, lead to disastrous consequences when detected late. Not only do these infections disrupt the physiological sequence of the reproductive system, but they also pose danger during pregnancy. Early diagnosis makes it possible to receive timely treatment, which can prevent infection from developing into more severe diseases like pelvic inflammatory disease or sterility. In addition, rapid uptake of effective interventions can also alleviate physical and psychological stress on women, hence leading to better overall outcomes. Thus, the early diagnosis of female RTIs is not only a matter of individual health but also an important public health matter that requires support and investment. Advances in technology through diagnostic devices have significantly enhanced early detection of RTIs, such that the treatment of such infections can be more efficient. Techniques such as loop-mediated isothermal amplification (LAMP) coupled with microfluidics are potential technologies to detect multiple pathogens involved in RTIs simultaneously, as supported by emerging evidence. These technologies have the potential to increase specificity and sensitivity with more robust results compared to traditional culture, which fails to detect some pathogens, resulting in treatment delays. This is particularly the case given that infections like Streptococcus agalactiae have significant implications on pregnancy outcomes. Through the utilization of advanced diagnostic methods, health care professionals are able to diagnose and treat infections more efficiently and in a timely manner, with the ultimate goal being improved reproductive health and pregnancy experience for women, particularly those who are high-risk. The impact of early detection extends not just to individual health but also to general public health implications. The rising incidence and implications of RTIs underscore the necessity for standardized screening and early diagnosis. Early detection programs can arrest the development of long-term sequelae, thereby reducing treatment costs at advanced levels. Moreover, enhanced awareness and education on the value of early detection can motivate women to be more proactive about their reproductive health. This forward-thinking approach can lead to improved health-seeking behavior, ultimately dwindling the prevalence and burden of RTIs at the community level. As seen in recent nanoparticle-based imaging reagents clinical trials, the promise of emerging technologies offers a promising path towards more effective early detection techniques, which can ultimately redefine the complexion of women's reproductive health care (Luo *et al.*, 2023; Xu *et al.*, 2022).

Test Your Knowledge

1. What are the common symptoms associated with female reproductive tract infections?
2. Which diagnostic methods are commonly used to identify reproductive tract infections in females?

11.4. Treatment Options

Learning Outcome

1. Define antibiotics and antifungal medications
2. Explain the home remedies and lifestyle changes
3. Define the importance of medical consultation

The treatments of choice for female reproductive tract infections (FRTIs) are many and can be combined, depending on the nature of the infection as well as its severity. Early treatment is crucial since, if not treated, infection outcomes can lead to severe long-term effects such as infertility and increased cancer risk. Antibiotic therapy has, in most instances, remained the treatment of choice for bacterial infections of the reproductive tract. However, antimicrobial resistance necessitates a new approach to conventional methods. While antibiotics act effectively in the majority of pathogens, patients have high rates of recurrence. This has prompted medical practitioners to seek out new therapy and preventive measures, such as vaccines and novel medicinal herbs, that target various pathogenic processes, thereby improving patient outcomes and inhibiting the use of traditional antibiotics, which could soon become obsolete as resistance accelerates, as referenced in Zhou *et al.*, (2023). In addition to antibiotics, advances in immunotherapy provide promising avenues for treating more developed or more complex infections of the female reproductive tract, particularly those involving cancer. For example, genetically engineered immune cells such as chimeric antigen receptor (CAR) T-cells are being studied for their ability to activate the immune system to destroy malignant cells in reproductive tract cancers. These new treatments are all aimed at utilizing the body's immune system to recognize and destroy cancer cells efficiently. Personalized medicine further goes a step ahead by tailoring interventions based on the unique genetic and molecular profile of an individual patient's tumor so that more targeted and effective therapeutic strategies can be used. With expanding research, the application of engineered immune cell-based treatments as part of the therapy regimen in FRTIs is highly promising for producing improved short-term outcomes as well as increased long-term survival rates, just as was stated in Nazeer *et al.*, (2024). Lastly, preventative treatments and measures are the solution to managing female reproductive tract infections. Health education campaigns regarding safe sexual practices, cleanliness, and regular screening are aimed at lessening the prevalence of FRTIs. For instance, vaccination with a particular focus on immunization against human papillomavirus (HPV) and hepatitis B significantly reduces the incidence of infection and its related cancers.

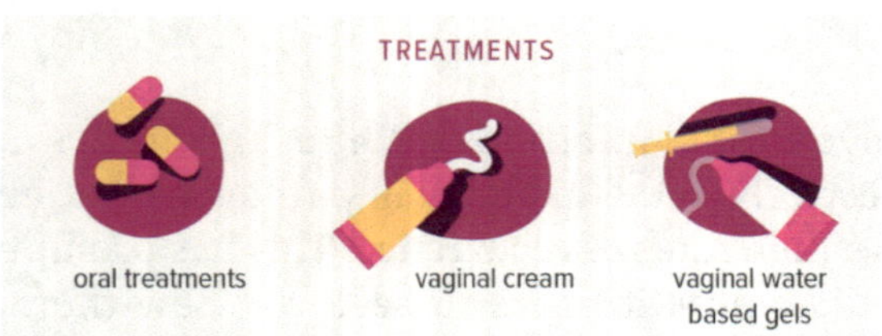

Figure 11.10. Treatment of bacterial vaginosis (BV).

Source: https://i0.wp.com/images-prod.healthline.com/hlcmsresource/images/topic_centers/2020-1/13014-Tips_to_Treat_and_Prevent_Bacterial_Vaginosis-1296x2196-Infographic.jpg?w=1155&h=4611

Moreover, continuing research into the contribution that microbiomes make to reproductive health indicates the potential for using probiotics and other natural treatments to restore balance and prevent the onset of infection. This preventive approach, incorporated into healthcare planning, not only covers the treatment of acute infection but also promotes a general strategy to female reproductive health wherein patient education and anticipatory care management are the keys to reducing infection rates and maximizing outcomes.

11.4.1. Antibiotics and Antifungal Medications

The role of antibiotics in the management of infections involving the female reproductive system cannot be overstated, given their high efficacy against most bacterial pathogens. Such day-to-day infections as bacterial vaginosis (BV) and pelvic inflammatory disease (PID) commonly necessitate antibiotic therapy. While very effective, the use of antibiotics is not without complications. The challenge of antibiotic resistance is a significant concern, as bacterial pathogens evolve to resist conventional methods of treatment. This resistance is traditionally demonstrated by the presence of a high prevalence of *Prevotella* species, which have in the past been associated with a host of genitourinary infections and antibiotic resistance (Faisal, 2025). Hence, medical practitioners must walk carefully and cautiously apply antibiotic stewardship to eliminate unwanted side effects but effectively manage infections. Antifungal agents also play a significant role in the treatment of infections in the female reproductive tract, particularly those caused by Candida species, such as vulvovaginal candidiasis. Such infections are very widespread and have a tendency to be painful presentations, such as itching and discharge. Antifungal agents, such as fluconazole and clotrimazole, are typically used to cure such infections effectively. However, as with antibiotics, overuse of antifungals may lead to resistance, and treatment regimens become burdensome with the need for alternative therapeutic interventions. Furthermore, disruption of vaginal microbiota following antifungal therapy predisposes to the recurrence of infections. Knowledge of the delicate equilibrium of the reproductive tract flora and the incorporation of preventive strategies through dietary as well as lifestyle modifications can optimize the cure and decrease the dependence on antifungal drugs in the long run (Faisal, 2025).

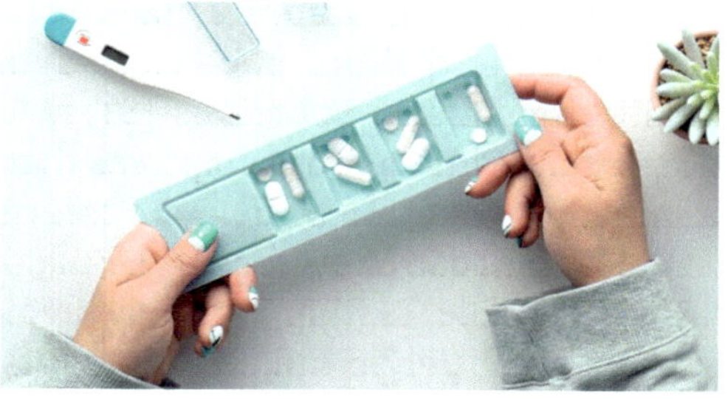

Source: https://www.caritashospital.org/static/media/images/RTIS.png

Apart from conventional antibiotics and antifungals, interest is increasingly being taken in exploring other forms of therapy, including herbal medicine, as a potential treatment for female reproductive tract infections. While such natural treatments are capable of curing certain infections and reducing antibiotic use, care must be exercised in their handling. The efficacy and safety of many herbal preparations are currently inadequately researched, and they can interact with prescribed medications to pose serious health risks. Yet some studies suggest that medicinal plants can be valuable adjuncts, particularly in the prevention of recurrent urinary tract infections. As emerging evidence is produced, there is a growing need for healthcare professionals to consider the efficacy and limitations of incorporating such alternatives within general treatment patterns, balancing efficacy against patient safety in the management of female reproductive tract infections (George *et al.*, 2024).

11.4.2. Home Remedies and Lifestyle Changes

Home care and lifestyle change offer other avenues to manage female reproductive tract infections (RTIs) where the conventional medical interventions have not worked. Certain women are unable to be treated of recurring bacterial vaginosis (BV) with antibiotic treatment, whereby non-prescription alternatives are being investigated. These include dietary changes to reconstruct the natural vaginal microbiome balance by incorporating probiotics and fiber-containing foods. Evidence indicates that the enhancement of good microbial diversity can inhibit the recurrence of RTIs. In addition, behavior modifications such as smoking cessation and consistent condom use significantly reduce the risk factors associated with infection and improve women's reproductive health. Since harmful impacts of RTIs could lead to serious conditions, such as preterm labor and pelvic inflammatory disease, treatment of such problems with holistic lifestyle interventions is increasingly valuable in current healthcare discourse (Abbe *et al.*, 2023).

In addition, lifestyle adjustments extend beyond basic dietary modifications to encompass holistic self-care methods that could mitigate symptoms and promote healing. Exercise on a daily basis, for example, can improve immune function as well as good circulation, both of which are very important in combating infection. Stress control processes such as yoga or meditation can also prove to be useful for hormonal balance and all-around health and may even lower the risk of RTIs by strengthening the body's defenses. Alternative medicine, such as herbal medicine, has similarly gained popularity among women as they search for holistic therapy. However, it is important to receive these treatments with caution, as they may interact with conventional medications or have undesirable side effects. By encouraging a proactive approach through informed lifestyle choices, women can not only manage existing infections but also promote their reproductive health more generally (N/A, 2023).

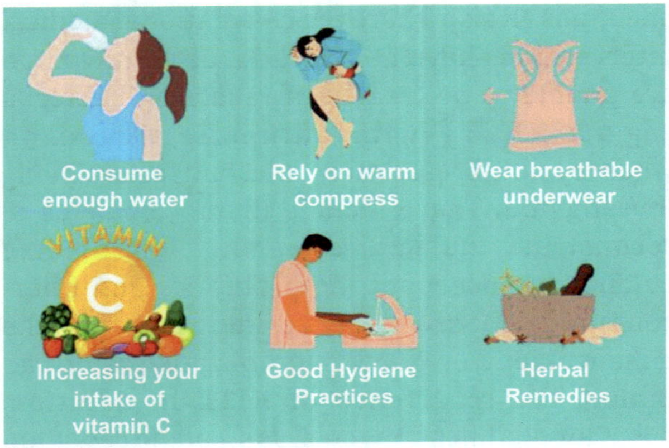
Consume enough water
Rely on warm compress
Wear breathable underwear
VITAMIN
C
Increasing your intake of vitamin C
Good Hygiene Practices
Herbal Remedies

Figure 11.11. Home remedies for treat urinary tract infections.

Source: https://ilioshealth.com/wp-content/uploads/2024/06/home-remedies-treat-urinary-tract-infections-768x768.jpg

Finally, the integration of these home remedies into mainstream medical practice forms a comprehensive management plan for female reproductive tract infection. Health care providers increasingly realize that an empowering patient paradigm that educates and informs women regarding options for holistic treatment is optimal. This paradigm can enhance compliance with preventive interventions since women become more engaged in their health process. By incorporating routine gynecological testing in conjunction with lifestyle change, women can achieve optimum reproductive health outcomes. T

he evolving nature of research concerning bacterial vaginosis treatment, defined by the present investigation of probiotics and microbiome health, testifies to the potential for these integrative interventions. Lastly, enabling women to gain knowledge about and practice such domestic treatments as well as lifestyle adjustments can enhance their agency and effectiveness in combating female reproductive tract infections (Abbe *et al.*, 2023).

11.4.3. Importance of Medical Consultation

The most important aspect of the treatment of female reproductive tract infections (RTIs) is medical consultation because it illustrates the interconnectedness of accurate diagnosis and effective treatment. From bacterial vaginosis to sexually transmitted infections (STIs), these infections come with unclear symptoms that may lead to misinterpretation or delay in treatment. Early medical care can allow for proper diagnosis by way of suitable testing, thereby avoiding sequelae such as pelvic inflammatory disease (PID), which can have long-term implications on fertility. In the absence of expert advice, women might use over-the-counter therapy, which might not treat the causal infection, making it more likely for them to develop chronic health problems. Therefore, the inclusion of medical consultation in reproductive health services not only educates women with knowledge but also enhances the well-being and health status of women as a whole in the case of RTIs. Moreover, the importance of medical consultation extends beyond immediate diagnosis and treatment since it provides an essential avenue for preventive care and health education. With consultations, healthcare providers can give crucial information regarding safe sex and hygiene that are vital in reducing the rate of RTIs. They can offer details regarding vaccination for STIs such as HPV and hepatitis B, giving women access to tools that will enable them to exercise control over their sexual health. In addition, consultation creates an environment in which the patient is not hesitant to share his/her concerns and ask questions, hence de-mythologizing RTIs. The process facilitates two-way communication, enhancing health literacy and the likelihood of seeking help in the future. Medical consultation, therefore, is an integral component, not just in the treatment of active infection, but also in maintaining reproductive health in the long term. Last but not least, the economic impact of medical consultation for

RTIs cannot be underestimated. The expense of untreated infection can be high, leading to more serious health issues that require lengthy medical care. A case in point would be the effects of PID or recurrent RTIs that would necessitate expensive hospitalization, operations, and prolonged health care management. By giving top priority to medical consultations, women can cure infections at an early stage, thereby saving the healthcare system and the infected people the monetary burden. Moreover, long-term medical surveillance can ensure efficient resource allocation in healthcare to allow for proactive rather than reactive treatment interventions. As in the larger context of medical care, where protocol and correct communication are everything to ensure quality care (N/A, 2023; Baumgartner *et al.*, 2020), the proactive approach through medical consultation in women's reproductive health demonstrates its central contribution to individual healthcare and public health economics.

Test Your Knowledge

1. How does the treatment approach differ between sexually transmitted and non-sexually transmitted infections?
2. Why is it important to complete the full course of prescribed treatment for reproductive tract infections?

11.5. Prevention Strategies

Learning Outcome

1. Explain the safe sexual practices
2. Discuss the regular health check-ups
3. Define education and awareness programs

Effective prevention strategies against female reproductive tract infections (RTIs) play a critical role in reducing the public health threat caused by these conditions. Most prevention methods are massive education and sensitization campaigns with the goal of encouraging safe sex, reducing the prevalence of sexually transmitted diseases (STDs), and promoting the practice of regular health check-ups. Health education interventions must reach women of reproductive age, emphasizing the importance of consistent condom use, along with the need for regular gynecological check-ups in order to detect infections at an early stage. Furthermore, community-level interventions can make discussions on reproductive health a matter of routine so that women will be encouraged to seek medical services at the appropriate moment. These preventive measures not only decrease the rate of RTIs but also improve general reproductive health by decreasing the chances of complications like infertility or long-term health complications such as pelvic inflammatory disease. Prevention of female RTIs through intervention of social determinants of health is also vital. A multi-dimensional approach that includes increasing access to health facilities, particularly in low- and middle-income countries, can make preventive practices more powerful. Barriers of socioeconomic status, education, and attitudes can all be barriers to women's access to safe reproductive health practices. By combating these barriers, healthcare policy can encourage equitable access to STI and RTI information and services. The inclusion of fertility services under national health schemes, as emphasized by WHO, also highlights the relationship between comprehensive reproductive health care and the prevention of infection. Postpartum sepsis and unsafe abortion hazard training can actually avert many cases of RTIs, highlighting the need for an integrated approach to women's health. Another cornerstone of effective prevention efforts is the development and supply of vaccines against prevalent pathogens that cause RTIs. Investing in the research and development of vaccines against sexually transmitted infections such as human papillomavirus (HPV) and others could go a long way in curbing RTI cases. Not only does immunization directly protect an individual, but it also aids in developing herd immunity, thus reducing levels of overall transmission across populations. Private sector and government health agency partnerships and global cooperation can ensure these vaccines are deployed faster and reach more people. Further, integrating vaccine programs in existing healthcare systems ensures that women receive the best preventive healthcare at the most critical junctures of a woman's life. Through the provision of effective prevention methods with education, health care access, and vaccination programs, female reproductive tract health can be improved extensively, with improved health care outcomes for women globally.

11.5.1. Safe Sexual Practices

Practice of safe sex is essential in avoiding the spread of female reproductive tract infections (RTIs). Safe, protected, and consensual sex significantly reduces the risk of transmitting sexually transmitted infections (STIs), which can grow to develop into more serious health conditions. Numerous protection methods, such as barrier methods like condoms, also block the exchange of fluids and are protective against STIs as well as undesired pregnancy. Screening regularly and treating STIs early in sexually active individuals is also critical to preventing long-term illness from infection that is not treated. This is an initiative at the forefront emphasizing the need for safe sexual behavior education, which is important in maintaining perfect reproductive health and lowering the rate of RTIs among women (Sarkar *et al.*, 2020).

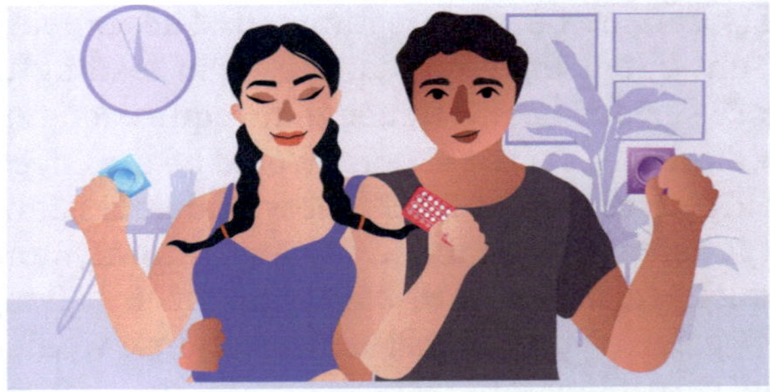

Source: https://kayakalpinternational.com/wp-content/uploads/2024/03/Sexual-Health.jpg

In addition to using protection, communication between partners is crucial in the development of safe sex. Open and honest discussions on sexual health history, such as past STIs or reproductive problems, enable partners to make informed decisions about their sex. Honesty fosters trust and empowers an individual to exercise caution, for example, screening or immunization against preventable infections like human papillomavirus (HPV) and hepatitis B. Information about reproductive health, including the awareness of how RTIs affect general health, is central in encouraging safe behavior. People individually, these habits create a platform where both of them will feel comfortable speaking about what they want and are afraid of, hence bringing better sexual health results (Christy E Manyi-Loh *et al.*, 2018). The understanding of the consequences of reproductive tract infections also helps to put into perspective the significance of safe sex. RTI-endemic females can be predicted to experience such complications as infertility, chronic pelvic pain, or adverse pregnancy outcomes, which can detract significantly from their quality of life. Education interventions for the interaction between safe sex and reduced rates of RTIs can encourage people to make healthier life choices. Moreover, control of structural determinants such as stigma and myths regarding sexual health can allow for prevention in a community-based program. For these objectives to be achieved productively, collaboration between medical professionals, educators, and advocacy organizations is required to make information and resources available. Thus, promotion of safe sex practice not only ensures individual health but also has strategic relevance for public health in reducing the incidence and overall disease burden of reproductive tract infections (Sarkar *et al.*, 2020).

11.5.2. Regular Health Check-Ups

Regular check-ups for health play a vital role in early detection and management of Female Reproductive Tract Infections (FRTIs). FRTIs have significant implications on women's reproductive well-being, and their complications may involve infertility, chronic pain, or pregnancy complications. With the incorporation of regular screening in the health practice, women are able to detect infections at an early point, facilitating timely intervention and tailored treatment plans.

Preventative measures through regular check-ups assist medical professionals to more clearly spot individual risk factors in terms of lifestyle, sexual history, and family background, all of which contribute significantly towards formulating customized healthcare plans. The periodic monitoring of reproductive health can thus not only enhance individual well-being but also contribute to larger public health programs towards minimizing FRTIs among women. Apart from the early recognition of reproductive tract infection, regular check-ups for health are sources of learning experiences for women regarding the nature and risks of reproductive tract infection. These are experiences where health workers can educate them with key information on prevention, such as safe sex and immunization needs, such as the HPV vaccine that successfully prevents the onset of certain infections and diseases.

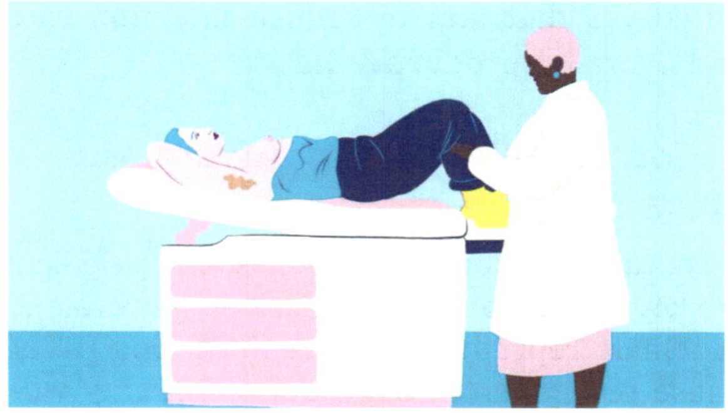

Source: https://i.ytimg.com/vi/RyuMqB0GOrg/maxresdefault.jpg

Moreover, through encouraging honest discussion between patients and health professionals, regular check-ups can potentially enhance women's capacity to express concern about their reproductive health and seek assistance as soon as needed. Such empowerment would be vital in demystifying the stigmatization of reproductive health ailments, compelling women to put their sexual welfare at the top of their priorities, and putting things into perspective for routine surveillance and assessment in averting risks related to FRTIs. Yet another significant aspect of regular health check-ups is their capability to improve the compliance of patients diagnosed with FRTIs, along with the other concomitant conditions. With the aid of advanced drug delivery systems, doctors can eliminate some of the most common barriers to compliance, such as complex dosing regimens or side effects. As has been demonstrated in recent studies, drug delivery systems of the new generation can improve acceptability and compliance rates among patients for many conditions, including FRTIs. The systems also enable women to gain more control over their reproductive health, thereby providing continuity of care and augmented health benefits. Finally, incorporating regular health check-ups into an overall plan for Female Reproductive Tract Infections care fortifies not just individual health but also public health initiatives that aim to reduce infection rates and overall reproductive health.

11.5.3. Education and Awareness Programs

Practical education and awareness campaigns are the key to overcoming the increasing prevalence of female reproductive tract infections (RTIs). These programs, through disseminating wide-ranging information about the reproductive system, help women identify symptoms and visit a doctor in time. It is observed that a vast majority of research studies reveal substantial knowledge gaps about reproductive health among men that have the cascading effect of undermining women's health indirectly. For instance, in one study, a significant number of men—62.50%—did not want to accompany their spouses for antenatal care and hence it was imperative to involve men in health education outreach (Gaikwad *et al.*, 2012). Hence, specially tailored interventions that enhance male awareness and build supportive behavior in reproductive health can enhance health outcomes among women. The inclusion of education and awareness interventions among men and women has been shown to increase reproductive health behaviors among populations. Adolescent reproductive and sexual health in India was the theme of research that yielded significant findings on why locally acceptable messages and community mobilization work (Kurz *et al.*, 2006). Interventions may de-myth RTIs, make people aware of safe sexual practice, and highlight the requirement for check-ups from time to time. By creating a culture in which free discourse regarding reproductive health is the norm, these programs are able to significantly decrease stigmatization of RTIs and enable people to maintain their health and well-being as a priority. In addition, education campaigns that incorporate information regarding symptoms and treatments of RTIs are vital in order to ensure that people will be at ease in seeking help when necessary. Also, the success of education and sensitization campaigns can be measured not only by increased knowledge but also by changes in health-seeking behavior. For instance, data prove that out of men with reproductive health issues, 72.73% of them sought treatment, which shows the potential efficacy of awareness initiatives (Gaikwad *et al.*, 2012). Community-based interventions that encourage community participation and foster a supportive culture can go a long way in enhancing treatment-seeking behavior and reducing the disease burden of untreated RTIs. Reducing both knowledge gaps and behavior barriers, these programs can effectively work against the transmission of female reproductive tract infections, ultimately yielding health gains. Engaging men and women both in the conversation that pertains to reproductive health, thus, becomes critical in the making of a healthier society that sees and values reproductive rights.

Test Your Knowledge

1. What role does personal hygiene play in preventing vaginal infections?
2. Why are regular gynecological check-ups important in the prevention of reproductive tract infections?

SUMMARY

The prevalence of female reproductive tract infections (RTIs), namely urinary tract infections (UTIs), emphasizes major health concerns that necessitate intensive awareness and preventive interventions. In agreement, research has established that recurrent UTIs rank as a significant burden in the context of females, with studies mirroring the rate of 22.30% among working female reproductive age personnel in a cross-sectional study in central Kerala (Johny *et al.*, 2025). This number not only indicates the incidence of such infections, but it also indicates with alarm the resultant impact on the quality of life in women's health. The understanding that a recurrent UTI is capable of creating chronic disease ensures early detection, management, and prevention measures are a priority to tackle associated risks efficiently. Moreover, the relationship between one's personal hygiene routine and RTI incidence cannot be overstressed. Poor personal hygiene has also been identified as a key determinant in the vulnerability of girls in adolescence to reproductive organ infections (Akbar, 2020). This indicates that education-based health interventions promoting the practice of good hygiene would be successful in increasing levels of health among women in youth. The implication of such data is that bridging gaps in education pertaining to personal hygiene, particularly among socioeconomically disadvantaged groups, is the starting point in reducing RTIs. By means of preventive education, health care providers can enable women to take charge of their own reproductive well-being. Finally, the management of female reproductive tract infections must address the issue in a multi-faceted manner with special emphasis on awareness, hygiene education, and preventive healthcare strategies. The findings on recurring UTIs form a clarion call for intervention with specific strategies to enhance awareness among women about risk factors as well as preventive methods. These programs, coupled with socioeconomic determinants, will not only decrease the rate of infection but also enhance the overall quality of life in those infected (Johny *et al.*, 2025). Prioritizing hygiene on a personal level through programs of health education underlines the importance of equipping women with knowledge to combat infections, which will lead to healthier generations to come.

The knowledge of the burden of female reproductive tract infections (RTIs) mandates balanced assessment of their etiology, prevalence, and impact on women's health globally. RTIs are a significant public health issue because they are associated with both chronic reproductive health morbidity as well as acute genital infections. Epidemiological data reveal that an overwhelming majority of women are suffering from various RTIs, which have significant repercussions, including infertility, pelvic pain, and increased risk of HIV infection. The causative factors for the infections are multifactorial, including bacterial, viral, and parasitic causes. Effect measures to curb the RTI burden include a combined strategy aiming at prevention, early diagnosis, and treatment, with special focus on public education and information to prevent RTI spread. The interaction between antimicrobial resistance (AMR) and the treatment of RTIs gives good insights into how to challenge the issues of effective management of RTIs. It has been decades since resistant bacterial strains re-emerged and made the clinical environment more challenging, reducing the effectiveness of traditional treatment. According to Murray *et al.*, (2022), the estimated global burden of bacterial AMR deaths is an indicator of how significant it is that such a threat be curbed across the world. With regards to RTIs, increasing resistance towards common antibiotics is not only a risk to personal health but also to the overall public health consequences. An understanding of these dynamics will enable healthcare professionals to make informed decisions regarding treatment protocols and highlight the necessity for the development of new therapies and guidelines to combat these resistant infections. Furthermore, the socio-economic impact of female RTIs is considerable and affects women's quality of life, productivity, and mental well-being. RTIs disproportionately target women in low-resource settings where access to education and quality health care is weak. This is also compounded by the stigmatisation of reproductive tract infections, leading to delayed treatment and under-reporting. Reflections on long-term impacts of untreated RTIs emphasize the importance of developing targeted interventions to the advantage of concerned groups. The environments and systems driving the transmission of these infections must be tackled, as identified in Dharmage *et al.*, (2019), a complete understanding of environmental and genetic determinants will form the foundation for more efficient modes of prevention and management. Hence, public health facility investment and expanding access to healthcare resources for women are essential steps towards the mitigation of female RTIs' burden.

KEY TERMS FROM THIS CHAPTER

- Bacterial Vaginosis
- Chlamydia
- Syphilis
- Ureaplasma
- Opportunistic Infections
- Antimicrobial Resistance
- Reproductive tract infections (RTIs)
- Dysbiosis
- Candidiasis
- Gonorrhea
- Pelvic Inflammatory Disease (PID)
- Chorioamnionitis
- Sexually Transmitted Infections (STIs)
- Condom
- Fallopian tubes
- Ectopic pregnancy

CRITICAL THINKING QUESTIONS

1. **Which of the following organisms is the most common cause of bacterial vaginosis in women?**
   a. Gardnerella vaginalis
   b. Candida albicans
   c. Neisseria gonorrhoeae
   d. Trichomonas vaginalis
2. **Pelvic Inflammatory Disease (PID) is most commonly caused by:**
   a. Chlamydia trachomatis and Neisseria gonorrhoeae
   b. Staphylococcus aureus and Streptococcus pyogenes
   c. Escherichia coli and Pseudomonas aeruginosa
   d. Candida albicans and Trichomonas vaginalis
3. **Which infection is characterized by a "strawberry cervix" on examination?**
   a. Herpes simplex virus infection
   b. Trichomoniasis
   c. Bacterial vaginosis
   d. Candidiasis
4. **A thick, white, curd-like vaginal discharge with itching and irritation is most commonly caused by:**
   a. Trichomonas vaginalis
   b. Candida albicans
   c. Gardnerella vaginalis
   d. Neisseria gonorrhoeae
5. **Which virus is responsible for causing genital warts in females?**
   a. Herpes simplex virus
   b. Human papillomavirus (HPV)
   c. Cytomegalovirus
   d. Epstein-Barr virus

Short Answer Questions

1. What are some common types of reproductive tract infections (RTIs)?
2. List two major causes and risk factors for reproductive tract infections.
3. What symptoms typically indicate a reproductive tract infection?
4. Which diagnostic tests are commonly used to detect reproductive tract infections?
5. What treatment options are available for managing reproductive tract infections?
6. Name three prevention strategies to reduce the risk of reproductive tract infections.

Answer to Critical Thinking Questions

1. (a) 2. (a) 3. (b) 4. (b) 5. (b)

REFERENCES

1. Abbe, C., & Mitchell, C. M. (2023). Bacterial vaginosis: A review of approaches to treatment and prevention. *Frontiers in Reproductive Health, 5*. https://doi.org/10.3389/frph.2023.1100029 (accessed on 14th June 2025).
2. Adams, K., Li, X., Rohan, L., & Bies, R. R. (2025). PBPK models of the female reproductive tract: Current and future analysis. *Expert Opinion on Drug Metabolism & Toxicology, 21*, 429–444. https://www.semanticscholar.org/paper/c38712364d8506db2c1a0f87f3c39dd6aef96812 (accessed on 14th June 2025).
3. Akbar, H. (2020). Faktor yang Brukunga denga personal hygiene pada romaji Putri di SMA Negeri 1 Kutanoglu. *Journal Kesehatan, 11*, 23–28. https://www.semanticscholar.org/paper/ad5cde3cd6e18bd64c713fb3d2fceb7cea00cd66 (accessed on 14th June 2025).
4. Amabebe, E., & Anumba, D. (2018). The vaginal microenvironment: The physiologic role of lactobacilli. *Frontiers in Medicine, 5*. https://doi.org/10.3389/fmed.2018.00181 (accessed on 14th June 2025).
5. Baryakova, T., Pogostin, B. H., Langer, R., & McHugh, K. J. (2023). Overcoming barriers to patient adherence: The case for developing innovative drug delivery systems. *Nature Reviews Drug Discovery, 22*, 387–409. https://doi.org/10.1038/s41573-023-00670-0 (accessed on 14th June 2025).
6. Batkoska, M., & Pečlin, P. (2025). Multidisciplinary management of pregnancy in bladder exstrophy: A case report. *The American Journal of Case Reports, 26*. https://www.semanticscholar.org/paper/d8a20f4f64fb92dfe6b47a5f10af367413f17725 (accessed on 14th June 2025).
7. Baumgartner, H., De Backer, J., Babu-Narayan, S. V., Budts, W., Chessa, M., Diller, G. P., Lung, B., *et al.* (2020). 2020 ESC Guidelines for the management of adult congenital heart disease. *European Heart Journal, 42*, 563–645. https://doi.org/10.1093/eurheartj/ehaa554 (accessed on 14th June 2025).
8. Butt, R. L., & Volkoff, H. (2019). Gut microbiota and energy homeostasis in fish. *Frontiers in Endocrinology, 10*. https://doi.org/10.3389/fendo.2019.00009 (accessed on 14th June 2025).
9. Chen, X., Lu, Y., Chen, T., & Li, R. (2021). The female vaginal microbiome in health and bacterial vaginosis. *Frontiers in Cellular and Infection Microbiology, 11*. https://doi.org/10.3389/fcimb.2021.631972 (accessed on 14th June 2025).
10. Collar, A. L., Jamus, A. N., Flanagan, J., Core, S., Geisler, W. M., Wheeler, C., & Frietze, K. M. (2025). Immunization against *Chlamydia trachomatis* polymorphic membrane protein D tetrapeptide motifs limits early female reproductive tract infection in a mouse model. *Vaccines, 13*. https://www.semanticscholar.org/paper/48f2010ca4cfa43a0878829ecf15f88129ecf49e (accessed on 14th June 2025).
11. Collins, M. K., McCutcheon, C. R., & Petroff, M. G. (2022). Impact of estrogen and progesterone on immune cells and host–pathogen interactions in the lower female reproductive tract. *The Journal of Immunology, 209*, 1437–1449. https://doi.org/10.4049/jimmunol.2200454 (accessed on 14th June 2025).
12. Dharmage, S. C., Perret, J. L., & Ćustović, A. (2019). Epidemiology of asthma in children and adults. *Frontiers in Pediatrics, 7*. https://doi.org/10.3389/fped.2019.00246 (accessed on 14th June 2025).

13. Faisal, M. S. (2025). The healing power of nature: Herbal medications in treating urinary tract infections. *International Journal of Pathology*. https://www.semanticscholar.org/paper/9174f78cfe9e254877f29ad5d616b72b96685353 (accessed on 14th June 2025).

14. Gaikwad, V. S., Murthy, T. S. M., & Sudeepa, D. (2012). A qualitative study on men's involvement in reproductive health of women among auto-rickshaw drivers in Bangalore Rural. https://core.ac.uk/download/pdf/13598720.pdf (accessed on 14th June 2025).

15. George, S. D., Van Gerwen, O. V., Dong, C., Sousa, L. G. V., Cerca, N., Elnaggar, J., Taylor, C. M., *et al.* (2024). The role of *Prevotella* species in female genital tract infections. *Pathogens, 13*. https://www.semanticscholar.org/paper/3835540c29e7d3321fd7f23ebf67b86b53896ddf (accessed on 14th June 2025).

16. Johny, F., Menon, V. T. K., Georgy, S., Saju, C., & Jini, M. P. (2025). Prevalence of recurrent urinary tract infections and its associated factors in female staff of reproductive age group in a medical college in central Kerala: A cross-sectional study. *BMC Infectious Diseases, 25*. https://www.semanticscholar.org/paper/5eb0c392f74dfd96118c4e7cd77328f16c8e8a1e (accessed on 14th June 2025).

17. Kümpfel, T., Giglhuber, K., Aktaş, O., Ayzenberg, I., Bellmann-Strobl, J., Häußler, V., Havla, J., *et al.* (2023). Update on the diagnosis and treatment of neuromyelitis Optica spectrum disorders (NMOSD) – Revised recommendations of the Neuromyelitis Optica Study Group (NEMOS). Part II: Attack therapy and long-term management. *Journal of Neurology, 271*, 141–176. https://doi.org/10.1007/s00415-023-11910-z (accessed on 14th June 2025).

18. Kurz, K., MacQuarrie, K., Pande, R., Jain, S., & Walia, S. (2006). Improving the reproductive health of married and unmarried youth in India. https://core.ac.uk/download/71352223.pdf (accessed on 14th June 2025).

19. Li, T., Liu, Z., Li, K., & Bai, H. (2019). Evaluation of the vaginal microbiome in clinical diagnosis and management of vaginal infectious diseases. *Chinese Medical Journal, 132*, 1100–1103. https://doi.org/10.1097/cm9.0000000000000211 (accessed on 14th June 2025).

20. Luo, L., Zhou, H. L., Wang, S., Mei, P., Zhang, J., Hu, Y., & You, J. (2023). The application of nanoparticle-based imaging and phototherapy for female reproductive organs diseases. *Small*. https://doi.org/10.1002/smll.202207694 (accessed on 14th June 2025).

21. Manyi-Loh, C. E., Mamphweli, S., Meyer, E. L., & Okoh, A. I. (2018). Antibiotic use in agriculture and its consequential resistance in environmental sources: Potential public health implications. *Molecules, 23*, 795. https://doi.org/10.3390/molecules23040795 (accessed on 14th June 2025).

22. Murray, C. J. L., Ikuta, K. S., Sharara, F., Swetschinski, L. R., Robles Aguilar, G., Gray, A. P., Han, C., *et al.* (2022). Global burden of bacterial antimicrobial resistance in 2019: A systematic analysis. *The Lancet, 399*, 629–655. https://doi.org/10.1016/s0140-6736(21)02724-0 (accessed on 14th June 2025).

23. Nazeer, N., Manna, R., Shukla, S., Patil, A., & Bhargava, A. (2024). Engineered immune cell-based therapeutics for female reproductive tract cancers: Advances and future prospects. *Journal of Reproductive Healthcare and Medicine*. https://www.semanticscholar.org/paper/007cf553af734839b61be2199a1060d8cecc06c2 (accessed on 14th June 2025).

24. Paluch, M., Tomkiewicz, M., Olko, P., Radulski, J., Sałata, P., Żuchnik, M., Szczuraszek, H., *et al.* (2023). HPV virus as the main cause of cervical cancer, vaccination–Literature review.

Journal of Education, Health and Sport. https://www.semanticscholar.org/paper/26c3aed49279a30934aebe8b39e7216cf0263c86 (accessed on 14th June 2025).

25. Patnaik, N., Sarkar, U., Jojula, M., Vaddiraju, H., & Dey, R. J. (2025). Comprehensive assessment of genital infections and reproductive health in women visiting a fertility clinic in Warangal, India—A case-control study. *Health Science Reports, 8.* https://www.semanticscholar.org/paper/809ad512d559cc578f0cbef2333075094bfc55fc (accessed on 14th June 2025).

26. Rodríguez-García, M., Patel, M. V., Shen, Z., & Wira, C. R. (2021). The impact of aging on innate and adaptive immunity in the human female genital tract. *Aging Cell, 20.* https://doi.org/10.1111/acel.13361 (accessed on 14th June 2025).

27. Sarkar, M., Brady, C. W., Fleckenstein, J., Forde, K. A., Khungar, V., Molleston, J. P., Afshar, Y., *et al.* (2020). Reproductive health and liver disease: Practice guidance by the American Association for the Study of Liver Diseases. *Hepatology, 73,* 318–365. https://doi.org/10.1002/hep.31559 (accessed on 14th June 2025).

28. Semet, C. (2024). Descriptive characteristics, etiological agents, and risk factors for mortality of urinary tract infections in older adults. *Kocatepe Tıp Dergisi.* https://www.semanticscholar.org/paper/8a581c0c13f8ff330560c27edb0f62105e1f4bb4 (accessed on 14th June 2025).

29. Sethi, S., Sharma, N., Sharma, M., Dadwal, R., Singh, C., Chaudhary, H., Malhotra, S., *et al.* (2022). Prevalence of nonviral reproductive tract infections/sexually transmitted infections in female patients with cervicovaginal discharge: Excerpts from a regional reference center in North India. *Indian Journal of Sexually Transmitted Diseases and AIDS, 43,* 135–140. https://www.semanticscholar.org/paper/c0f31ec9be6412ae9373365eef4ea33da5095881 (accessed on 14th June 2025).

30. Ul Haq, F., Riaz, A., Ali, N., Shafiq, S. F., Wahab, Q. M. F., Uddin, T. M., Shah, M. I., *et al.* (2024). Lornoxicam induced toxic epidermal necrolysis (TEN) in a 54 years old female: A case report and its systematic literature review with respect to its causes and treatment overview. *World Journal of Advanced Research and Reviews.* https://www.semanticscholar.org/paper/40e99a153d03611b56dcc12686e6deb9e47f259b (accessed on 14th June 2025).

31. Verma, N., Awasthi, S., & Pankaj, K. (2024). Assessment of knowledge and behavioral risk factors of reproductive tract infections among married women of 15–49 years in rural areas of Halwani block, Uttarakhand. *Journal of Family Medicine and Primary Care, 13,* 4706–4711. https://www.semanticscholar.org/paper/e1ac0bdebfdd00337a0086bbad01657351cf4b9d (accessed on 14th June 2025).

32. Vinitha, G., Balakrishnan, J., Nagarajan, P., & Kannan, S. (2025). Reconnoitering the association of vaginal microbiota composition in the female reproductive tract with health and disease. *The Open Microbiology Journal.* https://www.semanticscholar.org/paper/54375e69c799e6e82d903d0adf1e1a9616168389 (accessed on 14th June 2025).

33. Xu, X., Jia, Y., Li, R., Wen, Y., Liang, Y., Lao, G., Liu, X., *et al.* (2022). Rapid and simultaneous detection of multiple pathogens in the lower reproductive tract during pregnancy based on loop-mediated isothermal amplification–microfluidic chip. *BMC Microbiology, 22.* https://doi.org/10.1186/s12866-022-02657-0 (accessed on 14th June 2025).

34. Yadav, A., Chaudhary, S., Kaur, S., Nagarrgoje, M. M., & Chauhan, S. (2025). Health-seeking behavior and its challenges for reproductive tract infections among married women of reproductive age group residing at urban slums of Agra: A cross-sectional study. *Healthline.*

https://www.semanticscholar.org/paper/d4bc6f6255118abaee2858db6a5c43c88698d0db (accessed on 14th June 2025).

35. Zeng, J., Wu, T., Wang, L., Yu, L., Lin, H., & Chen, Z. (2024). Characteristics of reproductive tract infections caused by common pathogens among the outpatients of reproductive medicine center in Putina: Retrospective study. *BMC Infectious Diseases, 24*. https://www.semanticscholar.org/paper/15ae8c3527a6a0fad97f62d818d7a31c70023b40 (accessed on 14th June 2025).

36. Zhou, Y., Zhou, Z., Zheng, L., Gong, Z., Li, Y., Jin, Y., Huang, Y., *et al.* (2023). Urinary tract infections caused by uropathogenic *Escherichia coli*: Mechanisms of infection and treatment options. *International Journal of Molecular Sciences, 24*. https://www.semanticscholar.org/paper/379caae8ee37e13217dcffd031d485a1779f895e (accessed on 14th June 2025).

ENDOCRINE DISORDERS IN GYNECOLOGY

12

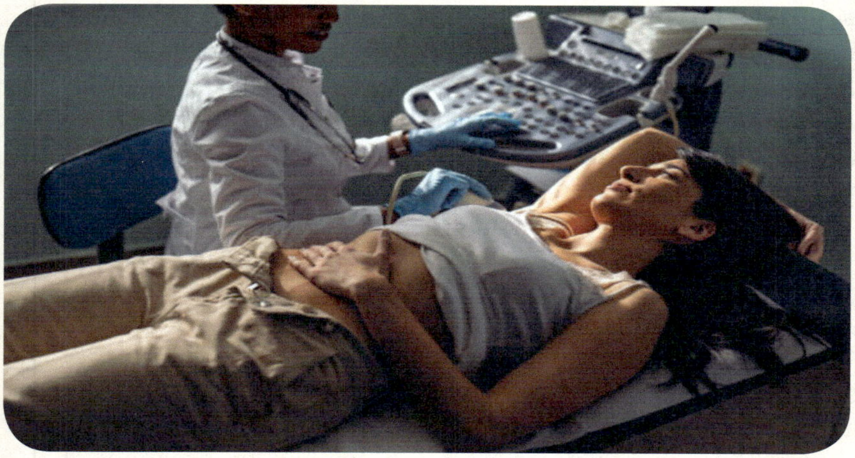

LEARNING OBJECTIVES

After studying this chapter, you will be able to:

1. Understand the endocrine system
2. Identify common endocrine disorders that affect women
3. Explain the symptoms and diagnostic approaches for endocrine disorders
4. Analyze the impact of endocrine disorders on female reproductive health
5. Evaluate available treatment options for managing endocrine disorders in women

Introduction

The intricate area of gynecological health is intimately related to the endocrine system, a very important regulator of various physiological processes. Endocrine disorders such as polycystic ovary syndrome (PCOS) and menopause-related hormonal disorders have severe impacts on women's reproductive health and well-being. As these hormonal changes become evident, they can influence a wide variety of symptoms, ranging from irregular menstrual cycles to infertility, ultimately affecting the quality of life of the woman. Furthermore, interconnectivity between gynecological disease and endocrine malfunction calls for a thorough understanding of the two systems. This chapter attempts to lay out the complications of endocrine disease in gynecology and its implications on treatment and diagnosis. Identification of the prevalence and potential impact of endocrine disorders in gynecology entails consideration of social and psychological factors involved. Pregnancy, in turn, typically a welcome milestone to be coveted, can be overshadowed by elevated health risks tied to malignancies not diagnosed because of a lack of awareness on the patient and healthcare provider levels. The psychological cost of this neglect also tends to lead to delays in diagnosis, exacerbating health problems. Furthermore, the increasing trend towards delayed childbearing to advanced ages is also associated with greater risks of acquiring conditions such as breast cancer during or post-pregnancy. It becomes relevant to note these subtleties in framing effective clinical approaches to prevent risks and enhance patient outcomes, as highlighted by recent research. Recent guidelines emphasize the urgency for individualized treatment regimens for women experiencing various stages of hormone-related changes, particularly menopause. The Treatment of Symptoms of the Menopause Task Force has underlined that while menopausal hormone therapy (MHT) is the most effective form of treatment for symptom management, it needs to be approached cautiously. Health care providers are prompted to assess all patients' cardiovascular well-being and risk for breast cancer in depth prior to prescribing MHT. Low-dose vaginal estrogen and non-hormonal therapy are available alternatives for women who are unwilling participants in hormone therapy. This greater understanding of endocrine disease in gynecology underscores the necessity for continuing clinical practice improvement, ultimately for the benefit of women's health and well-being across their lifespan.

Definition of Endocrine Disorders

Endocrine disorders are a general term describing a variety of disease states resulting from disturbances in hormone production and regulation in the endocrine system. The system is composed of a few glands, including the pituitary gland, thyroid gland, adrenal glands, and ovaries, which secrete hormones that influence numerous physiological processes. Whenever there is an imbalance in the levels of hormones, it can lead to disease states of metabolism, growth, reproduction, and mood. Endocrine disorders are also expressed in all forms, from the hyperthyroid syndrome of excess hormone production to disorders such as PCOS that are aggregations of signs based on hormonal imbalance. Endocrine disorders are typically complex and require a multidisciplinary intervention in order to correctly diagnose and manage them, particularly in gynecological settings where they have far-reaching implications for women's health. Interactions between various endocrine states and reproduction highlight the intricate nature of hormonal regulation. In the case of anorexia nervosa (AN), an illness common to young women, endocrine adaptation leads to functional amenorrhea and disrupted reproduction due to dysregulation of the hypothalamic-pituitary-ovarian axis. These types of disruptions in the endocrine system can have serious consequences concerning fertility as well as overall reproductive function. Specifically, while most of these effects are reversed by good treatment and nutritional recovery, long-term effects persist and affect maternal and fetal outcomes in pregnancy. Recognition of the influence of nutritional and psychological factors on endocrine function is critical to an understanding of the complete health importance of disorders like AN in female patients. Polycystic ovary syndrome (PCOS) is a second crucial example of the confluence between endocrine disease and gynecology. This condition not only leads to irregular menstrual periods and endocrine disturbances but also poses severe challenges in terms of physical and mental well-being. PCOS has the potential to profoundly affect women's quality of life, rendering supportive counseling and interventions essential components of optimal management. Recent evidence highlights the importance of integrative approaches in favoring wellness in women with PCOS, both physical and psychological well-being. With healthcare professionals and researchers expanding their knowledge of the intricacies of endocrine disorders, it is progressively evident that initiating holistic care is at the heart of addressing the challenges posed by these diseases and enhancing the outcome of affected women.

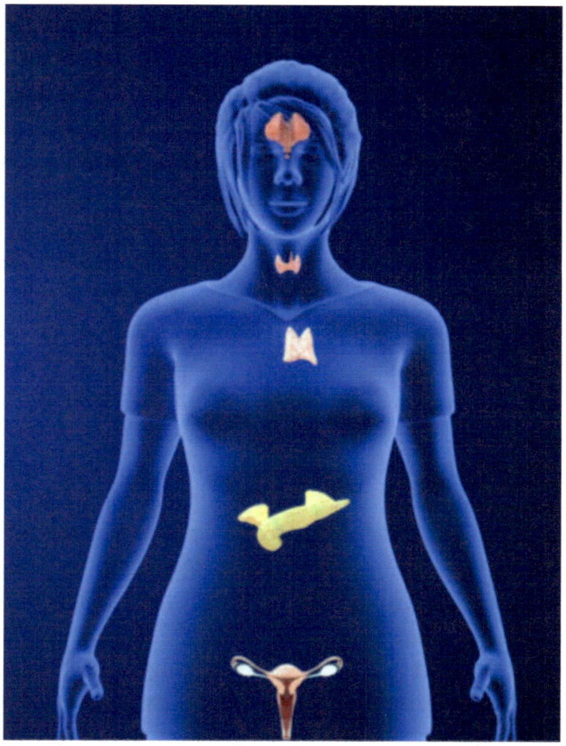

Source: https://mdaquest.org/wp-content/uploads/2024/05/iStock-1475501653-scaled-e1716303221369-1024x512.jpg

Importance of Studying Endocrine Disorders in Gynecology

Endocrine gynecological disorders represent a critical field of inquiry for comprehending the intricate balance between hormone regulation and female reproductive health. By exploring how hormonal dysregulation may result in a variety of gynecological syndromes, clinicians are better able to diagnose and treat conditions such as polycystic ovary syndrome (PCOS), oligomenorrhea, and menopause. The reason that endocrine disorders and symptoms such as metabolic and reproductive failure are increasing calls for extensive education and awareness among gynecologists. Also, the importance of stressing the link between gestational diabetes, obesity and endocrine disorders is critical to address the health of females at different phases of life, pointing out the fact that medical professionals need to keep up with the latest research advancements in this sector. Along with this, the adverse impact caused by environmental factors on hormonal well-being increases the importance of studying endocrine disorders in gynecology. Studies in recent times suggest that the use of some industrial chemicals as endocrine disruptors can aggravate reproductive health complications.

Phthalates and perfluorinated compounds are some industrial chemicals whose association has been found with various unfavorable health outcomes, such as low birth weight and developmental disorders. Therefore, gynecologists play vital roles as intermediaries between medical practice and science, enabling them to educate women about potential risks of environmental contaminants. By promoting regulatory changes and advocating for healthier living, gynecologists are able to reduce the effects of these endocrine disruptors on women's health, thus promoting individual and public health outcomes (N/A).

Also, sexual health concerns in gynecology directly relate to endocrine disorder examination, and this opens up a facet of women's overall health that is always overlooked. Woman's sexual dysfunction, frequently triggered by hormonal imbalance, indicates that healthcare providers need to proactively engage patients in discussions about their sexual health. Given the high incidence of sexual dysfunction among gynecologic patients, research has demonstrated that gynecologists do not often address sexual health, largely because there are psychophysiological barriers to discussion by patients. It is essential to include sexual health screening as a part of routine gynecologic practice to facilitate increased integrated care of the patient. By standardizing discussions of sexual health and its connection with endocrine function, gynecologists can considerably enhance the quality of their patients' lives with the assurance that women's health is not simply concerned with reproductive function but embraces a complete picture of their endocrine welfare as well (Ancane *et al.*, 2013).

12.1. Overview of the Endocrine System

Learning Outcome

1. Identify and describe the key components of the endocrine system
2. Explain the role of hormonal regulation and its significance in maintaining physiological balance
3. Define the interaction between the endocrine system and reproductive health

The endocrine system is a complex network of glands that are tasked with the synthesis and secretion of hormones, which play a critical role in the regulation of an array of physiological functions in the human system. The glands, including the pituitary, thyroid, adrenal, and gonads, coordinate to maintain homeostasis and regulate functions such as growth, metabolism, and mood control. The hormones released into the bloodstream travel to the various target tissues and organs, needing precise timing and balance for optimal health. Any interference with the production or transmission of the hormones can bring significant physiological effects. An understanding of the complexity of the endocrine system is crucial, particularly to comprehend how disruption can be manifested as endocrine disorders more relevant to gynecology in conditions such as menstrual dysfunction, infertility, and mood disorders secondary to hormonal fluctuations. In females, some hormonal fluctuations throughout various stages of life, like menarche, pregnancy, and menopause, illustrate the function of the endocrine system in gynecology. The combination of estrogen and progesterone, for example, is responsible for reproductive well-being, determining everything from menstrual cycles to pregnancy. On top of that, shifts in these hormones are the cause of mood disorders, a category of Reproductive Mood Disorders, that primarily burden women of childbearing age. As women are more prone to depression than men, particularly in the context of hormone shifts, there is a need to consider how the endocrine system not only directly affects physical health but also psychological well-being. This is further reinforced if one considers that reproductive hormones enter into complex relationships with steroid stress-related systems, which means women's healthcare is an interdisciplinary affair with both endocrinology and psychology being part of it. The impact of endocrine illness falls outside the scope of gynecology and impacts overall health outcomes, contributing to women's quality of life. Data from research indicate high comorbidity among depressive disorders and medical conditions, validating the contention that health should be examined comprehensively. For instance, (Berk *et al.*, 2023) points out the compounded challenges that arise with both physical illness and mental illness simultaneously because they may trigger and exacerbate each other and complicate treatment. Moreover, heightened vulnerability to fluctuations in reproductive hormones may enhance vulnerability to emotional events, which could elicit the onset of mood disorders in vulnerable individuals. This establishes a priority for health practitioners to consider the intricate dynamic of endocrine change and emotional health, necessitating integrated treatment strategies that consider not just endocrine functionality but also psychological counseling, with the ultimate advantage of improved outcomes for women exposed to these multifaceted conditions (Schweizer-Schubert *et al.*, 2021).

12.1.1. Key Components of the Endocrine System

The endocrine system is a highly developed system responsible for regulating various physiological functions by way of hormone secretion. The key components of this system are glands such as the pituitary, thyroid, adrenal, and gonads (ovaries and testes). These glands release and seep hormones that regulate everything from growth and metabolism to reproduction and stress.

The relationship between these glands matters, as they talk to one another in feedback loops to maintain homeostasis within the body. A good example of this is the function of the hypothalamus within the endocrine system by serving as a liaison between the nervous and endocrine systems and coordinating the discharge of pituitary hormones that govern other glands, thereby highlighting the fine balance of this system. Gynecological disorders of the endocrine system can have substantial consequences on the female reproductive system.

Polycystic ovary syndrome (PCOS) is only one illustration of the effect of hormonal imbalance on menstruation, ovulation, and overall metabolic health. Hormones such as insulin, estrogen, and progesterone need to be in balance in order to facilitate normal reproductive function, and dysregulation can lead to symptoms of abnormal menstruation, infertility, and cardiovascular vulnerability. The importance of these hormonal interactions becomes clear when one considers how imbalances can cause disorders that need to be carefully managed and treated, impacting women's quality of life and their sexual well-being, a multidisciplinary problem drawing on both physiological and psychological realms, which may be further complicated by social influences (Kaundal *et al.*, 2024).

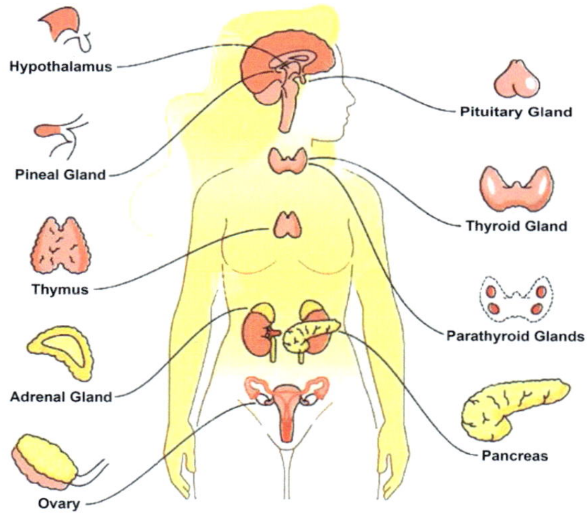

Figure 12.1. Female endocrine system.

Source: https://thumbs.dreamstime.com/z/female-endocrine-system-inner-glands-pancreas-ovary-outline-concept-physiological-body-parts-as-educational-anatomy-209957864.jpg

Understanding the predominant components of the endocrine system is important in the diagnosis and management of disorders that involve the gynecologic tract. Clinicians often employ multifactorial approaches in managing conditions, cognizant of the reality that sexual dysfunction and endocrine dysfunction often co-exist, complicating the care of the patient. Baseline hormonal screening, followed by a comprehensive workup, can detect possible issues early on. Besides, awareness and education of such disorders are necessary during the treatment process, as many women may feel stigmatized or uncomfortable discussing their symptoms. By embracing a multidisciplinary treatment approach, healthcare providers can ensure that a majority of women receive integrated care that addresses both the physiological and emotional dimensions of sexual health concerns, thus enhancing therapeutic outcomes and patient satisfaction (Behboudi-Gandevani *et al.*, 2020).

12.1.2. Hormonal Regulation and Its Significance

The delicate hormonal regulation is the focus of management of endocrine disorders in gynecology. Estrogen, progesterone, and androgen are three hormones that are pivotal to the normal function of the female reproductive system. Their balance regulates a range of reproductive processes, including menstrual cycles, fertility, and pregnancy maintenance. Disturbance of the balance of these hormones can lead to a range of endocrine disorders, including polycystic ovarian syndrome (PCOS) and thyroid disorders. For instance, a disruption of estrogen and progesterone hormone balances can disrupt the menstrual cycle, leading to irregularities that may affect a woman's overall health as well as fertility outcomes. Advances in reproductive endocrinology have illuminated the manner in which targeted hormonal therapy can significantly contribute to these hormone balances, eventually enhancing reproductive health and therapeutic outcomes (Laddad et *al.*, 2023). Moreover, the significance of hormone regulation extends into the area of reproductive technology. Enhanced understanding of hormone profiles has led to biomarker-based methods that optimize ovarian stimulation protocols in ART.

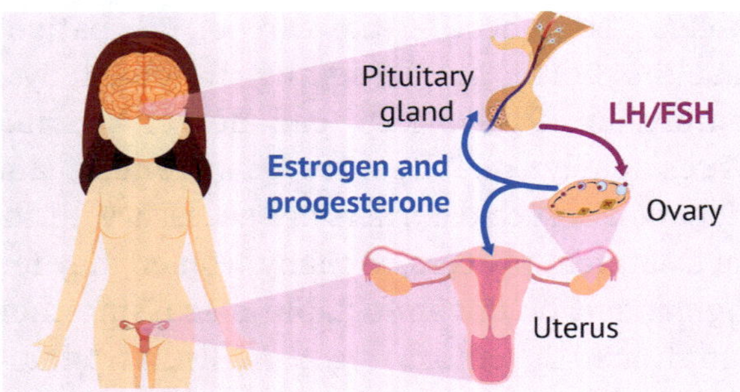

Figure 12.2. Hormonal regulation of endocrine disorders.

Source: https://www.invitra.com/en/female-hormone-check/hormonal-regulation-of-the-menstrual-cycle/

Individualized hormonal treatment may permit better ovarian stimulation, which results in higher oocyte yields and enhanced male and female factors with resultant improved implantation potential. Such intricacy underscores the need for reproductive health personalized medicine strategies, where the individual's estrogenic, androgenic, and ovarian reserve profiles influence the treatment to be delivered. These advances in hormonal control aim not only to repair endocrine disorders but to render reproductive therapy more effective and therefore offer hope for individuals with fertility disorders. This specificity is transforming the treatment of gynecology and promises bright prospects for future clinical use (Laddad *et al.*, 2023). External factors like environmental pressures and psychosocial interactions also account for the modulation of hormonal control. For instance, nutrition, stress, and exposure to endocrine-disrupting chemicals are the variables that can regulate levels of hormones, thus affecting the age of menarche onset as well as the regularity of menstruation. It has been noted through research that changes in societal exposures and influences have produced earlier menarche ages, showing the relationship between societal influences and hormonal control. Understanding these interactions is essential in addressing hormonal dysregulations and designing integral treatment strategies for endocrine gynecologic disorders. As science evolves, increasing importance is being given to integrative strategies that include evidence from genetics, environmental health, and psychosocial research, eventually augmenting intervention effectiveness in promoting hormonal balance in women's health.

12.1.3. Interaction Between the Endocrine System and Reproductive Health

The interaction between the endocrine system and reproductive health is complex and vital to a woman's overall well-being. Hormones produced by the endocrine system, like estrogen, progesterone, and testosterone, play pivotal roles in regulating most reproductive functions. The hormones play a significant role in regulating the menstrual cycle, ovulation, and maintaining pregnancy. Hormone balance changes can lead to severe health complications, including menstrual disorders, infertility, and menopause complications. For instance, the endocrine disruption that underlies conditions such as polycystic ovary syndrome (PCOS) can adversely affect both endocrine function and fertility. Furthermore, the prevalence of endocrine disorders in gynecology speaks to the imperative for clinicians to understand these associations in order to treat and manage patients afflicted by them effectively. According to research, adolescent girls with a history of extreme changes in body weight are at risk of having reproductive health issues associated with endocrine disorders. Findings show that girls born to low or high body weights during infancy may have increased risks of extragenital diseases, which are, in fact, precursors to the reproductive system disorder (Kachaylo *et al.*, 2022). For example, some infections, such as mumps, can potentially damage the ovarian follicles and hence significantly impact fertility prospects. It is because of this that endocrine balance is so important and that early checks and interventions need to be undertaken in young women in order to prevent the eventual effects of such imbalances. Resolution of such complications not only improves the health condition of individuals but also plays a crucial role in reducing infant and maternal mortality, hence public health at a greater level. As females pass various stages of life, particularly menopause, the impact of the endocrine system becomes more powerful. HRT is necessary to treat menopausal symptoms in the majority of women since it improves quality of life by alleviating vasomotor symptoms and preserving overall reproductive health (Davis *et al.*, 2015). The decision to initiate HRT, however, should be individualized according to age, duration since menopause, and co-existing health risk history. The guideline is presently of the view that for women with symptoms below 60 years of age, the risk may be offset by the advantages of hormone therapy if only cardiovascular as well as breast cancer risk is carefully screened (Davis *et al.*, 2015). In addition, such in-depth understanding and management of endocrine disorders within gynecology reinforce the pivotal role played by the endocrine system in relation to reproductive health over a woman's lifetime.

Test Your Knowledge

1. What are the primary glands involved in the endocrine system, and what hormones do they secrete?
2. How does hormonal regulation contribute to maintaining reproductive function?

12.2. Common Endocrine Disorders Affecting Women

Learning Outcome

1. Discuss the polycystic ovary syndrome (PCOS)
2. Define thyroid disorders (hypothyroidism and hyperthyroidism)
3. Explain the adrenal gland disorders (Cushing's syndrome and Addison's disease)

Endocrine disorders significantly impact women's health, as diseases such as Polycystic Ovary Syndrome (PCOS) and menopause have unique challenges. PCOS is characterized by a disturbance of hormones that can lead to manifestations such as irregular menstrual bleeding, acne, and hirsutism. The disorder is typically also associated with metabolic disturbances, including obesity and insulin resistance. Greater visceral fat, which is common in women with PCOS, increases the risk of type 2 diabetes and cardiovascular conditions, so the importance of early detection and management is emphasized according to each patient's requirements. Nonetheless, the severity and incidence of obesity related to PCOS phenotypes are variable, suggesting an exquisite therapeutic and intervention strategy should be given to treat this condition effectively in females with this syndrome (Akbaezadeh *et al.*, 2017).

Another prevalent endocrine disorder in women is the one related to menopause, a normal physiological process typified by the cessation of menstruation and decline in estrogen production. This transition may result in vasomotor symptoms such as hot flashes and night sweats, significantly impacting quality of life. The challenge is that these symptoms must be managed effectively without regard to the risks of hormone replacement therapy (HRT). Current guidelines suggest that low-dose menopausal hormone therapy (MHT) remains the most effective treatment for alleviating vasomotor symptoms, with regard to cardiovascular and cancer risks (Davis *et al.*, 2015). Importantly, treatment plans need to be tailored, particularly for women who are likely to have hormone therapy contraindications, in which practitioners need to make thorough risk evaluations and patient-centered consultations regarding therapeutic options. Besides PCOS and menopause, thyroid disease, such as hypothyroidism and hyperthyroidism, has significant consequences for women's health. These conditions are capable of inducing a wide range of symptoms with similar signs and symptoms to other illnesses, making diagnosis difficult. Hypothyroidism, for example, can cause weight gain, depression, and fatigue, while hyperthyroidism can result in heightened anxiety and hyperactivity. The interaction between thyroid gland function and fertility and menstrual cycles is particularly notable, as hypothyroidism and hyperthyroidism are capable of causing menstrual irregularities and infertility. Such comprehension of endocrine-related issues influencing reproductive health is, thus, essential for complete gynecological care. Therapeutic control of thyroid disease and interactions with sex hormones constitute a basic aspect of enhancing well-being for women involved, and this highlights the need for early screening and balanced therapy.

12.2.1. Polycystic Ovary Syndrome (PCOS)

Polycystic Ovary Syndrome (PCOS) is a serious health problem that plagues a significant number of women throughout their reproductive years. It is defined by the presence of a combination of disturbances in hormones, insulin resistance, and other reproductive abnormalities. PCOS can lead to a host of psychological and somatic issues. Irregular menses, weight gain, and infertility are prominent among them. Apart from the reproductive arena, PCOS has an enormous influence on women's mental health as well. Women with this condition may experience difficulties that affect personal as well as social functioning, and this underscores the need for coordinated care planning aimed at addressing mental as well as physical health. Special education and information tailored to PCOS women are instrumental to enhancing their quality of life and general health (Annagur *et al.*, 2018). Effective interventions must be comprehensive, addressing simultaneously medical, psychological, and social health. The metabolic subtleties implicated in PCOS add to the health outcomes of the condition.

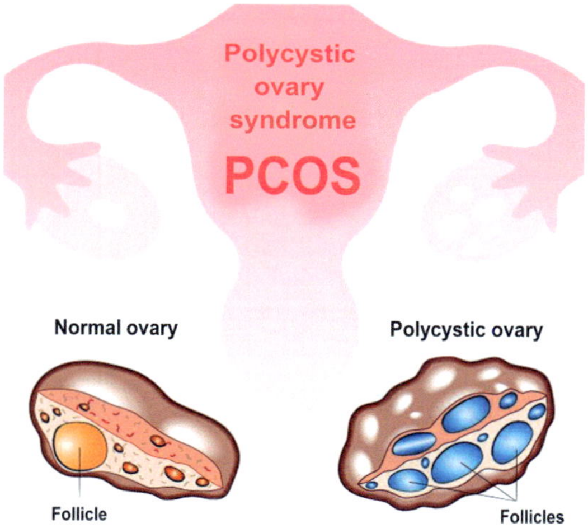

Figure 12.3. PCOS (Polycystic Ovary Syndrome).

Source: https://atlashealthmedicalgroup.com/wp-content/uploads/2021/11/PCOS-3.png

Evidence indicates that patients with the condition are at greater risk of experiencing a multitude of metabolic disorders, including type 2 diabetes, cardiovascular disease, and metabolic syndrome. The risks increase the importance of clinical practitioners adopting evidence-based approaches in treatment and diagnosis. Understanding the metabolic comorbidities of PCOS allows medical doctors to tailor their interventions to a greater degree. Specifically, guidelines that have been formulated by professional organizations like The Endocrine Society and the American Society of Reproductive Medicine stand out because they emphasize the importance of early risk identification and intervention. With the application of evidence-based algorithms in clinical care, clinicians can better facilitate the long-term health of PCOS women, hence limiting the contribution of these extreme comorbidities to their general well-being (Christopherson *et al.*, 2016).

The treatment of PCOS holistically is imperative in order to improve health outcomes in affected women. As research evolves, the focus on patient-centered and integrative care is all the more significant. Interventions not only need to address physical health but also mental health concerns and quality of life. Wellness programs that involve counseling and lifestyle modification, for instance, may have a profound impact and allow women to deal with the issues provoked by PCOS. Development of an in-depth appreciation of PCOS's multi-dimensional nature can help with the development of specific clinical practice informed by more than symptomatic treatment. Via ending collaborations with gynecologists, and mental health practitioners, a holistic approach to managing PCOS can be developed. This integrative approach is crucial in empowering women with the ability to reclaim their health and wellbeing regardless of this prevalent endocrine disorder (Annagur *et al.*, 2018).

12.2.2. Thyroid Disorders (Hypothyroidism and Hyperthyroidism)

Thyroid disorders, i.e., hypothyroidism and hyperthyroidism, are significant conditions in women's health, particularly in reproductive years. Hypothyroidism, which is low thyroid hormone production, is extremely prevalent during pregnancy, in which it can lead to severe obstetric complications. In a study, subclinical hypothyroidism (SCH) was present in approximately 9.5% of pregnant women, with risk factors such as anemia, gestational diabetes mellitus (GDM), and preeclampsia. These complications underscore the importance of routine thyroid screening and appropriate management in pregnant women to avoid maternal and neonatal morbidity. An awareness of the significant prevalence of thyroid diseases can raise the rate of detection and treatment of these conditions, promoting improved maternal and infant outcomes as well as establishing a vital preventive health measure within gynecological practice (Garag *et al.*, 2017). Conversely, pregnancy hyperthyroidism, most often caused by Graves' disease, has equally severe effects if left untreated. The most frequent presentation in patients with hyperthyroidism is weight change, nervousness, and tachycardia that are confused with normal pregnancy. Hyperthyroidism poses a risk of adverse outcomes, including premature delivery and low birth weight. Studies state that untreated hyperthyroidism may also cause dire fetal complications, such as cardiac arrhythmia and abnormalities of growth. In these, physicians must take extra care in monitoring thyroid levels during pregnancy to avoid the complications caused by hyperthyroidism. Early detection and treatment are the solution to achieve maximal mother and child health, noting a significant interaction between endocrine and gynecologic health (Radi *et al.*, 2010).

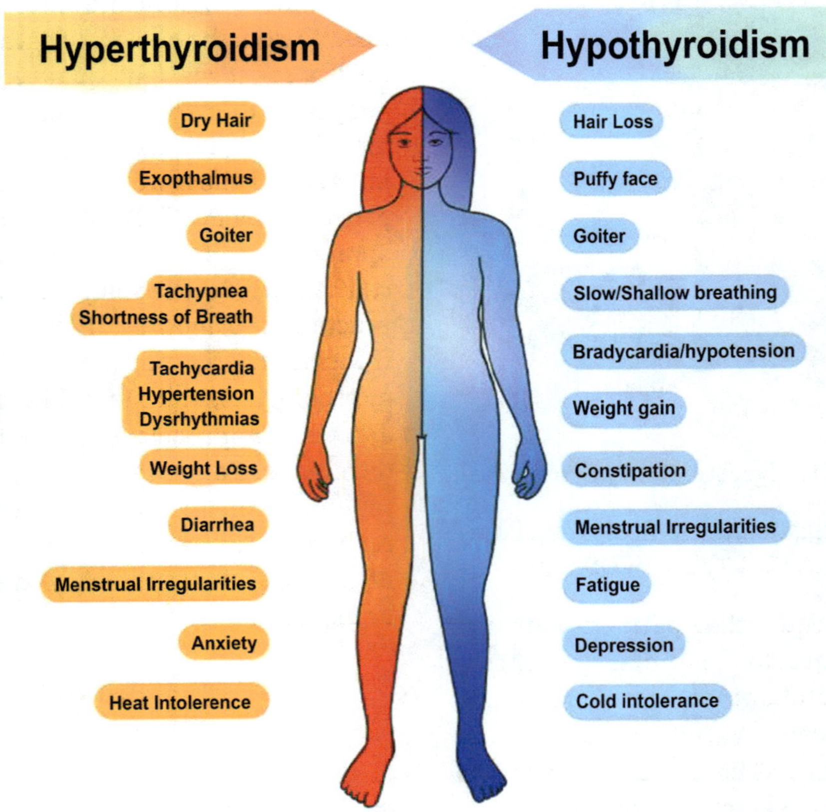

Figure 12.4. Comparison of the clinical manifestations of hyperthyroidism and hypothyroidism.

Source: https://wtcs.pressbooks.pub/app/uploads/sites/47/2024/02/HyperthyroidismHypothyroidism-1-1024x1024.png

The effects of thyroid disease extend beyond pregnancy to influence broader aspects of women's reproductive health. Thyroid dysfunction is associated with menstrual dysfunction, such as oligomenorrhea or amenorrhea, that may complicate issues related to fertility. Women with such interruptions typically undergo thorough workups to rule out disturbances in endocrine, including thyroid hormone profiles. Hypothyroidism and hyperthyroidism may disrupt the hypothalamic-pituitary-ovarian axis and result in conception challenges and maintenance of pregnancy. In addition, the impact of these disorders on pregnancy emphasizes the necessity of specific healthcare interventions to address women with thyroid abnormalities. By recognizing and intervening in these diseases within the realm of gynecological health, practitioners are able to ensure improved health outcomes for women during their reproductive lifespan (Garag *et al.*, 2017; Radi *et al.*, 2010).

12.2.3. Adrenal Gland Disorders (Cushing's Syndrome and Addison's Disease)

Cushing's syndrome and Addison's disease, which are adrenal gland diseases, have enormous gynecological consequences. Cushing's syndrome, in which there is an excess of cortisol, disrupts other endocrine pathways and leads to conditions like obesity, hirsutism, and menstrual irregularities in women. The surplus of cortisol can also suppress the activity of sex hormones, resulting in infertility. Furthermore, the resultant increase in cortisol levels may exacerbate the risk of developing such conditions as polycystic ovary syndrome (PCOS), contributing to the clinical presentation that is experienced in gynecological practice. Accurate diagnosis is contingent upon recognizing the underlying causes of Cushing's syndrome that range from adrenal tumors to pituitary adenomas and thus tailoring treatment regimens responsive to each patient's condition and reproductive health complications (Yanholenka *et al.*, 2011). Conversely, Addison's disease features a diametrically contrasting clinical presentation, characterized by adrenal hypofunction in generating some adrenal hormones, such as cortisol and aldosterone. The condition is likely to lead to adrenal insufficiency, and patients may present with fatigue, weight loss, and low blood pressure, all of which may overpower gynecological findings. Importantly, females with Addison's disease can observe alterations in their menstrual cycles, typically consisting of amenorrhea or irregular menstrual cycles, thus complicating reproductive planning. The relationship between adrenal insufficiency and gynecological function requires a comprehensive treatment plan that may include hormone replacement therapy and close monitoring of endocrine function. Also, the treatment of Addison's disease requires prompt detection and intervention for the prevention of adrenal crises, which have significant consequences for overall health and quality of life (Cheng *et al.*, 2017).

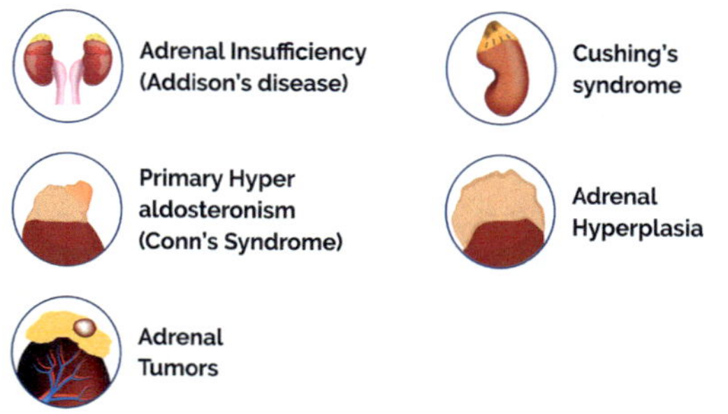

Figure 12.5. Common adrenal gland disorders.

Source: https://drshreyaendocrinologist.com/assets/img/treatment/disorders-of-the-adrenal-gland/disorders-of-the-adrenal-gland02.jpg

Cushing's syndrome and Addison's disease underscore the intricate relationship between reproductive health and adrenal function in gynecology. Both cases underscore the necessity for interdisciplinary management strategies, such as those involving endocrinologists, gynecologists, and general physicians, in order to give complete care. Educating the patient regarding the potential impact of these adrenal disorders on fertility, as well as reproductive health, needs to be done, along with increasing awareness of the psychosocial concomitants of these endocrine disorders. Furthermore, advancing studies on the minimal effects of adrenal gland states on women's health will be advantageous for medical practitioners in terms of delivering preparedness and effective treatment protocols, thus promoting overall results for the infected patients (Yanholenka *et al.*, 2011).

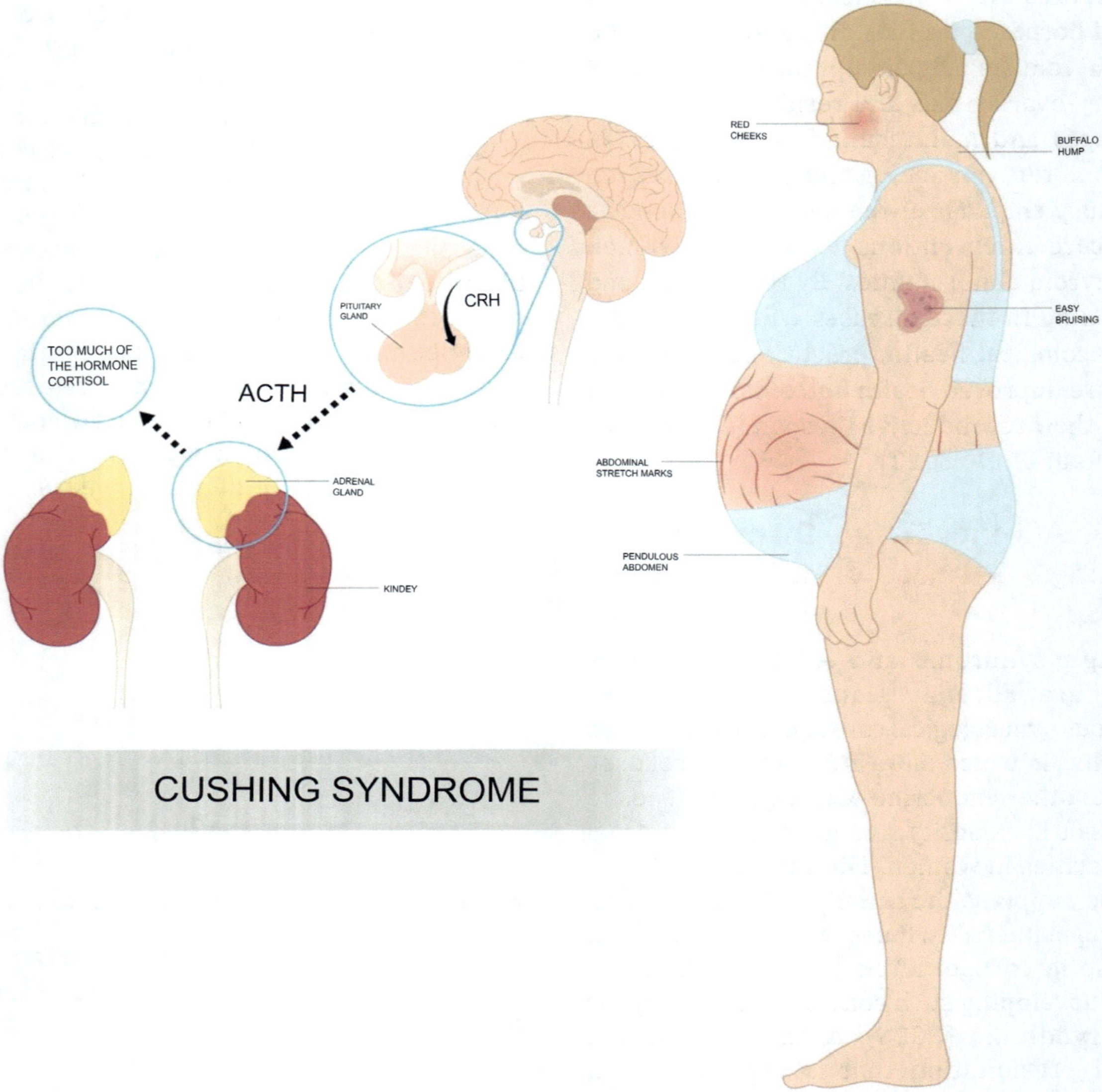

Figure 12.6. Cushing syndrome is characterised by an overproduction of cortisol hormone.

Source: https://acesurgery.sg/service/adrenal-gland-disorders-and-surgery/

Test Your Knowledge

1. What are the main hormonal imbalances involved in polycystic ovary syndrome (PCOS)?
2. How do hypothyroidism and hyperthyroidism affect the female reproductive system?

12.3. Symptoms and Diagnosis of Endocrine Disorders

Learning Outcome

1. Identify the common symptoms associated with endocrine disorders
2. Discuss the diagnostic tests and procedures
3. Explain the importance of early diagnosis in gynecological health

The clinical manifestations of endocrine disorders in gynecology are often multifaceted, reflecting the complex interplay between hormonal disturbances and various physiological processes. The most frequent endocrine disorder in women is PCOS, with its hallmark features of irregular menses, hirsutism, and infertility. Diagnosis typically comes after the Rotterdam criteria, wherein two of three manifestations must be present: oligo-ovulation, clinical or biochemical hyperandrogenism, or transvaginal ultrasound (TVUS) polycystic ovarian morphology. The significance of accurate diagnosis is evidenced by the potential adverse outcomes of a lack of diagnosis of PCOS, including long-term impacts such as type 2 diabetes and cardiovascular disease.

Early detection of symptoms is crucial as it allows for appropriate interventions in the form of addressing both short-term problems and long-term health outcomes. Endocrine diseases are typically diagnosed by combining clinical evaluation, imaging studies, and biochemical examinations. In PCOS, the traditional application of TVUS to assess polycystic ovarian morphology is compromised by inter-operator and machine variability. More recent evidence indicates that serum concentrations of anti-Müllerian hormone (AMH) may represent a useful substitute for diagnosing polycystic morphology and correlate well with the antral follicle count on ultrasound. The use of AMH as a diagnostic marker can potentially make the diagnosis of PCOS much simpler without the requirement for interventions and enhance the overall accuracy of diagnosis (Piltonen *et al.*, 2024). Ongoing research means that the introduction of new biomarkers into general clinical practice has the potential to revolutionize the appearance of endocrine disorder diagnosis in gynecology. The prevalence and presentation of endocrine disorders differ among different populations, underscoring the need for context-based research to guide diagnosis. In a recent Tobago study, PCOS-like symptoms were found to be highly prevalent, with a rate of 19.7% in a chiefly Afro-Caribbean population. Notably, the research also revealed drastic age-dependent differences in presenting symptoms, such as increased rates of abnormal menstrual function and infertility among older groups. These observations emphasize the need for customized diagnostic criteria that consider ethnic and environmental factors, as well as an entire series of biochemical tests to fully delineate endocrine disorders in certain populations (Talbott, 2024). By understanding these disparities, doctors can enhance diagnostic specificity and ultimately improve management plans for women who are afflicted with endocrine disorders.

12.3.1. Common Symptoms Associated With Endocrine Disorders

Endocrine disorders are usually manifested by a variety of generalized symptoms that have a significant impact on the welfare and health of individuals, particularly women. One of the most significant areas of concern is the disturbance of hormonal balance that may lead to a variety of clinical states. For instance, disorders such as polycystic ovary syndrome (PCOS) are likely to occur with manifestations such as menstrual irregularities, obesity, and hirsutism caused primarily due to elevated levels of androgens. Similarly, thyroid illness such as hypothyroidism can cause fatigue, weight changes, and depression that have a direct impact on a woman's quality of life. These results highlight the importance of detection and knowledge of the myriad of signs and symptoms of endocrine disease, particularly in the gynecologic clinic. Without adequate information, these disorders will remain undiagnosed, leading to unnecessary issues and a decreased level of well-being among sufferers. In addition, menopausal transition is a pivotal period during which endocrine changes may lead to profound symptoms impacting gynecological health. When estrogen declines at menopause, females commonly experience vasomotor symptoms, namely hot flashes and nocturnal sweats, which are of clinical significance and may interfere with function and sleep quality. In addition to these somatic manifestations, mood changes and depressive disorders may appear as psychological symptoms, which are the outcome of the complex interaction between sex hormones and neurotransmitters. As has been reviewed in evidence-based guidelines, these treatments for reducing symptoms, particularly menopausal hormone therapy (MHT), are effective. However, initiation of therapy should be adapted to clinical necessity and personal risk for health, according to the latest recommendations of The Endocrine Society (Davis *et al.*, 2015).

Moreover, care for endocrine disorders extends into the realm of breast cancer survival, where women may face unique hormonal issues following cancer therapy. Symptoms of deficiency in estrogen, such as vulvovaginal atrophy (VVA), sleep impairment, and risk of osteoporosis, are of specific concern among survivors of breast cancer. Though routine hormone therapy is generally contraindicated in this group of patients, alternatives are available. Non-hormonal pharmacologic interventions, such as selective serotonin/noradrenaline reuptake inhibitors, have been reported to alleviate vasomotor symptoms and improve quality of life (Davis *et al.*, 2017). The individualized approach to menopausal symptom control in this population emphasizes monitoring close choice of endocrine and non-endocrine therapy based on the unique profile of each woman's health, further defining the subtlety associated with endocrine illness in gynecology.

12.3.2. Diagnostic Tests and Procedures

Evaluation of endocrine disease in gynecology often involves a thorough series of diagnostic testing and treatment. These tests are crucial in making accurate diagnoses, particularly in diseases such as polycystic ovary syndrome (PCOS) and thyroid disease, which significantly affect women's reproductive health. Detailed hormonal profiles, including tests of estrogen, progesterone, testosterone, and insulin levels, allow clinicians to determine hormonal imbalance. Furthermore, imaging studies, such as ultrasound or magnetic resonance imaging (MRI), can show structural ovarian or uterine abnormalities that may be the cause of endocrine dysfunction. Coupled together, the synergy of laboratory testing with imaging techniques forms a robust foundation for diagnosing the etiology of gynecologic symptoms, enabling individualized treatment planning and management. Where a routine blood test and imaging are not enlightening, more invasive techniques can be employed to gain a clearer insight into endocrine function.

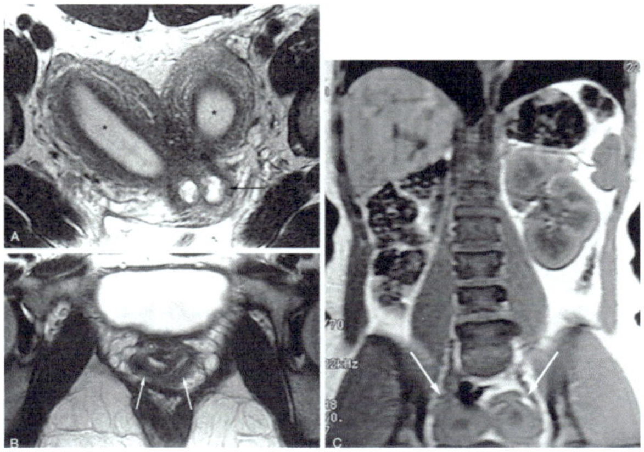

Figure 12.7. Role of magnetic resonance imaging in the evaluation of gynecologic disorders.

Source: https://radiologykey.com/wp-content/uploads/2019/02/f036-007ac-9780323328340.jpg

For instance, fine-needle aspiration of tissue from the ovaries is a method used to identify the presence of endocrine tumors, and endometrial biopsy can be performed to ascertain how hormones influence the uterine lining. These procedures are vital since, in addition to creating diagnoses, they provide information regarding therapeutic decisions, particularly in complex cases involving the presence of two or more endocrine illnesses. A judicious observance of these diagnostic processes can improve patient outcomes significantly by enabling individually defined treatment regimens to correct not just the hormonal imbalance but also the consequences of such imbalance on the reproductive system. More insight from these methods is required to address the clinical practice of gynecological endocrinology more effectively. Furthermore, the development of new equipment for diagnosis continues to refine the treatment of endocrine disorders in gynecology. For example, advances in biomarkers and genetic testing have shown the capability of detecting specific endocrine abnormalities at the molecular level, allowing for the provision of more personalized therapy. Use of such higher-level diagnostics can identify predispositions for diseases such as endometriosis or adrenal hyperplasia that would normally obfuscate the clinical picture. By integrating traditional testing with cutting-edge research and methods, doctors can create a more comprehensive understanding of the interrelationships between endocrine function and gynecological health. This expansive diagnostic process is of most significance as the field advances further, so that women are treated with the optimal type of care in successfully addressing their endocrine illness.

12.3.3. Importance of Early Diagnosis in Gynecological Health

Prompt gynecological wellness diagnosis is of the highest priority, particularly where endocrine diseases critically affect women's reproductive health and overall well-being. Endocrine diseases such as PCOS and autoimmune endocrine disorders tend to present with easily overlooked or blamed symptoms of more common disorders. Correct identification precedes proper management steps to be taken that may or may not prevent or reduce long-term effects such as infertility or metabolic disease. For instance, a successful understanding of the underlying pathology in relation to infertility caused by endocrine abnormality can enable an interdisciplinary intervention that not only cures the reproductive disease but also the general health implications for women afflicted with these conditions as well. Early diagnosis is therefore able to ensure that women receive appropriate care that addresses reproductive as well as overall health. Infertility, which affects approximately 10-15% of all couples, is so widespread that early detection of potential endocrine disorders that are the underlying cause is critical. Autoimmune disease of the hypothalamus, pituitary gland, and other endocrine glands can have a devastating impact on a woman's fertility. In addition to the direct impact on reproductive function, endocrine disorders not treated can cause as much emotional and psychological damage. Early diagnosis offers the chance for targeted interventions where medical professionals can provide targeted advice and measures to preserve fertility in at-risk women. As noted in the literature, there is a need to value the contribution made by endocrine autoimmunity to cause infertility, as it brings into perspective studies and adoption of new diagnostic approaches to integrated daily clinical practice (Josephine *et al.*, 2023).

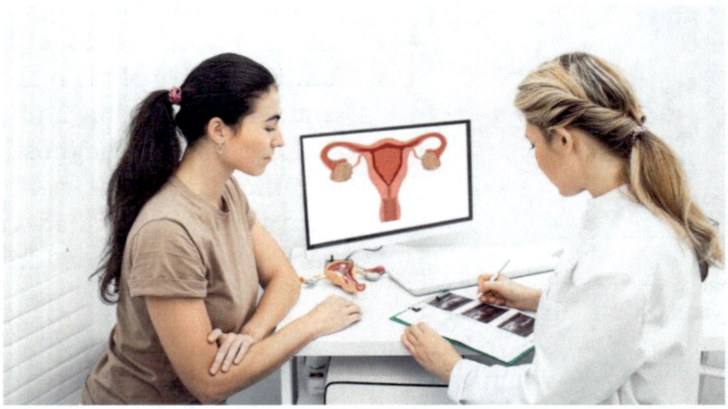

Source: https://d18unesthp5g3j.cloudfront.net/www.southshorehealth.org/assets/styles/responsive_image/s3/2021-10/gynecologist-discussing-case-with-a-woman.jpg?VersionId=yZohquNkZ.9AubR1ms_iITp7RW3g8osV&h=119335f7&itok=oWGRJzjp

This firm attitude can enable women to assume control of their reproductive lives. Moreover, the importance of early detection even extends beyond infertility to the broader area of gynecological well-being, particularly about diseases like PCOS. This endocrine disorder not only disturbs hormonal balance but also endangers mental health and quality of life, and therefore, it is essential that medical professionals remain vigilant in diagnosing its signs in time. By the practice of wellness-oriented integrative interventions, PCOS women can see enhancements in physical and psychological functioning. Education and counseling focused on lifestyle modifications can boost the provided care, ultimately leading to enhanced long-term outcomes. As more research continues to break down the complexities of PCOS and how it impacts, the importance of an early diagnosis becomes critical, highlighting the development of a solid framework in detecting such endocrine illnesses in gynecology (Annagur *et al.*, 2018). Intervention in the initial stages continues to be an underlying pillar in promoting women's health and providing them with the tools to effectively control their reproductive future.

Test Your Knowledge

1. What are some common symptoms associated with endocrine disorders affecting female reproductive health?
2. Which diagnostic tests are commonly used to identify endocrine disorders in gynecology?

12.4. Impact of Endocrine Disorders on Reproductive Health

Learning Outcome

1. Identify the effects on the Menstrual Cycle and Fertility
2. Explain the relationship between endocrine disorders and pregnancy complications
3. Discuss the long-term health implications for women

Endocrine disorders have a severe impact on reproductive health, typically leading to many complications in fertility and menstrual cycle regularity. The disruption of hormonal balance in polycystic ovary syndrome (PCOS) is a quintessential manifestation of endocrine disorders leading to infertility and irregular menstruation. The intricate interplay between hormones and reproduction is exemplified by the role of insulin and androgens in PCOS, leading to metabolic dysfunctions such as obesity and diabetes. Alongside, the psychological impact of infertility and the physical impact of irregular menstruation can contribute to more health problems, and hence a multi-dimensional treatment plan is required. Aiding these hormonal imbalances through medical therapy or lifestyle modification forms part and parcel of the exercise to achieve the return of reproductive health, thereby emphasizing the prime relationship between endocrine well-being and overall good health (Davis *et al.*, 2015). Menopause is another stage wherein reproductive health is severely affected by endocrine disorders. Menopause transition entails a physiological decline in estrogen and progesterone, oftentimes leading to symptoms that vary from hot flashes and mood changes to pain in the vulvovaginal area. The effect of these endocrine changes extends beyond physical complaints; they can severely impair sexual function and quality of life for a majority of women. HRT is now an over-the-counter drug but must be managed with an intellectual balancing of risk against benefit, particularly with regard to cardiovascular risk and cancer risk. Tailoring therapy based on individual health status and preference must be done in the best management of menopausal symptoms, as shown by newer guidelines on requesting individualized therapeutic practices adapted to the unique profiles of each patient (Davis *et al.*, 2015). Complicating reproductive health are conditions like endometriosis, that presents unique challenges to hormonal imbalance. The condition, which is the growth of endometrial tissue outside the uterus, affects approximately 30–40% of women presenting with infertility. Prior research has indicated genetic susceptibility, with point mutations in genes like NAT2 having the potential to exacerbate by interfering with metabolic routes and creating oxidative stress. The three-dimensional character of endometriosis requires a comprehensive therapeutic approach, traditionally consisting of surgical repair coupled with therapies for the reversal of attendant biochemical abnormalities, e.g., therapeutic plasmapheresis. These treatment modalities not only repair the physical defects but enhance reproductive outcomes as well, thus supporting the necessity to understand the hormonal underpinning of endocrine conditions to achieve effective control in gynecologic practice.

12.4.1. Effects on Menstrual Cycle and Fertility

These endocrine disorders influence the menstrual cycle very strongly and may disturb the delicate balance of the endocrine function necessary for normal ovulation and menstruation. Dysfunctions of thyroid glands and polycystic ovary syndrome are good examples of endocrine imbalance leading to irregular menstruation, anovulation, and ultimately affecting a woman's fertility. Research also indicates that PCOS women may experience irregular menstrual cycles due to elevated androgenic activity, disrupting proper follicular maturation and ovulatory feedback mechanisms. As documented in the literature, this can lead to long-term fertility issues for the subject. In addition, the biochemical underpinnings of such disorders are necessary to explore because they underscore the interplay between hormonal control and reproductive function, placing emphasis on early diagnosis and specially aimed interventions in an attempt to restore normal menstrual function as well as enhance fertility outcomes. As health practitioners, when investigating the relationship between menstruation and fertility, they now turn to a variety of diagnostic techniques in an effort to assess ovulatory cycles. One of the older techniques, basal body temperature (BBT) monitoring, has been a technique long used by couples desiring conception. BBT monitoring is an indication of ovulation, as slight increases in body temperature after ovulation occur since progesterone levels are elevated. But recent controversy questioned the validity and applicability of BBT in the modern view, most significantly in the context of emerging fertility studies. Such research supports the necessity of contemporary practice that unifies both historical knowledge and current discovery to provide comprehensive reproductive counseling, highlighting the role that accurate knowledge plays in aiding successful conception attempts in couples with endocrine problems, adding depth to the gynecological discussion of menstrual health (Barron *et al.*, 2005).

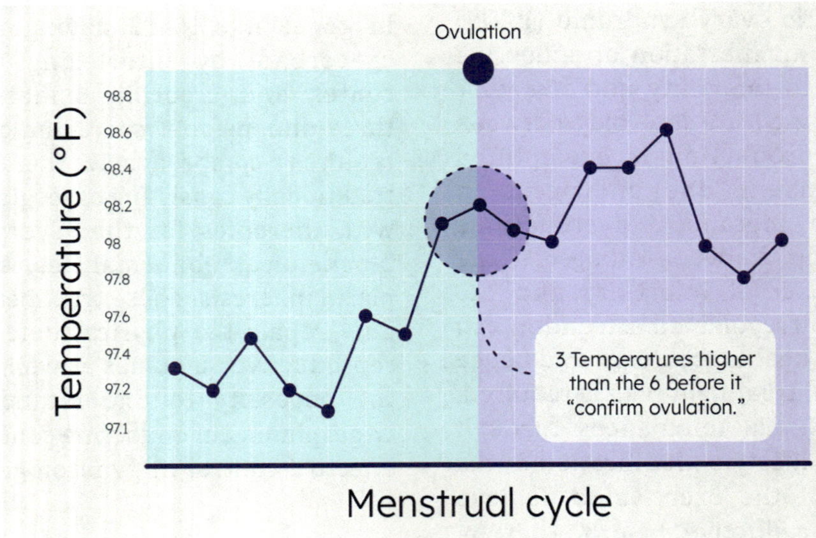

Figure 12.8. Basal Body Temperature.

Source: https://cdn.shopify.com/s/files/1/0038/5417/2275/files/October_Fertility_Blog_Content-02.png?v=1727467056

In spite of progress achieved in knowledge acquisition regarding the menstrual cycle, there are still scientific knowledge gaps that exist concerning its complex interactions with broader physiologic systems. The lack of comprehensive studies hinders effective public health planning to maximize menstrual wellness and fertility rates for women worldwide. As has been underscored in a key report, a systematic review of the ways in which menstruation affects and is affected by various conditions of health is vital to designing women's health programs. This not only involves looking at the interrelationships between menstrual disorders and overall health but also identifying research priorities that can close existing gaps in knowledge. Developing an integrated research agenda will refine our understanding of menstrual cycle dynamics and their implications for fertility, ultimately leading to better health interventions and education materials empowering women to manage their reproductive health efficiently (Ephross *et al.*, 1995).

12.4.2. Relationship Between Endocrine Disorders and Pregnancy Complications

The interplay of the endocrine disorders with pregnancy complications is a critical topic of interest in the gynecology field, as these disorders are significant in their influence on the health of both the mother and the fetus. Endocrine disorders such as diabetes, thyroid disease, and adrenal insufficiency pose the possibility of inducing several pregnancy complications such as gestational diabetes, preeclampsia, and fetal growth issues. For instance, pregnant women with poorly controlled diabetes during pregnancy and before gestation are likely to develop severe neonatal complications, including macrosomia and congenital malformations, which can complicate delivery and postpartum recovery. Furthermore, thyroid disorders, particularly hypothyroidism, also pose increased risks of miscarriage and preterm labor, thus the need for screening and management of such conditions in a proactive manner to secure optimal pregnancy outcomes. Secondly, endocrine disorder treatment in pregnant women has to be multidirectional to both cover maternal well-being as well as fetal safety. Physicians have to balance carefully when handling the endocrine disorder while not exacerbating complications for pregnancy. This can involve continuous monitoring of hormone levels, regular screening for associated complications, and modifying treatment procedures that will not negatively affect the unborn child. The evidence supports an anticipatory plan; healthcare providers should familiarize themselves with the current literature related to these disorders to make informed clinical practice decisions (Conde-Agudelo *et al.*, 2007). The application of evidence-based practice and systematic reviews in prenatal care can help minimize some of the risks of endocrine disorders, thereby leading to improved fetal and maternal health. Current reports emphasize the necessity for high-quality systematic reviews in maternal medicine to address knowledge gaps regarding the relationship between endocrine disease and pregnancy complications. Hugely varying in review methodology is how one can describe the published reviews, with Cochrane reviews generally having more methodological quality than their non-Cochrane counterparts (Bauerfeind *et al.*, 2006). This gap highlights the urgent need for robust evidence that can be used in clinical decision-making in the management of endocrine disorders during pregnancy. Without high-quality and methodologically sound systematic reviews, physicians may be disabled from making well-informed decisions that have the potential to avoid serious complications of uncontrolled or untreated endocrine diseases. Hence, it is important to enhance the quality of systematic reviews to ensure that inferences are robust that translate into quantifiable improvement in maternal and fetal health outcomes within the context of endocrine disorders.

12.4.3. Long-Term Health Implications For Women

The long-term health implications of endocrine disorders in women are multifaceted and can significantly impact their general well-being and quality of life Sexual dysfunction is one of the outstanding impacts of the disorders, particularly during menopause. Decreasing hormone levels mean that most women experience a variety of sexual health disorders, varying from lowered sexual desire to lubrication problems. The studies show that 40-55% of women are sexually averse, and 25-30% are poorly lubricated, highlighting the prevalence of these dysfunctions in menopausal women. These dysfunctions are directly related to the shifts in hormones, that is, the reduction of sex steroids, but psychological and relationship variables also contribute importantly. Management of such multifactorial complications needs individualized treatment modalities considering the intensity of the symptoms, potential side effects, and personal preference in an attempt to enhance women's sexual health and wellness during their lifetime (Stasi *et al.*, 2019).

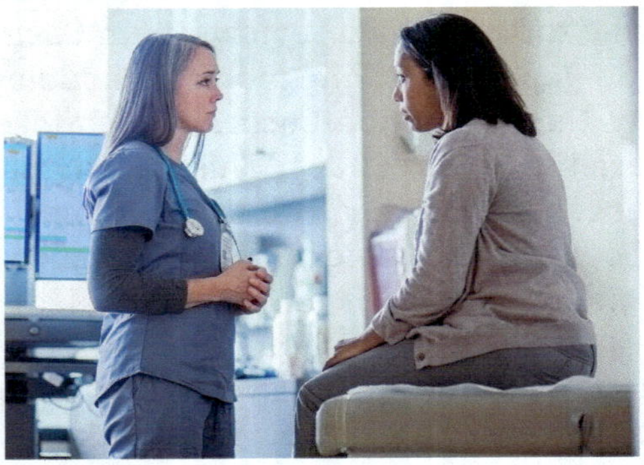

Source: https://img.lb.wbmdstatic.com/vim/live/webmd/consumer_assets/site_images/articles/health_tools/supplements_for_eczema_what_you_should_know_slideshow/1800ss_getty_rf_doctor_talking_with_female_patient.jpg

Infertility is another key element of women's long-term health complications, showing how endocrine diseases interact with reproductive health. The complexities of infertility are often exacerbated by a variety of gynecological diseases, including uterine fibroids and endometrial polyps. A recent study confirms that among women with infertility, the prevalence of uterine fibroids is 6.86%, with most found in women with primary infertility. Also, the prevalence of endometrial polyps is 96.15%, suggesting a high association between the conditions and reproduction challenges. With the multifactorial etiology of infertility, these results call for a complete and multidisciplinary diagnostic and treatment process with emphasis on resolving underlying gynecological pathology. In enhancing awareness and performing focused interventions, health workers can more effectively assist women with infertility and the long-term impacts of its effects on their lives (Amza *et al.*, 2024).

In addition, the long-term health implications of endocrine disorders can evolve as various chronic diseases, including metabolic and cardiovascular disease. As women grow older during menopause, the reductions in estrogen levels are associated with increases in the comorbidities of these diseases. Based on the relationship between hormonal fluctuations and the development of such diseases as cardiovascular disease, the majority of women are ensnared in increased health risks later in life. The increasing incidence of metabolic syndrome—linked to a cluster of conditions including hypertension, high blood sugar, and dyslipidemia—prevents the health profile of women in this age category from being even more complicated. To minimize these risks, preventive care should be given top priority by healthcare systems, and lifestyle modifications that target endocrine health, as well as the prevention of chronic disease, should be promoted to enhance the quality and duration of life in women who experience endocrine disorders at reproductive as well as post-reproductive ages.

Test Your Knowledge

1. How do endocrine disorders affect the menstrual cycle and fertility?
2. What is the relationship between endocrine disorders and pregnancy complications?

12.5. Treatment Options for Endocrine Disorders

Learning Outcome

1. Explain the hormonal therapies and medications
2. Discuss the lifestyle modifications and their role in Management
3. Define surgical interventions when necessary

Treatment of endocrine disease in gynecology increasingly utilizes evidence-based practice to validate effective treatment strategies. For menopausal syndrome, hormone therapy is a popular, yet still prevalent, option. Menopausal hormone therapy (MHT) is very effective for alleviating vasomotor symptoms and improving the quality of life in women following menopause. The new recommendations emphasize that the benefits of MHT generally offset the risks for women under the age of 60 or who are beginning menopause, requiring individualized treatment regimens that consider individual risk factors like cardiovascular and breast cancer histories. But for females seeking alternatives or with contraindications to hormonal therapy, a number of non-hormonal treatments like low-dose vaginal estrogen and other pharmacologic interventions provide alternative forms of relief (Davis *et al.*, 2015).

Especially in the case of breast cancer survivors, the care of endocrine-related disorders necessitates a more complex management approach. Because mainstream hormone replacement therapies are contraindicated following diagnosis, lifestyle optimization is a universal recommendation by doctors as a first-line of treatment. In cases of severe symptoms, non-hormonal pharmacotherapy in the form of selective serotonin/norepinephrine reuptake inhibitors and gabapentinoids has been effective in alleviating vasomotor symptoms and enhancing quality of life. Particularly, management of vaginal atrophy and other symptoms of estrogen deficiency is a primary concern area that calls for careful consideration of the available treatments to avoid the risk of reactivating dormant breast cancer cells. Consequently, medical professionals must personalize treatments accordingly, weighed against the heterogeneity of available non-hormonal treatments and respecting the unique challenges facing breast cancer survivors (Davis *et al.*, 2017). In general, management of endocrine gynecologic disorders is multifaceted and calls for an individualized multi-modal management depending on patient-specific profiles. While hormone therapies remain a pillar for most patients, the widening trend towards personalized treatment has led the way to new non-hormonal therapies targeting personalized symptoms without subjecting patients to risks related to hormones. Healthcare practitioners must stay informed about the evolution of therapies, like the new treatments for vaginal atrophy and other estrogen-related symptoms. Through a shared decision-making culture, providers can help patients navigate the complexity of their healthcare choices, ultimately improving their quality of life as well as the effective control of endocrine conditions (Davis *et al.*, 2015; Davis *et al.*, 2017).

12.5.1. Hormonal Therapies and Medications

Hormonal medications and therapies have a central place in management in gynecology to relieve various endocrine ailments, particularly at some stages of life, such as menopause and the treatment of polycystic ovary syndrome (PCOS). Menopausal hormone therapy (MHT) becomes an upfront intervention for the relief of vasomotor symptoms and other menopausal complications. Specific guidelines set forth by The Endocrine Society stipulate that MHT is highly effective for symptomatic menopausal women, especially women under 60 years or fewer than ten years following the start of menopause. Importantly, the decision to initiate MHT must be tailored to each woman's clinical profile and individualized preferences, weighing benefits against potential risks, e.g., cardiovascular disease or breast cancer. Also, low-dose vaginal estrogen and non-hormonal options are introduced for the scenario of those who are unable to use or do not prefer MHT (Davis *et al.*, 2015).

In managing PCOS, which is a common endocrine disease in women of reproductive age, hormonal medications play an important role in managing the symptoms and also the associated metabolic impairments. The treatment is commonly achieved through the utilization of oral contraceptives, which can control menstrual cycles and reduce hirsutism and acne outbreaks. The utilization of insulin-sensitizing medications like metformin is also common to counteract insulin resistance, which is very prevalent in women with PCOS, further proving the intricacies of being able to manage it effectively. This complexity is revealed in the fact that PCOS can affect not only reproductive health but also emotional well-being, as depression symptoms might be encountered by women (Sahu *et al.*, 2024).

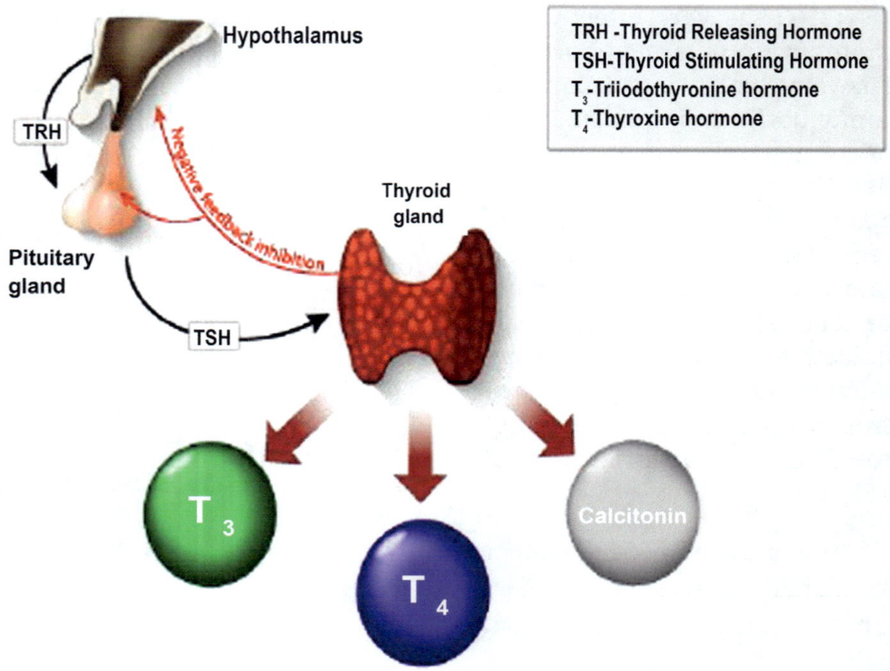

Figure 12.9. Hormonal Therapy for Endocrine Disorders.

Source: https://www.saintjohnscancer.org/endocrine/wp-content/uploads/sites/3/2018/08/thyroid-hormones.png

Thus, hormonal therapies need to be considered within an integrated clinical context that encompasses the different presentations of this endocrine condition. Coordination between caregivers is required in simplifying hormonal therapies in gynecology. Cooperation between endocrinologists, gynecologists, and family physicians can enhance patient care and result in more effective management approaches based on individual needs. Education plays a part in this interactive environment since healthcare workers must be current with the latest evidence-based practice, including hormone therapy comparison studies and their impact on health outcomes. Educating patients and involving them in discussions of treatment options provides them with the opportunity to become participants in their healthcare decisions. Through encouraging open dialogue and sharing the latest updates on hormonal therapies, medical practitioners are able to work together to improve the quality of life for women who must deal with the challenges offered by endocrine diseases (Davis *et al.*, 2015; Sahu *et al.*, 2024).

12.5.2. Lifestyle Modifications and Their Role in Management

Endocrine disease management, and by extension, in gynecology, necessitates a holistic strategy involving significant changes in lifestyle. Polycystic ovary syndrome (PCOS) is used to demonstrate the inter-relationship of metabolic health with reproductive health. Evidence suggests the potential for great alleviation of symptoms associated with PCOS by the integration of beneficial lifestyle interventions, that is, diet and exercise. Control for weight becomes an important intervention. It has been seen that even minimal weight loss has an effect on improving the sensitivity to insulin, and hence, the occurrence of metabolic complications in the disorder decreases. Control of endocrine disorders with a diet decreasing saturated fats with a balanced use of unsaturated fats, carbohydrates, and protein is necessary. These changes address not only weight management but also treat other conditions such as hirsutism and infertility, hence illustrating the central role of lifestyle in the holistic management of endocrine diseases such as PCOS (Ghazeeri *et al.*, 2021).

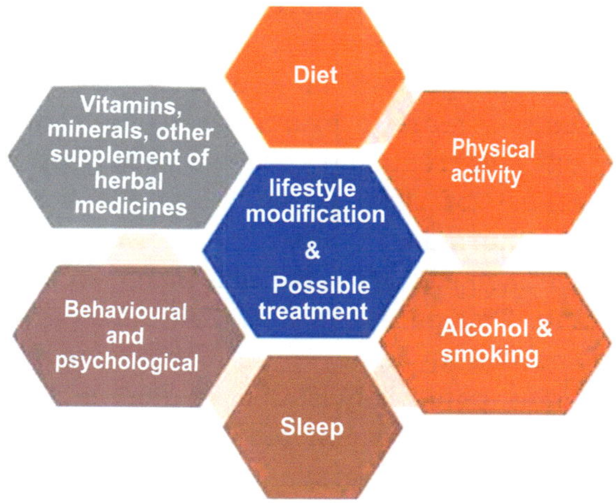

Figure 12.10. Probable modification of lifestyle and the possible treatment to overcome PCOS.

Source: https://www.researchgate.net/figure/Probable-modification-of-lifestyle-and-the-possible-treatment-to-overcome-PCOD-Cowan-et_fig3_376512356

For post-menopausal women and for women with signs of estrogen deficiency following breast cancer, lifestyle is also essential. It has been recommended that, rather than hormone replacement therapy, otherwise contraindicated, optimization of lifestyle can result in relief from symptomatic complaints for vasomotor symptoms (VMS), vulvovaginal atrophy (VVA), and similar concerns. Addition of activities such as exercise as frequently as reasonably possible, dietary intake in moderation, and stress management exercises can contribute to overall well-being and health as well as to quality of life. Non-pharmacologic hormone-free treatments remain, but lifestyle modifications are usually the first step in treating menopausal symptoms in breast cancer survivors. The fact that this is noted highlights the role of customizing treatment protocols involving both lifestyle modification and appropriate medical intervention, thereby highlighting the multi-faceted nature of endocrine disorder management

(Davis *et al.*, 2017). Moreover, the embedded relationship between lifestyle modification and global management of endocrine disorders suggests a more overarching trend toward preventative treatment strategies. The growing awareness of the role that lifestyle has in affecting hormonal health requires even greater emphasis on education and self-management of patients. This paradigm shift makes the patient become directly engaged in determining their outcomes, potentially leading to more effective long-term management of conditions such as PCOS and menopausal symptoms. Incorporation of lifestyle changes into treatment plans not only enhances patient autonomy but also overall health literacy as a result of improved comprehension of their conditions. Therefore, healthcare practitioners must advocate for the use of lifestyle modifications as part of management strategies that will ultimately reduce the burden of these disorders and improve the quality of life for women with endocrine diseases in gynecology (Ghazeeri *et al.*, 2021; Davis *et al.*, 2017).

12.5.3. Surgical Interventions When Necessary

In gynecology, surgery is most often required when conservative treatment of an endocrine disorder has failed or in the presence of urgent complications from such disorders. For instance, for insulinomas, which are the most frequent pancreatic neuroendocrine tumors, surgery for removal is the primary form of treatment. Surgical treatment has been very successful in benign insulinomas, as it can effectively eliminate the cause of hypersecretion of insulin and thus abolish symptoms of hypoglycemia. A prompt diagnosis and early surgical intervention are essential, especially in patients who have malignancies. As the occurrence of pancreatic neuroendocrine tumors has been on the rise, there is a need for surgical skill to be provided to enhance patient outcomes when it comes to endocrine disease, as evidenced by the increased emphasis on such methods as endoscopic ultrasound-guided radiofrequency ablation as an alternative for certain instances (Rychlewska-Duda *et al.*, 2025). Surgical treatment is not limited to insulinomas and can encompass a variety of endocrine gynecological conditions, such as Polycystic Ovary Syndrome (PCOS) and endometriosis. Surgery for these conditions, such as laparoscopy, can result in dramatic relief of chronic pelvic pain and improved fertility outcomes. The coexistence of PCOS and endometriosis poses challenges of a different sort; surgical removal of endometrial lesions or ovarian cysts not only symptomatically relieves but also restores reproductive function. Surgical intervention is particularly critical in avoiding the deleterious impact on quality of life, since both these disorders lead to debilitating pain and emotional distress. Therefore, a surgical approach is needed, tailored to the individual's particular medical profile, to maximize efficacy and safety and address the complexity of endocrine disorders in gynecology (Ramos *et al.*, 2024).

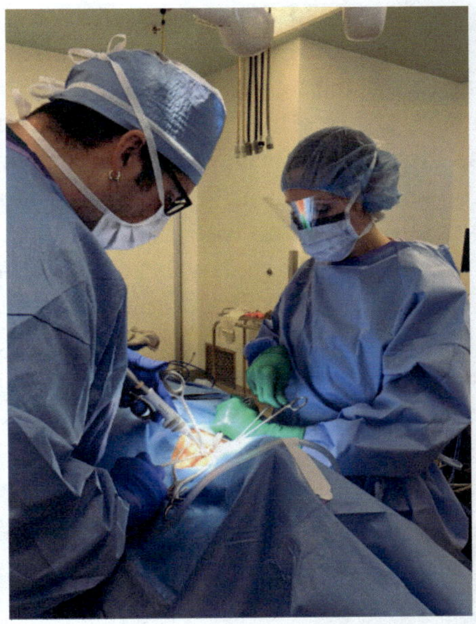

Source: https://www.westernsurgical.com/wp-content/uploads/thyroid.jpg

In addition, surgical appropriateness and timing must be carefully evaluated in terms of each patient's general health and disease course. Patient age, severity of the disease, and malignancy potential are also factors to consider. For instance, patients with severe endometriosis may occasionally be aided by early surgical treatment to prevent further difficulty and preserve reproductive capacity. Similarly, in insulinomas, whether surgery is performed hinges on tumor size and behavior and the need for understanding its pathophysiology. It is essential that practicing health professionals develop a common environment with patients to discuss risks, benefits, and realistic hope regarding surgical options. Such cautious consideration ensures that surgical interventions are not only necessary but also tactically well positioned to improve patient prognosis with gynecological endocrine disorders (Rychlewska-Duda *et al.*, 2025; Ramos *et al.*, 2024).

Test Your Knowledge

1. What types of hormonal therapies and medications are commonly used to treat endocrine disorders?
2. How do lifestyle modifications contribute to managing endocrine disorders?

SUMMARY

Finally, summarizing the research of endocrine disorders in gynecology, it must not be exaggerated how significant it is to identify the multifaceted impact of such disorders on women's welfare. Endocrine disorders such as Polycystic Ovarian Syndrome (PCOS) and thyroid disease not only interfere with the normal hormonal balance but also influence metabolic processes and welfare. The path of endocrine pathology to the concomitant gynecologic symptoms serves as an indicator of the need for a thorough understanding of the ways in which hormonal imbalance might yield emergent clinical issues. The prevalence of obesity in PCOS, for instance, is overwhelming and has been discovered by research to be amongst the major risk factors for diabetes and cardiovascular complications in the affected group, calling for urgent diagnosis and targeted intervention (Akbaezadeh *et al.*, 2017). Further complicating the challenge of endocrine disorders, the research indicates that women's experience of these conditions is often supplemented with inadequate, high-quality evidence to guide treatment. Systematic reviews play a crucial role in synthesizing available research and providing practitioners with reliable information; however, heterogeneity in methodological quality across reviews indicates a vast gap in the literature. The contrast between Cochrane and non-Cochrane reviews indicates that although there are high-quality studies out there, most of the reviews that exist lack adequate capacity to guide clinical practice (Conde-Agudelo *et al.*, 2007). The variability in evidence, therefore, creates a challenge for healthcare professionals trying to provide effective and well-informed care to patients. Lastly, this review calls for concerted efforts to achieve the enhancement of endocrine disorder research quality in gynecology. The synthesis of high-quality systematic reviews based on sound methodologies is vital in offering a rigorous guideline. Improved research findings have the potential to directly impact maternal mortality and morbidity, as well as equip healthcare practitioners with the mechanisms required for effective patient care. As the region grows, ongoing interactions among clinicians, researchers, and patients will be instrumental in building a broader body of evidence of endocrine disorders and enhancing improved health in women's healthcare (Conde-Agudelo *et al.*, 2007).

The identification of endocrine disorders in gynecology has been crucial in offering information on the nature of the complexity of polycystic ovary syndrome (PCOS). The disease, which ranges in its manifestations from an abnormal menstrual cycle to insulin resistance, has been a focus of recent discussion. Of note, the diagnosis of PCOS has been controversial, and therefore, there has been a need to standardize its evaluation and treatment. This need is compounded by inconsistent practice among providers, so that numerous women are under-supported. The incorporation of overseas evidence-based guidelines has attempted to bridge these discrepancies. The process of developing guidelines was guided through extensive consultation of multidisciplinary clinicians and consumer groups, providing a firm platform for promoting care and guiding future research in this prevalent condition. Furthermore, emphasizing the functions of education and lifestyle modification in the management of endocrine disorders, the new guidelines facilitate holistic treatment. Along with medical management, a greater focus on patient education, lifestyle change, and emotional well-being is central to enhanced health outcomes among PCOS women. The guidelines are based on recent evidence that lifestyle interventions can have an important role in minimizing symptoms and generally enhancing health. Because standard diagnostic criteria have often been a source of confusion, this integrated approach aims to simplify such criteria and rank highest the need for minimizing unnecessary testing. As such, emphasis has thereby shifted toward practical aspects such as emotional well-being and lifestyle modifications as integrated components of effective management strategies (Network, 2018). One of the major strengths of the new guidelines' contribution to gynecology is the formulation of these guidelines through teamwork. The recommendations were guided by pluralistic input from various disciplines, including gynecology, endocrinology, psychology, and public health, explicitly showing a multidisciplinary process. In addition to enriching the content of the recommendations, the collaborative work also makes them more sensitive to the needs and choices of various patients. Additionally, the guidelines lay the basis for future research studies with areas of focus highlighted, particularly for further clarification of diagnostic features of PCOS and evidence-based practice gap filling. Here, the guidelines are not only clinical practice guidelines but more so a fundamental resource that enables further illumination and creation of endocrine disorders in gynecology for eventual advantage in patient experience and health outcomes (Network, 2018).

KEY TERMS FROM THIS CHAPTER

- Anorexia nervosa (AN)
- Endocrine disruptors
- Environmental factors
- Hormonal disorders
- Hormonal imbalance
- Hormone production
- Menopausal hormone therapy (MHT)
- Menstrual cycle
- Optimal management
- Endocrine disorders
- Endocrine system
- Estrogen
- Hormonal dysregulation
- Hormonal regulation
- Hyperthyroid syndrome
- Menopause
- Metabolism
- Pituitary

CRITICAL THINKING QUESTIONS

1. **Which of the following is a common endocrine disorder associated with infertility and irregular menstruation in women?**
   a. Hypothyroidism
   b. Polycystic Ovarian Syndrome (PCOS)
   c. Diabetes mellitus
   d. Addison's disease
2. **Hyperprolactinemia in women most commonly presents with:**
   a. Menorrhagia
   b. Amenorrhea and galactorrhea
   c. Dysmenorrhea
   d. Hirsutism and acne
3. **Which of the following thyroid disorders is associated with menorrhagia (heavy menstrual bleeding)?**
   a. Hyperthyroidism
   b. Hypothyroidism
   c. Thyroid cancer
   d. Euthyroid goiter
4. **A woman with PCOS typically shows elevated levels of:**
   a. Follicle-stimulating hormone (FSH)
   b. Estrogen
   c. Androgens (testosterone)
   d. Progesterone
5. **Which endocrine disorder is most commonly associated with delayed puberty in females?**
   a. Cushing's syndrome
   b. Turner syndrome (gonadal dysgenesis)
   c. Acromegaly
   d. Hyperthyroidism

Short Answer Questions

1. What is the primary function of the endocrine system?
2. Name two common endocrine disorders that affect women.
3. What are the typical symptoms of endocrine disorders in women?
4. Which diagnostic methods are used to identify endocrine disorders?
5. How can endocrine disorders impact female reproductive health?
6. What are common treatment options for managing endocrine disorders?

Answer to Critical Thinking Questions

1. (b) 2. (b) 3. (b) 4. (c) 5. (b)

REFERENCES

1. Akbaezadeh, M., & Behbahani, B. M. (2017). Central obesity and BMI associated with different phenotypes of polycystic ovary syndrome in adolescent. https://core.ac.uk/download/480549992.pdf (accessed on 14th June 2025).
2. Amza, M., Balalau, O. D., Bobirca, A., Gorecki, A., *et al.* (2024). Infertility as a possible multifactorial condition; the experience of a single center. https://core.ac.uk/download/624145766.pdf (accessed on 14th June 2025).
3. Ancane, G., Ancans, A., Briedite, I., Erts, R., *et al.* (2013). Insufficient assessment of sexual dysfunction: A problem in gynecological practice. https://core.ac.uk/download/480425745.pdf (accessed on 14th June 2025).
4. Andersen, M., Azziz, R., Balen, A., Baye, A., *et al.* (2018). Recommendations from the international evidence-based guideline for the assessment and management of polycystic ovary syndrome. https://core.ac.uk/download/224640444.pdf (accessed on 14th June 2025).
5. Annagur, B., Beck, D., Benson, R., Cronin, K., Dennett, C., Dowdy, E., *et al.* (2018). Polycystic ovary syndrome across the life span of women: A wellness-based integrative intervention. https://core.ac.uk/download/213088882.pdf (accessed on 14th June 2025).
6. Barron, M. L., & Fehring, R. (2005). Basal body temperature assessment: Is it useful to couples seeking pregnancy? https://core.ac.uk/download/213076060.pdf (accessed on 14th June 2025).
7. Bauerfeind, I., Dian, D., Friese, K., Gerber, B., *et al.* (2006). Pregnancy-associated breast cancer–Special features in diagnosis and treatment. https://core.ac.uk/download/16432352.pdf (accessed on 14th June 2025).
8. Behboudi-Gandevani, S., & Tehrani, F. R. (2020). Cardio-metabolic risk factors in polycystic ovary syndrome. https://core.ac.uk/download/478050147.pdf (accessed on 14th June 2025).
9. Berk, M., Köhler-Forsberg, O., Turner, M., Penninx, B. W. J. H., Wrobel, A. L., Firth, J., Loughman, A., *et al.* (2023). Comorbidity between major depressive disorder and physical diseases: A comprehensive review of epidemiology, mechanisms and management. *World Psychiatry, 22*, 366–387. https://doi.org/10.1002/wps.21110 (accessed on 14th June 2025).
10. Cabral-Pacheco, G. A., Garza-Veloz, I., Castruita-De la Rosa, C., Ramirez-Acuña, J. M., Perez-Romero, B. A., Guerrero-Rodriguez, J. F., Martínez-Avila, N., *et al.* (2020). The roles of matrix metalloproteinases and their inhibitors in human diseases. *International Journal of Molecular Sciences, 21*, 9739. https://doi.org/10.3390/ijms21249739 (accessed on 14th June 2025).
11. Cheng, J. (2017). The mechanisms of psychological therapy with people with long-term physical health conditions. https://core.ac.uk/download/96838376.pdf (accessed on 14th June 2025).
12. Christopherson, R. (2016). Polycystic ovary syndrome metabolic comorbidities: A critical appraisal of the evidence with practice recommendations. https://core.ac.uk/download/162578547.pdf (accessed on 14th June 2025).
13. Ciobanu, C., Fica, S., Poterasu, M., Rowland, M., *et al.* (2020). Anorexia nervosa and reproduction: Connecting brain to gonads. https://core.ac.uk/download/304672903.pdf (accessed on 14th June 2025).

14. Conde-Agudelo, A., Coomarasamy, A., Oxman, A. D., Jadad, A. R., Dennis, C. L., *et al.* (2007). A review of the methodological features of systematic reviews in maternal medicine. https://core.ac.uk/download/pdf/18982.pdf (accessed on 14th June 2025).

15. Davis, S. R., Gompel, A., Lumsden, M. A., Murad, M. H., *et al.* (2015). Treatment of symptoms of the menopause: An Endocrine Society clinical practice guideline. https://core.ac.uk/download/42367511.pdf (accessed on 14th June 2025).

16. Davis, S. R., Gompel, A., Lumsden, M. A., Pinkerton, J. V., *et al.* (2017). Managing menopausal symptoms and associated clinical issues in breast cancer survivors. https://core.ac.uk/download/96884955.pdf (accessed on 14th June 2025).

17. Di Stasi, V., Maseroli, E., Scavello, I., Vignozzi, L., *et al.* (2019). Sexual health in menopause. https://core.ac.uk/download/326839410.pdf (accessed on 14th June 2025).

18. Diliz-Pere, H., Greene, D. A., Hakala, T. R., Iwatsuki, S., *et al.* (1984). Pancreaticoduodenal transplantation in humans. https://core.ac.uk/download/12203978.pdf (accessed on 14th June 2025).

19. Dubinskaya, E., Lapteva, N., & Lukyanova, Y. (2016). The use of plasmapheresis in treatment of patients with infertility, peritoneal endometriosis and Nat2 gene polymorphism. https://core.ac.uk/download/301580751.pdf (accessed on 14th June 2025).

20. Ephross, S. A., & Harlow, S. D. (1995). What we do and do not know about the menstrual cycle or, questions scientists could be asking. https://core.ac.uk/download/229803302.pdf (accessed on 14th June 2025).

21. Fox, M., Glynn, L. M., & Howland, M. A. (2018). Maternal programming: Application of a developmental psychopathology perspective. https://core.ac.uk/download/215784219.pdf (accessed on 14th June 2025).

22. Ramos Frattini, A. S. B., Bochini, L. L. M., Andrade, L. L., Fiúza, L. B., Silva, A. C. R., Vasconcelos, C. A., Santos, L. B. M., *et al.* (2024). Polycystic ovary syndrome and endometriosis: Impact on fertility and quality of life and surgical options. *Brazilian Journal of Implantology and Health Sciences*. https://www.semanticscholar.org/paper/5b32db7ad097d8455658da322271a5033429385b (accessed on 14th June 2025).

23. Garag, S., Krishnappa, S., Sannaboraiah, A., Upadhyaya, V., *et al.* (2017). Subclinical hypothyroidism in pregnancy and outcomes. https://core.ac.uk/download/543137100.pdf (accessed on 14th June 2025).

24. Ghazeeri, G., Hmedeh, C., *et al.* (2021). Nutritional management in polycystic ovary syndrome: Challenges and opportunities. https://core.ac.uk/download/161103740.pdf (accessed on 14th June 2025).

25. International PCOS Network. (2018). Recommendations from the international evidence-based guideline for the assessment and management of polycystic ovary syndrome. https://core.ac.uk/download/491176961.pdf (accessed on 14th June 2025).

26. Josephine, A., Renjith, K. R., Sindhu, K., Simi, N., *et al.* (2023). Endocrine autoimmunity in association with female infertility. https://core.ac.uk/download/591404113.pdf (accessed on 14th June 2025).

27. Kachaylo, I., Piontkovska, O., Pylypenko, N., Romanova, I., *et al.* (2022). Somatic status of adolescent girls with gynecological disorders born with low and excessive weight. https://core.ac.uk/download/587245399.pdf (accessed on 14th June 2025).

28. Kaundal, A., & Renjhen, P. (2024). Female sexual dysfunction: A review. https://core.ac.uk/download/613230341.pdf (accessed on 14th June 2025).

29. Laddad, M., *et al.* (2023). Recent advances in reproductive endocrinology: Implications for fertility treatment in gynecology. https://core.ac.uk/download/596247493.pdf (accessed on 14th June 2025).

30. McAuliffe, F. M., Killeen, S. L., Jacob, C. M., Hanson, M. A., Hadar, E., McIntyre, D., Kapur, A., *et al.* (2020). Management of prepregnancy, pregnancy, and postpartum obesity from the FIGO Pregnancy and Non-Communicable Diseases Committee: A FIGO (International Federation of Gynecology and Obstetrics) guideline. *International Journal of Gynecology & Obstetrics, 151*, 16–36. https://doi.org/10.1002/ijgo.13334 (accessed on 14th June 2025).

31. Mohapatra, I., & Samantaray, S. R. (2024). Exploring societal and environmental influences on decreasing monarchial age: A comprehensive review. https://core.ac.uk/download/613230461.pdf (accessed on 14th June 2025).

32. Piltonen, T., Allegranza, D., Hund, M., Buck, K., Sillman, J., & Arffman, R. (2024). Validation of an anti-Müllerian hormone cutoff for polycystic ovarian morphology in the diagnosis of polycystic ovary syndrome in the HARMONIA Study: Protocol for a prospective, noninterventional study. *JMIR Research Protocols, 13*. https://www.semanticscholar.org/paper/12e6a1ca843de24c7b700d92caa2fa91630f755c (accessed on 14th June 2025).

33. Radi, R. A. E. (2010). Assessment of thyroid function in pregnant women from Rimal Health Center, Gaza City. https://core.ac.uk/download/385927694.pdf (accessed on 14th June 2025).

34. Rychlewska-Duda, J., Lisiecka, J., Janik, M., Ufnalska, B., Konarska, A., Fabijański, A., Machowiak, A., *et al.* (2025). Insulinomas: Comprehensive review of epidemiology, pathophysiology, clinical manifestations, diagnostic approaches, and treatment options. *Quality in Sport*. https://www.semanticscholar.org/paper/64ae9c3faebfed938fe4398653fbd25356933417 (accessed on 14th June 2025).

35. Sahu, P., & Mishra, S. (2024). Ayurveda management of polycystic ovarian syndrome by single herbs & combinations–A case report. https://core.ac.uk/download/617189862.pdf (accessed on 14th June 2025).

36. Schweizer-Schubert, S., Gordon, J. L., Eisenlohr-Moul, T. A., Meltzer-Brody, S., Schmalenberger, K. M., Słopień, R., Zietlow, A. L., *et al.* (2021). Steroid hormone sensitivity in reproductive mood disorders: On the role of the GABAA receptor complex and stress during hormonal transitions. *Frontiers in Medicine, 7*. https://doi.org/10.3389/fmed.2020.479646 (accessed on 14th June 2025).

37. Skotnes, L. L. H. (2019). An exploratory view of female reproductive health issues: A case study in Norway. https://core.ac.uk/download/542326928.pdf (accessed on 14th June 2025).

38. Talbott, E. (2024). Prevalence of polycystic ovarian syndrome (PCOS) like symptoms in the general practice of an obstetrics and gynecological office on the island of Tobago: A retrospective chart analysis. *Epidemiology International Journal*. https://www.semanticscholar.org/paper/279426139f61702bb069aff78af4476d6dd27992 (accessed on 14th June 2025).

INDEX